Handbook of

Nurse
Anesthesia

Handbook of
Nurse
Anesthesia

Third Edition

John J. Nagelhout, PhD, CRNA
Director, School of Anesthesia
Kaiser Permanente/California State University, Fullerton
Southern California Permanente Medical Group
Pasadena, California

Karen L. Zaglaniczny, PhD, CRNA, FAAN
Director, Perioperative Services Education and Research
Director, Graduate Program of Nurse Anesthesia
William Beaumont Hospital
Royal Oak, Michigan

ELSEVIER
SAUNDERS

ELSEVIER
SAUNDERS

11830 Westline Industrial Dr.
St. Louis, MO 63146

HANDBOOK OF NURSE ANESTHESIA
Copyright © 2005, Elsevier Inc.

Notice

Nursing is an ever-changing field. Standard safety precautions must be followed, but as new research and clinical experience broaden our knowledge, changes in treatment and drug therapy may become necessary or appropriate. Readers are advised to check the most current product information provided by the manufacturer of each drug to be administered to verify the recommended dose, the method and duration of administration, and contraindications. It is the responsibility of the licensed prescriber, relying on experience and knowledge of the patient, to determine dosages and the best treatment for each individual patient. Neither the publisher nor the authors assume any liability for any injury and/or damage to persons or property arising from this publication.

Previous editions copyrighted 2001, 1997

ISBN-13: 978-0-7216-0362-9
ISBN-10: 0-7216-0362-9

Executive Editor: Michael Ledbetter
Senior Developmental Editor: Lisa P. Newton
Production Services Manager: John Rogers
Project Manager: Doug Turner
Design Project Manager: Bill Drone

Printed in the United States of America

Last digit is the print number: 9   8   7   6   5   4   3   2

PREFACE

The complexity of clinical anesthesia practice continues to increase as new procedures and drugs are introduced and as our methods of conceptualizing and managing diseases evolve. Anesthetists must stay abreast of current practices in a variety of disciplines, since our patients may arrive with an array of medical problems and surgical needs. When selecting the format of this handbook, we chose not to simply produce a condensed version of our text *Nurse Anesthesia*. We believe that there is a need for a single comprehensive source containing information on common diseases, procedures, and drugs, and that such a source, in a handbook format, would complement the larger text and provide an "in the operating room" guide for practice. This third edition of our handbook has been totally reviewed and revised to include the most up-to-date clinical information available on numerous topics, including SARS and diagnostic and therapeutic procedures. Today, many clinicians practice at more than one facility and thus may be called on to provide anesthesia care in a broader spectrum of operative and diagnostic situations. A comprehensive reference guide is an essential tool for hands-on management in the modern operating suite.

We compiled the *Handbook of Nurse Anesthesia* as a single source that provides the following:

- A thorough overview of the *common diseases* encountered in surgical patients
- A *procedure manual* and set of guidelines for anesthesia management for a wide variety of diagnostic and surgical procedures
- A convenient and comprehensive *drug reference* for clinical use

A standardized format was designed and customized for use throughout each of the three individual parts of the *Handbook*. The appendices at the end of the *Handbook* offer the clinician easy access to the difficult airway algorithm, hemodynamic formulas, guidelines for drug therapy, latex allergy guidelines, pulmonary function testing, preoperative laboratory values, AANA Standards of Practice, and much more.

In the 8 years since we produced the first edition of this handbook, we are consistently amazed and grateful for the professional contributions that Nurse Anesthetists make to academic medicine and nursing, clinical practice, and society as a whole. We are proud that this handbook has played a part in the continuous evolution of our specialty.

John J. Nagelhout
Karen L. Zaglaniczny

ACKNOWLEDGMENTS FOR THE THIRD EDITION

We are especially gratified with the comments and widespread acceptance of this handbook by the anesthesia community. Its extensive use as a clinical guide confirms our assumptions that a convenient and inclusive source such as this is essential in modern anesthesia practice. We have incorporated many of these comments in revising and updating this new edition. Each section has been thoroughly edited to include the latest information available on common diseases, procedures, and drugs encountered during daily practice.

We would like to thank the following individuals for their suggestions and review in the preparation of this third edition:

Ban Batu, MSN, CRNA
Julie Bean, MSN, CRNA
Kathy Bender, MSN, CRNA
Brad Brooke, MSN, CRNA
Jill Buist, MSN, CRNA
Abigail Callejo-Covacha, MSN, CRNA
Carrie Chmielewski, MSN, CRNA
Julie Cicerone, MSN, CRNA
Andrea Clearhout, MSN, CRNA
Suzanne Clickett, MSN, CRNA
Terry Durley, MSN, CRNA
Kritina Eiden, MSN, CRNA
Kathy Everts, MSN, CRNA
Rachel Facciolla, MSN, CRNA
Michelle Godlewski, MSN, CRNA
Barb Griffin, MSN, CRNA
Jody Grusser, MSN, CRNA
Michael Johnson, MSN, CRNA
Susan Kay, MSN, CRNA
Erin Kitchenmaster, MSN, CRNA
Chris LeBel, MSN, CRNA
Mary Lulgjuraj, MSN, CRNA

Tom Lyons, MSN, CRNA
Mark Meitzner, MSN, CRNA
Caryl Molton, MSN, CRNA
Mark Nold, MSN, CRNA
Kary Pinchek, MSN, CRNA
Karen Piper, MSN, CRNA
Dennis Poterek, MSN, CRNA
Jennifer Radtke, MSN, CRNA
Jamie Russell, MSN, CRNA
Denise Sarnacki, MSN, CRNA
Julie Skurnowicz, MSN, CRNA
Shannon Smith, MSN, CRNA
Janice Sosin, MSN, CRNA
Marlena Stankiewwicz, MSN, CRNA
Jackie Stefak, MSN, CRNA
Lindsay Thibert, MSN, CRNA
Trish Tuttle, MSN, CRNA
Susan Webb, MSN, CRNA
Tammie Williams, MSN, CRNA
Jessica Wisser, MSN, CRNA
Randy Wright, MSN, CRNA

We would also like to thank the following individuals who were also instrumental in the production of this handbook: the staff at Elsevier, Michael Ledbetter, Executive Editor; Lisa Newton, Senior Developmental Editor; John Rogers, Publishing Services Manager, and Doug Turner, Project Manager. Again, we would like to thank our professional colleagues, friends, and especially our families for their support.

CONTENTS

SECTION III
Endocrine System, 56

SECTION IV
Gastrointestinal System, 85

SECTION V
Hematologic System, 96

SECTION VI
Hepatic System, 107

SECTION VII
Musculoskeletal System, 116

SECTION VIII
Renal System, 129

SECTION IX
Respiratory System, 134

SECTION III
Genitourinary System, 242

SECTION IV
Head and Neck, 258

SECTION XI
Pediatrics, 382

SECTION XII
Anesthesia for Therapeutic and Diagnosis Procedures, 399

SECTION XIII
Vascular Surgery, 415

PART III
DRUGS: LISTED ALPHABETICALLY, 431

APPENDIXES

SECTION   I

CARDIOVASCULAR SYSTEM

A. Arrhythmias

The current drugs of choice for common arrhythmias are listed in the table provided. Several reports have indicated that when given to asymptomatic or mildly symptomatic patients, some antiarrhythmic agents may become pro-arrhythmic.

Drugs of Choice for Common Arrhythmias

Arrhythmia	Drug of Choice	Alternatives	Remarks
Atrial fibrillation or flutter	Calcium channel blockers (verapamil, diltiazem) (class I) β-blockers (class I) (esmolol) to slow ventricular response	Amiodarone (IIb) Ibutilide (IIa) Flecainide (IIa) Propafenone (IIa) Procainamide (IIb)	Consider DC cardioversion if the condition is <48 hours in duration or the patient is hemodynamically unstable. Conversion of atrial fibrillation/flutter to a normal sinus rhythm may cause embolization of atrial thrombi unless the patient has adequate anticoagulation.
	Digoxin (IIb)	Impaired heart function (ejection fraction <40% or evidence of congestive heart failure) Digoxin (IIb) Diltiazem (IIb) Amiodarone (IIb)	DC cardioversion is the safest and most effective treatment. For patients with atrial flutter, atrial pacing can also be effective. Patients with Wolff-Parkinson-White syndrome and atrial fibrillation should be treated with IV procain-amide if hemodynami-cally stable and, if not, with DC cardioversion.
Supraven-tricular tachy-cardias	Narrow complex: Amiodarone (IIb) Adenosine Verapamil Diltiazem (IIb)	Esmolol (class I), another β-blocker or digoxin for termination	DC cardioversion or atrial pacing may be effective for some patients. Vagotonic maneuvers (i.e., carotid sinus massage, gagging, Valsalva maneuver, or increasing venous return by straight leg raising) may first be attempted.

Continued

Drugs of Choice for Common Arrhythmias—cont'd

Arrhythmia	Drug of Choice	Alternatives	Remarks
Bradycardia	Symptomatic treatment: including atropine or transcutaneous pacing Nonsymptomatic bradycardia: observation and assessment for second-degree type II or third-degree heart block	Dopamine Epinephrine Isoproterenol	Consider causes, administer oxygen, and monitor blood pressure and pulse oximeter.
Premature ventricular complexes or nonsustained ventricular tachycardia	No drug therapy indicated for asymptomatic patients	Symptomatic patients: β-blocker	Sudden cardiac death may still occur, despite therapy. For patients after myocardial infarction, β-blocker therapy has decreased mortality.
Sustained ventricular tachycardia	Normal cardiac function: Amiodarone (IIb) Lidocaine (indeterminate) Procainamide (IIa) Sotalol (IIa)	Impaired cardiac function: Amiodarone (IIb) Lidocaine (indeterminate)	DC cardioversion is the safest and most effective treatment. It is preferred for sustained ventricular tachycardia causing hemodynamic compromise. Chest "thump" and/or IV medications should be attempted. Some ventricular tachycardias can be caused or exacerbated by bradycardia or heart block. In the presence of high-grade heart block, antiarrhythmic drugs can cause cardiac standstill. A temporary pacemaker should be inserted before using antiarrhythmic drugs in these circumstances; pacing may abolish the arrhythmia.
Ventricular fibrillation Pulseless ventricular tachycardia	Lidocaine (indeterminate) Amiodarone (IIb) Procainamide (IIa) Vasopressin Epinephrine Magnesium sulfate		Defibrillation is the treatment of choice; drugs are for prevention of recurrence.

Drugs of Choice for Common Arrhythmias—cont'd

Arrhythmia	Drug of Choice	Alternatives	Remarks
Torsades de pointes	Normal cardiac function: Magnesium sulfate Discontinuance of medications that prolong QT Correction of electrolytes Cardioversion Magnesium sulfate (indeterminate) Overdrive pacing with or without β-blocker Isoproterenol Phenytoin Lidocaine	Impaired cardiac function: Cardioversion Amiodarone (IIb) Lidocaine (indeterminate)	Causative agents (e.g., quinidine) should be discontinued. Magnesium sulfate in a dose of 1 g IV, repeated once if necessary, may be effective even in absence of hypomagnesemia. Potassium replacement should be given to raise serum potassium to between 4 and 5.5 mEq/L.
Digitalis-induced ventricular tachyarrhythmias	Digoxin-immune Fab (digoxin antibody fragments; Digibind)	Lidocaine, phenytoin	Self-limited if digoxin is stopped. Phenytoin may be effective. Avoid DC cardioversion except for ventricular fibrillation or sustained ventricular tachycardia. A β-blocker or procainamide can make heart block worse. Potassium chloride can be given carefully, 10–20 mEq/hr IV, to patients with low or normal serum potassium concentrations. Extreme care must be taken to keep serum potassium <5.5 mEq/L. In the presence of heart block not associated with paroxysmal atrial tachycardia, potassium should be withheld if the serum concentration is >4.5 mEq/L because high serum potassium may increase atrioventricular blockade.

B. Cardiomyopathy

DEFINITION

Cardiomyopathies are acute or chronic diseases of the myocardium that may also involve the endocardium and pericardium. They are characterized by myocardial dysfunction unrelated to coronary artery disease, valvular abnormalities, or hypertension. They ultimately affect contractile function, and life-threatening congestive heart failure (CHF) is common to all cardiomyopathies.

ETIOLOGY

Cardiomyopathies can be classified according to their associated hemodynamics and morphologies: dilated, restrictive, hypertrophic, and obliterative.

DILATED CARDIOMYOPATHY

Whereas the origin of dilated cardiomyopathies is usually idiopathic, other causes are attributed to nutritional deficits or alcohol abuse. In some patients in whom febrile illness occurs prior to the onset of cardiac dysfunction, a virus may be the cause. Dilated cardiomyopathies can be acute or chronic and can lead to a decrease in myocardial contractility, often involving both ventricles. This leads to decreased cardiac output (CO) and increased filling pressures. Mitral and tricuspid insufficiency may occur if dilation becomes severe. The electrocardiogram (ECG) may reveal left ventricular (LV) hypertrophy, ST and T-wave abnormalities, first-degree heart block, or bundle branch block. Arrhythmias can also be seen, such as premature ventricular contractions and atrial fibrillation. Chest x-ray study may show cardiac enlargement and interstitial pulmonary edema. Diagnosis by echocardiography requires an ejection fraction of less than 0.40, a dilated and hypokinetic left ventricle, and mild to moderate regurgitation. Mural thrombi often form (typically in the left atrium), and systemic embolization is common.

TREATMENT

Patients with dilated cardiomyopathy must avoid unnecessary physical activity and must exhibit total abstinence from alcohol. CHF is treated with digoxin and diuretics. Vasodilator treatment or an inotrope with vasodilator properties (amrinone or milrinone) may also be helpful. Ventricular arrhythmias are treated with procainamide or quinidine. Because of the increased risk of pulmonary embolism, these patients may be treated with anticoagulants (not proved to be of benefit). Patients with associated collagen vascular disease, sarcoidosis, or inflammation on endocardial biopsy are treated with corticosteroids preoperatively. Tachyarrhythmias can be treated with β-blockers. Patients with coronary artery disease and dilated cardiomyopathy may benefit from coronary revascularization to improve LV function. With advanced CHF, these patients may be candidates for heart transplantation, provided pulmonary hypertension does not exist.

ANESTHETIC CONSIDERATIONS

- Avoid drug-induced myocardial depression (i.e., avoid inhalational agents, if possible).
- Maintain normovolemia.

- Prevent increases in afterload.
- Invasive monitoring may be necessary if manipulation of pulmonary and systemic vascular resistances is needed.

Excess cardiovascular depression on induction of anesthesia in patients with a history of alcohol abuse may reflect undiagnosed dilated cardiomyopathy; however, failure of this expected response to intravenous induction agents may reflect a slow circulation time. During maintenance, myocardial depression produced by volatile agents must be considered. Opiates exhibit benign effects on cardiac contractility but may not produce unconsciousness. In addition, an opioid, nitrous, benzodiazepine technique may cause unexpected cardiac depression. Increases in heart rate associated with surgical stimulation may be treated with β-blockers. Nondepolarizing muscle relaxants that exhibit few cardiovascular effects are advised. Cardiac filling pressures should guide intravenous fluids; therefore, a pulmonary artery catheter aids in early recognition of the need for inotropes or vasodilators. Prominent "v" waves reflect mitral or tricuspid regurgitation. Intraoperative hypotension is treated with ephedrine. Phenylephrine could adversely affect afterload as a result of increased systemic vascular resistance (SVR). Regional anesthesia may be used in selected patients, although caution is indicated in avoiding abrupt sympathetic blockade as seen in spinal or epidural anesthesia.

PROGNOSIS

Prognosis of dilated cardiomyopathy is poor, with a 5-year survival rate of 25% to 40%. The cause of death in 75% of these patients is CHF. Pulmonary embolism or sudden death from arrhythmia is found in more than 50% of these patients on autopsy.

RESTRICTIVE CARDIOMYOPATHY

This condition manifests as impaired diastolic filling that produces increased filling pressures and decreased CO mimicking constrictive pericarditis. Restrictive cardiomyopathy causes a greater impairment of LV filling than right ventricular (RV) filling. LV filling pressures are usually greater than RV filling pressures, and the left ventricle becomes less compliant. There is no effective treatment for this disease, and death is often the result of cardiac arrhythmia or intractable CHF. Anesthetic management follows the same principles used in cardiac tamponade.

HYPERTROPHIC CARDIOMYOPATHY

This disease is an autosomal dominant hereditary condition. The peak incidence is in patients 50 to 70 years of age. Most elderly patients diagnosed with this condition are female.

The genetic defect involves increased density of calcium channels, thus affecting the contractile process of the heart. The disease manifests as unexplained myocardial hypertrophy, often with greater thickening of the interventricular septum compared with the wall of the left ventricle. Echocardiography reveals a large variation in the location and extent of the hypertrophy. The disease is therefore often referred to as *hypertrophic cardiomyopathy with or without LV outflow obstruction*. These patients should not participate in sports because of the risk of sudden death. There is hypertrophy of the left ventricle, which becomes slitlike and elongated. The ejection fraction is often greater than 0.80, reflecting the hypercontractile condition of the heart even with severe LV outflow obstruction. Mitral regurgitation (MR) may be present and indicates interference with movement of the septal leaflet of the mitral valve (systolic anterior motion) by the hypertrophied septum. The degree of ventricular outflow obstruction is influenced by contractility, preload, and afterload.

CLINICAL MANIFESTATIONS

The major symptoms include angina, syncope, tachyarrhythmias, and CHF. Angina that is relieved by placing the patient in the recumbent position is pathognomonic for this disease, because the increase in LV size in recumbency decreases the outflow obstruction. These patients are especially susceptible to coronary ischemia as a result of the marked LV hypertrophy, particularly when subendocardial blood flow is decreased from excessive pressure in the left ventricle.

To maintain CO, adequate atrial contribution to CO (usually 25%) is necessary; therefore, atrial fibrillation is poorly tolerated. In addition, tachyarrhythmias impair diastolic filling time, which also decreases CO. These patients are prone to systemic embolization, and even asymptomatic patients are at risk for sudden unexpected death from LV outflow obstruction or ventricular tachycardia.

Cardiac murmurs may indicate LV outflow obstruction or MR in patients with hypertrophic cardiomyopathy. These murmurs are characterized by their marked variation with different maneuvers. Valsalva maneuver decreases LV size, which increases the outflow obstruction; LV systolic pressures increase, causing the murmur of mitral regurgitation to intensify as well. Nitroglycerin and the standing position also intensify the murmur. Chest x-ray studies and ECG reveal LV hypertrophy, which may be the only sign in an asymptomatic patient. Abnormal Q waves may be seen in leads II, III, AVF, or V_4 to V_6, mimicking a pseudoinfarction pattern. This diagnosis should be considered in any young patient with an ECG suggestive of myocardial infarction. Cardiac catheterization will suggest MR or increased LV end-diastolic pressure. Decreased LV compliance causes increases in the height of the "a" wave to more than 30 mm Hg. If LV outflow obstruction exists, there will be a pressure gradient across the aortic valve.

TREATMENT

The goal of treatment in these patients is to relieve the obstruction to LV outflow. This is often achieved with β-blockers to lower the heart rate and decrease contractility. Calcium channel antagonists may also help. Caution should be taken to prevent drug-induced hypotension and negative inotropic effects; therefore, nitroglycerin should be avoided in these patients who present with angina. Should CHF also exist, treatment becomes more difficult. Diuretics can lead to hypovolemia, and digoxin can increase cardiac contractility, both of which may worsen the obstruction. Cardioversion may be necessary to maintain normal sinus rhythm. Patients with atrial fibrillation require anticoagulant treatment to prevent embolization. These patients are at risk for infective endocarditis and should receive prophylactic antibiotic treatment for dental or surgical procedures. Myotomy or myomectomy under cardiac bypass may be needed in 10% to 15% of patients. Mitral valve replacement may also be needed.

ANESTHETIC CONSIDERATIONS

Anesthetic management is directed at minimizing LV outflow obstruction. Any drug or event that decreases cardiac contractility or increases preload or afterload will decrease LV outflow obstruction.

Preoperative

Preoperative medications should minimize anxiety. Expansion of intravascular fluid volume will help to maintain intraoperative stroke volume and lessen the adverse effects of positive-pressure ventilation.

Induction

Intravenous induction is acceptable, provided sudden decreases in SVR are avoided. Some degree of myocardial depression can be tolerated. Ketamine is not a good choice because the increased myocardial contractility will enhance LV outflow obstruction and decrease the stroke volume. Laryngoscopy should be smooth and stress-free, and using a volatile anesthetic, opioid, or β-blocker before laryngoscopy may blunt responses.

Maintenance

During maintenance, mild cardiac depression while maintaining intravascular fluid volume and SVR is desirable. Opiates alone are not the best choice because they do not provide cardiac depression and can decrease SVR. Opiates combined with nitrous oxide, however, may be helpful in providing myocardial depression and a slight increase in SVR. Care should be taken if spinal or epidural anesthesia is used because of the hemodynamic changes that may occur with sympathectomy (it may increase the LV outflow obstruction). Nondepolarizing muscle relaxants with little effect on the circulation are best for skeletal muscle paralysis. Tachycardia associated with pancuronium is not desirable in these patients.

Invasive monitors, such as a pulmonary artery catheter, as well as transesophageal echocardiography may be useful. Intraoperative hypotension in response to decreased preload or afterload can be treated with an α-agonist (phenylephrine, 50 to 100 mcg intravenously). β-agonists, such as ephedrine, dopamine, or dobutamine, should be avoided because an increase in cardiac contractility or heart rate can worsen outflow obstruction. Most important in maintaining blood pressure is prompt replacement of blood loss and titration of fluids to the cardiac filling pressures. Persistent hypertension can be treated with titration of a volatile anesthetic. Vasodilators (sodium nitroprusside or nitroglycerin) should be used with caution because they decrease SVR and may worsen the problem. Maintenance of normal sinus rhythm is vital to optimize the atrial component to ventricular filling. β-Blockers may be needed to slow a persistently increased heart rate.

OBLITERATIVE CARDIOMYOPATHY

Obliterative cardiomyopathy is considered a variant of restrictive cardiomyopathy and is characterized by a marked decrease in ventricular compliance. This condition may occur in association with hypereosinophilic syndromes. Cardiac arrhythmias, conduction disturbances, systemic embolization, and valvular inefficiency are common. Treatment may include steroids.

C. Congestive Heart Failure

DEFINITION
Congestive heart failure (CHF) is the failure of the myocardium to function properly, causing pulmonary congestion and ultimately pulmonary edema. CHF may involve one or both sides of the heart.

ETIOLOGY
CHF is usually caused by impaired myocardial contractility (secondary to ischemic heart disease or cardiomyopathy), cardiac valve abnormalities, systemic hypertension, or pulmonary hypertension (*cor pulmonale*). CHF in the preoperative period is the most important contributor to postoperative cardiac morbidity and mortality. Normal adaptive cardiac mechanisms that allow the heart to maintain cardiac output (CO) are the Frank-Starling relation (i.e., an increase in stroke volume accompanies an increase in end-diastolic pressure); inotropic state, afterload, changes in heart rate and myocardial hypertrophy and dilation; sympathetic nervous system activity; and humorally mediated responses.

DIAGNOSTIC AND LABORATORY FINDINGS
- Cardiac index is less than 2.5 L/min in severe CHF.
- Ejection fraction is often less than 0.50 (50%).
- Left ventricular end-diastolic pressure parallels the end-diastolic volume and is increased in the presence of CHF. Left ventricular end-diastolic pressure is normally less than 12 mm Hg, and right ventricular end-diastolic pressure is normally less than 5 mm Hg.

CLINICAL MANIFESTATIONS
Left Ventricular Failure
- Fatigue
- Dyspnea resulting from interstitial pulmonary edema
- Orthopnea
- Paroxysmal nocturnal dyspnea
- Acute pulmonary edema
- Tachypnea and rales
- Tachycardia and peripheral vasoconstriction
- Oliguria
- Pleural effusion

Right Ventricular Failure
- Systemic venous congestion: jugular venous distention
- Hepatomegaly
- Ascites
- Peripheral edema: dependent and pitting edema

TREATMENT
Treatment of CHF includes the use of digitalis, diuretics, angiotensin-converting enzyme inhibitors, vasodilators, and/or inotropes.

Digitalis
Digitalis is the only orally effective positive inotropic agent currently in use. Digoxin is excreted mainly by the kidneys, and its elimination parallels

creatinine clearance. In the perioperative period, sensitivity to digoxin can be increased if there are decreases in renal function or hypokalemia. Prophylaxis with digitalis is controversial in those patients with CHF undergoing elective surgery. Elderly patients undergoing thoracic surgery, however, may benefit. Digitalis may be continued in the preoperative period, especially if it is used to control heart rate. Toxicity should be suspected if the patient complains of nausea and vomiting, if cardiac arrhythmias are present, and if the serum digitalis level is greater than 3 ng/mL. Treatment of digitalis toxicity includes correction of hypokalemia, treatment of arrhythmias, and insertion of a temporary pacemaker if complete heart block ensues. If surgery cannot be delayed in the patient with digitalis toxicity, it is important to avoid sympathomimetics (ketamine) and hyperventilation (leading to hypokalemia).

Diuretics

Loop diuretics (e.g., furosemide) are often given to patients with CHF. Long-term administration of these drugs can lead to hypovolemia, orthostatic hypotension, and hypokalemia. Monitoring serum electrolytes (i.e., potassium) is essential, especially if the patient is treated with digitalis preparations.

Vasodilators

Vasodilators are the mainstay in the treatment of CHF because they decrease the impedance against which the left ventricle must work. Hypotension can result, however, and is a limiting factor in treating CHF with these drugs. Invasive monitoring (arterial and pulmonary artery catheters) may become necessary when information regarding CO, filling pressures, and systemic, pulmonary, and peripheral vascular resistances are needed to treat these patients effectively. Commonly used vasodilators include the following drugs:

Nitroglycerin, 0.5 to 5 mcg/kg/min intravenously
Hydralazine, 25 to 100 mg orally
Nitroprusside, 0.5 to 5 mcg/kg/min intravenously
Prazosin, 1 to 5 mg orally
Captopril, 25 to 75 mg orally
Enalapril, 5 to 40 mg orally

Inotropes

Inotropic therapy is used cautiously because β-agonists can increase myocardial oxygen demand and can also increase heart rate via β_1 stimulation. Intravenous dopamine and dobutamine are used perioperatively to improve myocardial contractility. The combination of these two drugs provides beneficial renal effects (from dopamine) and β effects (from dobutamine) at doses that are unlikely to increase afterload. A phosphodiesterase inhibitor such as milrinone (Primacor) may also be used as an inotropic agent. The advantage of this drug is increased inotropic action with afterload reduction. Epinephrine is also a drug of choice for inotropic support secondary to its β effects. A pulmonary artery catheter should be used to monitor the effects of these drugs on CO, cardiac index, and filling pressures.

ANESTHETIC CONSIDERATIONS

If surgery is absolutely necessary, the goal is to optimize CO. Ketamine, etomidate, and midazolam, given slowly and sparingly, have all been used successfully to induce anesthesia in the patient with CHF. Volatile anesthetics must be used with caution because of their propensity to cause myocardial depression. Severe CHF requires careful titration of all anesthetic agents for maintenance. Positive-pressure ventilation may help by decreasing pulmonary congestion and improving arterial oxygenation but may also reduce venous return and lower blood pressure. Therefore, invasive monitoring should strongly be considered in these patients. CO can be supported with dopamine, dobutamine, or both as needed. Regional anesthesia may be used for extremity surgery in the patient with CHF. Anesthetic technique and agents should be individualized for each patient, with consideration of the medical history and surgical procedure.

D. Hypertension

DEFINITION

Hypertension (HTN) is a systolic blood pressure (SBP) greater than 160 mm Hg or diastolic blood pressure (DBP) greater than 90 mm Hg or both. Mortality and morbidity increase with increasing levels of either SBP or DBP.

INCIDENCE

HTN is the most common circulatory derangement, affecting more than 60 million Americans. The prevalence of HTN increases with age, and approximately two thirds of those older than 65 years of age have systolic or diastolic HTN.

ETIOLOGY

BP is regulated by baroreceptors and secretion of vasoactive hormones (renin, angiotensin, aldosterone, and catecholamines). Any abnormality in this system can lead to HTN. *Essential* HTN has no identifiable cause and accounts for more than 90% of HTN. *Secondary* HTN is caused by renal disease, coarctation, Cushing's syndrome, pheochromocytoma, primary aldosteronism, or pharmacologic agents.

DIAGNOSIS AND LABORATORY FINDINGS

Persistent elevation of SBP greater than 160 mm Hg and/or DBP greater than 90 mm Hg is seen. Renal disease, coarctation, hyperadrenocorticism, and pheochromocytoma are common secondary causes. Organ system involvement is determined through diagnostic testing.

TREATMENT

When DBP is greater than 90 mm Hg, drug treatment is usually employed, although isolated systolic HTN may respond to diet modification and weight loss. Patients with borderline HTN can decrease their BP with exercise and weight loss. If DBP exceeds 105 mm Hg, aggressive treatment is needed to decrease morbidity and mortality from myocardial infarction, congestive heart failure, cerebrovascular accident, and renal failure.

   Drugs used to treat HTN include diuretics, angiotensin-converting enzyme inhibitors, calcium antagonists, β-blockers, and vasodilators. Initial treatment is usually with a diuretic, an angiotensin-converting enzyme inhibitor, or a β-blocker. A combination of two antihypertensives is often used to minimize the undesirable physiologic responses to any one particular drug (e.g., a compensatory increase in renin activity). Serum potassium levels should be monitored, because hypokalemia or hyperkalemia may be a side effect.

ANESTHETIC CONSIDERATIONS

Preoperative

Reviewing the patient's medication and determining adequacy of BP control is essential. Associated organ dysfunction should be evaluated, particularly for orthostatic hypotension, ischemic heart disease, cerebrovascular disease, peripheral vascular disease, and renal dysfunction. Anti-HTN medications should be continued preoperatively. If emergency surgery is imminent, the patient with uncontrolled HTN should have BP maintained at or near 140/90 mm Hg, provided no evidence of cerebral ischemia or renal dysfunction is present. Patients with DBP of 110 mm Hg or greater have a significantly increased risk of perioperative cardiac morbidity.

Ideally, patients should be normotensive prior to surgery. During anesthesia and operation in the hypertensive patient, BP is more likely to decrease precipitously. Chronic HTN is frequently associated with hypovolemia and ischemic heart disease; therefore, a decrease in BP is more likely to result in myocardial ischemia.

Induction

During induction of anesthesia, the clinician should expect exaggerated changes in BP and hypotension as a result of drug-induced vasodilation in the presence of a decrease in intravascular fluid volume. Laryngoscopy and intubation may cause exaggerated rises in BP and should be performed as smoothly as possible. Methods used to attenuate HTN and tachycardia during induction of anesthesia include deepening anesthesia by including a volatile anesthetic, opioids, lidocaine, and β-blockers.

Maintenance

Intraoperatively, the goal is to maintain the patient's BP stability within 20% of the normal BP range. Intraoperative events that cause wide fluctuations in BP should be anticipated and treated immediately. Increases in BP in response to surgical stimulation are the most common intraoperative changes. A volatile anesthetic is ideal for allowing rapid adjustment of anesthetic depth in response to changes in BP. Volatile agents produce a dose-dependent decrease in BP. A nitrous oxide/opioid technique may also be used; however, a volatile anesthetic may be needed to control undesirable increases in BP. Vasoactive agents can be used intraoperatively to treat HTN or hypotension.

Monitors include routine use of electrocardiographic monitoring leads II and V_5 to detect cardiac ischemia most accurately. Direct arterial pressure monitoring may be warranted.

Postoperative

HTN in the postoperative period is common because of pain and an exaggerated sympathetic response. Hypervolemia related to intraoperative fluid management may also contribute to HTN seen postoperatively. Prompt assessment and treatment of postoperative HTN are necessary to decrease the potential for myocardial ischemia, arrhythmia, CHF, cerebrovascular accident, and bleeding. If HTN continues despite adequate analgesia, labetalol (0.1 to 0.25 mg/kg intravenously every 10 minutes), esmolol (0.5 to 1.0 mg/kg), or other β-blockers may be given. Hydralazine (2.5 to 10 mg intravenously every 10 to 20 minutes) may be considered; however, its potential to increase heart rate should be considered. In extreme cases of unmanageable HTN postoperatively, sodium nitroprusside or nitroglycerin may need to be considered.

E. Ischemic Heart Disease

DEFINITION
Ischemic heart disease (IHD) describes the condition in which atherosclerotic plaque is present in the coronary arteries, giving way to coronary artery disease (CAD).

INCIDENCE
More than 10 million adults in the United States have IHD, and it is the leading cause of death (500,000 deaths/year). The first manifestation of IHD is often acute myocardial infarction resulting in sudden death.

The overall prognosis of patients with IHD is dependent on the frequency and severity of cardiac arrhythmias, myocardial infarction, and left ventricular (LV) dysfunction. About 40 million people in the United States undergo anesthesia and operation each year; of these, 30% are considered to be at high risk because of the presence of IHD.

ETIOLOGY
IHD results from the presence of atherosclerotic plaque in the coronary arteries that causes narrowing and subsequently impedes blood flow. Angina pectoris is the presenting complaint of the patient experiencing a reduction in coronary artery blood flow. Dyspnea that occurs after the onset of angina indicates acute LV dysfunction, which can lead to congestive heart failure (CHF) from myocardial ischemia. The most important risk factors are advanced age and male gender. Other risk factors include hyperlipidemia, hypertension, cigarette smoking, diabetes, obesity, sedentary lifestyle, familial history of premature development of IHD, and other psychosocial characteristics. There are three types of angina: stable, variant, and unstable. *Stable angina* is chest pain that occurs predictably when there is an increase in cardiac work. As the heart rate increases (usually more than 100 beats/min), demand exceeds supply, and angina becomes evident. *Variant angina* is due to coronary artery spasm of unknown cause that gives way to ischemia and ultimately chest pain. *Unstable angina* is a combination of stable and variant angina and usually represents an advanced degree of CAD. These patients may have angina at rest.

DIAGNOSTIC AND LABORATORY FINDINGS
Cardiac Evaluation
A complete history and physical examination, chest x-ray study, and electrocardiogram (ECG) should be performed in the patient with known or suspected IHD. If the initial evaluation suggests IHD, stress testing may be indicated. An exercise ECG with or without concomitant administration of intravenous radionuclide (i.e., thallium) or pharmacologic echocardiography is usually performed. If the stress test is suggestive of IHD, cardiac catheterization may then be indicated. In addition, dobutamine stress

echocardiography is also available to evaluate overall cardiac function further (see the box on evaluation of LV function).

Evaluation of Left Ventricular Function

Poor Function	Good Function
1. History	1. History
a. Multiple MI	a. Angina
b. Symptoms of CHF	b. Hypertension and obesity
	c. No symptoms of CHF
2. Cardiac catheterization	2. Cardiac catheterization
a. EF <40%	a. EF >50%
b. LVEDP >18 mm Hg	b. LVEDP <12 mm Hg
c. Multiple areas of ventricular dyskinesia	c. No areas of ventricular dyskinesia
d. Decreased CO	d. Normal CO
e. Ventricular septal defect	
f. MI in progress	
g. Extreme age	

CHF, Congestive heart failure; *CO,* cardiac output; *EF,* ejection fraction; *LVEDP,* left ventricular end-diastolic pressure; *MI,* myocardial infarction.

History

The clinician should elicit the severity and functional limitations imposed by IHD. Evaluation of symptoms as they relate to exercise tolerance, dyspnea, angina, and peripheral edema will give a qualitative estimate of the degree of impairment. Symptoms in some patients may not be present at rest, so the patient's response to physical activity should be elicited through careful, appropriate questioning (e.g., Can the patient climb a flight of stairs?). One must be able to identify borderline CHF because the stress of anesthesia and operation may elicit overt heart failure perioperatively.

CLINICAL MANIFESTATIONS
Angina

Angina pectoris is substernal chest pain that often radiates to the neck, jaw, left shoulder, or left arm and is frequently precipitated by exertion. It may be relieved with rest or sublingual nitroglycerin (see the following table).

Manifestations of Angina

	Exercise-Induced	Occurs at Rest	Night Pain	ST Segment
Stable	Yes	No (yes with emotion)	Occasionally with dream	↓ ST
Unstable	Yes	Yes	Yes	↑ or ↓ ST
Variant	Rarely	Yes	Early in a.m.	↑ ST usually; can also be depressed

Classic
- The symptom is precipitated by exertion and is relieved by rest.
- It is a specific predictor for identification of patients with CAD, placing them at a higher risk for cardiac complications.

Atypical
- Signs and symptoms are different in type, location, precipitating events or character.

Unstable
- The progression of coronary stenosis is occurring more rapidly than the development of collateral circulation.

TREATMENT
Treatment goals are geared toward using those measures to decrease myocardial oxygen demand and increase supply (i.e., increase coronary blood flow). This can be achieved in various ways.

General Medical Methods
- Control of related pathology: CHF, hypertension
- Smoking cessation
- Weight loss
- Exercise
- Stress modification
- Antithrombotic medications: low-dose aspirin may prevent reinfarction
- Avoidance of heavy meals or cold prior to exertion

Drug Therapy
- Nitrates
- β-blockers
- Calcium channel blockers
- Antiplatelet drugs

Revascularization: When the Patient's Condition Is Refractory to Drug Therapy
- Coronary artery bypass graft
- Percutaneous transluminal coronary angioplasty
- Coronary artery stent

ANESTHETIC CONSIDERATIONS
Preoperative
The goal is to decrease anxiety and thus sympathetic stimulation, which may otherwise increase myocardial oxygen demand, causing ischemia. Benzodiazepines (e.g., midazolam) and/or narcotics may be administered for preoperative sedation and amnesia. Nitroglycerin may also be administered prophylactically to optimize coronary blood flow. Guidelines are included based on whether the patient has good or poor LV function (see the box provided).

Intraoperative
Prevent intraoperative events that adversely affect the balance between myocardial oxygen supply and demand. Factors that can *decrease*

Factors Influencing Oxygen Supply and Demand

Decrease Oxygen Supply	Increase Oxygen Demand
Decreased cerebral blood flow	Sympathetic stimulation
Tachycardia	Tachycardia
Increased diastolic pressure	Increased systolic pressure
Increased $PaCO_2$	Increased myocardial contractility
Coronary artery spasm	Increased afterload
Decreased CaO_2, anemia, PaO_2	
Increased preload	

oxygen supply and *increase oxygen demand* are listed in the box given here.

The goal is to maintain heart rate and blood pressure within 20% of normal. Although it is generally accepted that a heart rate higher than 100 beats/min is more likely to cause ischemia, it has been shown that ischemia may also develop at rates lower than 100 beats/min (see the box provided).

Preoperative Medication and Left Ventricular Function

Poor Function	Good Function
Light premedication	Heavy premedication
Intravenous sedation for line insertion	Intravenous sedation for line insertion
Slow narcotic/relaxant induction	Narcotic/relaxant/thiopental induction
	Inhalation agent may be used

Induction

Most induction drugs are acceptable, provided they are administered judiciously. Laryngoscopy and intubation time should be kept at a minimum (less than 15 seconds) to decrease sympathetic stimulation and its deleterious effects. If hypertension exists in the patient prior to anesthesia, the following drugs can be used to facilitate a smooth, stress-free induction.

Lidocaine, 1 to 2 mg/kg intravenously 90 seconds prior to laryngoscopy
Nitroprusside, 1 to 2 mcg/kg intravenously 15 seconds prior to laryngoscopy
Esmolol, 100 to 300 mcg/kg intravenously before induction
Fentanyl, 1 to 3 mcg/kg intravenously during induction

Maintenance

It is imperative to identify whether the patient has normal or poor LV function. In patients with normal LV function, it is important to avoid tachycardia and hypertension during periods of intense stimulation (laryngoscopy and surgical incision). Volatile anesthetics will minimize increases in sympathetic activity and oxygen demand. Inclusion of nitrous oxide with an inhalational agent or alone as part of a nitrous oxide/opioid technique is also acceptable. A high-dose narcotic technique with the addition of a volatile anesthetic to treat undesired increases in blood pressure is effective. In patients with poor LV function, agents that precipitate myocardial depression are not advocated. Opioids are the agent of choice, with low-dose volatile anesthetics, nitrous oxide, and benzodiazepines added as needed.

Muscle Relaxation

Any of several nondepolarizing muscle relaxants may be used. Intermediate-acting relaxants (vecuronium, cisatracurium) have been used successfully, as have longer acting relaxants (pancuronium). Choice of relaxant may be determined by its potential effect on heart rate, length of procedure, plan for emergence (i.e., Will the patient be mechanically ventilated postoperatively or is "fast tracking" to be considered?), and cost. Pancuronium can cause a dose-dependent increase in heart rate (which could potentially lead to myocardial ischemia); however, it can also be used to offset the bradycardia that ensues when high-dose narcotics are used. Mivacurium and atracurium should be used with caution because of the potential of histamine release.

Reversal Agents

Anticholinesterase drugs (pyridostigmine, neostigmine) and anticholinergics (atropine, glycopyrrolate, and scopolamine) are considered safe. Many clinicians prefer glycopyrrolate because of its tendency to preserve a somewhat "normal" heart rate when used in combination with an anticholinesterase.

Emergence

The same considerations apply here as for induction of anesthesia (i.e., prevent increases in myocardial oxygen demand and decreases in supply). Patients with severe IHD may need treatment for hypertensive episodes during emergence from anesthesia and into the postoperative period.

POSTOPERATIVE CARE

Maintenance of normal cardiac dynamics (blood pressure and heart rate), normal arterial oxygen and carbon dioxide pressure, and adequate pain relief are essential to prevent sympathetic stimulation and its deleterious effects on myocardial oxygen supply and demand.

F. Myocardial Infarction

DEFINITION

Myocardial infarction (MI) or myocardial cell death occurs when a portion of heart muscle is deprived of its blood supply as a result of blockage, acute thrombosis, or spasm of a coronary artery.

INCIDENCE AND PREVALENCE

The clinician should first determine whether the patient has a previous history of MI. The likelihood of perioperative reinfarction correlates with the time elapsed since prior MI. The average reinfarction rate is 6% if the time elapsed since the first MI is 6 months. Therefore, elective surgery, especially thoracic or abdominal, *should be delayed for 6 months following MI.* Even with a 6-month delay, these patients are still at greater risk than patients who have not suffered an MI. In high-risk patients, invasive hemodynamic monitoring, transesophageal echocardiograpy, and aggressive treatment of cardiac alterations have reduced the risk of reinfarction.

The incidence of reinfarction is also increased in patients undergoing intrathoracic or intraabdominal operations lasting more than 3 hours. Factors increasing the potential for reinfarction include hypotension (i.e., mean arterial pressure less than 60 mm Hg) lasting longer than 10 minutes, hypertension and tachycardia, diabetes, smoking, and hyperlipidemia.

ETIOLOGY

When myocardial oxygen supply (i.e., coronary blood flow) does not meet demand (myocardial oxygen consumption), ischemia or MI may occur. The risk for perioperative MI increases when a patient who has suffered a previous MI undergoes anesthesia and operation.

LABORATORY TESTS

Laboratory tests as indicated by the history and physical examination may include electrolytes, complete blood count, blood urea nitrogen, creatinine, cardiac enzymes (MB bands), and a coagulation profile. Twenty-four hour Holter monitoring may be necessary if the patient is at risk for ischemic episodes or arrhythmias. Echocardiography, stress testing, or cardiac catheterization may become necessary in the patient with cardiac disease. The approach must be individualized to the needs and risks of the patient.

CLINICAL MANIFESTATIONS

Many patients are asymptomatic following an MI. Common manifestations of coronary artery disease include poor exercise tolerance, angina (stable or unstable), dyspnea, congestive heart failure (CHF), and arrhythmias. These patients may be risk stratified according to the New York Heart Association functional classification and the American Society of Anesthesiologists classification.

TREATMENT AND ANESTHETIC CONSIDERATIONS

Anesthesia care begins with a thorough history and physical examination. The history reveals risk factors for ischemic heart disease, activity tolerance, determination of angina (stable or unstable), and use of coronary vasodilators (e.g., nitroglycerin). The physical examination may reveal extra heart sounds (i.e., S_3 and/or S_4), rales/rhonchi, jugular venous distention, peripheral edema, or other findings consistent with underlying cardiac disease. The anesthetist should communicate any findings with the primary physician and surgeon to weigh the risks and benefits of the proposed surgical procedure. The importance of minimizing stress (demand) and optimizing myocardial perfusion (supply) intraoperatively cannot be overemphasized. Reduction of stress begins in the preoperative area with the use of individualized sedation. Any increase in metabolic work during the perioperative period increases myocardial oxygen demand, which may result in myocardial ischemia or MI. Myocardial oxygen supply and demand must be balanced for an optimal outcome.

Four questions must therefore be answered before the patient proceeds to anesthesia and operation. The answers to these questions are often determined by careful history taking. The first three questions to be addressed are: *What is the extent of coronary artery disease? Is additional therapy indicated (e.g., cardiac catheterization, angioplasty, or coronary artery bypass grafting? What is the extent of ventricular compromise?* How the clinician determines the answers to these questions will inevitably affect the administration and titration of anesthetics. Finally, the fourth question to be asked is: *Will the patient tolerate surgery?*

Standard monitoring should always be considered in these patients. In addition, electrocardiographic (ECG) monitoring of lead II (inferior ischemia) and lead V_5 (anterior ischemia), ST-segment trend analysis, esophageal ECG (to identify P waves, posterior ischemia), and/or transesophageal echocardiography can be used perioperatively. Invasive intravascular lines, such as a central venous pressure (CVP) line, a pulmonary artery (PA) catheter (to evaluate right- and left-sided heart pressures, pulmonary capillary wedge pressure, pulmonary and systemic vascular resistances, and cardiac output/index), and an arterial line for beat-to-beat evaluation of blood pressure and frequent blood specimen analyses, may need to be considered. These measures should be used to optimize anesthetic care when the patient is at risk because of clinical history and/or the surgical procedure.

Recognition and aggressive treatment of ischemia are vital. Careful, vigilant monitoring perioperatively will allow rapid intervention in the patient at risk for cardiac complications. Likewise, interpretation of data and prompt initiation of treatment have been shown to improve outcome.

Fluid management in these patients should be individualized to the length and type of operation and the degree of left ventricular compromise. A CVP or PA catheter can offer useful information in these high-risk patients. Intraoperative overhydration (i.e., fluid overload) may lead to postoperative hypertension and CHF.

Urine output should be closely monitored in the cardiac patient (approximately 0.5 to 1.0 mL/kg/hour). It is believed to be a reflection of renal perfusion and thus cardiac output, provided renal function is normal. Urine output may also be an indicator of overall patient volume status.

Choice of anesthetic in these patients should be individualized to the patient and the proposed procedure. General, regional, and local anesthetic techniques have all been used successfully. It is important for the clinician to understand that patient outcome is based on *how* the agents are administered, rather than the specific technique used.

General anesthesia and spinal anesthesia are similar when the risk of perioperative MI and death is considered. A combined general-epidural technique for vascular surgery has been suggested to lower cardiac complications. The incidence and risk of CHF are higher with general anesthesia in patients with severe coronary artery disease.

Emergence from anesthesia should be smooth and stress-free, with special efforts made to maintain cardiac hemodynamics (myocardial oxygen supply and demand). Time of extubation may need to be delayed until cardiovascular stability is established.

Ongoing postoperative observation of high-risk patients is essential to identify and aggressively treat cardiac complications. Shivering, fever, pain, wide swings in blood pressure, tachycardia, arrhythmias, and CHF may alter cardiac dynamics, leading to ischemia (and MI). Careful fluid management may also minimize the potential for postoperative ischemic events and may improve outcome.

Recognizing the importance of complications and mortality related to anesthesia and surgery is the first step toward prevention. Patients at risk for perioperative cardiac complications can be risk stratified, and the information can be used to plan the safest anesthetic and intraoperative monitoring.

G. Peripheral Vascular Disease

DEFINITION

Peripheral vascular disease (PVD) is an inflammation or disease of the peripheral vasculature.

ETIOLOGY

PVD may manifest as systemic vasculitis or arterial occlusive disease. There are several types of PVD.

TAKAYASU'S ARTERITIS

Takayasu's arteritis is a chronic inflammation of the aorta and its major branches. It causes multiple organ dysfunction.

MANAGEMENT OF ANESTHESIA

Corticosteroid supplementation may be needed in patients already treated with these drugs. These patients also may be taking anticoagulants; therefore, regional anesthesia may be controversial. Blood pressure may be difficult to measure noninvasively in the upper extremities, so an arterial line may be necessary. Preoperatively, it is wise to evaluate range of motion of the cervical spine because hyperextension of the head during laryngoscopy may compromise cerebral blood flow (the carotid arteries are shortened as a result of the vascular inflammatory process). Finally, a major anesthetic goal intraoperatively is maintenance of adequate perfusion pressure.

THROMBOANGIITIS OBLITERANS

DEFINITION

Thromboangiitis obliterans is an inflammatory process of the wall and connective tissue surrounding the arteries and veins, especially in the extremities. It is often associated with the thrombosis and occlusion that commonly result in gangrene. Jewish men between the ages of 20 and 40 years seem to have a higher incidence.

MANAGEMENT OF ANESTHESIA

Prevention of cold-induced vasospasm is a major concern. Increasing the ambient room temperature and using convective warming devices (e.g., warming blankets, fluid warmers) will help maintain body temperature. Noninvasive blood pressure monitoring is preferable to invasive (arterial) monitoring in this patient population. Regional anesthesia is acceptable; however, the concomitant use of vasoconstrictors (i.e., epinephrine) should be avoided.

PROGNOSIS

The prognosis depends on the progression of the associated underlying disease. Raynaud's phenomenon (i.e., spasm of the digital arteries) is often associated with a period of "remission."

CHRONIC PERIPHERAL ARTERIO-OCCLUSIVE DISEASE

DEFINITION

Chronic peripheral arterio-occlusive disease is typically the result of peripheral atherosclerosis and often occurs in association with coronary or cerebral atherosclerosis.

ETIOLOGY AND CLINICAL MANIFESTATIONS

Occlusion of the distal abdominal aorta or the iliac arteries frequently presents as claudication of the hips and buttocks. Elderly patients often present with occlusion of the common femoral or superficial femoral arteries. This produces a syndrome of claudication from the calf area of the lower extremity.

TREATMENT

Treatment includes revascularization, such as femoral-femoral bypass or any of several different femoral-to-distal bypass procedures.

ANESTHETIC CONSIDERATIONS

The major risk for operative revascularization is associated ischemic heart disease. Although these procedures can be performed while the patient is under general anesthesia, regional (i.e., epidural) anesthesia prior to anticoagulant therapy has not been associated with untoward events. Infrarenal cross-clamping of the distal aorta in the patient with PVD is associated with minimal hemodynamic derangements. Typically, monitoring of right-sided heart pressures (i.e., central venous pressure) is sufficient unless left-sided heart disease requires the use of a pulmonary artery catheter. Thromboembolic complications, particularly in the kidneys, usually reflect dislodgement of atherosclerotic debris. Spinal cord damage is unlikely, and special monitoring is not mandatory.

SUBCLAVIAN STEAL SYNDROME

Occlusion of the subclavian or innominate artery by an atherosclerotic plaque proximal to the origin of the vertebral artery may result in reversal of blood flow from the brain, leading to syncopal episodes. The pulse in the ipsilateral arm is usually absent or diminished (10 mm Hg lower).

CORONARY-SUBCLAVIAN STEAL SYNDROME

This syndrome occurs when incomplete stenosis of the left subclavian artery leads to reversal of blood flow. The patient typically presents with angina and decreased systolic blood pressure (at least 20 mm Hg lower) in the ipsilateral arm. Bilateral brachial artery blood pressure measurement is helpful in the differential diagnosis and may be useful in the preoperative assessment in patients with an internal mammary–to–coronary artery bypass.

ANEURYSMS OF THE THORACIC AND ABDOMINAL AORTA

DEFINITION

Diseases of the aorta are frequently aneurysmal, whereas occlusive disease is most likely to affect the peripheral arteries.

ETIOLOGY

The primary event in aortic dissection is a tear in the intimal wall through which blood surges and creates a false lumen. The adventitia then separates up and/or down the aorta for various distances. Associated conditions include hypertension (which is present in 80% of these patients), Marfan's syndrome, blunt chest trauma, pregnancy, and iatrogenic surgical injury (e.g., resulting from aortic cannulation during cardiopulmonary bypass). Aortic dissections involving the ascending aorta are considered *type A*. Surgical repair is through a median sternotomy using profound hypothermia. Aortic dissections involving the descending aorta (i.e., beyond the origin of the left subclavian artery) are considered *type B*. Aneurysms can also be classified as saccular, fusiform, or dissecting.

CLINICAL MANIFESTATIONS

Signs and symptoms include the following: excruciating chest pain; a decrease or absence of peripheral pulses, stroke, paraplegia, and ischemia of extremities; vasoconstriction and hypertension; myocardial infarction; and cardiac tamponade.

TREATMENT

Early, short-term treatment includes the use of β-blockers or other cardio-active agents that decrease systolic blood pressure (to approximately 100 mm Hg) and aid in decreasing myocardial contractility and vascular resistance. Ultimately, surgical intervention is often necessary using aortic stent grafts or an open approach.

ANESTHETIC CONSIDERATIONS
Abdominal Aortic Aneurysm

History and physical examination with special focus on cardiac function are essential. Hypertension and diabetes mellitus may also be present. Preoperative analysis of important laboratory work should include hematology, chemistry, and coagulation profiles. Serum glucose levels should be kept lower than 200 mg/dL.

Anesthetic goals

To minimize morbidity and mortality, the anesthetic goals are to preserve myocardial (primary), renal, pulmonary, central nervous system, and visceral organ function. To meet these goals, one must ensure an adequate oxygen supply to the myocardium while meeting myocardial demand.

Monitors

Routine monitors should be employed, including leads II and V_5 of the electrocardiogram. In addition, blood pressure should be invasively monitored with an arterial catheter. This allows intraoperative monitoring of arterial blood gases, serum potassium, glucose, hemoglobin and hematocrit, and coagulation parameters. Transesophageal echocardiography and/or a pulmonary artery catheter may be used to enhance hemodynamic monitoring.

Induction

Most intravenous induction agents are acceptable, provided they are used judiciously in conjunction with a nondepolarizing muscle relaxant. The goal is to establish a deep level of anesthesia using a slow, controlled titration of anesthetic agents prior to induction to minimize hemodynamic fluctuations. Positioning of the patient for surgery is usually supine or lateral, depending on the location of the incision (transabdominal or retroperitoneal approaches).

Maintenance

General anesthesia or a combined technique (i.e., general and epidural) has been used successfully. Selection of appropriate agents will depend on the patient's physical status.

Intravenous fluids

Fluid volume deficits result from hemorrhage, insensible loss, and evaporative losses associated with large abdominal incisions. Surgically, an abdominal approach will typically require 10 to 15 mL/kg/hour of crystalloid (i.e., balanced salt solutions), and a retroperitoneal approach will require only 10 mL/kg/hour. Colloids may be necessary in volume-sensitive patients.

Aortic cross-clamping

Mannitol (25 g) and heparin (5000 to 10,000 units) are administered prior to cross-clamping. Activated coagulation times (ACT) are monitored (i.e., baseline before and then 5 minutes after heparin administration). The therapeutic goal is an ACT that is two to three times normal.

NOTE: Renal perfusion is at risk during cross-clamping and may lead to renal failure. *Adequate fluid replacement is the major factor in preventing renal failure.* It is important to monitor the hemodynamic parameters and urine output. Systemic blood pressure should be maintained 10 to 15 mm Hg higher than normal during aortic cross-clamping. Protamine may be given to reverse this effect.

Hemodynamics

Blood pressure is maintained slightly lower than normal before aortic cross-clamping. If the aorta is clamped *below* the renal arteries (infrarenal), elevations in afterload and blood pressure will be minimal. If the aorta is clamped *above* the renal arteries (suprarenal), a greater increase in afterload and blood pressure will be observed. Should the aorta be clamped above the supraceliac artery, an even greater increase in afterload and blood pressure can be expected. Systemic blood pressure should be maintained 10 to 15 mm Hg higher than normal during aortic cross-clamping. Have vasodilating drugs available (nitroglycerin or nitroprusside) prior to aortic cross-clamping in anticipation of hypertension.

Blood Loss

Surgical blood loss may be replaced with crystalloids, colloids, autologous blood, or packed red blood cells. Administration of fresh-frozen plasma and platelets depends on coagulation values and the number of packed red blood cells transfused.

Cross-clamp time

Cross-clamp time is usually minimized to 30 to 60 minutes. Prior to unclamping, give fluids to increase the central venous pressure 5 mm Hg higher than baseline. This helps to ensure cardiovascular stability, maintenance of blood pressure, and renal preservation.

Unclamping

- Anticipate a drop in afterload, preload, and blood pressure following removal of the aortic cross-clamp.
- Lighten the depth of anesthesia prior to unclamping, thus allowing the blood pressure to climb 30 to 40 mm Hg.

- Be prepared to transfuse 1 unit of blood.
- Should systemic blood pressure drop precipitously, the surgeon may reclamp until acceptable blood pressure is restored. Release of the clamp one limb at a time may also help with hemodynamic stability.
- Use vasopressors as necessary.
- As circulation to the lower extremities begins, a negative inotropic effect may be seen resulting from a washout of anerobic products and systemic acidosis. This response is dependent on the duration of cross-clamp time and the amount of collateral circulation.

Emergence

Consider the patient's preoperative physical status, the amount of intra-operative fluid administered, blood loss, the length of procedure, and the presence or absence of any untoward intraoperative events. The patient may require postoperative ventilation for a period of time to limit wide swings in hemodynamic parameters.

Complications

Complications include bleeding, infection, coagulation abnormalities, renal failure, and ischemia distal to the site of repair (visceral or spinal cord).

Emergency aortic abdominal aneurysm surgery

Signs and symptoms include back pain, syncope, vomiting, and severe hypotension. Primary goals of emergency surgery are rapid control of blood loss and reversal of hypotension, with secondary preservation of myocardial function.

Emergency, stable patients should proceed quickly through the preoperative area. Rapid sequence intubation following preoxygenation should be performed with hypnotic agents, opioids, and muscle relaxants.

Emergency, unstable patients require rapid intravascular volume replacement. Massive blood loss and hypotension can lead to myocardial infarction, acute renal failure, respiratory failure, or mortality in 40% to 50% of patients. Rapid surgical control of the bleeding is the first priority, and placement of invasive monitors should not delay definitive treatment.

Thoracic Aortic Aneurysm

Note: Systemic blood pressure should be monitored above the aneurysm (right or left radial artery, depending on the site at the arch). This will allow assessment of cerebral perfusion pressure as well as the perfusion pressure to the kidneys. During aortic resection, mean arterial pressure should be maintained at 100 mm Hg in the upper body and at more than 50 mm Hg distal to the aneurysm. Frequently, an endobronchial tube is required to facilitate surgical exposure.

These procedures are usually done with profound hypothermia, total circulatory arrest, or cardiopulmonary bypass. Large-bore venous access is necessitated to allow large volumes of blood or fluid to be replaced rapidly. Eight to 10 units of blood should be available. Heart rate and blood pressure should be maintained at lower than normal levels. The most common surgical approach is via a thoracotomy incision.

Prior to initiation of cardiopulmonary bypass, the aorta is cross-clamped proximal to the level of the left subclavian artery and distal to the aortic lesion. Doing so produces a mechanical decompression with the oxygenator. If cross-clamping is done without the benefit of a surgical bypass shunt, vasodilator therapy will be needed to control left ventricular after-load. A pulmonary artery catheter is typically used. The risk of spinal cord ischemia or damage increases as the cross-clamp period extends beyond 30 minutes. Postoperative complications are similar to those for abdominal aortic aneurysm. These patients are at greater risk of renal failure and of visceral and spinal cord ischemia.

H. Pericardial Processes/Tamponade

PERICARDITIS

DEFINITION
Pericarditis is an inflammatory process of the pericardium.

ETIOLOGY
Pericarditis is typically the result of a viral infection.

CLINICAL MANIFESTATIONS
There is a sudden onset of severe chest pain. Auscultation reveals a friction rub, which is "leathery" in quality and increases in intensity on exhalation. Sinus tachycardia and a low-grade fever are also common.

TREATMENT
Treatment is symptomatic with analgesics and corticosteroids. Acute pericarditis in the absence of pericardial effusion does not alter cardiac function.

PERICARDIAL EFFUSION

DEFINITION
Pericardial effusion is the accumulation of fluid in the pericardial space that is often associated with pericarditis.

ETIOLOGY
The pericardial space normally contains 20 to 25 mL of pericardial fluid; pressure here is subatmospheric, decreasing on inspiration and increasing on exhalation. Clinical effects depend on whether the fluid is creating a tamponade effect. If the fluid in the pericardium accumulates slowly, the pericardium can stretch to accommodate the increased volume without a concomitant increase in pressure. When the fluid volume increases rapidly, tamponade is possible.

DIAGNOSTIC AND LABORATORY FINDINGS
Whereas echocardiography is best at detecting pericardial effusion, computed tomography scans can also be beneficial.

CHRONIC CONSTRICTIVE PERICARDITIS

DEFINITION
Chronic constrictive pericarditis resembles cardiac tamponade. Venous pressure is increased, and stroke volume is decreased. Chronic constrictive pericarditis can interfere with filling of the heart during diastole.

ETIOLOGY

Most cases of chronic constrictive pericarditis are idiopathic; however, chronic renal failure, radiation, rheumatoid arthritis, and cardiac surgery are all possible contributing factors. Patients have fibrous scarring and adhesion of both pericardial layers, which lead to a somewhat rigid shell around the heart.

DIAGNOSTIC AND LABORATORY FINDINGS

Diagnosis depends on a history and physical examination that recognize the increase in venous pressure despite the absence of other signs of cardiac disease. Although both sides of the heart may be involved, the primary manifestations are those related to right ventricular failure with venous congestion, hepatosplenomegaly, and ascites. Atrial arrhythmias are common. Kussmaul's sign (i.e., exaggerated neck vein distention on inspiration) is also common, whereas pulsus paradoxus is more typical of cardiac tamponade. Chest x-ray study reveals a normal to small heart with calcium evident in the pericardium. Electrocardiography reveals low-voltage QRS complexes, inverted T waves, and notched P waves. Computed tomography scan and echocardiography will effectively reveal pericardial thickening.

TREATMENT

Treatment involves surgical removal of the constricting pericardium, which can result in bleeding from the epicardium. Cardiopulmonary bypass may be needed, especially if bleeding is difficult to control. Surgical correction is not immediately followed by decreases in right atrial pressure or increased cardiac output. Right atrial pressure normalizes within 3 months after surgery. Generally, myocardial function is normal.

ANESTHETIC CONSIDERATIONS

Provided hypotension does not exist as a result of pericardial tamponade, anesthetics used should not depress myocardial contractility, cause hypotension, lower the heart rate, or impede venous return. Maintenance is best accomplished by using a combination of benzodiazepines, opioids, and nitrous oxide, with or without a low concentration of volatile agent. Nondepolarizing muscle relaxants with minimal circulatory effects are best; however, the modest increase in heart rate with pancuronium is usually tolerated. Preoperative optimization of the patient's fluid status is important. If hemodynamic changes occur secondary to pericardial tamponade, an appropriate change in anesthetic management should follow.

A pulmonary artery catheter may provide beneficial information during the recovery period that is associated with wide swings in blood pressure and cardiac output. Arrhythmias are common during the procedure, and antiarrhythmic drugs, as well as a mechanical defibrillator, should be available. Patients may require postoperative ventilatory support; patients should be monitored for arrhythmias and low cardiac output, which may necessitate treatment.

CARDIAC TAMPONADE

DEFINITION

Cardiac tamponade is the accumulation of fluid in the pericardial space that elevates intrapericardial pressure.

INCIDENCE AND ETIOLOGY

The incidence varies, and cardiac tamponade may be characterized as acute or chronic. It is most commonly the result of trauma, infection, or neoplastic disease states. It can present following cardiac surgery.

DIAGNOSTIC AND LABORATORY FINDINGS

Echocardiography is the best method to detect pericardial fluid. Chest x-ray studies do not reveal a change in the cardiac silhouette until fluid accumulation reaches 250 mL.

CLINICAL MANIFESTATIONS

As pressure in the pericardial space rises, central venous pressure (CVP) also rises. Right atrial pressure may be monitored to determine whether tamponade is present. Other signs and symptoms include activation of the sympathetic nervous system (as manifested by sinus tachycardia), equalization of atrial and left ventricular filling pressures, decreased voltage and electrical alternans on electrocardiography, paradoxical pulse, hypotension, and muffled heart sounds (Beck's triad).

TREATMENT

Pericardiocentesis using local anesthesia may be used to release the tamponade surgically. Pericardiotomy using local or general anesthesia is recommended when tamponade develops from trauma or cardiac surgery and becomes symptomatic. Temporary measures to maintain stroke volume include administration of intravenous fluids, use of inotropes to increase contractility, and correction of metabolic acidosis if needed.

ANESTHETIC CONSIDERATIONS

If the intrapericardial pressure contributing to tamponade is not relieved before induction of anesthesia, the goal is to maintain cardiac output. A primary goal is to avoid decreases in contractility, systemic vascular resistance, and heart rate. Ketamine is a suitable choice for induction and maintenance. Although pancuronium is a logical choice for muscle relaxant because it maintains heart rate, other nondepolarizing muscle relaxants may be used as long as they do not contribute to decreasing the heart rate or systemic vascular resistance. Positive-pressure ventilation can also decrease venous return. Continuous CVP and invasive blood pressure monitoring can be instituted prior to anesthesia if the patient's condition permits. Maintenance of CVP with intravenous fluids should be used to maintain venous return. The surgeon should be prepared for emergency pericardiocentesis in the event of circulatory collapse after induction of anesthesia.

I. Shock

HEMORRHAGIC SHOCK

DEFINITION

Hemorrhagic shock is a complication that arises from acute blood loss, also referred to as hemodynamic or vascular collapse. There is a decreased intravascular fluid volume that leads to a decreased venous return and cardiac output (CO) and subsequently leads to inadequate organ and tissue perfusion.

ETIOLOGY

Hemorrhagic shock is a result of acute blood loss, frequently owing to trauma. Along with a decrease in intravascular fluid volume, sympathetic nervous system activity is increased, redirecting blood flow to the brain and heart. If this condition persists, a detrimental decrease in renal and hepatic blood flow occurs. Anaerobic metabolism is increased (lactate production), and metabolic (lactic) acidosis is manifested.

TREATMENT

Blood replacement therapy typically includes administration of whole blood or packed red cells. Crystalloids (balanced salt solutions) are also used because fluid shifts accompany hemorrhage, but controversy exists whether colloids (albumin, dextran, hetastarch) provide a better resuscitative fluid medium. Invasive monitoring, including arterial blood pressure, central venous pressure, and urinary drainage system to guide volume replacement, may become necessary. A pulmonary arterial catheter is helpful to determine CO, filling pressures, systemic and pulmonary vascular resistances, and oxygen extraction and delivery to the tissues. Dopamine may be useful in some cases, especially if the goals are a mild inotropic effect and an increase in renal blood flow. Vasopressors may be necessary as well to preserve cerebral and cardiac perfusion until intravascular fluid volume can be replaced. Other blood component therapy may need to be considered as more banked blood is given (e.g., fresh-frozen plasma and platelets).

ANESTHETIC CONSIDERATIONS

Induction (if possible) and maintenance typically require invasive monitoring of blood pressure. Ketamine is used to induce anesthesia because it stimulates the sympathetic nervous system. Additional anesthetic agents must be carefully titrated to the patient's hemodynamic status. Treatment of hemorrhagic shock includes control of bleeding and replacement of intravascular volume (with whole blood and/or packed red blood cells) while maintaining adequate perfusion pressures to the vital organs.

SEPTIC SHOCK

DEFINITION

Septic shock is shock resulting from the presence of pathogenic organisms or their toxins in the blood.

ETIOLOGY

Early Phase

The early phase is characterized by hypotension resulting from a decrease in systemic vascular resistance. An increase in CO, elevated temperature, and hyperventilation also manifest themselves. Vasodilation is probably caused by endotoxins from bacterial cell walls that release vasoactive substances (i.e., histamine) and can last up to 24 hours.

Late Phase

CO may also be increased in this phase. Dilation of peripheral vessels gives over to the shunting of blood away from vital organs, and lactic acidosis develops as a result of impaired tissue oxygenation. Intravascular fluid volume may fall because of damaged muscle. Oliguria is often present. Coagulation defects are common.

DIAGNOSIS AND LABORATORY FINDINGS

Septic shock is suggested by the development of hypotension in the presence of perioperative oliguria.

TREATMENT

Treatment includes intravenous antibiotics and restoration of intravascular fluid volume. Antibiotics should be started immediately. Typically, two antibiotics are used to cover both gram-positive bacteria (clindamycin) and gram-negative bacteria (gentamicin). Fluid replacement should be guided by pulmonary artery catheter measurements of cardiac filling pressures and urine output. Intravenous dopamine is effective when supportive function is needed.

ANESTHETIC CONSIDERATIONS

No specific anesthetic drug has been proven ideal in the presence of septic shock. The anesthetic management should be individualized to each patient.

J. Valvular Heart Disease

DEFINITION

Valvular heart disease is characterized by abnormalities that alter the normal flow of blood through the heart and may eventually affect cardiac loading conditions. The most frequently encountered cardiac valve lesions produce *pressure* overload (mitral stenosis [MS], aortic stenosis [AS]) or *volume* overload (mitral regurgitation [MR], aortic regurgitation [AR]) on the left atrium or left ventricle.

AORTIC STENOSIS

INCIDENCE AND PREVALENCE

Two types of AS are commonly identified: *congenital* and *acquired*. Provided there are no other cardiac lesions, congenital AS is the most common cardiac valvular abnormality, with rheumatic disease responsible for less than 5% of these cases. AS can also be acquired, in which calcific disease is the most common form. Valvular AS without accompanying mitral valve disease is more common in men.

ETIOLOGY AND PATHOLOGY
Congenital

The congenital (nonrheumatic) form of AS results from progressive calcification and tightening of a congenitally abnormal valve. These stenotic valves may have unicuspid, bicuspid, or tricuspid leaflet morphology, but the bicuspid variety is the most common (greater than 50%). AS resulting from rheumatic fever almost always occurs in association with mitral valve disease.

Acquired

The most common form of acquired AS is calcific AS, in which degeneration of the valve apparatus increases with age. Calcium deposits build up on normal cusps and prevent them from opening and closing completely.

The anatomic obstruction to left ventricular (LV) outflow produces an increase in LV pressure to maintain stroke volume. A pressure gradient across the stenotic valve develops, and there is increased workload on the ventricle. Increased wall tension contributes to LV hypertrophy. Cardiac output is maintained by the hypertrophied ventricle, which may sustain a large pressure gradient across the LV outflow tract for years without evidence of clinical symptoms. Over time, diastolic function is reduced so that small changes in volume give way to large changes in LV filling pressures.

Significant AS is associated with a peak systolic transvalvular pressure gradient exceeding 50 mm Hg and an aortic valve orifice area of less than 1 cm^2 (normal area, 2.6 to 3.5 cm^2). The atrial contribution to ventricular filling may be as high as 40% in patients with AS (about 20% normally). LV end-diastolic pressure (LVEDP) is often elevated, causing symptoms of pulmonary congestion despite normal LV contractility. LVEDP values that are normal may, in fact, represent a patient who is hypovolemic.

DIAGNOSIS

As mentioned, a long latency period exists (approximately 40 to 50 years) during which obstruction increases gradually and the pressure load on the myocardium increases while the patient remains asymptomatic. Patients with advanced AS may begin to have angina, syncope, and signs of congestive heart failure. They also have a characteristic systolic murmur, best heard in the second right intercostal space, which transmits sound to the neck. Cardiac catheterization will give vital information about intracavitary pressures, the gradient across the aortic valve, and contractility. In patients with calcific AS, echocardiography often shows thickening and calcification of the aortic valve and decreased mobility of the valve leaflets. The incidence of arrhythmias leading to severe hypoperfusion accounts for syncope and the increased incidence of sudden death in patients with AS.

TREATMENT

When significant symptoms develop, most patients die without surgical treatment within 2 to 5 years. Percutaneous transluminal valvuloplasty may be an alternative to surgery, but restenosis usually occurs within 6 to 12 months.

ANESTHETIC CONSIDERATIONS

- Maintain normal sinus rhythm (70 to 90 beats/min).
- Avoid tachycardia and hypotension (myocardial depression).
- Ensure adequate coronary perfusion by maintaining diastolic blood pressure levels.
- Ensure sufficient preload LV end = diastolic volume (LVEDV) to maintain cardiac output.

Regional anesthesia in the patient with AS should be limited to peripheral-type procedures. If conduction anesthesia is used (i.e, spinal or epidural), the sensory level of blockade should be limited to lower levels so that profound hypotension (from sympathectomy) does not occur. Treatment in this case would be to use a vasoconstricting drug.

PROGNOSIS

The 5-year survival rate for adults with aortic valve replacement is approximately 85%.

AORTIC REGURGITATION

INCIDENCE AND PREVALENCE

Rheumatic fever is a common cause of disease of the aortic valve that inevitably leads to valve incompetence (regurgitation). Other causes of AR include infective endocarditis, trauma, congenital bicuspid valve, and diseases of connective tissue.

ETIOLOGY AND PATHOLOGY

AR may be caused by disease of the aortic valve leaflets, the wall of the aortic root, or both. The fundamental problem is that part of the LV stroke volume is allowed to flow backward into the ventricle after being ejected during systole (i.e., regurgitation).

In *chronic* AR, the LV progressively dilates and becomes hypertrophied eccentrically. End-diastolic volume increases to maintain an effective stroke volume. Ventricular compliance increases initially, and LVEDP is usually normal or only slightly elevated.

In *acute* AR, the regurgitant volume fills a ventricle of normal size that cannot accommodate both the regurgitant volume and the left atrial inflow volume. The sudden rise in LVEDP is transmitted back to the pulmonary circulation, causing acute pulmonary congestion.

DIAGNOSIS

Most patients with chronic AR remain asymptomatic for 10 to 20 years. When symptoms develop, exertional dyspnea, orthopnea, and paroxysmal nocturnal dyspnea are the principal complaints. Diastolic murmur is often auscultated at the left sternal border. Angina is a late and ominous symptom.

In acute AR, patients develop sudden clinical manifestations of cardiovascular collapse, weakness, severe dyspnea, and hypotension. Chronic AR is recognized by its characteristic diastolic murmur (best heard in the second intercostal space, right sternal border), widened pulse pressure, decreased diastolic pressure, and bounding peripheral pulses.

TREATMENT

Arterial blood pressure should be decreased to reduce the diastolic gradient for regurgitation using afterload reduction via arterial vasodilators and angiotensin-converting enzyme inhibitors. Early surgery is indicated for patients with acute AR because medical management is associated with a high mortality rate. Patients with chronic AR should undergo surgery before irreversible ventricular dysfunction occurs.

ANESTHETIC CONSIDERATIONS

• Maintain heart rate slightly higher than normal (80 to 110 beats/min).
• Avoid increases in systemic vascular resistance.
• Minimize drug-induced myocardial depression.

Most patients tolerate spinal and epidural anesthesia, provided intravascular volume is maintained.

PROGNOSIS

Favorable clinical responses to valve replacement have been reported in patients with evidence of relatively severe preoperative ventricular dysfunction.

Aortic valve replacement significantly improves LV performance in most patients with chronic AR.

MITRAL STENOSIS

INCIDENCE AND PREVALENCE

Pure MS occurs in 25% of patients; MS and MR occur in 40% of patients.

ETIOLOGY AND PATHOLOGY

The predominant cause of MS is rheumatic fever, which occurs about four times more frequently in women. Less common causes are congenital MS (in children) and complications associated with carcinoid syndrome, systemic lupus erythematosus, and rheumatic arthritis.

After the initial episode of acute rheumatic fever, stenosis of the mitral valve takes about 2 years to develop. Symptoms appear after 20 to 30 years, when the mitral valve orifice is reduced from its normal 4 to 6 cm^2 to less than 2 cm^2. In MS, the anterior and posterior valve cusps fuse at their edges, followed by shortening of the chordae tendineae as they thicken, producing obstruction to flow into the LV. The narrowed valvular orifice causes an increase in left atrial volume and pressure. LV filling and stroke volume in the presence of mild MS are usually maintained at rest by increased left atrial pressure. LV stroke volume may decrease when effective atrial contraction is lost or with tachycardia. Acute increases in left atrial pressure that subsequently result are transmitted to the pulmonary capillaries.

Pulmonary hypertension occurs from rearward transmission of the elevated left atrial pressure and irreversible increases in pulmonary vascular resistance. Chronic increases in pulmonary capillary wedge pressure (PCWP) are partially compensated by increases in pulmonary lymph flow; however, any acute increase in PCWP may result in pulmonary edema. Transudation of fluid into the pulmonary interstitial space, decreased pulmonary compliance, and increased work of breathing lead to dyspnea on exertion.

DIAGNOSIS

About 50% of MS patients present with an acute onset of congestive heart failure that is often associated with paroxysmal attacks of atrial fibrillation (this arrhythmia occurs in 40% of patients with MS). Stasis of blood in the left atrium predisposes to thrombus formation. The predominant symptom of MS is dyspnea from the reduced compliance of the lungs. Rupture of pulmonary-bronchial venous communications causes hemoptysis.

Cardiac catheterization allows quantification of the mitral valve orifice and transmitral gradients. Angiography is important in those patients with angina. Two-dimensional echocardiography can also provide information about orifice size. MS is recognized during auscultation by an opening snap that occurs early in diastole and by a rumbling diastolic heart murmur best heard at the cardiac apex. The chest x-ray study may show left atrial enlargement and evidence of pulmonary edema.

TREATMENT

Medical management is primarily supportive and includes limitation of physical activity, diuretics, and sodium restriction. Digoxin is useful in patients with atrial fibrillation, and β-blockers may control heart rate in some patients. Anticoagulation therapy is used in patients with a history of emboli and in those at high risk (i.e., those older than 40 years of age with a large atrium and chronic atrial fibrillation). Surgical correction is undertaken once significant symptoms develop. Recurrent MS following valvuloplasty is usually managed with valve replacement. Catheter-balloon valvuloplasty using a percutaneous venous introduction and a transseptal approach to the mitral valve may be used to decrease the degree of MS in selected patients.

ANESTHETIC CONSIDERATIONS
- Maintain sinus rhythm (70 to 90 beats/min).
- Maintain LV end-diastolic volume high enough to ensure adequate cardiac output without increasing pulmonary congestion.
- Avoid extreme decreases in contractility.
- Reduction in both right ventricular and LV afterload may improve hemodynamics.

If hypotension occurs, fluid administration may benefit these often fluid-depleted patients. Vasoconstrictors should be avoided, and early use of positive inotropes (e.g., epinephrine, dopamine, dobutamine) may be helpful.

Regional anesthesia is acceptable in the patient with MS, provided higher levels of sensory/sympathetic blockade are avoided during conduction blockade (resulting hypotension may be difficult to treat, based on the pathophysiology of MS).

PROGNOSIS
When MS produces total incapacity, 20% of patients die within 6 months without surgical correction.

MITRAL REGURGITATION

INCIDENCE AND PREVALENCE
Severe MR requiring surgical repair occurs in about 5% of men and in less than 1.5% of women.

ETIOLOGY AND PATHOLOGY
Abnormalities of the mitral annulus, leaflets, chordae tendineae, and papillary muscles may cause MR. *Chronic* MR is usually the result of rheumatic fever, congenital abnormalities, or dilatation, destruction, or calcification of the mitral annulus. *Acute* MR is most often the result of myocardial ischemia or infarction, infective endocarditis, or chest trauma.

The mitral valve orifice lies adjacent to the aortic valve. At the onset of ventricular contraction, about half the regurgitant volume is ejected into the left atrium before aortic valve opening. The total volume of regurgitant flow into the left atrium depends on the systemic vascular resistance and forward stroke volume. Effective cardiac output will be effectively diminished in symptomatic patients, whereas "total" LV output (forward and regurgitant) is usually elevated.

Interestingly, there is typically little enlargement of the left atrial cavity; however there is a significant rise in mean atrial pressure that leads to pulmonary congestion. The degree of atrial compliance will determine the clinical manifestations. Patients with normal or reduced atrial compliance (e.g., acute MR) demonstrate pulmonary congestion and edema. Those with increased atrial compliance (i.e., chronic MR with a large, dilated atrium) demonstrate signs of decreased cardiac output. Most patients fall between these two extremes and exhibit symptoms of both pulmonary congestion and low cardiac output.

DIAGNOSIS

Symptoms of MR can take up to 20 years to develop. Chronic weakness and fatigue secondary to low cardiac output are prominent features. On auscultation, the cardinal feature of MR is a blowing pansystolic murmur, best heard at the cardiac apex and often radiating to the left axilla. The regurgitant flow is responsible for the "v" wave present on the recording of the pulmonary artery occlusion pressure. The size of the v wave correlates with the magnitude of the regurgitant flow.

TREATMENT

Medical treatment typically includes digoxin, diuretics, and vasodilators. Reduction of afterload increases the forward stroke volume and decreases the regurgitant volume. Surgical treatment is usually reserved for patients with moderate to severe symptoms.

ANESTHETIC CONSIDERATIONS

- Avoid sudden decreases in heart rate.
- Avoid sudden increases in systemic vascular resistance.
- Minimize drug-induced myocardial depression.
- Monitor the size of the v wave as a reflection of regurgitant flow.

Prophylactic antibiotics are recommended. Spinal anesthesia and epidural anesthesia are tolerated well, provided bradycardia is avoided.

PROGNOSIS

In most patients with MR, the clinical course and the quality of life improve following valve replacement. The original cause of MR that warranted the operation is also important to the outcome following surgical treatment. In patients in whom mitral dysfunction is secondary to ischemic heart disease, the 5-year survival rate is approximately 30%; in rheumatic MR, the 5-year survival rate is approximately 70%.

TRICUSPID REGURGITATION

ETIOLOGY AND PATHOLOGY

Tricuspid regurgitation (TR) is commonly a result of right ventricular enlargement secondary to pulmonary hypertension. Pulmonary hypertension may itself be indirectly the result of chronic LV failure, because chronic LV failure often leads to sustained increases in pulmonary vascular pressures. This chronic increase in afterload causes the right ventricle to dilate progressively, and excessive dilation of the tricuspid annulus eventually results in tricuspid incompetence or regurgitation. TR can also be secondary to infective endocarditis, rheumatic fever, carcinoid syndrome, chest trauma, or congenital malformations. Fortunately, the right atrium and vena cava are compliant and accommodate the volume overload with a minimal increase in right atrial pressure.

DIAGNOSIS

Patients with isolated TR are often totally asymptomatic for many years (greater than 20 years). Some physical signs may be present early, such as pulsatile neck veins and systolic heart murmurs heard throughout the cardiac cycle. Other complaints that the patient may give are fatigue, weakness, and a feeling of fullness in the abdomen, probably from congestion in the liver (positive hepatojugular reflex). Some patients report cyanosis, which may result from blood flow from the right to the left atrium in those with a patent foramen ovale.

TREATMENT

TR is generally well tolerated, and some degree of regurgitation has been reported in many physiologically normal persons during echocardiography. Even surgical removal of the tricuspid valve is usually well tolerated. Treatment of the underlying disease process is more important than the TR itself.

ANESTHETIC CONSIDERATIONS

Many patients with clinically significant TR who undergo surgery and anesthesia also have pulmonary hypertension and possibly mitral or aortic valve disease.

- Maintain intravascular fluid volume and central venous pressure in the high-normal range.
- Avoid increases in pulmonary vascular resistance.
- Avoid positive end-expiratory pressure and high mean airway pressures because they reduce venous return and increase right ventricular afterload.
- Most patients tolerate spinal and epidural anesthesia well.
- Prophylactic antibiotics are recommended.

PROGNOSIS

Excellent results have been reported with the use of tricuspid annuloplasty in patients with moderate TR. Management of severe TR entails annuloplasty or valve replacement. Durability of more than 10 years has been established with valvular prostheses.

CENTRAL NERVOUS SYSTEM

A. Alzheimer's Disease/Dementia

DEFINITION

Dementia is the clinical syndrome characterized by acquired persistent impairment of cognitive and emotional abilities severe enough to interfere with daily functioning and quality of life.

INCIDENCE AND PREVALENCE

Dementia occurs primarily late in life, the prevalence being about 1% at age 60 years, and it doubles every 5 years, reaching 30% to 50% by 85 years of age. Alzheimer's disease is the most common of the progressive cortical dementias, accounting for about 70% of the dementias in persons older than 55 years of age.

ETIOLOGY

A specific cause or pathologic process is not identified for dementia.

LABORATORY RESULTS

No specific laboratory test exists for the disease. Assess for alterations in values normally associated with the elderly population or those for specific coexisting disease states.

CLINICAL MANIFESTATIONS

Multiple diseases are representative of the disorder. Cortical dementias include Alzheimer's disease, Pick's disease, and frontal lobe degeneration. Subcortical dementias are associated with Parkinson's disease, Huntington's disease, and Creutzfeld-Jakob disease. Dementia is associated with intellectual, language, memory, and judgment impairment.

Alzheimer's disease is the most common cortical dementia and is characterized by progressive memory loss, predominantly loss of short-term memory. Language impairment manifests as difficulty in finding words for spontaneous speech. Performance of daily tasks such as meal preparation and personal hygiene becomes impaired. In addition, symptoms of mental depression and anxiety may be prominent.

Diagnosis is probable when associated with an insidious onset, progressive worsening of memory, and a normal level of consciousness. Computed tomography often displays ventricular dilation and marked cortical atrophy. A definitive diagnosis can be made only after examination of brain tissue demonstrating amyloid and fibrillar protein aggregates.

TREATMENT

No proven preventive therapies for dementia or Alzheimer's disease are known. Drug therapy is on consistently effective for prevention of progression. Symptomatic therapy is helpful during the early stages, especially if mental depression is prominent.

Drugs with anticholinergic effects are avoided when treating mental depression. Anticholinesterase drugs such as tacrine or donepezil appear to have beneficial effects for some patients early in the disease.

ANESTHETIC CONSIDERATIONS

Management of this disease state is influenced by the pathophysiology of Alzheimer's disease. Preoperative challenges are related to dealing with patients who are unable to comprehend their environment. Sedatives should rarely be administered, because mental confusion could result. Centrally acting anticholinergic drugs are also not recommended for inclusion in preoperative medication. Maintenance of anesthesia can be acceptably achieved with standard inhalation and intravenous agents.

PROGNOSIS

The course of the disease is one of progressive decline, and the median survival after the onset of dementia is 3.3 years.

B. Autonomic Hyperreflexia/Dysautonomia

DEFINITION

Autonomic dysreflexia (or autonomic hyperreflexia) is a disorder that appears after resolution of spinal shock.

INCIDENCE AND PREVALENCE

The incidence and prevalence depend on the level of spinal cord transection. About 85% of patients with spinal cord transection above T6 may exhibit this syndrome. Autonomic dysreflexia is unlikely to be associated with spinal cord transection below T10. The stimulation of a surgical procedure, however, is a potent trigger of autonomic dysreflexia, even in patients with no previous history of this response.

ETIOLOGY

Autonomic dysreflexia can be initiated by cutaneous or visceral stimulation below the level of spinal cord transection. Distention of a hollow viscus (bladder or rectum) is a common stimulus. This stimulus initiates afferent impulses that enter the spinal cord below that level. These impulses elicit reflex sympathetic activity over the splanchnic outflow tract. This outflow is isolated from inhibitory impulses such that generalized vasoconstriction persists below the level of injury. Vasoconstriction results in increased blood pressure, which is then perceived by the carotid sinus. Subsequent activation of the carotid sinus results in decreased efferent outflow from the sympathetic nervous system. Activity from the central nervous system is manifested as a predominance of parasympathetic nervous system activity at the heart and peripheral vasculature. This predominance cannot be produced below the level of spinal cord transection (this part of the body remains neurologically isolated). Therefore, vasoconstriction persists below the level of spinal cord transection. If spinal cord transection is above the level of splanchnic outflow (T4 to T6), vasodilation in the neurologically intact portion of the body is insufficient to offset the effects of vasoconstriction (reflected by persistent hypertension).

LABORATORY RESULTS
No tests are available.

CLINICAL MANIFESTATIONS
The hallmark symptoms of autonomic dysreflexia are hypertension and bradycardia, which result from stimulation of the carotid sinus and cutaneous vasodilation above the level of spinal cord transection. Hypertension persists because vasodilation cannot occur below the level of injury. Nasal stuffiness reflects vasodilation. Other symptoms may include headache, blurred vision (from hypertension), increased operative blood loss, loss of consciousness, seizures, cardiac arrhythmias, and pulmonary edema.

TREATMENT
Treatment includes ganglionic blockers (trimetaphan, pentolinium), α-adrenergic antagonists (phentolamine, phenoxybenzamine), and direct-acting vasodilators (nitroprusside). General or regional anesthesia can be used. Drugs that lower blood pressure by central action alone are not predictably effective.

ANESTHETIC CONSIDERATIONS
Airway control and ventilation with large tidal volumes (10 to 15 mL/kg) are necessary to avoid hypercarbia and atelectasis. Special care should be taken when moving patients with chronic spinal cord injury. Preoperative hydration helps to prevent hypotension during induction and aids in maintenance of anesthesia. Prevention of autonomic hyperreflexia is key in the treatment of autonomic dysreflexia. Use nondepolarizing muscle relaxants to facilitate intubation and prevent reflex skeletal muscle spasms. Avoid using succinylcholine. Have nitroprusside and other cardioactive agents readily available to treat precipitous hypertension.

C. Cerebrovascular Disease

DEFINITION
Cerebral vascular disorders are characterized by sudden neurologic deficits resulting from ischemia or hemorrhagic events. Cerebrovascular disease is any of a collection of disorders that affects the vasculature of the brain, the primary disorder being cerebrovascular accident (CVA or "stroke") as a result of hemorrhage and ischemia.

INCIDENCE AND PREVALENCE
Cerebrovascular disease is the third leading cause of death and the leading cause of disability in the United States. Women have lower stroke rates than men.

ETIOLOGY
The major risk factors for the development of cerebrovascular disease are hypertension and diabetes. Other risk factors include atherosclerosis,

inflammatory processes, dissecting aneurysm, disorders affecting the myocardium, congestive heart failure, polycythemia, cigarette smoking, use of oral contraceptives, and postpartum infection. The different manifestations of cerebrovascular disease can be classified as

- *Transient ischemic attack (TIA):* A temporary, focal episode of neurologic dysfunction that develops suddenly and lasts a few minutes to hours, but usually never more than 24 hours. Approximately 41% of these persons may eventually suffer a stroke.
- *Reversible ischemic neurologic deficit (RIND):* Neurologic symptoms that persist up to 6 to 8 weeks before resolving.
- *Progressive stroke:* A stroke in progress. Neurologic symptoms and deficits develop slowly and are not reversible.
- *Complete stroke:* Neurologic deficits are permanent.
- *Amaurosis fugax:* A sudden, temporary, or fleeting blindness caused by a decrease in cerebral perfusion to the retina.

DIAGNOSTIC AND LABORATORY FINDINGS

Computed tomography, magnetic resonance imaging, cerebral angiography, and clinical examination are useful.

CLINICAL MANIFESTATIONS

Clinical manifestations involve numerous neurologic deficits. See the classification of symptoms in the section on etiology.

TREATMENT

Treatment includes risk-factor reduction (i.e., controlling hypertension, avoiding a high-fat diet, smoking cessation, and decreasing obesity).

ANESTHETIC CONSIDERATIONS

Preoperative evaluation should include a careful analysis of cardiovascular, neurologic, and pulmonary systems, as well as laboratory results and current medications. As expected, patients with cerebral vascular occlusive disease often have peripheral, renal, and cardiac occlusive disease as well. If the patient is scheduled for carotid endarterectomy, consider the benefits and risks associated with regional versus general anesthesia. Selection of anesthetic agents is based on the patient's need and the surgeon's desires. The goal is to ensure a smooth induction, maintenance, and emergence, with avoidance of wide swings in blood pressure. Moreover, an awake, extubated patient is the desired outcome so that immediate neurologic assessment can be performed. Cardioactive agents such as sodium nitroprusside, nitroglycerin, and phenylephrine (Neo-Synephrine) should be readily available.

D. Demyelinating Disease

DEFINITION

Demyelinating diseases share features of inflammation and selective destruction of central nervous system myelin, with sparing of the peripheral nervous system.

INCIDENCE AND PREVALENCE
Incidence is specific to the cause of demyelination.

ETIOLOGY
Specific diseases that cause nerve demyelination include multiple sclerosis, neuromyelitis optica, Devic's syndrome, acute disseminated encephalomyelitis, systemic lupus erythematosus, Behçet's syndrome, sarcoidosis, Lyme borreliosis, meningovascular syphilis, and infection with human immunodeficiency virus.

LABORATORY RESULTS
No specific tests for the demyelinating diseases exist, and diagnosis is based on clinical manifestations.

CLINICAL MANIFESTATIONS
Demyelinating diseases are evidenced by varying nerve conduction abnormalities.

TREATMENT
Treatment depends on the underlying cause.

ANESTHETIC CONSIDERATIONS
Preoperative evaluation of the patient with a demyelinating disease should include specific documentation of signs and symptoms. Other anesthetic care should take into consideration the underlying disease process.

E. Hydrocephalus

DEFINITION
Hydrocephalus is an abnormal accumulation of cerebrospinal fluid (CSF) resulting either from an excessive production or from decreased absorption that leads to an increase in pressure in the ventricles of the brain. The rise in intraventricular pressure causes adjacent brain tissue compression and progressive enlargement of the cranium.

INCIDENCE AND PREVALENCE
Hydrocephalus in newborns occurs in 3 of every 1000 births and is usually secondary to meningomyelocele. Hydrocephalus is common after subarachnoid hemorrhage because of impaired CSF circulation through the basal cistern. It is often a complication of a ruptured brain aneurysm. Hydrocephalus may occur in neonates as a result of obstruction of CSF circulation within the brain's ventricular system or at a site of reabsorption.

ETIOLOGY
Hydrocephalus can be divided into two main types: obstructive and nonobstructive.

• *Obstructive:* This results from obstruction to CSF flow; depending on the site, it can be further divided into *communicating* or *noncommunicating*.

- *Communicating obstructive (extraventricular hydrocephalus):* This results from obstruction to CSF absorption by the arachnoid villi, usually from remote inflammatory disease or traumatic subarachnoid hemorrhage.
- *Noncommunicating obstructive (extraventricular hydrocephalus):* This is secondary to obstruction to CSF flow between the lateral and fourth ventricles (the ventricles dilate proximal but not distal to the obstruction).

Obstructive hydrocephalus results from congenital malformation, scar tissue, fibrin deposits following intraventricular hemorrhage or infection, tumors, or cysts. Nonobstructive hydrocephalus results from excessive CSF production by the choroid plexus. Choroid plexus papillomas or benign tumors of the glomus of the lateral ventricles are common causes.

DIAGNOSTIC AND LABORATORY FINDINGS

Hydrocephalus can be diagnosed by computed tomography, by magnetic resonance imaging, and by signs of increased intracranial pressure.

CLINICAL MANIFESTATIONS

- *Early signs and symptoms:* Apnea, bradycardia, nausea and vomiting, increasing head circumference, headaches (most common), mentation changes, nystagmus, and decreased reflexes are noted.
- *Late signs and symptoms:* Bulging fontanelle, pupillary areflexia, nuchal rigidity, "setting sun" eyes, palsy of cranial nerve VI, limb spasticity, decreased level of consciousness leading to nonresponsiveness, widened pulse pressure, altered heart rate, visual changes, and hypertension are noted.

ANESTHETIC CONSIDERATIONS

With hydrocephalus, intracranial pressure is elevated. Hypoventilation, hypoxia, and hypertension are to be avoided. Baseline neurologic status must be established, and minimal to no premedication must be administered. Intravenous induction should be rapid and smooth with cricoid pressure. Once the airway is secure, hyperventilate the patient until ventricles are decompressed. The patient is maintained on nitrous oxide/oxygen and increments of thiopental if needed until intracranial pressure is reduced, then an inhalation agent or opioid can be added. Sudden removal of large CSF volumes may lead to bradycardia and hypotension that can be prevented by rapid replacement with saline and/or gradual removal of CSF. Although heat is lost by surgical exposure, some degree of hypothermia may be appropriate in these patients. Narcotics are given in small amounts (or not given at all) to enable rapid neurologic assessment on awakening from anesthesia.

TREATMENT

A bypass shunt is inserted to allow CSF to flow from the lateral ventricles to the peritoneal cavity (ventriculoperitoneal shunt). This type of shunt is preferable because of the lower incidence of complications and need for revision with growth. Ventriculoatrial and ventriculopleural shunts are less popular because of the risk of infection, microemboli, and hydrothorax. The lumboperitoneal shunt (between the lumbar subarachnoid space and the peritoneal space) may be used.

F. Intracranial Hypertension

DEFINITION

Intracranial hypertension occurs with a sustained increase in intracranial pressure (ICP) higher than 15 to 20 mm Hg. Intracranial hypertension develops with expanding tissue or fluid mass, interference with normal cerebrospinal fluid absorption, excessive cerebral blood flow (CBF), or systemic disturbances promoting brain edema.

ETIOLOGY

Head injury, stroke, intracranial hemorrhage, infection, tumor formation, postischemic or posthypoxic states, hydrocephalus, osmolar imbalances, and pulmonary disease can all cause increases in ICP. As ICP progressively increases, cerebral perfusion pressure (CPP) is diminished, and focal ischemia occurs. If ICP is already high, even small increases in intracranial volumes result in marked intracranial hypertension and global ischemia. When space-occupying lesions are present, intracranial tissue shifts and localized pressure gradients develop, causing vascular compression and regional ischemia.

LABORATORY RESULTS

Magnetic resonance imaging and computed tomography are the two most prominent tests to evaluate tumors, hemorrhage, stroke, and areas of ischemia. Lumbar puncture is used to diagnose infections and hydrocephalus.

CLINICAL MANIFESTATIONS

Symptoms of increased ICP include headache, nausea and vomiting, mental changes, and disturbances in consciousness and vision. During the early stages of intracranial hypertension, symptoms are most common in the early morning hours. Increased arterial carbon dioxide pressure and the associated cerebral vasodilation that occurs during sleep may produce an increase in intracranial contents that exceeds the limits of compensation, and ICP increases. Progressive increases in ICP eventually result in unexplained fatigue and drowsiness. Papilledema may be seen, which is accompanied by visual disturbances. A first-time seizure in an adult with no apparent cause should arouse suspicion of increased ICP. Systemic blood pressure may be elevated to maintain CPP in the presence of intracranial hypertension (i.e., CPP = mean arterial pressure – ICP).

TREATMENT

Patients with intracranial hypertension or reduced intracranial elastance can be managed using various interventions. All therapies are based on the concept that ICP can be reduced or intracranial elastance can be improved by reducing one of the three intracranial constituents. See specific interventions in the next section.

ANESTHETIC CONSIDERATIONS

Cerebral blood volume can be manipulated in various ways. Endotracheal intubation will allow prompt management of those conditions that could increase CBF and consequently increase ICP, related to hypoxemia and hypercarbia. Neuromuscular blockade often prevents increases in cerebral venous volume (and ICP) that result from coughing, straining, or actively exhaling. Cerebral venous drainage is facilitated by elevating the head of the bed; however, this maneuver may also decrease venous return and cardiac output (i.e., mean arterial blood pressure), thereby reducing CPP. Appropriate analgesia and sedation prevent increases in the cerebral metabolic rate for oxygen ($CMRO_2$) and any increases in CBF. Hyperventilation acutely reduces CBF, although CBF usually returns to its original level even with prolonged hyperventilation. Barbiturates in sufficient doses suppress both the $CMRO_2$ and CBF in association with profound electroencephalographic suppression. Caution should be used when barbiturate therapy is implemented because of concomitant vasodilation and myocardial depression. Brain tissue volume is usually reduced by diuresis. Osmotic diuresis with mannitol reduces brain water. Mannitol can be used as a continuous infusion or as treatment for acute episodes of increased ICP. Maximum reduction of ICP is accomplished with large doses of mannitol administered rapidly, then followed by furosemide. When a patient emerges from anesthesia, increased ICP caused by any coughing or bucking (especially on the endotracheal tube) must be considered. Extubation while the patient is still anesthetized and the concomitant use of intravenous lidocaine are possible ways to ameliorate these potential problems.

G. Mental Disorders

MENTAL DEPRESSION

DEFINITION

Mental depression is a psychiatric disorder distinguished from normal sadness and grief by severity and duration of the mood disturbances and by the presence of fatigue, loss of appetite, and insomnia.

INCIDENCE AND PREVALENCE

Depression is the most common psychiatric disorder, affecting 2% to 4% of the population.

ETIOLOGY

Pathophysiologic causes of major mental depression are unknown, although abnormalities of amine neurotransmitter pathways are the most likely etiologic factors. Cortisol hypersecretion is present in many of these patients.

LABORATORY RESULTS

Testing is as dictated by other coexisting morbidities.

CLINICAL MANIFESTATIONS

Diagnosis of major mental depression is based on the persistent presence of at least five characteristics and the exclusion of organic causes or a normal emotional reaction. Alcoholism and major depression often occur together, and it is presumed that toxic effects of alcohol on the brain are responsible. As stated earlier, this disease is characterized by mood disturbances and by the presence of fatigue, loss of appetite, and insomnia.

TREATMENT

Treatment of mental depression is with antidepressant drugs and/or electroconvulsive therapy (ECT). Common drug therapies include selective serotonin reuptake inhibitors, tricyclic antidepressants, and monoamine oxidase inhibitors (MAOIs). ECT is indicated for treating severe mental depression in patients who are unresponsive to drugs or who become acutely suicidal. Increased intracranial pressure is a contraindication to ECT.

ANESTHETIC CONSIDERATIONS

Treatment with tricyclic antidepressants need not be discontinued before administration of anesthesia for elective operations. Increased availability of neurotransmitters in the patient's central nervous system can result in increased anesthetic requirements. Increased level of norepinephrine at postsynaptic receptors in the peripheral sympathetic nervous system can be responsible for exaggerated systemic blood pressure responses following administration of indirect-acting vasopressors. Long-term treatment with tricyclic antidepressants may alter the responses to pancuronium, and the combination has been associated with tachyarrhythmias.

Anesthesia can be safely conducted despite earlier recommendation that these drugs be discontinued 14 to 21 days before elective operations. Careful consideration is needed when selecting drugs and the doses administered.

During anesthesia and surgery, it is important to avoid stimulating the sympathetic nervous system, so as to decrease the incidence of systemic hypertension and cardiac dysrhythmias.

Although uncommon, adverse interactions between MAOIs and opioids have been observed. Systemic hypertension, hypotension, hyperthermia, depression of ventilation, seizures, and coma may follow administration of opioids with these agents. Meperidine has been the opioid most often incriminated, but the same syndrome can occur with other opioids.

SCHIZOPHRENIA

DEFINITION

Schizophrenia is a psychotic disorder characterized most often with delusions and hallucinations.

INCIDENCE AND PREVALENCE

Schizophrenia is the most common psychotic disorder. It accounts for about 20% of all patients treated for mental illness.

LABORATORY RESULTS

Testing is as dictated by other coexisting morbidities.

CLINICAL MANIFESTATIONS

Features of the illness include an array of symptoms, such as delusions, hallucinations, flattened affect, and social or occupational dysfunction, including withdrawal and changes in appearance and hygiene. Some patients experience exacerbations and remissions.

TREATMENT

Treatment of schizophrenia is with antipsychotic drugs, which most likely exert their effects by inhibiting dopamine binding at postsynaptic dopamine receptors. These agents have an array of adverse effects; their therapeutic index is high, and side effects are rarely serious or irreversible.

ANESTHETIC CONSIDERATIONS

Neuroleptic malignant syndrome is a rare, potentially fatal complication of antipsychotic drug therapy that is presumed to reflect drug-induced interference with dopamine's role in central thermoregulation. This syndrome usually manifests during the first few weeks of treatment or following an increased drug dose. Clinical manifestations usually develop over a 24- to 72-hour period and include high fever, severe skeletal muscle rigidity, autonomic nervous system instability, altered consciousness, and increased serum creatine kinase concentrations reflecting skeletal muscle damage. Treatment is with immediate cessation of antipsychotic drug therapy, administration of bromocriptine (5 mg orally every 6 hours) or dantrolene (up to 6 mg/kg daily as a continuous intravenous infusion) in attempt to decrease skeletal muscle rigidity, and supportive therapy. These patients are vulnerable to developing malignant hyperthermia secondary to similarities between the pathophysiologies of the syndromes. This correlation is an important factor when planning for general anesthesia.

ANXIETY DISORDERS

Anxiety disorders can be responses to exogenous stimuli or endogenous stimuli. Anxiety resulting from identifiable stresses is usually self-limited and rarely requires pharmacologic treatment.

Panic disorders appear to be inherited and are characterized as discrete periods of intense fear that are not triggered by severe anxiogenic stimuli. This disorder is often accompanied by dyspnea, tachycardia, diaphoresis, paresthesias, nausea, chest pain, and fear of dying. An unexplained observation is that infusion of lactate may provoke panic attacks in susceptible persons. Tricyclic antidepressants and MAOIs are effective for treating panic attacks. Delayed recovery from anesthesia has been attributed to coexisting hysteria.

H. Multiple Sclerosis

DEFINITION

Multiple sclerosis (MS) is a demyelinating, acquired disease of the central nervous system characterized by random and multiple sites of demyelination of the corticospinal tract neurons in the brain and spinal cord.

ETIOLOGY

Although the exact cause is unknown, the major pathologic change consists of a loss of myelin covering axons in the form of demyelinative plaques. MS does not affect the peripheral nervous system.

INCIDENCE AND PREVALENCE

There seems to be an increased risk of developing MS (1:1000) in those persons living in northern temperate zones such as North America, Europe, and southern portions of New Zealand and Australia. The incidence is greater among inner city dwellers and affluent socioeconomic groups. Evidence for a genetic factor is demonstrated by a 12- to 15-fold increase among first-degree relatives. MS is a disease of young adults. Women have a 2:1 greater incidence than men, and women tend to develop MS at a younger age. The development of symptoms later in life (after 35 years of age) is associated with a slower progression of symptoms. There may be a viral or inflammatory component. A transmissible agent has not been identified.

DIAGNOSTIC AND LABORATORY TESTS

Visual, brain stem, auditory, and somatosensory evoked potentials can be used to elicit the slow nerve conduction that occurs as a result of demyelination in specific areas. Computed tomography and magnetic resonance imaging may demonstrate demyelinative plaques.

CLINICAL MANIFESTATIONS

Clinical manifestations reflect the site of demyelination in the central nervous system and spinal cord. "Ascending" spastic paresis of skeletal muscle is often prominent. Presenting symptoms may include unilateral vision impairment. Of all patients with demyelination, 10% to 15% develop full-blown MS. Symptoms develop over the course of a few days, remain stable for a few weeks, then improve. The incidence of seizure disorders increases, and the course of MS is characterized by exacerbations and remissions of symptoms at unpredictable intervals over a period of several years. Residual symptoms persist during remission.

TREATMENT

There is no cure for MS, and treatment is symptomatic. Corticosteroids are used to shorten the durations of attack, and skeletal muscle spasticity is treated with baclofen (Lioresal), dantrolene, and benzodiazepines (Valium). Immunosuppressive therapy and plasmapheresis may benefit some patients. Patients should avoid stress and fatigue.

ANESTHETIC CONSIDERATIONS

A baseline neurologic examination must first be documented. The impact of surgical stress on the natural progression of MS should also be considered. Any postoperative increase in body temperature may be more likely than drugs to be responsible for exacerbation of MS. Spinal anesthesia has been implicated in postoperative exacerbation of MS, whereas epidural or peripheral nerve block has not. General anesthesia is most often chosen. The use of succinylcholine should be avoided because of the possible exaggerated release of potassium. The response to nondepolarizing muscle relaxants may be prolonged because of coexisting muscle weakness and decreased muscle mass.

PROGNOSIS

The course of MS is unpredictable. Exacerbations and remissions are common. In the late-onset type, the course is generally progressive.

I. Myasthenia Gravis

DEFINITION

Myasthenia gravis is an acquired, chronic autoimmune disease involving the neuromuscular junction in skeletal muscle. Myasthenia gravis is manifested by increasing skeletal muscle weakness, fatigability on effort, and at least partial restoration of function after rest.

INCIDENCE AND PREVALENCE

In the United States, at least 1 in 7500 people has myasthenia gravis. In persons younger than 50 years, the ratio of women to men with the disease is 3:2; however, in those older than 50 years, the disease is equally distributed between the sexes. Myasthenia gravis can begin spontaneously at any age, but it occurs most frequently at about the age of 30 years. The onset may be abrupt or insidious, and the course is fluctuating, marked by periods of exacerbation and remission. Spontaneous remissions do occur and sometimes persist for years.

ETIOLOGY

Myasthenia gravis is a prototype autoimmune disease. Circulating antibodies react with myoneural acetylcholine receptor (AChR) proteins, leading to varying degrees of dysfunction. Anti-AChR antibodies are found in the sera of 85% to 90% of patients with myasthenia gravis, but the antibody level does not necessarily correlate with severity of disease. Most patients in clinical remission continue to show elevated serum levels of AChR antibodies.

The initiating stimulus for the production of anti-AChR immunoglobulin G antibodies is still unclear. A genetic cause or induction by microbial antigens has been postulated. The thymus gland seems to play a central role in the pathogenesis.

LABORATORY RESULTS

Patients suspected to have the disease should undergo clinical evaluation, including an edrophonium (Tensilon) test and electromyography.

CLINICAL MANIFESTATIONS

The clinical hallmarks of myasthenia gravis include generalized muscle weakness, which improves with rest, and an inability to sustain or repeat muscular contractions. Enhanced effort produces enhanced weakness. The severity of myasthenia gravis can range from mild (slight ptosis only) to severe (respiratory failure). Environmental, physical, and emotional factors seem to affect the disease process, although unpredictably.

Mouth, eyes, pharynx, proximal limb, and shoulder girdle musculature are most often affected. Visual symptoms (ptosis and diplopia) from extraocular muscle weakness occur in more than 50% of patients with myasthenia gravis. The disease is restricted to the extraocular muscles in 20% of patients. Sensation and cognition are not affected by the disease process.

Thymus gland abnormalities are detectable in about 75% of patients with myasthenia gravis. Autoimmune disorders, such as thyroid disease, collagen vascular diseases, polymyositis, and rheumatoid arthritis, occur more frequently in patients with myasthenia gravis.

Myocarditis may complicate myasthenia gravis, especially in patients with thymomas. The myocardial inflammation produces dysrhythmias, particularly atrial fibrillation and atrioventricular block. Myasthenia gravis is classified on the basis of the skeletal muscles involved and the severity of the symptoms.

TREATMENT

Therapy for patients with myasthenia gravis is directed toward improving neuromuscular transmission and includes cholinesterase inhibitors, corticosteroids and other immunosuppressants, plasmapheresis, intravenous immunoglobulin, and thymectomy. Treatment with cholinesterase inhibitors can dramatically reduce the symptoms of myasthenia gravis by inhibiting the hydrolysis of ACh and therefore increasing the neurotransmitter's concentration at the neuromuscular junction. Increasing the synaptic concentration of ACh enhances the possibility of postsynaptic AChR occupation, which is critical for the production of a threshold-reaching end-plate potential for muscle contraction. Anticholinesterase treatment is particularly successful in patients with milder disease. The most commonly used anticholinesterase agent in the United States is oral pyridostigmine. A 60-mg oral dose of pyridostigmine lasts 3 to 4 hours and is equivalent to an intramuscular or intravenous dose of 2 mg of pyridostigmine or 1 mg of neostigmine.

Titration of the anticholinesterase dose is challenging. Underdosing does not sufficiently retard the muscle weakness and can result in *myasthenic crisis,* a severe exacerbation of myasthenic symptoms. Overmedicating with a cholinesterase inhibitor can produce a surplus of ACh at the myoneural junction, causing a depolarizing block and augmenting skeletal muscle weakness. This situation is called *cholinergic crisis.* Muscarinic side effects (e.g., abdominal cramping, diarrhea, salivation, bradycardia, and miosis) predominate in a cholinergic crisis.

Corticosteroid therapy produces an 80% remission rate in patients with myasthenia gravis, in part by reducing AChR antibody levels. The use of steroid therapy is limited by the severe side effects (e.g., osteoporosis, gastrointestinal bleeding, suppression of endogenous cortisol release, cataracts, increased susceptibility to acute infections, hypertension, and glucose intolerance) observed with long-term administration.

In patients with more debilitating, widespread disease, the antimetabolite azathioprine (Imuran) may induce remission by interfering with the production of AChR antibodies. Side effects of azathioprine include severe hemopoietic depression, infection, and, in rare cases, malignancy.

Excision of the thymus gland is recommended for adults with generalized disease and for patients with thymomas, thymus gland hyperplasia, or drug-resistant myasthenia gravis. Thymectomy effectively arrests or reverses the myasthenic process by removing a major source of antibody production. Clinical improvement of myasthenic symptoms is seen in 75% to 96% of patients within weeks to months after surgery.

Plasmapheresis (plasma exchange) arrests severe refractive myasthenia gravis by reducing the concentration of circulating antibodies. It is used primarily as a short-term treatment because the improvement that it produces in symptoms is generally short-lived. Intravenous immunoglobulin may also be used for short-term control of symptoms before surgery.

ANESTHETIC CONSIDERATIONS

Several days before the operation and again immediately beforehand, the surgical candidate with myasthenia gravis should be evaluated for disease control and, if applicable, for stabilization of anticholinesterase dose.

The use of anticholinesterase medication in the immediate preoperative period is controversial. Some experts believe that an awareness of drug mechanisms can enable anticholinesterase therapy to be safely continued into the preoperative period, especially in patients who depend on this therapy for their well-being. Others recommend discontinuing or tapering anticholinesterase medication before surgery, to avoid complicating the anesthetic management. Patients with mild myasthenia gravis can usually tolerate the temporary disruption in treatment. The presence of cholinesterase inhibitors may potentiate vagal responses and may alter the intraoperative administration of muscle relaxants and the differential diagnosis and treatment of postoperative muscle weakness.

Emotional stress and surgery may precipitate or worsen skeletal muscle weakness. Pharyngeal and laryngeal muscle weakness, difficulty in eliminating oral secretions, and risk of pulmonary aspiration should be considered in the anesthesia plan of care. Swallowing and respiratory muscle dysfunction account for much of the morbidity and potential mortality in patients with myasthenia gravis.

With careful monitoring, regional or local anesthesia is preferred when appropriate. If general anesthesia is indicated, the respiratory depressant effects of barbiturates, sedatives, narcotics, and volatile anesthetic agents, compounded by the presence of an already weakened respiratory system, must be carefully considered. Additionally, administration of calcium channel antagonists or aminoglycoside antibiotics in large doses is capable of exacerbating myasthenic neuromuscular weakness.

In many patients, the relaxant effects of a volatile anesthetic in combination with the patient's preexisting skeletal muscle weakness can be sufficient to facilitate intubation of the trachea. Enhanced muscle relaxation may be seen with the administration of all the potent volatile anesthetics.

Succinylcholine may be used to facilitate tracheal intubation, but the response may be unpredictable. Untreated patients with myasthenia gravis appear to be two to three times more resistant to succinylcholine. Normal dosages of succinylcholine may not effectively depolarize the end plate because of the deficiency of viable AChRs. Conversely, patients treated with cholinesterase inhibitors exhibit a normal or prolonged response to succinylcholine. Cholinesterase inhibitors block the effects of plasma cholinesterase, as well as those of true cholinesterase; hence, succinylcholine and other medications metabolized by plasma cholinesterase (e.g., ester local anesthetics) may have a delayed hydrolysis and a prolonged duration of action. Mivacurium also is hydrolyzed by plasma cholinesterase, but it has been used successfully, with careful titration, in myasthenic patients. The ester hydrolysis of atracurium is independent of plasma cholinesterase activity.

The deficient number of functioning AChRs in patients with myasthenia gravis produces an extraordinary sensitivity to nondepolarizing muscle relaxants. Small doses of nondepolarizing agents can produce a profound block with a prolonged effect, even in patients being treated with cholinergic drugs. Some patients require no medication for surgical muscle relaxation at all.

Generally, muscle relaxant requirements are widely variable in patients with myasthenia gravis, a characteristic that makes neuromuscular blockade monitoring an essential and integral part of the anesthetic management. The orbicularis oculi muscle may overestimate the degree of muscle relaxation in patients with myasthenia gravis. This site may be the most ideal site to monitor neuromuscular blockade to avoid the possibility of undetected residual muscle weakness. When needed, the use of smaller doses (one half to two thirds the normal dose) of shorter-acting nondepolarizing relaxants is the prudent choice.

Reversal of neuromuscular blockade with an acetylcholinesterase inhibitor should be performed cautiously in patients with myasthenia gravis. Overtreatment with an anticholinesterase agent can precipitate a cholinergic crisis and can aggravate rather than reverse the muscle weakness.

In many circumstances, the neuromuscular block can be titrated to allow complete spontaneous recovery, thus avoiding the use of reversal.

Complete, sustained return of muscle strength must be demonstrated before extubation and resumption of spontaneous ventilation. The patient should be informed that postoperative tracheal intubation and ventilatory support may be required. Skeletal muscle strength may appear to be adequate shortly after surgery but may deteriorate a few hours later.

For patients undergoing transsternal thymectomy, duration of the disease longer than 6 years, a daily pyridostigmine dose greater than 750 mg, the presence of chronic obstructive pulmonary disease, and a preoperative vital capacity less than 2.9 L predict a higher likelihood for postoperative ventilation.

J. Neuropathy/Myopathy

DEFINITION

Neuropathy is a general term indicating nerve disorders of any kind. Myopathy is defined as any disorder with structural changes or functional impairment of muscle.

INCIDENCE AND PREVALENCE

These are variable, depending on the cause.

ETIOLOGY

Neuropathies may be caused by certain drugs, diabetes mellitus, human immunodeficiency virus, Lyme disease, leprosy, herpes zoster, Bell's palsy, sarcoidosis, and Guillain-Barré syndrome, among others.

Myopathies may be caused by periodic paralyses (hypokalemic, hyperkalemic, and paramyotonia congenita), metabolic alterations of glycolysis (e.g., myophosphorylase deficiency) and fatty acid utilization (e.g., carnitine palmitoyltransferase deficiency), muscular dystrophy, polymyositis, dermatomyositis, fibromyalgia, and polymyalgia rheumatica, among others.

LABORATORY RESULTS

Electrodiagnosis is used to diagnose neuropathies. Findings include slowing of nerve conduction velocity, dispersion and reduction in amplitude of evoked action potentials, or conduction block. Nerve biopsy may also be done to determine the cause of the neuropathy.

Muscle biopsy may be used to diagnose specific myopathies. Creatine kinase, which is the preferred muscle enzyme to measure in the evaluation of myopathies, may be elevated. Aspartate aminotransferase, alanine aminotransferase, and lactic dehydrogenase, enzymes in both muscle and liver, may also be elevated. Erythrocyte sedimentation rate may be elevated in patients with certain myopathies.

CLINICAL MANIFESTATIONS

Manifestations of neuropathy include tingling, prickling, burning, or pansensory loss, areflexia, muscle atrophy, and motor weakness in the affected nerve distribution. Specific manifestations are specific to the type of neuropathy, such as autonomic neuropathy, pure motor neuropathy, pure sensory neuropathy, or mixed motor and sensory, and the location of the affected nerve.

Manifestations of myopathy include intermittent or persistent muscle weakness. Fatigue is a common complaint. Muscle pain associated with involuntary muscle activity, cramps, contractures, and stiff or rigid muscles may also occur. In most myopathies, muscle tissue is replaced by fat and connective tissue, but the size of the muscle is usually not affected.

TREATMENT

Treatment of neuropathies depends on the cause and may include use of antidepressants, anticonvulsants, neuroleptics, or corticosteroids for pain control.

Glucocorticoids may be used to relieve the pain associated with myopathies.

ANESTHETIC CONSIDERATIONS

Preoperative evaluation of the patient with neuropathy should include specific documentation of signs and symptoms. Possible effects of medications should be considered. Intraoperatively, careful positioning and padding of bony prominences to avoid further damage are imperative. Regional anesthesia is not contraindicated in patients with neuropathies. However, some practitioners choose to avoid regional to avoid confusion if new deficits appear postoperatively. The risks and benefits of general versus regional anesthesia should be weighed in deciding a plan of care. Other anesthetic care should take into consideration the underlying disease process.

Anesthetic management of the patient with myopathy should take into account the affected muscle groups. Respiratory muscle involvement may diminish pulmonary reserve. Pulmonary function testing may be helpful if significant pulmonary disease is evident. History of dysphagia, regurgitation, or recurrent pulmonary infections may signal a risk of aspiration necessitating premedication with a histamine (H_2) antagonist and prokinetic agent and rapid sequence induction. Patients with myopathies are at an increased risk of malignant hyperthermia. Therefore, the anesthesia provider may want to avoid use of triggering agents. Anesthetic technique should be determined by the procedure and other coexisting diseases. Muscle relaxants should be avoided, if possible, because of the possibility of increased block. If muscle relaxation is necessary, a short-acting nondepolarizing agent should be used. In addition, succinylcholine should be avoided because of the risk of an unusual response (myotonic contractions, prolonged block, or phase II block), severe hyperkalemia, or malignant hyperthermia.

K. Guillain-Barré Syndrome

DEFINITION

Guillain-Barré syndrome is an acute form of idiopathic polyneuritis characterized by a sudden onset of weakness or paralysis. Typically seen first in the lower extremities, it spreads cephalad the next few days to involve skeletal muscles of the arms, trunk, and head.

INCIDENCE

Guillain-Barré syndrome occurs in 1 to 2 persons per 100,000.

ETIOLOGY

Central nervous system bulbar involvement is most frequently manifested as bilateral facial paralysis. The most common symptoms are difficulty in swallowing because of pharyngeal muscle weakness and impaired ventilation resulting from intercostal muscle paralysis. Lower motor neuron involvement gives way to flaccid paralysis, and corresponding tendon reflexes are diminished. Sensory disturbances occur as paresthesias in the distal extremities and generally precede the onset of paralysis. Pain occurs in different forms, such as headache, backache, or tenderness to deep pressure. Wide fluctuations in blood pressure (orthostatic), abnormalities on electrocardiogram (e.g., conduction disturbances, tachycardia), diaphoresis, peripheral vasoconstriction, and thromboembolism may be seen as a result of autonomic nervous system dysfunction. Complete recovery can occur within weeks when "segmental" demyelination in the central nervous system is the primary pathologic change. A mortality rate of 3% to 8% is the result of sepsis, respiratory distress syndrome, and pulmonary embolism.

DIAGNOSIS

Diagnosis is based on clinical findings of progressive bilateral weakness in the extremities. Examination of cerebrospinal fluid by lumbar puncture reveals increased levels of protein, although cell counts remain normal. A viral origin is supported by the observation that this syndrome develops after a respiratory or gastrointestinal infection in about half of all cases.

TREATMENT

Treatment is symptomatic. Monitor vital capacity; if it is less than 15 mL/kg, ventilatory support may be necessary. Corticosteroid therapy is not considered useful in these patients. Plasma exchange or infusion of gamma globulin may be of some benefit.

ANESTHETIC CONSIDERATIONS

As a result of the lower motor neuron and subsequent autonomic nervous system dysfunction, these patients may have an exaggerated response to noxious stimuli during operation and anesthesia. Regurgitation or aspiration during induction of anesthesia is a very real concern; however, succinylcholine should also be avoided (i.e., use a nondepolarizing muscle relaxant). Blood pressure should be monitored invasively (arterial line) because of compensatory cardiovascular responses to changes in posture, blood loss, or positive pressure. Postoperative mechanical ventilatory support may be needed. The presence of any neurologic deficits before surgery should be documented appropriately on the preanesthetic evaluation.

PROGNOSIS

The prognosis varies by individual patient.

L. Parkinson's Syndrome

DEFINITION

Parkinson's syndrome is also known as paralysis agitans. It is characterized by the onset of degenerative disease of the central nervous system (specifically the extrapyramidal system), where there is loss of dopamine cell bodies in the substantia nigra in the brain. The dopamine deficiency causes the clinical signs and symptoms.

INCIDENCE AND PREVALENCE

Parkinson's syndrome occurs generally between 60 and 80 years of age. Distribution in men and women is equal.

ETIOLOGY

The exact cause is unknown. There is no hereditary component. The syndrome has been observed to develop after encephalitis, intoxication with carbon monoxide, and long-term ingestion of antipsychotic drugs.

DIAGNOSTIC AND LABORATORY FINDINGS

None are currently available.

CLINICAL MANIFESTATIONS

Clinical manifestations include slow resting tremors, bradykinesia, rigidity, a slow, shuffling gait, and an expressionless face. The patient may present with a unilateral tremor or rigidity of an upper extremity.

TREATMENT

The goal is to increase the activity of the remaining dopaminergic cells in the substantia nigra. This can be accomplished in three ways.

1. Administer L-dopa (a dopamine precursor that crosses the blood-brain barrier) orally, thereby increasing the concentration of dopamine in the substantia nigra.
2. Administer an oral medication such as bromocriptine, which increases the dopamine receptor activity in the substantia nigra. Other similar medications used occasionally are trihexyphenidyl hydrochloride (Artane) and amantadine, but these are less effective.
3. Administer selegiline (Deprenyl) orally, which works by inhibiting the enzymes that break down dopamine in the substantia nigra.

ANESTHETIC CONSIDERATIONS

Those patients being treated with L-dopa should continue to receive their medication throughout the perioperative period, including the usual morning dose the day of operation. Because of the short elimination half-life of L-dopa and dopamine, interruption in therapy for greater than 6 to 12 hours can result in loss of therapeutic effect. Abrupt withdrawal of L-dopa may lead to skeletal muscle rigidity that interferes with ventilation. L-Dopa also sensitizes the cardiovascular system and may predispose the patient to perioperative arrhythmias. Long-term L-dopa therapy can cause blood pressure fluctuations because of autonomic instability; therefore, invasive blood pressure monitoring may be necessary. L-Dopa therapy causes an increase in renal blood flow and sodium excretion. It also causes a concomitant decrease in renin release, intravascular fluid volume, and systemic blood pressure during induction of anesthesia. These swings in blood pressure often require aggressive fluid administration with crystalloids and/or colloids. Drugs that block dopamine uptake (e.g., phenothiazines, butyrophenones) or dopamine receptor antagonists (metoclopramide) may exacerbate symptoms and should therefore be avoided. Anticholinergics or antihistamines may be useful during acute exacerbations. Diphenhydramine (Benadryl) is also very useful as a sedative in these patients. Ketamine may provoke an exaggerated sympathetic nervous system response and its use is questionable.

M. Seizures

DEFINITION
Seizures are the result of abnormal electrical discharges in the brain.

INCIDENCE AND PREVALENCE
Seizures are one of the most common neurologic disorders and may occur at any age. Seizures affect approximately 0.5% to 1% of the population in the United States. Numerous types of seizures exist, but most are generalized tonic-clonic seizures. The likelihood of a recurrent seizure after a single seizure is approximately 50% in the following 3 years, with the greatest incidence during the first 6 months.

ETIOLOGY
Seizures are caused by transient, paroxysmal, and synchronous discharge of groups of neurons in the brain. Most seizures are idiopathic. Idiopathic seizure disorders usually begin in childhood. Seizure onset in adults may indicate an expanding intracranial hematoma, tumor, intracranial hemorrhage, metabolic disturbance, infection, trauma, alcohol or addictive drug withdrawal, eclampsia (in pregnant women), previous trauma causing an irritative phenomenon in the brain, and local anesthesia toxicity.

DIAGNOSTIC AND LABORATORY FINDINGS
Seizures can be detected with electroencephalography (signals can be augmented with methohexital, etomidate, or ketamine), electrolyte abnormalities and examination of the cerebrospinal fluid for infection. Magnetic resonance imaging is better than computed tomography in detecting focal intracranial lesions.

CLINICAL MANIFESTATIONS
Clinical manifestations depend on location, number of neurons involved in the seizure, discharge, and duration of the seizure. Clinical manifestations include focal or generalized tonic-clonic seizures and an increase in the cerebral metabolic rate for oxygen. Cerebral metabolic decompensation occurs after 30 minutes of uncontrolled seizure activity. Therefore, the window for treatment is limited.

TREATMENT
The first priority is to protect and secure the airway, oxygenate, and ventilate. Supportive care and treatment of the underlying problem are needed.

Grand Mal Seizures
Appropriate drug therapy for grand mal seizures includes midazolam, 1 mg/min by intravenous push, until seizures stop or a total of 10 mg. Phenytoin (Dilantin), with an intravenous load of 15 mg/kg over 20 minutes, is also used. No more than 50 mg/min is infused (in an adult), followed

by daily maintenance doses of 300 to 500 mg orally or intravenously for adults. The therapeutic serum level is 10 to 20 mcg/mL. Phenobarbital can also be used to control seizures with an intravenous dose of 100 mg/min up to a total of 20 mg/kg. The therapeutic serum level is 20 to 40 mcg/mL.

Eclamptic Seizures

Magnesium sulfate, a mild central nervous system (CNS) depressant and vasodilator, is used for eclamptic seizures. An initial intravenous loading dose is 2 to 4 g administered over 15 minutes, followed by a continuous infusion of 1 to 3 g/hour. The therapeutic serum level is 4 to 8 mEq/L.

Local Anesthesia Toxicity

Thiopental (50 to 100 mg), midazolam (1 to 5 mg), or diazepam (5 to 20 mg by intravenous push) is used to treat local anesthesia toxicity resulting from increased vascular absorption or direct intravascular injection.

ANESTHETIC CONSIDERATIONS

Electrolytes, cultures, and serum drug levels should be obtained preoperatively. All current medications should be considered, and particular attention should be paid to any anticonvulsant drugs being taken and their possible cardiopulmonary effects and interactions with anesthetics, as well as consideration of protein-bound properties. When phenytoin (Dilantin) is administered intravenously, particular care should be taken to infuse and flush with normal saline; infusion should be no faster than 50 mg/min. Arrhythmias, hypotension, and cardiac arrest can occur if administration is too rapid. The intraoperative requirement for nondepolarizing muscle relaxants (NDMRs) may be increased. Other anticonvulsant medications used are phenobarbital, primidone, carbamazepine (increases requirement for NDMRs), valproic acid, and ethosuximide. Metrizamide, a water-soluble contrast agent, can produce seizures if it is allowed to enter the intracranial compartment in a high concentration.

Patients receiving antiepileptic drugs build a resistance to the effects of neuromuscular blocking agents and opioids because of changes in the number of receptors (up-regulation), altered drug metabolism, and interaction with endogenous neurotransmitters. A "paralyzing" dose of muscle relaxant stops peripheral but not CNS manifestations of seizure activity.

Methohexital can activate epileptic foci, and ketamine can potentially lower seizure threshold. Atracurium possesses a laudanosine metabolite that is a CNS stimulant. Magnesium sulfate may increase sensitivity to all muscle relaxants. Hyperventilation of the lungs decreases delivery of additional local anesthesia to the brain; respiratory alkalosis and hyperkalemia result in hyperpolarization of nerve membranes.

N. Spinal Cord Injury

DEFINITION

The spinal cord is vulnerable to trauma, compression by intradural or extradural tumors, and vascular injuries.

INCIDENCE AND PREVALENCE

Approximately 10,000 persons each year suffer acute spinal cord injuries that result in paraplegia and quadriplegia. Two thirds are male, and 70% to

80% are ages 11 to 30 years. The mortality rate before reaching the hospital is 30% to 40%; the mortality rate during the first year decreases to 10%.

ETIOLOGY

Spinal cord injuries result from motor vehicle accidents, falls, sport injuries (especially diving), and penetrating injuries (especially gunshot wounds). The spinal cord itself is not usually severed but is injured by compression from bone, foreign body, hematoma, and edema and by ischemia.

DIAGNOSTIC AND LABORATORY RESULTS

A clinical examination is needed.

CLINICAL MANIFESTATIONS

Clinical manifestations include changes in cardiopulmonary responses, fluids and electrolytes, temperature control function, and abnormal responses to drugs. Injuries at levels T2 to T12 cause paraplegia but leave the upper extremities and diaphragm intact. Injuries at levels C5 to T1 cause varying degrees of upper extremity paralysis as well.

TREATMENT

For acute injury, the ABCs of resuscitation are used (i.e., A = airway, B = breathing, C = circulation). Provide cervical spine protection by avoiding neck motion and subsequent further spinal cord damage. Maintain spinal cord perfusion with volume and vasoactive drugs. If the spinal cord is compressed by bone or hematoma, decompression is necessary. High-dose corticosteroid therapy (methylprednisolone, 30 mg/kg over 1 hour, followed by 5 mg/kg for 23 hours) is begun soon after injury to improve neurologic outcome.

ANESTHETIC CONSIDERATIONS

Cervical ("halo") traction sometimes necessitates fundamental changes in airway management of the patient with a cervical spine injury. Airway reflex impairment may be present. An assistant may be needed to help maintain neck immobility during laryngoscopy or intubation. Alternative techniques for securing the airway (e.g., fiberoptic intubation) are sometimes necessary. Nasal intubation is contraindicated in the presence of basilar skull fracture. Be prepared for emergency cricothyroidotomy, if necessary. Succinylcholine can be used safely within the first 24 hours after injury. Use anticholinergic agents to reduce secretions. Ventilate the patient with large tidal volumes (10 to 15 mL/kg) to avoid hypercarbia and atelectasis. Move the patient carefully to prevent injury to the limbs and trunk. Check pressure areas to prevent breakdown. Some cardioacceleration and vasoconstrictor tone is lost as a result of cord injuries that involve levels T1 to T4. Spinal cord shock is present. Respiratory compromise is possible, depending on the level of spinal injury.

ENDOCRINE SYSTEM

A. Acromegaly

DEFINITION

Acromegaly is the result of excessive secretion of growth hormone in an adult, most often from an adenoma in the anterior pituitary gland. The condition occurs with equal frequency in both sexes. If hypersecretion of growth hormone occurs before puberty, that is, before closure of the growth plates, the individual grows very tall (8 to 9 feet), a rare condition known as *gigantism.*

LABORATORY RESULTS

A skull radiograph and computed tomography scan are useful in detecting enlargement of the sella turcica, which is characteristic of an anterior pituitary adenoma.

PATHOPHYSIOLOGY

The excessive production of growth hormone associated with acromegaly does not induce bone lengthening but rather enhances the growth of periosteal bone. The unrestrained bone growth in patients with acromegaly produces bones that are massive in size and thickness. Bones of the hands and feet *(acral)* become particularly large. Overgrowth of vertebrae may cause kyphoscoliosis and arthritis.

Soft tissue changes are also prominent with growth hormone hypersecretion. The patient develops coarsened facial features *(acromegalic facies)* including the following: a large, bulbous nose; supraorbital ridge overgrowth; dental malocclusion; and a prominent prognathic mandible. The changes in appearance are insidious, and many patients do not seek treatment until the diagnosis is obvious and the disease course is advanced. Overgrowth of internal organs is less apparent clinically but no less serious. The liver, heart, spleen, and kidneys become enlarged. Lung volumes increase, which may lead to ventilation-perfusion mismatch. Exercise tolerance may be limited because of increased body mass and skeletal muscle weakness.

Cardiomyopathy, hypertension (28% of cases), and accelerated atherosclerosis in patients with acromegaly can lead to symptomatic cardiac disease (congestive heart failure, arrhythmias). Echocardiography often shows left ventricular hypertrophy. Resting electrocardiograms are abnormal in 50% of acromegalic patients. ST-segment and T-wave depression, conduction defects, and evidence of prior myocardial infarction may be present. The insulin antagonistic effect of growth hormone produces glucose intolerance in up to 50% of patients with acromegaly and frank diabetes mellitus in 10% to 25% of patients.

CLINICAL MANIFESTATIONS

Clinical manifestations resulting from the local effects of the expanding tumor may include headaches (55%), which reflect extrasellar extension of the tumor, papilledema, and visual field defects (19%), which are caused by compression of the optic nerves and chiasm. Significant increases in intracranial pressure are uncommon. Compression or destruction of normal pituitary tissue by the tumor may lead to panhypopituitarism. Common features of acromegaly are summarized in the following section.

Common Features of Acromegaly

- Skeletal overgrowth (enlarged hands and feet, prominent prognathic mandible)
- Soft tissue overgrowth (enlarged lips, tongue, and epiglottis; distortion of facial features)
- Visceromegaly
- Osteoarthritis
- Glucose intolerance
- Peripheral neuropathy
- Skeletal muscle weakness
- Extrasellar tumor extension (headache, visual field defects)

TREATMENT

Treatment of acromegaly is aimed at restoring normal growth hormone levels. The preferred initial therapy for active acromegaly is microsurgical removal of the pituitary tumor with preservation of the gland. The surgical approach to the pituitary tumor most often is by a transsphenoidal route. Surgical ablation usually is successful in rapidly reducing tumor size, inhibiting growth hormone secretion, and alleviating some symptoms. Administration of octreotide (a long-acting somatostatin analogue) or bromocriptine and gland irradiation are treatment options for patients who are not surgical candidates and are useful adjunctive forms of therapy.

ANESTHETIC CONSIDERATIONS

Preanesthetic assessment of patients with acromegaly should include a careful examination of the airway. Facial deformities and the large nose may hamper adequate fitting of an anesthesia mask. Endotracheal intubation may be a challenge because of these patients's large and thick tongue (macroglossia), enlargement of the thyroid, obstructive teeth, hypertrophy of the epiglottis, and general soft tissue overgrowth in the upper airway. Subglottic narrowing and vocal cord enlargement may dictate the use of a smaller-diameter endotracheal tube. Nasotracheal intubation should be approached cautiously because of possible turbinate enlargement.

Preoperative dyspnea, stridor, or hoarseness should alert the anesthetist to airway involvement. Indirect laryngoscopy and neck radiography may be performed for thorough assessment. If difficulties in maintaining an adequate airway are anticipated, a fiberoptic-guided intubation in an awake patient is of proven value. The endotracheal tube should remain in place until the patient is fully awake and has total return of reflexes. The predisposition to airway obstruction in these patients makes assiduous postoperative monitoring of the patient's respiratory status a wise precaution.

The frequent occurrence of cardiac arrhythmias, coronary artery disease, and hypertension in acromegalic patients warrants a thorough preanesthetic cardiac evaluation. The increased risk of diabetes mellitus in these patients mandates careful perioperative monitoring of blood glucose and electrolyte levels.

If preoperative assessment reveals impairment of the adrenal or thyroid axis, stress-level glucocorticoid therapy and thyroid replacement should be implemented in the perioperative period.

Entrapment neuropathies, such as carpal tunnel syndrome, are common in patients with acromegaly. An Allen test should be performed before placement of a radial artery catheter because hypertrophy of the carpal ligament may cause inadequate ulnar artery flow.

B. Addison's Disease

DEFINITION

Primary adrenal insufficiency (Addison's disease) reflects the absence of cortisol and aldosterone owing to the destruction of the adrenal cortex. The most common cause is adrenal hemorrhage in the patient in whom coagulation is hindered, but insufficiency can also develop as a result of sepsis or accidental or surgical trauma. In the United States, approximately 70% to 80% of cases of primary adrenocortical insufficiency are autoimmune mediated. Diagnosis of hypoadrenocorticism requires measurement of the plasma cortisol concentration within 1 hour of administration of adrenocorticotropic hormone (ACTH).

CLINICAL MANIFESTATIONS

Clinical symptoms of Addison's disease reflect glucocorticoid and mineralocorticoid deficiency. Weakness and fatigue are common clinical features. Reduced appetite with weight loss, vomiting, abdominal pain, and diarrhea are frequently reported. Hypoglycemia is often present.

Volume depletion is a common feature of the disease and may be manifested by orthostatic hypotension. Laboratory screening commonly reveals hyponatremia and hyperkalemia.

The adrenal-pituitary axis is intact in primary adrenal insufficiency. ACTH concentrations are elevated as a result of the reduced production of cortisol. Increased melanin formation in the skin and hyperpigmentation of the knuckles of the fingers, toes, knees, elbows, lips, and buccal mucosa may be evident. Women with adrenal insufficiency may experience oligomenorrhea or amenorrhea.

LABORATORY RESULTS

Laboratory findings include hyperkalemia and hypoglycemia. Lack of catecholamines may result in hypotension, which is often indistinguishable from shock from loss of intravascular fluid volume.

TREATMENT

Normal adults secrete 15 to 25 mg of cortisol (hydrocortisone) and 50 to 250 mcg of aldosterone per day. Therapeutic replacement dosages of glucocorticoids are typically 50% greater than basal adrenal output so that the patient is covered for mild stress. A typical oral replacement dose may consist of prednisone, 5 mg in the morning and 2.5 mg in the evening; or hydrocortisone, 20 mg in the morning and 10 mg in the evening. Mineralocorticoid replacement may consist of 0.05 to 0.2 mg/day of fludrocortisone. Standard glucocorticoid doses are increased during periods of increased stress. Treatment for primary adrenal insufficiency entails both glucocorticoid and mineralocorticoid replacement. Acute adrenal insufficiency (addisonian crisis) is a medical emergency, and treatment includes fluids, steroid replacement, inotropes as necessary, and electrolyte correction (see the following table).

Comparative Pharmacology of Endogenous and Synthetic Corticosteroids

	Antiinflam-matory Potency	Sodium-Retain-ing Potency	Equi-valent Dose (mg)	Elimi-nation Half-Time (hr)	Duration of Action (hr)	Route of Adminis-tration
Cortisol	1	1	20	1.5–3	8–12	Oral, IV, IM, IA
Cortisone	0.8	0.8	25	0.5	8–36	Oral, IM
Prednisolone	4	0.8	5	2–4	12–36	Oral, IV, IM, IA
Prednisone	4	0.8	5	3–4	18–36	Oral
Methylpred-nisolone	5	0.5	4	2–4	12–36	Oral, IV, IM, IA
Betametha-sone	25	0	0.75	5	36–54	Oral, IV, IM, IA
Dexametha-sone	25	0	0.75	3.5–5	36–54	Oral, IV, IM, IA
Triamcinolone	5	0	4	3.5	12–36	Oral, IM, IA
Fludro-cortisone	10	125	–	–	24	Oral

IA, Intraarticular; *IM,* intramuscular; *IV,* intravenous.

ANESTHETIC CONSIDERATIONS

Anesthetic management for patients with primary adrenal insufficiency should provide for exogenous corticosteroid supplementation. Etomidate should be avoided because it transiently inhibits synthesis of cortisol in physiologically normal patients. Doses of anesthetic drugs should be minimized because these patients may be sensitive to drug-induced myocardial depression. Invasive monitoring (arterial line and pulmonary artery catheter) is indicated. Because of skeletal muscle weakness, the initial dose of muscle relaxant should be reduced, and further doses should be governed by peripheral nerve stimulator response. Plasma concentrations of glucose and electrolytes should be measured frequently during surgery.

C. Cushing's Disease

DEFINITION

Cushing's syndrome is a diverse complex of symptoms, signs, and biochemical abnormalities caused by excess glucocorticoid hormone. Women manifest a degree of masculinization (hirsutism, hair thinning, acne, oligomenorrhea, amenorrhea), and men manifest a degree of feminization (gynecomastia, impotence) as a result of the androgenic effects of glucocorticoid excess. The most common cause of Cushing's syndrome today is the therapeutic administration of supraphysiologic doses of glucocorticoids for conditions such as arthritis, asthma, various autoimmune disorders, allergies, and a myriad of other diseases. Endogenous Cushing's syndrome is most often the result of one of three distinct pathogenic disorders: pituitary tumor (Cushing's disease), adrenal tumor, or ectopic hormone production.

Cushing's disease specifically denotes an anterior pituitary tumor cause of the syndrome. The pituitary tumor produces excessive amounts of adrenocorticotropic hormone (ACTH) and is associated with bilateral adrenal hyperplasia. Patients often develop skin pigmentation as a result of excess ACTH. Cushing's disease is the most common cause of endogenous Cushing's syndrome.

Adrenal Cushing's syndrome is caused by autonomous cortisol production (ACTH independent) by an adrenal tumor. This form of hyperadrenalism accounts for 20% to 25% of patients with Cushing's syndrome and is associated with suppressed plasma ACTH levels.[88] The tumors are usually unilateral. Adrenal tumors that are malignant are usually large by the time Cushing's syndrome becomes manifest.

Ectopic Cushing's syndrome results from autonomous ACTH production by extrapituitary malignancies, producing markedly elevated plasma levels of ACTH. Bronchogenic carcinoma accounts for most of these cases. Malignant tumors of the kidney and pancreas also can cause ectopic production of ACTH. Cushing's disease (hyperadrenocorticism) may reflect overproduction of ACTH by the anterior pituitary (about two thirds of cases), ectopic production of ACTH by malignant tumors (especially carcinoma of the lung, kidney, or pancreas), excess production of cortisol by a benign or malignant tumor of the adrenal cortex, or exogenous (pharmacologic) administration of cortisol or related drugs.

LABORATORY RESULTS

The most widely used test for the diagnosis of hyperadrenocorticism is measurement of the plasma cortisol concentration in the morning after a dose of dexamethasone. Dexamethasone suppresses plasma cortisol secretion in physiologically normal patients, but not in those with hyperadrenocorticism. Diagnosis of Cushing's syndrome is also based on elevations of plasma and urinary cortisol levels and of urinary 17-hydroxycorticosteroids.

CLINICAL MANIFESTATIONS

Clinical features reflect cortisol excess, either from overproduction by the adrenal cortex or from exogenously administered glucocorticoid. The clinical picture includes central obesity, hypertension, glucose intolerance, plethoric facies, purple striae, muscle weakness, bruising, and osteoporosis. The catabolic effects of cortisol result in skin that is thin and atrophic and unable to withstand the stresses of normal activity. Patients with Cushing's syndrome typically gain weight and develop a characteristic redistribution of fat in a yokelike pattern over the clavicles, neck, trunk, abdomen, and cheeks. Mineralocorticoid effects include fluid retention and hypokalemic alkalosis. Signs and symptoms include hypertension, hypokalemia, hyperglycemia, skeletal muscle weakness, osteoporosis, obesity, hirsutism, menstrual disturbances, poor wound healing, and susceptibility to infection.

TREATMENT

Treatment for Cushing's syndrome depends on the cause. Transsphenoidal hypophysectomy is a primary treatment option for Cushing's disease. Complications occur in about 5% of patients and include diabetes insipidus (usually transient), cerebrospinal fluid rhinorrhea, and hemorrhage. Adrenal Cushing's syndrome may be treated by surgical removal of the adrenal adenoma. Because the contralateral adrenal gland is preoperatively suppressed, glucocorticoid replacement may be necessary for several months until adrenal function returns. Bilateral adrenalectomy in the patient with Cushing's syndrome is associated with a high incidence of postoperative complications. Permanent glucocorticoid and mineralocorticoid deficiency results.

The treatment of choice for an ectopic ACTH-secreting tumor is surgical removal, but this may not always be feasible because of the nature of the underlying process (e.g., metastatic carcinoma). Metyrapone, an 11β-hydroxylase inhibitor, and ketoconazole, an agent that blocks steroidogenesis at several levels, may be used to help normalize cortisol levels.

ANESTHETIC CONSIDERATIONS

Perioperative considerations for the patient with Cushing's syndrome include normalizing blood pressure, blood glucose levels, intravascular fluid volume, and electrolyte concentrations. Spironolactone is an effective diuretic for decreasing extracellular fluid volume and correcting hypokalemia.

Osteoporosis is a consideration in positioning the patient for the operative procedure. Special consideration must be given to the patient's skin, which can easily be abraded by tape or minor trauma. Glucocorticoids are lympholytic and immunosuppressive, placing the patient at increased risk of infection and mandating particular enforcement of aseptic techniques where indicated.

The choice of drugs for induction and maintenance of anesthesia is not specifically influenced by the presence of hyperadrenocorticism. Muscle relaxants may have a more exaggerated effect in patients with preexisting muscle weakness, and a conservative approach to muscle relaxant dosing is warranted when significant skeletal muscle weakness is present.

If unilateral or bilateral adrenal resection is planned, glucocorticoids can be administered at doses equivalent to adrenal output for maximum stress (hydrocortisone, 100 mg intravenously every 8 hours). This dose can be reduced over 3 to 6 days postoperatively until a maintenance dose is reached.

Thromboembolic phenomena occur more frequently in patients with Cushing's syndrome, with an 11% incidence of deep venous thrombosis, and a 2% to 3% incidence of pulmonary embolus postoperatively. The thromboembolic events are believed to be secondary to the prevalence of obesity, hypertension, elevated hematocrit, and increased factor VIII levels.

Anesthetic management should account for the effects of excess cortisol secretion, especially as reflected in blood pressure, electrolyte balance, and blood glucose concentration. Osteoporosis is a consideration in positioning for the operative procedure. Plasma cortisol concentration decreases promptly after microadenomectomy or bilateral adrenalectomy. Intra-operative replacement therapy (cortisol, 100 mg intravenously) should be initiated.

D. Diabetes Insipidus

DEFINITION

Diabetes insipidus (DI) reflects the absence of antidiuretic hormone owing to the destruction of the posterior pituitary (neurogenic DI) or failure of the renal tubules to respond to antidiuretic hormone (nephrogenic DI).

ETIOLOGY

Neurogenic DI can be caused by intracranial trauma, hypophysectomy, neoplastic invasion, or sarcoidosis. Nephrogenic DI can be caused by hypokalemia, hypercalcemia, sickle cell anemia, obstructive uropathy, chronic renal insufficiency, or long-term use of lithium.

CLINICAL MANIFESTATIONS

Clinical features include polydipsia and polyuria with poorly concentrated urine despite increased plasma osmolarity. Neurogenic and nephrogenic DI are differentiated on the basis of response to desmopressin, which produces concentration of the urine in neurogenic, but not nephrogenic, DI.

TREATMENT

Treatment includes careful monitoring of urine output, plasma volume, and plasma osmolarity. Isotonic fluids may be administered until osmolarity is greater than 290; then hypotonic fluids are necessary. Neurogenic DI may be treated with desmopressin at 3 mcg/kg. Nephrogenic DI may be treated with chlorpropamide, an oral hypoglycemic drug that potentiates the effect of antidiuretic hormone on renal tubules.

ANESTHETIC CONSIDERATIONS

Anesthetic management for the patient with DI should include monitoring urine output and plasma electrolyte concentrations during the perioperative period. If emergency surgery is needed, central venous pressure monitoring may aid in the evaluation of volume status.

E. Diabetes Mellitus

DEFINITION

Diabetes mellitus (DM) is a complex metabolic derangement caused by relative or absolute insulin deficiency.

ETIOLOGY

Today, DM affects nearly 17 million people in the United States, about 6% of our population. The rise can be attributed to a combination of three factors: (1) an overweight population, (2) more sedentary life-styles, and (3) a rise in the number of elderly persons. As more of our population advances in age into the decades in which most cases of diabetes occur, the impact of the disease will become even more alarming.

Insulin-dependent DM (IDDM or type 1 DM) typically develops before the age of 16 years, and evidence points to a genetic predisposition to the disease. Resulting from autoimmune destruction of pancreatic beta cells, IDDM may be precipitated by a viral infection. About 15% of these patients have other autoimmune diseases such as hypothyroidism, Graves' disease, Addison's disease, or myasthenia gravis. The genetic predisposition is more of a reflection of susceptibility to the disease, rather than its inheritance. These patients depend on exogenous insulin to prevent ketoacidosis.

The other form of DM, non–insulin-dependent DM (NIDDM, adult-onset DM, or type 2 DM), most often develops after the age of 35 years, and evidence suggests a genetic predisposition. The prevalence increases with age, particularly among black women. Although many of these patients may require insulin therapy, they are not usually prone to ketoacidosis. Nevertheless, NIDDM may progress to the extent that insulin is needed to prevent ketoacidosis. Patients with NIDDM, who are typically overweight, constitute 90% of all diabetic patients. Obese nondiabetic persons require two to five times more insulin than do nonobese nondiabetic persons; thus, obesity may unmask latent DM.

Complications of DM are numerous. The most serious acute metabolic complication is ketoacidosis, defined as hyperglycemia in the presence of metabolic acidosis. The symptoms include nausea, vomiting, lethargy, and signs of hypovolemia from dehydration, which is the result of the osmotic effect of glucose. Causes of ketoacidosis include poor patient compliance with insulin therapy, insulin resistance because of infection, and silent myocardial infarction. Administration of a β_2-agonist to inhibit labor in the presence of IDDM has been reported to precipitate ketoacidosis abruptly, even with prior subcutaneous insulin administration. Complications of prolonged DM include macroangiopathies such as coronary artery disease, cerebrovascular disease, and peripheral vascular disease. These complications are more common in the patient with NIDDM; sequelae such as premature myocardial infarction, angina pectoris, or peripheral vascular insufficiency often are the presenting symptoms in an undiagnosed diabetic patient. However, in the patient with IDDM, microvascular complications and disorders of the nervous system predominate. Retinopathy, nephropathy, and autonomic and peripheral nervous system neuropathies are common. Diabetic retinopathy occurs in 80% to 90% of those with IDDM for longer than 20 years. Autonomic nervous system dysfunction may affect more than 15% of patients with DM. Delayed wound healing and postoperative infection are more likely in these patients. Stiff joint syndrome affects 30% to 40% of patients with IDDM and often affects all joints. Most important to anesthesia, the atlanto-occipital joint may be involved, making hyperextension of the head and subsequently, laryngoscopy, difficult.

Diabetics are subject to long-term complications that confer substantial morbidity and premature mortality. These complications include extensive arterial diseases, cataracts, peripheral neuropathies, and autonomic nervous system dysfunctions.

Arterial thrombotic lesions in the diabetic population are widely distributed in the extremities, kidneys, eyes, skeletal muscle, myocardium, and nervous system. As a result of these diffuse lesions, DM carries a serious risk for the development of nephropathy, atherosclerosis, stroke, retinopathy, and coronary artery disease.

TREATMENT

Treatment includes a diabetic diet, oral hypoglycemic drugs, and exogenous insulin. NIDDM is prevented primarily by avoidance or treatment of obesity. Transplantation of pancreatic tissue may be considered in selected patients.

ANESTHETIC CONSIDERATIONS

DM is the most common endocrine disorder encountered in surgical patients. Long-standing DM predisposes the patient to many diseases that require surgical intervention. Cataract extraction, kidney transplantation, ulcer débridement, and vascular repair are some of the operations frequently performed on diabetic patients. It is estimated that approximately 50% of diabetic patients have major surgery during their lifetimes.

Diabetic patients have higher morbidity and mortality in the perioperative period compared with nondiabetic persons of similar age. Increased complications are not because of the disease itself but primarily because of organ damage associated with long-term disease. Ischemic heart disease is the most common cause of perioperative mortality in the diabetic patient.

The diabetic surgical patient's operation should be scheduled early in the day if possible, to minimize disruptions in treatment and nutrition regimens. Day-stay for minor surgery may be used for patients with well-controlled DM who are knowledgeable about their disease and treatment and who have proper home support.

Preoperative Considerations

The diabetic patient may come to the operating room with a spectrum of metabolic aberrations and end-organ complications that warrant careful preanesthetic assessment.

Cardiovascular complications account for most of the surgical deaths in patients with DM. The presence of hypertension, coronary artery disease, or autonomic nervous system dysfunctions can result in a labile cardiovascular course during anesthesia. It is essential that the cardiovascular and volume status of the patient be thoroughly evaluated before surgery. Preoperative electrocardiography is necessary for all adult diabetic patients because of the high incidence of cardiac disease.

Autonomic nervous system dysfunction may result in delayed gastric emptying. It is estimated that gastroparesis occurs in 20% to 30% of all - diabetic patients. These patients are prone to aspiration, nausea and vomiting, and abdominal distention. Many authorities recommend routine preoperative aspiration prophylaxis with histamine (H_2) receptor blockers, metoclopramide, and/or preinduction antacids for patients with DM. Intubation during general anesthesia is a logical choice for the patient with gastroparesis.

Patients with significant autonomic neuropathy may have an impaired respiratory response to hypoxia. These patients are especially sensitive to the respiratory-depressant effects of sedatives and anesthetics and require particular vigilance in the perioperative period.

Peripheral neuropathies (paresthesias, numbness in the hands and feet) should be adequately documented in the preanesthetic evaluation. Their presence may affect the decision to use regional anesthesia.

An estimated 30% to 40% of patients with IDDM demonstrate restricted joint mobility. Limited motion of the atlanto-occipital joint can make endotracheal intubation difficult. Demonstration of the "prayer sign," an inability to approximate the palms of the hands and fingers, may help identify patients with tissue protein glycosylation and potentially difficult airways.

Evidence of kidney disease should be sought, and basic tests of renal function (urinalysis, serum creatinine, blood urea nitrogen) should be performed preoperatively. The presence of renal impairment may influence the choice and dosage of anesthetic agents. The use of potentially nephrotoxic drugs should be avoided.

The anesthetist should examine the patient's history of glycemic control to ensure preoperative optimization of the patient's metabolic state. A recommended target blood glucose range for the perioperative period is 120 to 180 mg/dL. Glycosylated hemoglobin levels provide an "averaged" estimate of glucose control.

Sustained hyperglycemia, with attendant osmotic diuresis, should alert the anesthetist to possible fluid deficits and electrolyte depletion. Preoperative levels of electrolytes should be determined for all diabetic patients, and adequate hydration and a good urine output should be maintained. Lactate-containing solutions are generally avoided because lactate conversion to glucose may contribute to hyperglycemia. An important part of the preoperative evaluation is a review of oral hypoglycemic and insulin regimens.

Oral hypoglycemic agents

Oral hypoglycemic agents are used as adjuncts to diet therapy for treating type 2 DM (NIDDM). Currently available oral hypoglycemic agents fall into the following classifications: (1) sulfonylureas, (2) α-glucosidase inhibitors, (3) thiazolidinediones, (4) biguanides, and (5) nonsulfonylurea secretagogues. *Sulfonylureas* increase the secretion of insulin from the pancreas and improve tissue sensitivity to insulin. These agents require the presence of functioning beta cells and thus are not efficacious in patients with IDDM. Hypoglycemia is the most important adverse side effect of sulfonylureas. Sulfonylurea therapy also is associated with a low incidence of cholestatic jaundice, rashes, and gastrointestinal symptoms. The syndrome of inappropriate antidiuretic hormone secretion and hyponatremia has been associated with chlorpropamide.

Acarbose (Precose) and miglitol (Glyset) are α-*glucosidase inhibitors*. These medications block the intestinal enzymes that digest starches into absorbable monosaccharides, resulting in a slower and lower rise in plasma glucose.

Rosiglitazone (Avandia) and pioglitazone (Actos) are *thiazolidinedione derivatives*. Thiazolidinediones decrease hepatic glucose output and reduce insulin resistance in the patient with type 2 DM by sensitizing the insulin receptor for glucose uptake. Liver enzymes must be monitored closely with these agents. The thiazolidinedione troglitazone (Rezulin) was withdrawn from the market in March 2000 for serious liver complications associated with the drug.

Metformin, a *biguanide*, decreases hepatic glucose production and increases peripheral insulin sensitivity. Lactic acidosis, a rare but potentially fatal problem, has been reported with biguanides. Lactic acidosis is precipitated by drug accumulation; therefore, even mild renal impairment is a contraindication to metformin therapy. Metformin is also not prescribed to patients with conditions that predispose to acidosis (e.g., liver failure, major surgery).

Newer oral hypoglycemic drugs such as the *meglitinides* (repaglinide) and D-*phenylalanine* (nateglinide) increase insulin production by pancreatic beta cells in a manner similar to the sulfonylureas. Repaglinide and nateglinide must be taken before each meal, and if a meal is missed, the drug should be omitted.

Insulin preparations

Insulin preparations differ in onset and duration after subcutaneous administration. In addition to subcutaneous injections, insulin delivery devices (implantable pumps, mechanical syringes) are used to facilitate exogenous administration. The greatest risk with all forms of insulin is hypoglycemia. The three major classes of exogenous insulin: short-acting, intermediate-acting, and long-acting are described in the following table.

Characteristics of Insulin Preparations

Insulin Type	Onset of Action	Peak Activity	Duration	Route
Short-acting				
Regular	30–60 min	1–2 hr	5–12 hr	IV, SC, IM
Rapid-acting				
Aspart (Novolog)	10–30 min	30–60 min	3–5 hr	SC
Lispro (Humalog)	10–30 min	30–60 min	3–5 hr	SC
Intermediate-acting				
NPH/Lente	1–2 hr	4–8 hr	10–20 hr	SC
Long-acting				
Ultralente	2–4 hr	8–20 hr	16–24 hr	SC
Glargine	1–2 hr	No peak	24 hr	SC

IM, Intramuscular; *IV,* intravenous; *NPH,* neutral protamine Hagedorn; *SC,* subcutaneous.
Time course is based on subcutaneous administration.

It is imperative to know the surgical patient's normal insulin dosage regimen and treatment compliance. Most diabetic patients are on a fixed regimen that consists of a mixture of rapid- and intermediate-acting insulins taken before breakfast and again at the evening meal. Multiple injection regimens are designed to give tight control. Insulin glargine (Lantus) is a recombinant DNA analogue of human insulin, taken once a day. It forms microprecipitates in subcutaneous tissue that delay its absorption and prolong its effects. Unlike NPH (neutral protamine Hagedorn) and ultralente insulin, it has no peak effect, but rather behaves like an insulin infusion.

The use of long-acting insulins (e.g., ultralente, glargine) is discouraged in the perioperative period because the dosage cannot be adjusted quickly for changes in blood glucose levels. Long-acting insulin regimens are often switched to intermediate- or short-acting insulin regimens for perioperative glucose control. Because glargine insulin maintains a stable level throughout the day, more experience with its use may demonstrate its safety as a basal insulin throughout the perioperative period.

Intraoperative Management

Surgery produces a catabolic stress response and elevates stress-induced counterregulatory hormones. The hyperglycemic, ketogenic, and lipolytic effects of the counterregulatory hormones in the diabetic patient compound the state of insulin deficiency. For this reason, perioperative hyperglycemia and other metabolic aberrations are common in the surgical diabetic patient.

No specific anesthetic technique is superior overall for diabetic patients. Both general anesthesia and regional anesthesia have been used safely. General anesthesia, however, has been shown to induce hormonal changes that accentuate glycogenolysis and gluconeogenesis, compounding the diabetic patient's hyperglycemic state. Regional anesthesia may produce less deleterious changes in glucose homeostasis.

The certified registered nurse anesthetist must be especially careful in positioning and padding the diabetic patient on the operating table. Decreased tissue perfusion and peripheral sympathetic neuropathy may contribute to the development of skin breakdown and ulceration.

Diabetic patients represent a heterogeneous group requiring individualized perioperative care. The specific approach to metabolic management depends on the type of DM (type 1 or type 2), the history of glycemic control, and the type of surgery being performed. Frequent blood sugar determinations should be an integral part of any diabetic management technique. A glucose meter or other accurate and rapid means of monitoring blood glucose levels should be available. Blood glucose should be routinely monitored in the preoperative and postoperative periods. An hourly intraoperative blood glucose measurement is the prudent course for the patient with brittle DM during a long surgical procedure or for major surgery.

Persistent hyperglycemia has been shown to impair wound healing and wound strength. In addition, reports suggest that postoperative infection is more prevalent in diabetic patients with uncontrolled blood glucose levels. Studies also provide evidence that hyperglycemia worsens the neurologic outcome after ischemic brain injury. Avoiding hyperglycemia is advisable, especially in the patient at risk for acute neurologic insult (carotid endarterectomy, intracranial surgery, cardiopulmonary bypass).

Various regimens have been tendered on how to best manage the metabolic changes that occur in the surgical diabetic. Experts differ on optimal protocols for case management. Current debate centers on the value of intensive or "tight" blood glucose control versus "nontight" control during surgery. The universal goal with all techniques is to avoid hypoglycemia and to minimize metabolic derangements. Patients under anesthesia are generally maintained with mild transient hyperglycemia to avoid the potentially catastrophic effects of hypoglycemia. Frequent blood glucose determinations during surgery and in the immediate postoperative period are central to safe practice.

Three different approaches to the metabolic management of the surgical diabetic patient are described here; however, the reader should note that there are numerous variations.

Nontight Control of Blood Glucose Levels in the Perioperative Period

Nontight control of blood glucose levels refers to diabetic management techniques that involve less intensive control of plasma glucose but avoid marked hyperglycemia and dangerous hypoglycemia. This is a traditional method of managing the surgical diabetic patient, and variations of this technique are used for stable diabetics undergoing elective operative procedures.[7,9,11,14]

Technique for nontight management of the diabetic patient

- On the morning of surgery, fasting blood glucose level is measured.
- An intravenous infusion containing 5% dextrose is started at 125 mL/hour/70 kg body weight.
- After the intravenous infusion is started, 30% to 50% of the patient's normal morning intermediate insulin (NPH or Lente) dose is administered subcutaneously.
- The glucose-containing intravenous infusion is continued throughout surgery. Additional fluid requirements are met with the administration of a second, glucose-free infusate.
- Blood glucose levels are checked every 1 to 2 hours during surgery.
- If the blood glucose level exceeds an established maximum level, commonly 200 mg/dL, a bolus of regular insulin is administered intravenously, according to an established "sliding scale." Insulin sensitivity varies markedly from one patient to the next, but on the average, 1 unit of regular insulin can be expected to decrease the blood glucose level 40 to 50 mg/dL.[47]

This time-tested regimen is easy to implement, and it usually is successful in preventing significant hypoglycemia and the other metabolic extremes, diabetic ketoacidosis, and hyperosmolar states.

The disadvantages of nontight control are as follows:

- Absorption of preoperatively administered subcutaneous insulin is unpredictable and erratic in the surgical patient because of blood pressure, blood flow, and temperature variations that occur with anesthesia.
- The onset and the peak effect of the preoperative intermediate-acting insulin may not correspond to the time of surgical stress, especially if the operation is delayed or prolonged.
- The half-life of regular insulin is short, and a "roller coaster" glucose profile may occur. Plasma glucose levels will vary considerably.

Tight Control of Blood Glucose Levels in the Perioperative Period

Tight control of plasma glucose refers to diabetic management techniques in which the blood glucose concentration is maintained within relatively narrow boundaries, commonly 100 to 180 mg/dL. These regimens require the use of infusion pumps. Tighter control of blood glucose levels requires more frequent blood glucose assays. Intensive perioperative regulation of blood glucose prevents hyperglycemia, but it carries the risk of hypoglycemia.

Insulin infusion during surgery is advised for the patient with type 1 DM who is having major surgery and for the patient with poorly controlled DM (type 1 or type 2). A combined insulin/glucose infusion regimen is advised to prevent hypoglycemia caused by inadvertent blockage of a glucose infusion when separate glucose and insulin infusions are used. An example of this regimen follows:

- An infusion of 5% dextrose with 0.32 units regular insulin/g of dextrose (16 units/L), with 20 mEq potassium/L is administered at 100 mL/hour.

- The glucose/insulin-containing intravenous infusion is started only when the patient's blood glucose level is 200 mg/dL or greater.
- Blood glucose levels should be measured every hour during an insulin infusion, and potassium levels should be checked after the first hour of the infusion.
- For patients with higher insulin needs, 1 to 2 units additional insulin can be added to the infusate bag.
- Additional fluid requirements are met with the administration of a second, glucose-free infusate.

Blood glucose levels less than 80 mg/dL may be treated with 50% dextrose in water ($D_{50}W$) and remeasured in 30 minutes. In a 70-kg patient, 15 mL of $D_{50}W$ can be expected to raise the blood glucose concentration by about 30 mg/dL. Surgical patients undergoing renal transplantation or coronary artery bypass graft procedures, obese and septic patients, and patients receiving steroid therapy usually have higher insulin infusion requirements.

The advantages of tight glucose management in the perioperative period are as follows:

- The insulin infusion can be finely regulated to correspond to hourly variations in blood glucose levels.
- Periods of hyperglycemia are less likely. Deleterious effects of hyperglycemia (hyperosmolarity, osmotic diuresis, impaired wound healing, infection) may be prevented.[78]
- The insulin/glucose infusion can be continued into the postoperative period until the patient is ready to eat, at which time subcutaneous insulin or an oral hypoglycemic agent can be reinstated.

Type 2 Diabetes and Oral Hypoglycemic Agents

Patients treated with oral hypoglycemic agents demand the same individualized perioperative management as those with type 1 DM. The duration of action of the patient's oral agent must be noted. Discontinuing long-acting agents 2 to 3 days before surgery and converting to shorter-acting agents or insulin affords better perioperative glucose control. Metformin should be discontinued 2 days or more before surgery because the surgical risks of hypotension and renal hypoperfusion place patients who are taking this drug at increased risk for lactic acidosis.

For the well-controlled type 2 DM patient who is scheduled for minor to moderate surgery, the patient's oral hypoglycemic agent may be continued until the evening before surgery. Glucose-containing fluids may be administered intraoperatively to protect against possible residual effects of oral hypoglycemic agents. Other experts adhere to a "no glucose, no insulin" technique for patients with well-controlled type 2 DM. Regardless of the technique chosen, plasma glucose should be measured regularly throughout the procedure and hyperglycemia treated with insulin on a "sliding scale."

F. Hyperaldosteronism

DEFINITION

Primary hyperaldosteronism (Conn's syndrome) is excess secretion of aldosterone from a functional tumor independent of a physiologic stimulus.

Secondary hyperaldosteronism is when increased renin secretion is responsible for the excess secretion of aldosterone.

ETIOLOGY

Hyperaldosteronism should be suspected in a patient with diastolic hypertension (100 to 125 mm Hg) and a plasma potassium concentration of less than 3.5 mEq/L. Hypertension reflects aldosterone-induced sodium retention and the resultant increased extracellular fluid volume. Hypokalemic metabolic acidosis is present secondary to aldosterone-induced renal excretion of potassium. Skeletal muscle weakness is presumed to reflect hypokalemia. Hypokalemic nephropathy can result in polyuria and the inability to concentrate urine optimally.

LABORATORY RESULTS

Diagnosis of hyperaldosteronism is confirmed by increased plasma concentration of aldosterone and increased urinary potassium excretion (greater than 30 mEq/L) despite coexisting hypokalemia. Measurement of plasma renin activity permits classification of the disease as primary (low renin activity) or secondary (increased renin activity).

TREATMENT

Treatment consists of supplemental potassium and administration of competitive aldosterone antagonists, such as spironolactone. Hypertension may require treatment with antihypertensive drugs. Hypokalemia from drug-induced diuresis is minimized with a potassium-sparing diuretic such as triamterene. The definitive treatment for aldosterone-secreting tumor is surgical excision.

ANESTHETIC CONSIDERATIONS

Anesthetic management begins with preoperative correction of hypokalemia and treatment of hypertension. Unsuspected hypovolemia is evidenced by orthostatic hypotension during preoperative evaluation. Invasive monitoring (central venous pressure, pulmonary arterial catheter) may be necessary in these patients to monitor intraoperative filling pressures. Supplementation with exogenous cortisol is also a consideration.

G. Hypoaldosteronism

DEFINITION

Hypoaldosteronism is suggested by hyperkalemia in the absence of renal insufficiency. Isolated deficiency of aldosterone secretion may reflect congenital deficiency of aldosterone synthetase or hyporeninemia resulting from a defect in the juxtaglomerular apparatus or treatment with an angiotensin-converting enzyme inhibitor leading to loss of angiotensin stimulation.

ETIOLOGY

Hyporeninemic hypoaldosteronism typically occurs in patients older than 45 years with chronic renal disease, diabetes mellitus, or both. Indomethacin-induced prostaglandin deficiency is a reversible cause of this syndrome.

CLINICAL MANIFESTATIONS

Symptoms include heart block secondary to hyperkalemia and postural hypotension with or without hyponatremia. Hyperchloremic metabolic acidosis is common.

TREATMENT

Treatment of hypoaldosteronism includes liberal sodium intake and daily administration of hydrocortisone.

ANESTHETIC CONSIDERATIONS

Begin anesthetic management with preoperative monitoring of the serum potassium level, which should be less than 5.5 mEq/L before elective surgery. Electrocardiographic monitoring for effects of hyperkalemia (tall, tentlike T waves; heart block) is recommended. Hypoventilation should be avoided to prevent an additional increase in serum potassium. Succinylcholine should be avoided when possible to prevent potassium release. Intravenous fluids should be free of potassium. If hypovolemia is suspected, fluid replacement should be initiated, possibly governed by invasive (i.e., central venous pressure) monitoring.

H. Hyperparathyroidism

DEFINITION

Hyperparathyroidism is present when the secretion of parathormone is increased. Serum calcium concentration may be increased, decreased, or unchanged. It is classified as primary, secondary, or ectopic.

INCIDENCE

Primary hyperparathyroidism may result from a parathyroid adenoma, gland hyperplasia, or parathyroid cancer. In 85% to 90% of the cases, hyperparathyroidism is caused by hypersecretion of a single parathyroid adenoma. Hyperplasia of one or more parathyroid glands accounts for about 10% of the cases. Carcinoma of the parathyroid gland is found in less than 1% of patients and is associated with particularly high serum calcium levels. Hyperparathyroidism may also exist as part of a multiple endocrine neoplastic (MEN) syndrome.

The incidence of primary hyperparathyroidism in the United States is approximately five cases per 10,000 people per year, with a higher occurrence in female patients and the elderly. Stimulation of the parathyroid gland during pregnancy or lactation, prior neck irradiation, and a family history of parathyroid disease are predisposing factors.

ETIOLOGY

Primary hyperparathyroidism results from excessive secretion of parathormone by a benign parathyroid adenoma, from carcinoma of a parathyroid gland, or from hyperplasia of the parathyroid glands. Secondary hyperparathyroidism reflects an appropriate compensatory response of the parathyroid glands to secrete more parathormone to counteract a disease process that produces hypocalcemia. Finally, ectopic hyperparathyroidism is caused by secretion of parathormone by tissues other than the parathyroid glands. This can occur with carcinomas of the lung, breast, pancreas, or kidney and lymphoproliferative diseases.

LABORATORY RESULTS

Sustained overactivity of the parathyroid glands is characterized by high serum calcium levels. Most patients remain asymptomatic until the total serum calcium level rises to more than 11 to 12 mg/dL. A concentration greater than 14 mg/dL may be life-threatening and demands immediate treatment. Patients with carcinomas usually have markedly increased calcium levels greater than 7.5 mEq/L.

CLINICAL MANIFESTATIONS

Hypercalcemia is responsible for a broad spectrum of signs and symptoms that accompany primary hyperparathyroidism and that affect multiple organ systems. Early signs and symptoms include nausea and vomiting, skeletal muscle weakness, and hypotonia. Persistent increases can interfere with urine-concentrating ability, and polyuria results. Oliguric renal failure can occur in advanced cases. Renal stones, peptic ulcer disease, hypertension, bone pain, pathologic fractures, hallucinations, mood disturbances, and acute or chronic pancreatitis can also occur.

The effect of hyperparathyroidism on bone becomes clinically apparent when osteoclastic absorption of bone overwhelms osteoblastic deposition. With severe and protracted disease, the weakened bones become filled with decalcified cavities, making them painful and susceptible to fracture. The destructive bone disease associated with sustained hyperparathyroidism is called *osteitis fibrosa cystica*.

Many of the nonskeletal manifestations of primary hyperparathyroidism are related to the accompanying hypercalcemia. Sustained hypercalcemia may produce deleterious effects in the pancreas (pancreatitis), in the kidney (nephrolithiasis, nephrocalcinosis, polyuria), in blood vessels (hypertension), in the heart (shortened ventricular refractory period, bradyarrhythmias, bundle branch block, heart block), and in the acid-producing areas of the stomach (peptic ulcer). The mnemonic "stones, bones, and groans" summarizes features of advanced, untreated hyperparathyroidism. Profound muscle weakness, anorexia, confusion, nausea, vomiting, and lethargy are additional features of the disorder.

Despite increased mobilization of phosphorus from bone, serum phosphate concentration usually is normal or low in hyperparathyroidism as a result of increased urinary excretion.

Patients with chronically low levels of serum calcium, such as those with chronic renal failure and gastrointestinal malabsorption, may develop compensatory parathyroid gland hyperplasia or *secondary hyperparathyroidism* in response to the hypocalcemia. Their clinical course is marked by the same parathyroid hormone–mediated skeletal assault seen in the primary form of the disorder, but because it is an adaptive response, secondary hyperparathyroidism is seldom associated with hypercalcemia.

TREATMENT

Saline infusion (150 mL/hour) is the basic treatment for all patients with symptomatic hypercalcemia. This calcium-lowering effect of saline hydration is limited and it is often necessary to add loop diuretics (furosemide [Lasix], 40 to 80 mg intravenously). Thiazide diuretics are not administered because these drugs may enhance renal tubular reabsorption of calcium. Bisphosphonates such as disodium etidronate is the drug of choice for life-threatening hypercalcemia. These drugs bind to hydroxyapatite in bone and act as potent inhibitors of osteoclastic bone resorption. Hemodialysis can also be used to lower serum calcium concentrations promptly, as can calcitonin, but its effects are transient. The usual treatment for symptomatic primary hyperparathyroidism is surgical removal of abnormal parathyroid tissue. Surgical treatment for asymptomatic hyperparathyroidism is more controversial.

ANESTHETIC CONSIDERATIONS

Parathyroidectomy is commonly performed with the patient under general anesthesia, although a cervical plexus block technique has been used, especially for elderly and medically compromised patients. Parathyroid tissue resembles brown fat, and this feature can occasionally make it difficult for the surgeon to locate this tissue. Further, parathyroid tissue sometimes can be found in such ectopic places as the deep recesses of the mediastinum, the carotid sheath, or the thymus gland.

Blood loss from parathyroid surgery is usually minimal, and advanced monitoring is not required based on the surgical procedure. Serum calcium, magnesium, and phosphorus levels should be monitored in the postoperative period until stable. In most cases, serum calcium levels return to normal within 3 to 4 days after surgery. With current methods of detection, most patients with hyperparathyroidism are asymptomatic; however, erosive effects of elevated parathyroid hormone on bone and the systemic effects of chronic hypercalcemia should be considered in the anesthetic plan for these patients.

Severely hypercalcemic (greater than 14 mg/dL) or symptomatic patients should be treated preoperatively. Isotonic saline hydration and loop diuretics (furosemide, 40 to 80 mg every 2 to 4 hours) can rapidly decrease serum calcium levels by 2 to 3 mg/dL. Less frequently, drugs that inhibit osteoclastic bone resorption (mithramycin, bisphosphonates, and calcitonin) are used. Loop diuretics promote calciuresis by decreasing tubular reabsorption of calcium. Thiazide diuretics increase renal tubular calcium reabsorption and will not effectively correct hypercalcemia.

The hypercalcemic patient may be dehydrated because of anorexia, vomiting, and the impaired ability of the kidneys to concentrate urine. Hydration with non–calcium-containing solutions should be maintained throughout the perioperative period to dilute serum calcium, maintain adequate glomerular filtration and calcium clearance, and ensure adequate intravascular volume. Vigorous hydration dictates the use of bladder catheterization, central venous pressure monitoring, and frequent determinations of serum electrolytes.

Elevated calcium levels may depress the central and peripheral nervous systems. The use of preoperative sedatives in the hypercalcemic patient who appears lethargic or confused should be avoided. General anesthetic requirements may be decreased as well.

Careful review of the patient's renal status is especially crucial in patients with secondary hyperparathyroidism. Associated complications of renal impairment (volume overload, anemia, electrolyte derangements) may affect anesthetic medication dosages and selection.

Cardiac conduction disturbances such as a shortened QT interval and a prolonged PR interval are observed with hypercalcemia. Dysrhythmias and hypertension may respond to calcium channel antagonists (e.g., verapamil, 5 to 10 mg intravenously).

Awareness of the effects of pH on the ionized portion of plasma calcium is important. Alkalosis protects against hypercalcemia by shifting the ionized calcium to the protein-bound form. Periodic determinations of serum ionized calcium levels help to guide management.

The response to neuromuscular blockade may be unpredictable. Muscle weakness, hypotonia, and muscle atrophy may increase the patient's sensitivity to nondepolarizing skeletal muscle relaxants. Careful titration of muscle relaxants with use of a peripheral nerve stimulator is prudent. The surgeon may sometimes request no muscle relaxation to facilitate identification of the recurrent laryngeal nerve during parathyroid surgery.

Enhanced osteoclastic bone resorption produces clinically significant bone disease in 10% to 15% of patients with hyperparathyroidism. These patients are susceptible to fractures, and care must be exercised in positioning and padding. Hyperparathyroid patients are prone to postoperative nausea and vomiting. Prophylactic antiemetic medications are advisable.

I. Hypoparathyroidism

DEFINITION

Hypoparathyroidism is the deficient or absent secretion of parathyroid hormone or a peripheral resistance to its effect. Pseudohypoparathyroidism is a congenital disorder in which the release of parathormone is intact but the kidneys are unable to respond to the hormone.

ETIOLOGY

Absence or deficiency of parathormone is almost always iatrogenic. Inadvertent removal of parathyroid tissue, parathyroid gland injury from irradiation or autoimmune destruction, and chronic severe magnesium deficiency (alcohol abuse, poor nutrition, malabsorption) are possible causes of hypoparathyroidism.

LABORATORY RESULTS

Patients with hypoparathyroidism typically have low serum calcium levels. The blood phosphate concentration may be elevated because of the decreased renal excretion of phosphate.

Serum calcium concentrations and the ionized fractions of calcium are the most valuable diagnostic indicators. Diagnosis is made with serum calcium concentrations less than 4.5 mEq/L and ionized calcium concentrations lower than 2 mEq/L.

CLINICAL MANIFESTATIONS

Clinical signs of hypoparathyroidism reflect the degree of hypocalcemia and the rapidity of calcium decline. A sudden drop in ionized calcium usually produces more severe symptoms than does a slow decline.

Cardinal features of the neuromuscular excitability are muscle spasms and hypocalcemic tetany. Symptoms vary in severity and may take the form of muscle cramps, perioral paresthesias, numbness in the feet and toes, or hyperactive deep tendon reflexes. The patient may feel restless or hyperirritable. Life-threatening laryngeal muscle spasm may occur, producing stridor, labored respirations, and asphyxia.

Two classic manifestations of latent hypocalcemic tetany are *Chvostek's sign* and *Trousseau's sign.* Chvostek's sign is a contracture or twitching of ipsilateral facial muscles produced when the facial nerve is tapped at the angle of the jaw. Trousseau's sign is elicited by the inflation of a blood pressure cuff slightly above the systolic level for a few minutes. The resultant ischemia aggravates the muscle irritability in hypocalcemic states and causes flexion of the wrist and thumb with extension of the fingers *(carpopedal spasm)*.

Chronic hypocalcemia is associated with complaints of fatigue and skeletal muscle cramps that may be associated with a prolonged QT interval on the electrocardiogram. The QRS complex, PR interval, and cardiac rhythm usually remain normal. Neurologic changes include lethargy, cerebration deficits, and personality changes reminiscent of hyperparathyroidism. Chronic hypocalcemia is associated with formation of cataracts, calcification involving the subcutaneous tissues and basal ganglia, and thickening of the skull. Chronic renal failure is the most common cause of chronic hypocalcemia.

TREATMENT

Treatment of acute hypocalcemia consists of an infusion of calcium (10% calcium gluconate intravenously) until signs of neuromuscular irritability disappear. Correction of any coexisting respiratory or metabolic alkalosis is indicated. For treatment of hypoparathyroidism not complicated by symptomatic hypocalcemia, the approach is administration of oral calcium and vitamin D. An exogenous parathyroid hormone preparation is not yet practical for clinical use. Thiazide diuretics may be useful, because these drugs cause sodium depletion without proportional potassium excretion, thereby tending to increase serum calcium concentrations.

ANESTHETIC CONSIDERATIONS

Management of anesthesia is designed to prevent any further decrease in the serum calcium concentrations and to treat the adverse effects of hypocalcemia, especially those on the heart. Avoid iatrogenic hyperventilation. Temporary hypocalcemia often is observed after successful parathyroid surgery for hyperparathyroidism. This may occur within a few hours after surgery or 1 to 2 days postoperatively. The transient postoperative hypocalcemia is the result of parathyroid gland suppression (by preoperative hypercalcemia) and rapid bone uptake of calcium ("hungry bone syndrome"). Inadvertent removal of all parathyroid gland tissue induces a decline in the serum calcium concentration from a normal level to 6 to 7 mg/dL. Even a small amount of remaining parathyroid tissue usually is capable of sufficient hypertrophy to preserve normal calcium-phosphate balance.[27]

Assiduous observation for signs of musculoskeletal irritability and frequent measurement of serum ionized calcium levels should be performed following parathyroid surgery. The threshold for the development of signs of hypocalcemia is variable; however, manifestations of neuromuscular compromise often are observed at serum calcium levels of 6 to 7 mg/dL.

Laryngeal muscles are especially sensitive to tetanic spasm, and laryngospasm may cause life-threatening airway compromise in the hypocalcemic patient. Respiratory distress following parathyroid surgery may be secondary to laryngeal muscle spasm, edema or bleeding in the neck, or bilateral recurrent laryngeal nerve injury. Unilateral recurrent laryngeal nerve injury produces hoarseness and usually requires only close observation. Bilateral recurrent laryngeal nerve injury causes aphonia and requires immediate airway support and intubation.

Hypocalcemia may be apparent on electrocardiographic tracings as a prolonged QT interval, reflecting delayed ventricular repolarization and a predisposition to ventricular dysrhythmias. The cardiac rhythm usually remains normal. Decreased cardiac contractility and hypotension may occur. Congestive heart failure, although rare, is a danger.

Circulating levels of ionized calcium can decline abruptly in the perioperative period. Precipitous increases in the circulating levels of anions such as bicarbonate, phosphate, and citrate lower ionized calcium levels. Hyperventilation, the rapid transfusion of citrated blood, or the rapid administration of bicarbonate may induce overt tetany in a previously asymptomatic hypocalcemic patient. Vigorous diuresis can augment calcium loss. Patients with hypocalcemia may have an altered response to muscle relaxants.

Patients with confirmed, symptomatic hypocalcemia require prompt therapy. Acute hypocalcemia can be treated with an initial intravenous bolus of 100 to 200 mg of elemental calcium administered over 10 minutes (10 mL of 10% calcium gluconate = 93 mg elemental calcium; 10 mL of 10% calcium chloride = 272 mg elemental calcium). Relief of symptoms is usually prompt but may be transient. For maintenance of normal levels, the initial bolus may be followed by an infusion of 1 to 2 mg/kg per hour of elemental calcium, diluted in 50 to 100 mL of saline. Calcium, magnesium, phosphate, potassium, and creatinine levels should be monitored diligently during calcium replacement.

J. Hyperthyroidism

Hyperthyroidism is an increase in thyroid function resulting from an excess supply of thyroid hormones and is associated with Graves' disease, thyroid-stimulating hormone (TSH) overproduction, and pregnancy. In subacute thyroiditis, excess thyroid hormone leaks out of the gland owing to inflammation. Ovarian tumors or metastatic thyroid carcinoma may also produce extrathyroid gland hormone. Exogenous consumption of thyroid hormone can also lead to hyperthyroidism.

ETIOLOGY

TSH is released from the anterior pituitary, causing iodine to be taken up into the thyroid gland. The iodine is then incorporated into tyrosine residues, and the hormones triiodothyronine (T_3) and thyroxine (T_4) are formed and stored. Peripheral tissues convert T_4 to T_3, which is three times more potent than T_4 and has a shorter half-life. Both T_4 and T_3 are partially bound to the plasma protein thyroid-binding globulin (TBG), although only the unbound forms are pharmacologically active. TBG levels can increase with acute liver disease, pregnancy, acute intermittent porphyria, and medications (oral hypoglycemics, exogenous estrogens, clofibrate, opioids). They can decrease with chronic liver disease, nephrotic syndrome, anabolic steroids, and acromegaly. TBG has no direct role in cell metabolism, but its concentration can alter diagnostic test results when checking for thyroid disease.

LABORATORY RESULTS

Laboratory findings in hyperthyroidism include elevated levels of T_3 and T_4. Because TBG concentration may affect the measured T_4, a resin T_3 uptake test may be performed to distinguish between protein-binding abnormalities and true metabolic changes associated with hyperthyroidism. TSH levels may be normal or decreased.

CLINICAL MANIFESTATIONS

Clinically, hyperthyroid patients present with nervousness, tachycardia, goiter, tremors, muscle weakness, heat intolerance, and weight loss despite high caloric intake. Exophthalmos occurs in approximately 7 of 10 cases of hyperthyroidism. Worsening of angina pectoris or unexpected onset of congestive heart failure or atrial fibrillation may reflect undiagnosed hyperthyroidism, especially in elderly patients in whom the increased amount of thyroid hormones is sufficient only to aggravate underlying heart disease.

Thyroid storm (thyrotoxicosis) is an abrupt exacerbation of hyperthyroidism caused by the sudden excessive release of thyroid gland hormones into the circulation. Hyperthermia, tachycardia, congestive heart failure, dehydration, and shock commonly occur. Thyroid storm may be precipitated by surgical stress but is usually seen 6 to 18 hours postoperatively. It may mimic malignant hyperthermia, sepsis, hemorrhage, or a transfusion or drug reaction.

TREATMENT

Treatments for hyperthyroidism include antithyroid drugs, subtotal thyroidectomy, or radioactive iodine. Thyroid storm therapy includes active cooling, hydration, β-adrenergic blockade, use of steroids if there is any indication of adrenal insufficiency, and institution of long-term therapy with antithyroid drugs or iodine. Six weeks are required to become euthyroid. Only emergency surgery should be performed in thyrotoxic patients. Premedication, including β-blockers, should be given generously. Sympathetic stimulation (pain, ketamine, pancuronium) should be avoided. Eyes should be protected well, especially if exophthalmos is present. Drug metabolism and anesthetic requirements are increased. Because of muscle weakness, muscle relaxants should be titrated carefully. Hypotension should be treated with direct-acting agents, such as phenylephrine. Regional anesthesia may be beneficial in thyrotoxic patients because it blocks the sympathetic response. Local anesthetics with epinephrine may lead to further arrhythmias.

K. Hypothyroidism

Hypothyroidism can be classified as either *primary* (because of destruction of the thyroid gland, where there is an adequate level of thyroid-stimulating hormone [TSH]) or *secondary* (because of central nervous system dysfunction leading to decreased levels of TSH). Causes of primary hypothyroidism include chronic thyroiditis, subtotal thyroidectomy, radioactive iodine therapy, and irradiation of the neck. Thyroid hormone deficiency may occur because of antithyroid drugs, excess iodide, or a dietary iodine deficiency. Causes of secondary hypothyroidism include hypothalamic dysfunction (leading to thyrotropin-releasing hormone deficiency) and anterior pituitary dysfunction (leading to TSH deficiency).

LABORATORY RESULTS

Laboratory findings in primary hypothyroidism include decreased levels of triiodothyronine (T_3) and thyroxine (T_4), with an increased concentration of TSH. Secondary hypothyroidism exhibits decreased levels of T_3, T_4, and TSH. Resin T_3 uptake is decreased in both instances.

CLINICAL MANIFESTATIONS

The onset of clinical symptoms in the adult patient is insidious and may go unrecognized. Patients experience lethargy, constipation, cold intolerance, facial edema with an enlarged tongue, reversible cardiomyopathy, pericardial effusion, ascites, anemia, and adynamic ileus with delayed gastric emptying. There may be adrenal atrophy with decreased cortisol production, dilutional hyponatremia, and decreased water excretion. There is a decreased cardiac output, bradycardia, hypovolemia, and diminished baroreceptor reflexes. Myxedema coma (profound hypothyroidism) may be triggered by trauma, infection, and central nervous system depressants, leading to respiratory depression, congestive heart failure, and depressed consciousness.

TREATMENT

Treatment for hypothyroidism involves the exogenous supplementation of thyroid hormone. T_4 requires 10 days to have an effect. T_3 begins to have an effect in 6 hours. Treatment for myxedema coma includes intravenous administration of T_3, and, if adrenal insufficiency is suspected, cortisol. Digitalis should be used sparingly to treat congestive heart failure because the drug increases myocardial contractility, and this is not well tolerated by patients with hypothyroidism. Careful fluid replacement is important, because these patients may be vulnerable to water intoxication and hyponatremia.

Elective surgery must be postponed in any patient who is clinically hypothyroid. In patients with hypothyroidism who must undergo emergency procedures, anesthetic considerations should include avoidance of preoperative sedation because of profound central nervous system and respiratory sensitivity to depressants. Cortisol supplementation should be considered, intravascular volume should be optimized, and anemia should be corrected. Anesthetic techniques must take into consideration airway problems associated with a large tongue, poor gastric emptying, and increased sensitivity to all depressant medications.

L. Pheochromocytoma

DEFINITION

Pheochromocytomas are catecholamine-secreting tumors derived most commonly (90%) from adrenomedullary chromaffin cells or less commonly from extraadrenal chromaffin cells. Pheochromocytomas involve both adrenal glands in 10% of adult patients with the tumor. Extraadrenal pheochromocytomas have been found anywhere from the pelvis to the skull base. Malignant spread of pheochromocytomas occurs in approximately 10% of cases. These pheochromocytomas are more often extraadrenal and often secrete dopamine. Malignant pheochromocytomas usually spread through venous and lymphatic channels to the liver.

ETIOLOGY

Pheochromocytomas are rare, occurring in less than 0.5% of all hypertensive patients. These tumors may be associated with neurocutaneous syndromes such as von Hippel–Lindau disease, tuberous sclerosis, Sturge-Weber syndrome, and as a component of multiple endocrine neoplasia (MEN) type 2A or 2B. Patients with a family history of MEN syndrome should be regularly screened for pheochromocytoma. Five to 10% of pheochromocytomas occur as part of an inherited autosomal dominant trait. Five percent of patients with pheochromocytomas have neurofibromatosis, but only 1% of patients with neurofibromatosis have pheochromocytomas.

Pheochromocytomas can occur at any age, but usually within the third to the fifth decade of life. They occur with equal frequency in both sexes in adults.

Pheochromocytomas produce, store, and secrete catecholamines, mostly norepinephrine and epinephrine. Unlike in a normal adrenal medulla, norepinephrine is the predominant catecholamine secreted by most of these tumors. In the majority of cases, however, it is impossible to predict the pattern of catecholamine secretion from the clinical features.

LABORATORY RESULTS

Diagnosis requires chemical confirmation of excessive catecholamine release. Measurement of "free" norepinephrine from a 24-hour urine test is thought to be a more sensitive index of pheochromocytoma than measures of catecholamine metabolites (normetanephrine, metanephrine, vanillylmandelic acid). Normotension despite increased plasma concentration of catecholamines is thought to reflect a decrease in the number of α-receptors (down-regulation) in response to increased circulating concentrations of the neurotransmitter. Clonidine (0.3 mg orally) suppresses the plasma concentration of catecholamines in patients with essential hypertension but not in patients with pheochromocytoma, reflecting the drug's ability to suppress increases in plasma catecholamine concentration resulting from neurogenic release but not from diffusion of excess catecholamine from a pheochromocytoma into the circulation. Computed tomography is the initial localizing procedure in the diagnosis of pheochromocytoma (see the following box).

Values for Catecholamines and Catecholamine Metabolites

Hormone/Metabolite	Normal Value
Vanillylmandelic acid, urine	2–7 mg/24 hr
Metanephrines, urine	<1.3 mg/24 hr
Norepinephrine, urine	<100 mcg/24 hr
Norepinephrine, plasma	150–450 pg/mL
Epinephrine, plasma	<35 pg/mL
Catecholamines, free urinary	<110 mcg/24 hr

CLINICAL MANIFESTATIONS

Manifestations of a pheochromocytoma reflect massive and sustained catecholamine release and include hypertension, diaphoresis, headache, tremulousness, palpitations, and weight loss. Symptoms may be paroxysmal or sustained. The combination of diaphoresis, tachycardia, and headache in the hypertensive patient is a frequently recognized and highly specific triad.

A catecholamine-mediated paroxysm typically consists of a sudden and alarming increase in blood pressure, a severe throbbing headache, profuse sweating, palpitations with or without tachycardia, a sense of doom, anxiety, pallor (rarely flushing), nausea, abdominal pain, and orthostatic hypotension. Orthostatic hypotension is a result of plasma volume deficit. Additionally, the postural reflexes that defend upright blood pressure may lose their tone with sustained excesses of catecholamines. Paroxysmal symptoms may last several minutes to days and are often followed by exhaustion.

A paroxysm may be triggered by acute physical stress, abdominal palpation, defecation, hypotension, activation of the sympathetic nervous system, or micturition if pheochromocytoma is present in urinary bladder wall. In other patients, no clearly defined precipitating factor can be found. Mental or psychological stress does not usually initiate a crisis.

The symptoms associated with a pheochromocytoma reflect the usual predominance of α-adrenergic activity over β-adrenergic effects. As a result of α-adrenergic inhibition of insulin, mild hyperglycemia may be present. The cardiac output and heart rate may be significantly increased. An overall increase in metabolism increases oxygen consumption and can cause hyperthermia. Vasoconstriction in the extremities may produce pain, paresthesias, intermittent claudication, or ischemia.

Hypertension is the most common symptom, occurring in more than 90% of patients. Paroxysmal hypertension is present in 40% to 50% of patients and it is a distinctive manifestation of the disease. Sustained hypertension is often resistant to conventional treatment. When pheochromocytomas are predominantly epinephrine secreting, hypertension can alternate with periods of hypotension associated with syncope. This may result from the surges of epinephrine causing disproportionate β-adrenergic stimulation with vasodilation in the presence of a contracted vascular space.

A catecholamine-induced increase in myocardial oxygen consumption, hypertension, and possibly coronary artery spasm can precipitate myocardial infarction or congestive heart failure even in the absence of coronary artery disease. Electrocardiographic (ECG) changes are common. Nonspecific ST-segment and T-wave changes and prominent U waves may be seen. Sinus tachycardia, sinus bradycardia, supraventricular tachycardias, and premature ventricular contractions have been noted. Right and left bundle branch blocks and ventricular strain sometimes occur. Ventricular tachycardia has been reported. The ECG is abnormal in as many as 75% of patients with pheochromocytoma. The classic symptom of pheochromocytoma is paroxysmal hypertension. The triad of tachycardia, diaphoresis, and headache in a hypertensive patient is highly suggestive of pheochromocytoma. Conversely, absence of this triad virtually rules out the presence of pheochromocytoma. Tremulousness, palpitations, and weight loss are common, especially in young to middle-aged patients. Symptoms may last from minutes to several hours and are often followed by fatigue. Decreased intravascular fluid volume associated with sustained hypertension may manifest as orthostatic hypotension. A hematocrit greater than 45% may reflect hypovolemia caused by this mechanism. Death resulting from pheochromocytoma is often the result of congestive heart failure, myocardial infarction, or intracerebral hemorrhage.

TREATMENT

Treatment consists of surgical excision of the catecholamine-secreting tumor only after medical control is optimized. α-Blockade (phentolamine, prazosin) should be instituted and blood pressure normalized before surgery. Return to normotension facilitates an increase in intravascular fluid volume as reflected by a decrease in the hematocrit. If cardiac arrhythmias or tachycardia persist after α-blockade, β-blockade is indicated in the absence of congestive heart failure (see the following table).

Drugs Used in the Management of Pheochromocytoma

Drug	Action	Blood Pressure Crisis Route	Dose	Preoperative Blood Pressure Control Route	Dose	Comments
Phentolamine	α-Blocker	IV	30–70 mcg/kg bolus			Rapid onset (2 min); short acting (10–15 min)
Phenoxybenzamine	α-Blocker			Oral	0.5–1 mg/kg/day	Long half-life; may accumulate
Prazosin	α₁-Blocker			Oral	1-mg single dose, increasing to tid regimen	First-dose phenomenon; may cause syncope
Propranolol	β-Blocker	IV	1-mg bolus to total of 10 mg	Oral	40 mg bid; increase to 480 mg/day	Introduce only after adequate α-blockade
Atenolol	β₁-Blocker			Oral	50–200 mg/day	Long acting; eliminated unchanged by kidney
Esmolol	β₁-Blocker	IV	100–300 mcg/kg/min			Ultrashort-acting; may be used during anesthesia
Labetalol	α₁- and β-Blocker	IV	0.1–0.5 mg/kg	Oral	200 mg tid	α-Blockade weaker than β-blockade; may increase blood pressure in patient with pheochromocytoma
Magnesium sulfate	Vasodilator	IV	40–60 mg/kg bolus followed by 2 g/hr			May potentiate neuromuscular blockade
Nicardipine	Calcium channel blocker	IV	2–6 mcg/kg/min			Most potent vasodilator of all calcium entry blockers
Nitroprusside	Vasodilator	IV	Infusion initially 0.5–2 mcg/kg/min			Short acting; may be used during anesthesia; risk of cyanide toxicity
α-Methyl-tyrosine	Inhibits catecholamine biosynthesis			Oral	1–4 g/day	Suitable for patients not amenable to surgery; may be nephrotoxic

bid, Twice daily; *IV*, intravenous; *tid*, three times daily.

ANESTHETIC CONSIDERATIONS

Preoperative Management

The pharmacologic effects of released catecholamines present major anesthetic challenges. Medical management, before tumor excision, aims to reverse the effects of excessive adrenergic stimulation. Preoperative anti-hypertensive therapy and volume replacement have helped to decrease the surgical mortality rate from 40% to 60% down to 1% to 3%. The preoperative use of α-adrenergic antagonists or calcium channel blockers and reexpansion of the intravascular fluid compartment greatly improve cardiovascular stability intraoperatively. Myocardial infarction, congestive heart failure, cardiac dysrhythmias, and cerebral hemorrhage decrease in frequency when the patient has been treated preoperatively with α-adrenergic antagonists.

The following criteria may be used as end points for the patient awaiting surgery for pheochromocytoma resection:

- No in-hospital blood pressure reading should be higher than 165/90 mm Hg, evident 48 hours before surgery.
- Blood pressure on standing should not be lower than 80/45 mm Hg.
- The ECG should have no ST-segment or T-wave abnormality before surgery that cannot be attributed to a permanent defect.
- The patient should have no marked symptoms of catecholamine excess and no more than one premature ventricular contraction every 5 minutes.

Anesthetic Management

Effective anesthetic management is based on selecting drugs that do not stimulate catecholamine release, avoiding sympathetic nervous system activation, and implementing monitoring techniques that facilitate early and appropriate intervention when catecholamine-induced changes in the cardiovascular function occur.

Most pheochromocytomas are excised by open laparotomy, but successful laparoscopic removal of pheochromocytoma has also been performed. It is generally recommended that laparoscopic removal be reserved for small, solitary, and hormonally latent tumors. During pneumoperitoneum, significant catecholamine release has been reported.

Certain drugs and conditions can precipitate hypertension in the surgical patient with pheochromocytoma. Dopamine antagonists (metoclopramide, droperidol), radiographic contrast media, indirect-acting amines (ephedrine), drugs that block neuronal catecholamine reuptake (tricyclic antidepressants, cocaine), histamine, glucagon, and pancuronium can trigger catecholamine release from the tumor. Hypoxia and hypercapnia can elicit a catecholamine response by stimulating the sympathetic nervous system.

Preoperative sedation is advised to decrease anxiety and to prevent activation of the sympathetic nervous system. Benzodiazepines are especially useful. Preoperative atropine should be avoided because of its potential for inducing tachydysrhythmias.

Large-bore intravenous lines and a peripheral arterial catheter should be established preoperatively. A central venous pressure or pulmonary artery catheter should be placed to help guide fluid management and intervention with inotropes or vasodilating drugs. Arterial blood gases, electrolyte concentrations, and blood glucose levels should be assessed regularly during the anesthetic regimen.

Critical intraoperative junctures are as follows: (1) during induction and intubation of the trachea, (2) during surgical manipulation of the tumor, and (3) after ligation of the tumor's venous drainage.

Induction can be accomplished with barbiturates, benzodiazepines, or propofol. Anesthetic depth can be enhanced by mask ventilation of the lungs with a volatile anesthetic and nitrous oxide before laryngoscopy and intubation of the trachea. Lidocaine (1 to 2 mg/kg, intravenously) administered 1 minute before intubation may attenuate the hemodynamic response to laryngoscopy. Rapid-acting vasodilating drugs such as nitroprusside and phentolamine should be readily available to treat persistent hypertension.[9] Short-acting opioids, such as fentanyl or sufentanil, administered before intubation may help attenuate blood pressure responses to intubation.[9] Morphine sulfate should be avoided because of its propensity for histamine release.

Selection of a volatile anesthetic should be based on its ability to decrease sympathetic nervous system activity and a low likelihood of sensitizing the myocardium to the dysrhythmic effects of catecholamines. Halothane is not recommended because of the potential for causing ventricular irritability in the presence of an increased catecholamine concentration. Sevoflurane and isoflurane provide cardiovascular stability and possess the ability to change anesthetic depth rapidly, attractive features in the anesthetic management of the patient with pheochromocytoma. The tachycardia associated with desflurane makes it an undesirable choice for these cases.

The use of succinylcholine has been questioned because compression of an abdominal tumor by drug-induced skeletal muscle fasciculations may provoke catecholamine release. However, a predictable adverse effect of succinylcholine has not been supported clinically when it is administered to patients with pheochromocytoma. Skeletal muscle paralysis with a non-depolarizing muscle relaxant devoid of vagolytic or histamine-releasing effects is desirable. Pancuronium should be avoided because of its known chronotropic effect.

Particular efforts should be made to keep the rate of fluid replacement equal to the rate of loss. Hypotension generally responds to volume replacement. Adequate preparation should be in place for the hypertension and cardiac dysrhythmias that occur, especially during tumor manipulation. Hypertension can be treated with intravenous nitroprusside or phentolamine and high concentrations of inhaled anesthetic. Propranolol, lidocaine, labetalol, or esmolol may be given intravenously to decrease tachydysrhythmias. β-Adrenergic antagonists must be used cautiously in patients with catecholamine-induced cardiomyopathy because even minimal β-adrenergic blockade can accentuate left ventricular dysfunction. The short half-life of esmolol makes it an advantageous choice for β-adrenergic blockade. Dysrhythmias associated with hypertension may be resolved by simply lowering an abnormally high blood pressure. Norepinephrine or phenylephrine administration is usually satisfactory when a vasopressor is needed. Indirect-acting sympathomimetics have an unpredictable pressor effect in these patients and should be avoided.

Magnesium sulfate appears to be a useful addition to the armamentarium available for anesthetic management of patients with pheochromocytoma. Rationale for its use is based on its ability to inhibit catecholamine release from both the adrenal medulla and peripheral adrenergic nerve terminals, to decrease the sensitivity of α-adrenergic receptors to catecholamines, and to exert a direct vasodilator effect.

After surgical ligation of the veins that drain a pheochromocytoma, the rapid decrease in circulating catecholamines and the associated down-regulation of adrenergic receptors may precipitate a decrease in blood pressure. During this juncture, close communication with the surgical team is important. Decreasing the inhaled anesthetic agent concentration and increasing the administration of intravenous crystalloid or colloid solution should adequately increase blood pressure. Intravenous administration of phenylephrine or norepinephrine may be needed until the peripheral vasculature can adapt to the decreased level of endogenous α-stimulation.

Hyperglycemia is common before excision of the pheochromocytoma. With tumor removal, the sudden withdrawal of catecholamine stimulation can result in hypoglycemia. Further, β-adrenergic blockade impairs both hepatic glucose production and the glucagon secretion mechanism. β-Adrenergic blockers may also mask hypoglycemic signs by preventing tachycardia and tremor. Blood glucose levels should be monitored at frequent intervals intraoperatively and postoperatively.

Regional anesthesia has been used successfully for the excision of pheochromocytomas. A specific disadvantage of this technique for this procedure is the blockade of sympathetic nervous system activity if hypotension accompanies vascular isolation of the pheochromocytoma. Additionally, spontaneous alveolar ventilation may be impaired during intraabdominal manipulation and retraction.

Some pheochromocytomas may first present as a hypermetabolic state during anesthesia for unrelated surgery. The hypertension, tachycardia, hyperthermia, and respiratory acidosis of a pheochromocytoma may mimic light anesthesia, thyroid crisis, malignant hyperthermia, or sepsis.

Postoperative Management

Fluid shifts, pain, hypoxia, hypercapnia, autonomic instability, urinary retention, and residual tumor are all potential causes of postoperative hypertension. Invasive monitoring is indicated during the initial postoperative period to assess blood pressure changes and cardiac status keenly. Fifty percent of patients remain hypertensive during the postanesthesia recovery period despite removal of the pheochromocytoma. Transient hypertension postoperatively usually reflects fluid shifts and autonomic instability. Postoperative catecholamine levels decrease to normal over several days. Normal blood pressure returns within about 10 days after surgery in 75% of patients.

Relief of postoperative pain can be accomplished with neuraxial opioids and may contribute to early tracheal extubation in otherwise healthy patients.

GASTROINTESTINAL SYSTEM

A. Carcinoid Tumors/Syndrome

DEFINITION

Carcinoid tumors are slow-growing malignancies composed of enterochromaffin cells usually found in the gastrointestinal tract. About 75% are gastrointestinal and 22% are in the lung. They have also occurred in the pancreas, thymus, and liver. A high incidence of carcinoid tumor is found in the appendiceal region. Carcinoid tumors have also been noted to occur in the bronchi and rarely from an ovarian site. Carcinoid tumors release vasoactive substances such as serotonin, bradykinin, histamine, tachykinins, kallikrein, adrenocorticotropic hormone, prostaglandins, vasoactive peptide, and others. These substances are capable of producing profound deleterious effects on cardiovascular homeostasis, although under normal circumstances the effects of the release of these substances are usually insignificant because of their hepatic metabolism.

INCIDENCE AND PREVALENCE

Approximately 5% to 10% of patients with carcinoid tumors develop carcinoid syndrome.

ETIOLOGY

Carcinoid syndrome is produced by metastatic tumors that secrete excessive amounts of vasoactive substances, such as histamine, bradykinin, serotonin, and various prostaglandins. Vasoactive peptides released from carcinoid tumors located in the bronchi and ovaries exert a faster effect because of their direct drainage into the portal vein. Carcinoid tumors are also functionally autonomous. Two factors that enhance release of carcinoid hormones are direct physical manipulation of the tumor and β-adrenergic stimulation.

LABORATORY RESULTS

Levels of those vasoactive substances mentioned earlier are increased.

CLINICAL MANIFESTATIONS
Signs and Symptoms of Carcinoid Syndrome

- Episodic cutaneous flushing (kinins, histamine)
- Diarrhea (serotonin, prostaglandins E and F)
- Heart disease

Tricuspid regurgitation and/or pulmonic stenosis
Supraventricular tachydysrhythmias (serotonin)
- Bronchoconstriction (serotonin, bradykinin, substance P)
- Hypotension (kinins, histamine)
- Hypertension (serotonin)
- Abdominal pain (small bowel obstruction)
- Hepatomegaly (metastases)
- Hyperglycemia
- Hypoalbuminemia (pellagra-like skin lesions due to niacin deficiency)

TREATMENT

Patients with carcinoid syndrome may undergo primary resection of the carcinoid tumor. Examples of other procedures that these patients often undergo include cardiac valve replacement and hepatic resection (e.g., lobectomy) for excision of metastases. Treatment consists of fluid resuscitation, histamine-1 and histamine-2 (H_1 and H_2) antagonists, steroids, and ketanserin (a serotonin antagonist). Bronchodilation is used. Histamine release is treated with bronchodilation and epinephrine.

Octreotide, a somatostatin analogue, is used to blunt the vasoactive and bronchoconstrictive effects of carcinoid tumor products. Octreotide mimics the inhibitory action of somatostatin on the release of several gastrointestinal hormones, as well as those derived from carcinoid tumors. Treatment for 2 weeks preoperatively with a dose of 100 mcg subcutaneously three times a day is standard. If prior therapy was not used, a dose of 50 to 150 mcg subcutaneously is given preoperatively. Intraoperative infusion may be continued at 100 mcg/hour. Intravenous bolus doses of 100 to 200 mcg may be used for intraoperative carcinoid crises.

Aprotinin, an inhibitor of kallikrein, has been reported to be effective in reversal of carcinoid-induced bronchospasm and hypotension. Used in conjunction with octreotide and methylprednisolone, aprotinin (2,000,000-kilounit bolus; 50,000 kilounit/hour infusion) has been reported to be effective prophylaxis for hypotension in a patient with carcinoid syndrome who is undergoing cardiac surgery.

ANESTHETIC CONSIDERATIONS

Many anesthetic techniques have been used successfully in the treatment of patients with carcinoid syndrome. Preoperative preparation of the patient requires correction of deficiencies in circulating volume and electrolyte levels. Use of histamine-releasing agents, such as morphine, thiopental, atracurium, and mivacurium, should be avoided. Fasciculations may induce release of carcinoid hormones and are thus prevented by avoidance of succinylcholine, although this drug has been used successfully many times, especially for rapid sequence induction.

Etomidate may be used for induction, while avoiding thiopental because of associated histamine release. Propofol, both in bolus doses and infusion, has also been frequently used. Because it may produce hypotension, judicious use is advised. Vecuronium and *cis*-atracurium may be safely used for neuromuscular blockade. Rocuronium is an attractive alternative when rapid onset is desired.

Vecuronium, *cis*-atracurium, and rocuronium are virtually devoid of activity invoking histamine release or hemodynamic changes. The piperidine-derivative opioids fentanyl, sufentanil, alfentanil, and remifentanil are suitable for use because of their lack of histamine-releasing properties and their innocuous effect on hemodynamics.

Isoflurane, desflurane, and sevoflurane may all be safely used. No one anticholinesterase neuromuscular relaxant reversal agent is thought to be advantageous over any other. However, glycopyrrolate, used as an adjunct to attenuate vagolysis, may be more desirable than atropine, to avoid a significantly increased heart rate.

Ketamine activates the sympathetic nervous system, and catecholamine release may activate the kallikreins and other vasoactive substances and thus should be avoided. The desire to avoid the use of sympathomimetics such as ephedrine to treat hypotension makes the use of regional anesthesia controversial. Epidural anesthesia, cautiously administered, may be a reasonable technique for lower extremity and abdominal procedures. Severe and possibly refractory hypotension resulting from sympathectomy makes spinal anesthesia relatively contraindicated for use in carcinoid syndrome.

Hypotension should be treated with an α-adrenergic agonist (e.g., phenylephrine infusion) to avoid hormone release by β-adrenergic stimulation. Bronchospasm resulting from histamine or bradykinin release has been shown to be resistant to ketamine and inhalation anesthetics. Low-dose β_2-agonists are effective in bronchodilation and have relatively little influence on carcinoid hormone release. In the presence of high levels of serotonin in carcinoid syndrome, adjustments in anesthetic selection and dosage must be considered if further compromise of cardiovascular function is to be prevented. Anesthetic management is reviewed in the following list.

- Most common clinical signs are flushing, wheezing, blood pressure and heart rate changes, and diarrhea.
- Preoperative assessment should include complete blood count, electrolytes, liver function tests blood glucose, electrocardiogram (echocardiogram if indicated), and urine 5-hydroxyindoleacetic acid levels.
- Optimize fluid and electrolyte status and pretreat with octreotide as noted. Continue octreotide throughout the postoperative period. Interferon-α has shown success in controlling some symptoms.
- Both H_1- and H_2-receptor blockers must be used to counteract histamine effects fully.
- Ovoid histamine releasing agents such as morphine, thiopental, atracurium and mivacurium. Avoid sympathomimetic agents such as ketamine and ephedrine.
- Treat hypotension with an α receptor agonist such as phenylephrine.
- General anesthesia is preferred over regional. Patients with high serotonin levels may exhibit prolonged recovery; therefore, desflurane and sevoflurane, with rapid recovery profiles, may be beneficial.
- Aggressively maintain normothermia to avoid catecholamine-induced vasoactive mediator release.
- Monitor intraoperative plasma glucose because these patients are prone to hyperglycemia. Treat with insulin as is customary.

B. Diaphragmatic Hernia

DEFINITION
Diaphragmatic hernia is an incomplete embryologic closure of the diaphragm with herniation of abdominal contents into the thorax. Normal lung maturation is impaired because abdominal contents compress developing lung tissue. Lungs develop with varying degrees of pulmonary hypoplasia.

INCIDENCE AND PREVALENCE
Diaphragmatic hernia occurs in 1 of 4000 live births. The mortality rate is approximately 50%.

ETIOLOGY
Diaphragmatic hernia is caused by incomplete embryologic closure of the diaphragm.

LABORATORY RESULTS
Antenatal diagnosis shows that polyhydramnios is present 30% of the time. Abdominal ultrasonography is used to detect these hernias.

CLINICAL MANIFESTATIONS
Clinical manifestations depend on the degree of the hernia and interference with ventilation. They include scaphoid abdomen, reduced or absent breath sounds on the affected side, a barrel-shaped chest, arterial hypoxia, abdominal contents in the thorax (as shown on chest and/or abdominal x-ray study), increased pulmonary vascular resistance, and congenital heart disease.

TREATMENT
Treatment consists of prompt decompression of the stomach and oxygenation with endotracheal intubation.

ANESTHETIC CONSIDERATIONS
The airway should be secured and anesthesia administered after awake endotracheal intubation. Invasive monitoring of blood pressure should be considered. In some patients, delaying surgery for 24 to 48 hours may be possible to allow some degree of stabilization in their condition. Anesthetic induction may then be used by raising the head of the bed and using a rapid sequence approach.

C. Gallstone/Gallbladder Disease

GALLSTONES

DEFINITION
Gallstones are cholesterol-containing stones that form in the gallbladder or bile ducts. They usually form when the bile contains more cholesterol than can be held in solution.

The gallbladder, which has a capacity of approximately 40 to 50 mL, concentrates bile and delivers it to the duodenum. Surgically removing the gallbladder has little effect on the body's ability to digest fat.

INCIDENCE AND PREVALENCE

The prevalence of gallstones is high in the United States. In women, gallstones tend to form at 20 to 30 years of age; in men, they form at 30 to 60 years.

ETIOLOGY

The two most common types of gallstones are cholesterol and mixed (containing bile pigment, calcium bilirubinate, or calcium and copper). Cholesterol stones are more likely in women.

LABORATORY RESULTS

Ultrasonography and cholangiography are used to identify stones and obstruction.

CLINICAL MANIFESTATIONS

The formation of gallstones begins with excessive cholesterol secreted into the bile. Cholesterol eventually precipitates into stones. The stones can block the cystic duct, resulting in inflammation cholelithiasis with or without jaundice.

GALLBLADDER DISEASE: CHOLANGITIS

DEFINITION

Cholangitis is an inflammation of the biliary duct that presents as Charcot's triad: epigastric, upper abdominal pain; jaundice; and fever and chills.

ETIOLOGY

Cholangitis is caused by obstruction or bacterial growth in the biliary tract.

LABORATORY RESULTS

The white blood cell count is $\geq 10,000/mm^3$, and the bilirubin concentration is 2 mg/dL. Hepatic alkaline phosphatase and blood urea nitrogen are elevated. Prerenal azotemia is the result of dehydration. Ultrasonography, computed tomography, and x-ray studies are used for diagnosis.

TREATMENT

- Cholecystectomy, common duct exploration with open or closed surgical approach
- Mechanical removal with forceps or baskets
- Disintegration (dissolving of stones with chemicals)
- Endoscopia removal

ANESTHETIC CONSIDERATIONS

The patient may require preoperative pain relief if emergency surgical intervention is required. If the patient is vomiting, fluids and electrolytes should be evaluated and imbalances corrected.

D. Hiatal Hernia/Gastric Reflux

DEFINITION
Hiatal Hernia
Hiatal hernia is bulging of the stomach and other abdominal viscera through an enlarged esophageal hiatus in the diaphragm. A hiatal hernia consists of a defect in the diaphragm that allows a portion of the stomach to migrate upward into the thoracic cavity. Two types of esophageal hiatal hernias are the sliding type (type I), which is formed by the movement of the upper stomach through an enlarged hiatus, and the paraesophageal type (type II), in which the esophagogastric junction remains in normal position but all or part of the stomach moves into the thorax and assumes a para-esophageal position. A third type of hiatal hernia (type III) has been identified that combines the features of a sliding and a paraesophageal hernia. A fourth type of hiatal hernia (type IV) occurs when other organs, such as the colon or small bowel, are contained in the hernia sac that is formed by a large paraesophageal hernia.

Gastric Reflux
Gastric reflux relates to a reduced lower esophageal sphincter tone, which can increase the risk for regurgitation and aspiration. Reflux can occur without the presence of hiatal hernia. The lower sphincter is a physiologic sphincter with no specialized musculature. Tone is 15 to 35 mm Hg.

INCIDENCE AND PREVALENCE
Types I to IV hiatal hernias are present in 10% of the population, usually without symptoms. Only 5% of the population has reflux symptoms along with a hiatal hernia.

ETIOLOGY
In most cases, the cause is unknown, whether the condition is congenital, traumatic, or iatrogenic.

LABORATORY TESTS
Chest or abdominal x-ray studies and "barium swallow" can be used.

CLINICAL MANIFESTATIONS
Hiatal hernia and peptic esophagitis often exist concurrently, although one does not cause the other. The major symptom is retrosternal pain of a burning quality that commonly occurs after meals. It is assumed that patients with a hiatal hernia are predisposed to developing peptic esophagitis, thus providing a rationale for surgical correction of this condition. Most patients with hiatal hernia do not have symptoms of reflux esophagitis, however, and do not require histamine-2 (H_2)-antagonist and oral antacid therapy. Other symptoms typically involve heartburn, regurgitation, esophageal stricture, bleeding with a large hernia, sensation of food "sticking," fullness or bloating after eating, and sharp pain.

TREATMENT
The primary goal in the surgical correction of hiatal hernia consists of reestablishment of gastroesophageal competence. This usually entails repair

of the sliding hernia, reduction by 2 cm or more of the tubular distal esophagus below the diaphragm, and valvuloplasty. An abdominal, a thoracic, or a thoracoabdominal surgical approach may be selected. Common procedures for correction of hiatal hernia include the Nissen, Belsey, and Hill operations. Laparoscopic fundoplication techniques are also more commonly being used. A gastroplasty may be performed (the Collis procedure) in association with repair of the hiatal hernia when indicated, usually in patients with a shortened esophagus. If a thoracic approach is selected, the patient must be assessed for ability to tolerate one-lung anesthesia because this method may be used to enable surgical exposure.

ANESTHETIC CONSIDERATIONS

Symptomatic patients require pretreatment with a nonparticulate antacid and an H_2 blocker. For induction of anesthesia, elevation of the head of the bed or stretcher and rapid sequence induction to prevent aspiration should be considered. If the hernia is large, one-lung anesthesia may be used to improve surgical access during repair. Communication with the surgical team is imperative when the thoracoabdominal approach is being considered.

E. Inflammatory Bowel Disease

DEFINITION

Inflammatory bowel diseases include ulcerative colitis and Crohn's disease. Ulcerative colitis is an inflammatory disease of the colonic mucosa that primarily affects the rectum and distal colon. Crohn's disease is characterized by ileal and colonic involvement.

INCIDENCE AND PREVALENCE

Ulcerative colitis is most common in women between the ages of 25 and 45 years and in people of Jewish origin. Ulcerative colitis carries an increased risk of colon cancer. Crohn's disease most commonly occurs at about 30 years of age.

ETIOLOGY

The cause is unknown.

LABORATORY RESULTS

Electrolyte disturbances may be evident, especially during exacerbations. Complete blood count may reflect anemia resulting from chronic hemorrhage, iron deficiency, or vitamin B_{12} or folate deficiency. Hypoalbuminemia may result from protein loss from the diseased bowel mucosa.

CLINICAL MANIFESTATIONS

Inflammatory bowel disease is characterized by intermittent diarrhea and cramping abdominal pain.

Fatigue, low-grade fever, and weight loss may occur during exacerbations of ulcerative colitis. Toxic megacolon or intestinal perforation may occur with severe ulcerative colitis. Extracolonic manifestations of ulcerative colitis include erythema nodosum, iritis, ankylosing arthritis, fatty liver infiltration, pericholangitis, and cirrhosis of the liver.

Crohn's disease is often complicated by fistulas between the diseased intestinal loops and adjacent structures. Rectal fissures, rectocutaneous fistulas, and perirectal abscesses are common. Extracolonic manifestations include arthritis, iritis, renal stones, and gallstones.

TREATMENT

Inflammatory bowel diseases are treated with antidiarrheal drugs, sulfasalazine, and corticosteroids. Proctocolectomy with ileostomy is curative for ulcerative colitis, whereas surgery is rarely curative for Crohn's disease. Hyperalimentation may be indicated when exacerbations lead to weight loss and malnutrition.

ANESTHETIC CONSIDERATIONS

Preoperatively, the patient's volume status should be assessed, in addition to seeking evidence of extracolonic complications such as anemia, arthritis, and liver dysfunction. Supplementation with corticosteroids is indicated if the patient is being treated with steroids.

F. Pancreatitis

DEFINITION

Pancreatitis is differentiated into edematous and necrotizing types. Plasma amylase concentrations are increased in a patient experiencing intense midepigastric pain. Chronic pancreatitis is present in patients with alcoholism and in patients with diabetes mellitus or fatty liver infiltration.

INCIDENCE AND PREVALENCE

The incidence of pancreatitis varies in different countries, depending on the incidence of causative factors such as alcoholism, gallstones, and drug use. In the United States, acute pancreatitis is more commonly associated with alcohol abuse than with gallstones. It occurs in about 0.5% of the general population.

ETIOLOGY

The cause of *pancreatitis* is multifactorial. Common causes include alcohol abuse, direct or indirect trauma to the pancreas, ulcerative penetration from adjacent structures (e.g., the duodenum), infectious processes, biliary tract disease, metabolic disorders (e.g., hyperlipidemia and hypercalcemia), and certain drugs (e.g., corticosteroids, furosemide, estrogens, and thiazide diuretics). The patient who has undergone extensive surgery involving mobilization of the abdominal viscera is at risk for developing postoperative pancreatitis, as are patients who have undergone procedures involving cardiopulmonary bypass. Patients who have received large doses of calcium intraoperatively, particularly after cardiopulmonary bypass, have also been shown to be at risk for developing postoperative pancreatitis.

Enzymes implicated as major culprits in the syndrome of pancreatitis are those activated by trypsin, enterokinase, and bile acids. These enzymes are necessary for proteolysis, elastolysis, and lipolysis. The inappropriate elaboration of these enzymes results in pancreatic inflammation, which is caused by vascular breakdown, coagulation necrosis, fat necrosis, and parenchymal necrosis.

LABORATORY RESULTS

Computed tomography and ultrasonography are used. Complete blood count reveals leukocytosis (10,000 to 20,000/mm³). Serum amylase is normal. Serum lipase, urinary amylase, and urinary lipase are elevated. Pleural and peritoneal fluid should be analyzed. Blood glucose levels are elevated. Calcium levels lower than 7.5 mg/dL are associated with necrosis. Liver function enzymes are elevated. Coagulation studies, electrocardiogram, chest x-ray study, and levels of methemalbumin should be assessed.

CLINICAL MANIFESTATIONS

Clinical manifestations are based on etiologic factors that include an enlarged pancreas, pain, nausea, vomiting, diarrhea, bleeding, agitation, and fever.

Stages

- *Initiating process:* Bile reflux, duodenal reflux, lymphatic spread of inflammation
- *Initial pancreatic injury:* Edema, vascular drainage, rupture of pancreatic ducts, acinar damage
- *Activation of digestive enzymes:* Trypsin, lipase
- *Autodigestion*
- *Pancreatic necrosis:* Associated with abscesses, septicemia, pulmonary failure, acute renal failure, hyperglycemia

Cardiovascular complications of acute pancreatitis can lead to pericardial effusions, alterations in cardiac rhythmicity, signs and symptoms mimicking acute myocardial infarction, thrombophlebitis, and cardiac depression. Acute pancreatitis also predisposes the patient to the development of acute respiratory distress syndrome and disseminated intravascular coagulopathy.

TREATMENT

Treatment is supportive: pain should be relieved; shock should be overcome; metabolic, fluid, and electrolyte balances should be restored; and pancreatic secretion should be suppressed (give nothing by mouth, gastrointestinal suction, antacids, histamine-2 (H_2) blockers, calcitonin, and somatostatin). Secondary infection should be prevented. Optimal respiratory care should be instituted. Renal function should be preserved, and renin release should be neutralized.

ANESTHETIC CONSIDERATIONS

Laboratory results should be reviewed, and the patient should be evaluated for shock, hemorrhage, and pain relief (meperidine is the drug of choice). Fluid and electrolyte status is of concern because the patient should receive nothing by mouth. The patient will have a nasogastric tube, and H_2 blockers will be given. In addition, the patient should undergo typing and crossmatching for possible transfusion. Plasma expanders, crystalloids, and invasive monitoring may be used.

G. Splenic Disorders

DEFINITION

A palpable spleen is the major physical sign produced by diseases affecting the spleen and suggests enlargement of the organ. The normal spleen is said to weigh less than 250 g, decreases in size with age, normally lies entirely within the rib cage, has a maximum cephalocaudad diameter of 13 cm by ultrasonography or maximum length of 12 cm and/or width of 7 cm by radionuclide scan, and is usually not palpable.

INCIDENCE AND PREVALENCE

A palpable spleen was found in 3% of 2200 asymptomatic, male, freshman college students. Follow-up at 3 years revealed that 30% of those students still had a palpable spleen without any increase in disease prevalence. Ten-year follow-up found no evidence for lymphoid malignancies. Furthermore, in some tropical countries (e.g., New Guinea) the incidence of splenomegaly may reach 60%. Thus, the presence of a palpable spleen does not always equate with presence of disease.

ETIOLOGY

Hyperplasia or hypertrophy is related to a particular splenic function such as reticuloendothelial hyperplasia (work hypertrophy) in diseases such as hereditary spherocytosis or thalassemia syndromes that require removal of large numbers of defective red blood cells and to immune hyperplasia in response to systemic infection (infectious mononucleosis, subacute bacterial endocarditis) or to immunologic diseases (immune thrombocytopenia, systemic lupus erythematosus, Felty's syndrome). Passive congestion results from decreased blood flow from the spleen in conditions that produce portal hypertension (cirrhosis, Budd-Chiari syndrome, congestive heart failure). Infiltrative diseases of the spleen include lymphomas, metastatic cancer, amyloidosis, Gaucher's disease, and myeloproliferative disorders with extramedullary hematopoiesis.

The differential diagnostic possibilities are fewer when the spleen is "massively enlarged," that is, it is palpable more than 8 cm below the left costal margin or its drained weight is 1000 g or more. Most such patients have non-Hodgkin's lymphoma, chronic lymphocytic leukemia, hairy cell leukemia, chronic myelogenous leukemia, myelofibrosis with myeloid metaplasia, or polycythemia vera.

LABORATORY RESULTS

The major laboratory abnormalities accompanying splenomegaly are determined by the underlying systemic illness. A complete blood count is the diagnostic examination needed with any patient presenting with splenic disorders. It is vital for a differential diagnosis. A complete blood count also identifies platelet or white blood cell dysfunction.

CLINICAL MANIFESTATIONS

The most common symptoms produced by diseases involving the spleen are pain and a heavy sensation in the left upper quadrant. Massive splenomegaly may cause early satiety. Pain may result from acute swelling of the spleen with stretching of the capsule, infarction, or inflammation of the capsule. Symptoms of hypersplenism include fatigue, malaise, recurrent infection, and easy or prolonged bleeding. These symptoms occur from a hyperfunctional spleen that removes and destroys normal blood cells. In portal hypertension, transmitted backpressure results in hypersplenism, which leads to congestive failure of splenic function.

Vascular occlusion, with infarction and pain, is commonly seen in children with sickle cell crises. Rupture of the spleen, either from trauma or infiltrative disease that breaks the capsule, may result in intraperitoneal bleeding, shock, and death. The rupture itself may be painless.

TREATMENT

Correction or amelioration of certain hematologic and immunologic disorders may be attempted through splenectomy. Commonly accepted medical disease processes for which splenectomy is considered include idiopathic thrombocytopenic purpura, thrombotic thrombocytopenic purpura, Hodgkin's disease, lymphoma, certain leukemias, hereditary spherocytosis, hereditary hemolytic anemia, idiopathic autoimmune hemolytic anemia, and hypersplenism. Splenectomy may also be performed in treatment of thalassemia and sickle cell disease when these diseases are refractory to medical management and when hypersplenism supervenes. The development of primary (with no identifiable underlying cause) or secondary (from a known cause) hypersplenism may warrant splenectomy. Treatment of the primary disease process usually provides relief of symptoms. Splenectomy, however, is often a necessary part of therapy; particularly in long-standing disorders.

HEMATOLOGIC SYSTEM

A. AIDS/HIV Infection

DEFINITION

Acquired immunodeficiency syndrome (AIDS) is not a single disease but rather the appearance of various opportunistic infections resulting from generalized depression of the immune system. Immunodeficiency is caused by infection of helper T lymphocytes with a retrovirus known as human immunodeficiency virus (HIV). This virus destroys T lymphocytes and leaves the host susceptible to the development of infection and neoplastic diseases.

INCIDENCE

In the United States, AIDS statistics are as follows. More than 90% of adult patients with AIDS are men; 70% are homosexual or bisexual men. Heterosexual intravenous drug users account for 15% of men with AIDS and 50% of affected women. Persons with hemophilia coagulation disorders account for 1% of all AIDS cases, and recipients of infected blood transfusions account for 2% of all cases.

ETIOLOGY

The virus is transmitted by sexual contact, inoculation by other body secretions, and transfusion of blood or blood products (especially factor VIII concentrates). Because HIV selectively infects lymphocytes, concentrations of the virus are probably highest in secretions containing lymphocytes, such as semen, vaginal secretions, and blood. There is no evidence of airborne transmission of HIV.

CLINICAL MANIFESTATIONS

Patients develop severe immunosuppression caused by the destruction of T lymphocytes, resulting in susceptibility to opportunistic infections. The most frequently encountered opportunistic, life-threatening infection is pneumonia resulting from the parasite *Pneumocystis carinii*. The most common malignant condition in patients with AIDS is Kaposi's sarcoma. Of all patients with AIDS/HIV infection, 50% develop some element of central nervous system dysfunction. Weight loss, fatigue, idiopathic thrombocytopenia, chronic diarrhea, and anemia are nonspecific findings. Milder manifestations of AIDS include a transient mononucleosis-like syndrome and persistent generalized lymphadenopathy.

LABORATORY RESULTS AND DIAGNOSTIC FINDINGS

Laboratory findings include lymphopenia and reduction in the ratio of helper T lymphocytes to suppressor T lymphocytes. Detection of HIV antibodies using an enzyme-linked immunoassay indicates that the patient has been infected with the virus. To increase reliability, a positive enzyme-linked immunoassay result is confirmed by a Western blot test. Persons infected with HIV usually develop antibody (seroconvert) against the virus within 6 to 12 weeks of being infected. A positive antibody test result does not mean that the person has AIDS or will develop the syndrome.

TREATMENT
Oral administration of zidovudine (formerly azidothymidine, or AZT) inhibits replication of some retroviruses, including HIV, and therefore may be useful in reducing the risk of developing opportunistic infections associated with AIDS. The drug is primarily eliminated by the kidneys following breakdown by the liver. Drugs such as probenecid, acetaminophen, aspirin, and indomethacin may competitively inhibit zidovudine's breakdown in the liver. Anemia and granulocytopenia are adverse effects of zidovudine therapy.

ANESTHETIC MANAGEMENT
Anesthetic management must assume that all patients are potentially infected with HIV or other bloodborne pathogens. Universal precautions must be followed. Disposable laryngoscope blades should be used if available and bacterial filters should be placed in the anesthesia circuit. The choice of anesthetic drugs and techniques depends on accompanying systemic manifestations of AIDS and related opportunistic infections. For example, oxygenation may be impaired in patients with *P. carinii* infection. Frequently, patients are malnourished and dehydrated. Anemia from chronic infection may require transfusion.

PROGNOSIS
The incubation period for AIDS may be 7 years or longer. The mortality rate approaches 70% within 2 years after diagnosis.

B. Anemia

DEFINITION
Anemia is a deficiency of erythrocytes caused by either too rapid a loss or too slow production of the cells. Therefore, numeric concentrations of hemoglobin are reduced, and the oxygen-carrying capacity of blood is decreased. This results in reduced oxygen delivery to peripheral tissues.

ETIOLOGY
Anemia may result from acute blood loss; however, iron-deficiency anemia from persistent blood loss is the most frequent form of chronic anemia. Anemia is also associated with many chronic diseases, such as persistent infections, neoplastic processes, connective tissue disorders, and renal and hepatic disease. Other forms of anemia include aplastic anemia, which involves bone marrow depression, and megaloblastic anemias, which are related to deficiencies of vitamin B_{12} or folic acid. Finally, various anemias can result from intravascular hemolysis of erythrocytes.

LABORATORY RESULTS
Erythrocyte production can be assessed from the reticulocyte count in peripheral blood. For instance, a low reticulocyte count in the presence of a

low hematocrit suggests an erythrocyte production defect, rather than blood loss or hemolysis as a cause of anemia. A decrease in hematocrit that exceeds 1% per day is most likely related to acute blood loss or intravascular hemolysis.

CLINICAL MANIFESTATIONS

A history of reduced exercise tolerance characterized as exertional dyspnea is a frequent clinical sign of chronic anemia. A functional heart murmur and evidence of cardiomegaly may be detected on physical examination. The decreased oxygen-carrying capacity of arterial blood is reflected in the arterial oxygen content equation (i.e., arterial oxygen content = [hemoglobin × 1.39] × oxygen saturation + [arterial oxygen tension × 0.003]).[2] This decrease is compensated for by a rightward shift oxyhemoglobin dissociation curve and an increase in the cardiac output. Decreased blood viscosity and vasodilation lower systemic vascular resistance and increase blood flow. Blood pressure and heart rate remain unchanged with increased cardiac output.[3] The decreased exercise tolerance reflects the inability of cardiac output to increase to maintain tissue oxygenation when these patients become physically active.

TREATMENT

Packed erythrocytes can be transfused preoperatively to increase hemoglobin concentrations (*but it should be remembered that about*) with peak effect at 24 hours (*are necessary*) to restore intravascular fluid volume and blood viscosity. Compared with a similar volume of whole blood, erythrocytes produce about twice the increase in hemoglobin concentration. Packed red blood cells have a hematocrit of 70%, and cell saver has a hematocrit of 45% to 65%.

ANESTHETIC CONSIDERATIONS

Transfusion guidelines include assessment of the patient's cardiovascular status, age, anticipation of further blood loss, arterial oxygenation, mixed venous oxygen tension, cardiac output, and infection risk. (*Minimum acceptable hemoglobin concentrations for elective surgery have changed over the years. The "old" value of 10 g/dL has been lowered to approximately 8 g/dL, depending on the patient, operation, institution, etc.*) If elective surgery is performed, the anesthetic regimen should be geared toward preventing changes that may interfere with tissue oxygen delivery. Adequate oxygenation can be obtained with a hemoglobin of 8 g/dL as long as the patient is normovolmic.[1] For example, myocardial depression produced by the volatile agents may reduce cardiac output and thus impair the patient's compensatory mechanisms. Likewise, leftward shifts of the oxyhemoglobin dissociation curve (as produced by hyperventilation resulting in respiratory alkalosis) can impair release of oxygen from hemoglobin to the tissues. It is also important to maintain body temperature, because hypothermia will cause a leftward shift of the curve. Intraoperative blood loss should be promptly replaced and closely monitored. Finally, it is important to minimize shivering or increases in body temperature postoperatively, because these changes can greatly increase total body oxygen requirements.

Rule of Thumb Transfusion Guidelines

Blood loss >20%
Hemoglobin <8 g/dL

Hemoglobin <10 g/dL with major disease and/or with autologous blood
Hemoglobin <12 g/dL when ventilator dependent[4]

C. Coagulopathies

HEMOPHILIA A

DEFINITION

Hemophilia A is a disorder of blood coagulation resulting from inadequate
activity of factor VIII. It is classified as severe (no factor), moderate (1% to
4% of factor), and mild (5% to 25% of the factor). Mild disease may be
recognized only after trauma or surgery.

INCIDENCE AND PREVALENCE

It is estimated that hemophilia A is present in 1 of 10,000 males because the
gene for factor VIII is carried on the X chromosome.

ETIOLOGY

Plasma concentrations of factor VIII and the severity of bleeding are
directly related. For example, spontaneous hemorrhage is likely when factor
VIII concentrations are less than 3% of normal values.

LABORATORY RESULTS

Classically, patients present with a prolonged partial thromboplastin time
(PTT) but a normal prothrombin time and bleeding time. These patients
have an instrinsic pathway deficiency.

CLINICAL MANIFESTATIONS

Deep tissue bleeding, hemarthrosis, and hematuria are common forms
of clinical bleeding associated with hemophilia A. The condition is often
associated with hemarthrosis and is first noticed when a child begins to
walk. Hemorrhage into closed spaces compresses nerves, vessels, and the
airway. Central venous system bleeding is a major cause of death in these
patients.

TREATMENT

Factor VIII levels should be increased to more than 50% before anesthesia
and operation. Treatment consists of transfusion of fresh-frozen plasma or
recombinant factor VIII. Recombinant factor VIII is stabilized in albumin
that is pooled from several donors, and methods to reduce viral infection
have made it relatively safe. Fresh-frozen plasma is considered to have 1 unit
of factor VIII activity per milliliter. Cryoprecipitate has 5 to 10 units of
activity per milliliter, whereas recombinant factor VIII concentrates 40 units
of activity per milliliter. Transfusions are given twice a day following surgery
because of the short half-life of factor VIII (8 to 12 hours).

ANESTHETIC CONSIDERATIONS

All intramuscular injections should be avoided. Regional anesthesia should
be avoided because of the risk of bleeding. Tracheal intubation should be
handled with care to avoid tongue bleeding and airway obstruction. The
possibility of coexisting liver disease from hepatitis that may have occurred

after blood or factor VIII transfusions should be considered. Universal precautions must always be followed. Prolonged and potentially fatal hemorrhage may occur both during and after surgery.

HEMOPHILIA B

DEFINITION

Hemophilia B, also known as Christmas disease, is a disorder of blood coagulation resulting from the absence or decreased activity of factor IX.

INCIDENCE AND PREVALENCE

Hemophilia B is similar to hemophilia A, but it is much less common (1 in 100,000 males).

LABORATORY RESULTS

The PTT is prolonged in these patients, who have an intrinsic pathway deficiency. Measurement of factor IX levels establishes the diagnosis. Factor IX activity should be maintained at more than 30% of normal.

CLINICAL MANIFESTATIONS

See the earlier discussion of hemophilia A.

TREATMENT

Fresh-frozen plasma is no longer considered adequate therapy for patients with hemophilia B. Specific procoagulant concentrates to raise plasma concentrations of factor IX are chosen.

VON WILLEBRAND'S DISEASE

DEFINITION AND ETIOLOGY

Von Willebrand's disease is a hematologic disease that is transmitted as an autosomal dominant characteristic affecting both sexes. It is most likely the result of the deficiency of a protein (von Willebrand's factor) important for adequate activity of factor VIII and optimal function of platelets.

LABORATORY RESULTS

The classic expression is prolonged bleeding time, impaired aggregation of platelets, and decreased plasma concentrations of factor VIII.

CLINICAL MANIFESTATIONS

Epistaxis, bleeding from mucosal surfaces, and superficial bruising are common. Pregnancy produces an increase in factor VIII and von Willebrand's factor in parturients with mild to moderate forms of this disorder. A differential diagnosis between von Willenbrand's disease and hemophilia A can be made by response from the transfusion of fresh-frozen plasma or cryoprecipitate. In hemophilia A, factor VIII reaches the maximum after transfusion, whereas in von Willenbrand's disease, factor VIII continues to elevate over the next 24 hours.

TREATMENT

Desmopressin, a synthetic analogue of antidiuretic hormone, is the treatment of choice. The dose is 0.3 mcg/kg over 15 to 30 minutes, and it will increase factor VIII and von Willebrand's factor by two to five times. Cryoprecipitate (40 units/kg) provides von Willebrand's factor as well as factor VIII.

ANESTHETIC CONSIDERATIONS

Drugs that interfere with optimal aggregation of platelets should be avoided. The patient should also be properly positioned to avoid bruising. Adverse reactions to desmopressin therapy may occur, such as seizures from hyponatremia, hypotension, and anaphylaxis.

DISSEMINATED INTRAVASCULAR COAGULATION

DEFINITION

Disseminated intravascular coagulation (DIC) is characterized by uncontrolled activation of the coagulation system, with consumption of platelets and procoagulants. Thrombi develop in the microcirculation, and bleeding results because of loss of coagulation factors into these thrombi.

ETIOLOGY

Normal mechanisms of controlling intravascular coagulation may be overwhelmed by extensive tissue damage in cases such as sepsis, burns, retained placenta after delivery, trauma to the central nervous system, and prolonged extracorporeal circulation. Large amounts of thromboplastic material are released into the circulation, with subsequent activation of the extrinsic coagulation pathway. Consumption of platelets and procoagulants, including factors I, II, V, VIII, and XIII, reflects generalized activation of the entire coagulation system. Furthermore, impaired perfusion of the liver interferes with extraction of activated clotting factors.

LABORATORY RESULTS

Platelet counts are often less than 150,000/mm^3 because of consumption. Prothrombin time (PT) and PTT are prolonged. Decreased fibrinogen (less than 150 mg/dL) reflects consumption of this procoagulant. Levels of fibrin degradation products are elevated.

CLINICAL MANIFESTATIONS

Patients often demonstrate hemorrhage from wound sites and around sites of placement of intravascular catheters. In some cases, thromboembolic phenomena may follow.

TREATMENT

The goal is correction of the underlying disorder responsible for initiating the widespread clotting process. Correct acidosis, hypovolemia, and hypoxemia first. Platelet concentrates and fresh-frozen plasma may be administered as determined by measurement of the platelet count and of the PT and PTT, respectively. Heparin has been recommended as therapy, but its use is controversial.

ANESTHETIC CONSIDERATIONS

Intramuscular injections and regional anesthesia should be avoided. Coagulation factors and the DIC screen should be monitored, and be prepared to administer the necessary blood products.

D. Polycythemia Vera

DEFINITION AND ETIOLOGY

Polycythemia vera is a myeloproliferative neoplastic disorder that generally occurs in patients between 60 and 70 years of age. Hyperactivity of myeloid progenitor cells results in increased production of erythrocytes, leukocytes, and platelets.

LABORATORY RESULTS

Hemoglobin concentrations typically exceed 18 g/dL, and platelet counts can be greater than 400,000/mm^3.

CLINICAL MANIFESTATIONS

Clinical symptoms are the result of hyperviscosity of the blood, which leads to stasis of blood flow and an increased incidence of vascular thrombosis, particularly in the cardiovascular and central nervous systems. Erythromelalgia (burning pain) in fingers and toes is caused by digital ischemia. Defective platelet function is the most likely mechanism for spontaneous hemorrhage, which may occur in these patients. Splenomegaly is often present.

TREATMENT

Treatment entails reducing the hematocrit to near-normal levels of about 40% by phlebotomy before elective surgery.

ANESTHETIC CONSIDERATIONS

Surgery in the presence of uncontrolled polycythemia vera is associated with a high incidence of perioperative hemorrhage and postoperative venous thrombosis. In emergency situations, viscosity of the blood can be reduced by intravenous infusions of crystalloid solutions or low-molecular-weight dextrans. NPO (nothing by mouth) replacement should be infused early to assist in decreasing the blood viscocity.

E. Leukemia

DEFINITION

Leukemia is the uncontrolled production of leukocytes because of cancerous mutation of lymphogenous cells or myelogenous cells. Lymphocytic leukemias begin in lymph nodes or other lymphogenous tissues and then spread to other areas of the body. Myeloid leukemias begin as cancerous production of myelogenous cells in bone marrow, with spread to extramedullary organs. Cancerous cells usually do not resemble other leukocytes and lack the usual functional characteristics of white cells. Leukemia cells may infiltrate the liver, spleen, and meninges and produce signs of dysfunction at these sites.

INCIDENCE, PREVALENCE, ETIOLOGY, CLINICAL MANIFESTATIONS, AND LABORATORY RESULTS

Acute lymphoblastic leukemia accounts for approximately 15% of all leukemias in adults. Central nervous system dysfunction is common.

These patients are highly susceptible to life-threatening infections, including those produced by *Pneumocystis carinii* and cytomegalovirus.

Chronic lymphocytic leukemia accounts for approximately 25% of all leukemias and is most common in elderly men. Diagnosis is confirmed by the presence of lymphocytosis (greater than 15,000/mm^3) and lymphocytic infiltrates in bone marrow. There may be neutropenia with an associated increased susceptibility to bacterial infections. Treatment is with cancer chemotherapeutic drugs classified as alkylating agents.

Acute myeloid leukemia can result in death in about 3 months if untreated. Patients present with fever, weakness, bleeding, and hepatosplenomegaly. Chemotherapy produces a temporary remission in about one half of patients.

Patients with chronic myeloid leukemia present with massive hepatosplenomegaly and white blood cell counts greater than 50,000/mm^3. Fever and weight loss reflect hypermetabolism. Anemia may be severe. Splenectomy is routine in these patients.

TREATMENT

Cancer chemotherapy is the best available therapy for irradiation of cancerous cells anywhere in the body. Adverse clinical effects of these drugs include bone marrow suppression (susceptibility to infection, thrombocytopenia, and anemia), nausea, vomiting, diarrhea, ulceration of the gastrointestinal mucosa, and alopecia. Destruction of tumor cells by chemotherapy produces a uric acid load that may result in urate nephropathy and gouty arthritis.[2] Bone marrow transplantation is also becoming an increasingly successful treatment for leukemia.

ANESTHETIC MANAGEMENT

Management of anesthesia for the patient with leukemia requires a clear understanding of the mechanisms of action, potential interactions, and likely toxicities associated with the use of cancer chemotherapeutic drugs. Patients taking doxorubicin or daunorubicin (antibiotics) may develop cardiomyopathy leading to congestive heart failure, which is often refractory to cardiac inotropic drugs. Cardiomegaly and/or pleural effusions may be found on chest x-ray studies. Marked left ventricular dysfunction was found to persist for as long as 3 years after the drug was discontinued. Nonspecific and usually benign electrocardiographic changes have been observed in 10% of patients. Bleomycin is an antibiotic that can cause pulmonary toxicity, with dyspnea and nonproductive cough being the initial manifestations. Pulmonary function tests demonstrate "restrictive" pulmonary disease. The inspired fraction of oxygen should be maintained at less than 30% during surgery because patients are susceptible to the toxic pulmonary effects of oxygen while they are receiving bleomycin therapy. (*Strict aseptic technique is important because of immunosuppression. Preoperatively, signs of central nervous system depression, autonomic nervous system dysfunction, and peripheral neuropathies should be noted. Renal or hepatic dysfunction should influence the choice of anesthesia and muscle relaxants. Volatile anesthetics may reduce myocardial contractility in patients with cardiotoxicity related to chemotherapeutic drugs. Arterial blood gases should be monitored. Replacing fluid losses with colloid rather than crystalloid solutions in patients with pulmonary fibrosis may be considered. In addition, possible postoperative ventilation, depending on the length of the procedure and the degree of fibrosis, should be considered.*)

Considerations

- A risk of infection from immunosuppression exists.
- Renal function is affected by uric acid production.
- A thorough neurologic assessment related to chemotherapy treatment is indicated.
- Patients with acute lymphoblastic leukemia may develop malignant hyperthermia.
- Nitrous oxide should be avoided in bone marrow transplantation. (The use of nitrous oxide in patients donating bone marrow or undergoing bone marrow transplantation should be avoided because of the potential for drug-induced adverse effects on the bone marrow itself. Donors may be given heparin before removal of bone marrow, and this influences the use of spinal or epidural anesthesia for this procedure.)

F. Sickle Cell Disease

DEFINITION

Sickle cell disease represents an inherited group of disorders, ranging in severity from the usually benign sickle cell trait to the often fatal sickle cell anemia. All the variants of the disease have in common various quantities of hemoglobin S. Hemoglobin S differs from normal hemoglobin A by the substitution of valine for glutamic acid at the sixth position on the β chain of hemoglobin molecules.

INCIDENCE AND PREVALENCE

The incidence of sickle cell trait among the black population of the United States is about 10%. Sickle cell anemia is present when patients are homozygous for hemoglobin S and affects approximately 0.3% to 1% of the African-American population in the United States. In the homozygous state, 70% to 98% of hemoglobin is of the S type that may "sickle," resulting in severe hemolytic anemia.

ETIOLOGY

Sickle cell trait is the heterozygote manifestation of sickle cell disease containing the hemoglobin genotype AS. Erythrocytes of patients with the trait contain 20% to 40% hemoglobin S; the remainder being hemoglobin A. Affected persons are usually asymptomatic. Sickle cell anemia occurs when deoxygenated forms of hemoglobin S result in the deformation of erythrocytes into sickle shapes instead of their usual biconcave shape. This damages the erythrocyte membranes, leading to their rupture and chronic hemolytic anemia. Formation of sickle cells is exaggerated by low oxygen partial pressures (less than 40 mm Hg). Formation tends to be greater in veins than in arteries, so maintenance of pH is important. Hypothermia also promotes formation of sickled cells from vasoconstriction, which leads to stasis of blood flow and deoxygenation of hemoglobin.

CLINICAL MANIFESTATIONS

Most commonly, the clinical manifestations are infarctive events resulting from occlusion of blood vessels with sickled cells and anemia resulting from hemolysis. The cardiac output is generally increased to compensate for chronic anemia. The oxyhemoglobin dissociation curve for hemoglobin S is shifted to the right (P_{50} = 31 mm Hg). Patients are susceptible to bacterial infections because splenic function is lost secondary to repeated thrombosis. Multiple organ dysfunction produced by infarctive events is the major reason that survival beyond 30 years of age is unlikely.

LABORATORY RESULTS

In steady state, hemoglobin concentrations are 5 to 10 g/dL. Arterial blood gases, electrolytes, liver function tests, and other tests should be watched, depending on the patient's clinical symptoms and possible organ involvement.

TREATMENT

Treatment of a painful infarctive crisis is with hydration and mild alkalinization of blood. Partial exchange transfusions with erythrocytes containing hemoglobin A reduce concentrations of hemoglobin S and decrease the incidence of further infarctive damage. The goal of exchange transfusions is to increase hemoglobin A concentrations to at least 40%.

ANESTHETIC CONSIDERATIONS

Hypoventilation of the lungs should be avoided, to prevent acidosis. Oxygenation should be maintained. To prevent circulatory stasis, improper body positioning or the use of tourniquets should be avoided. Intravascular fluid volume must be maintained to prevent increased blood viscosity. Normal body temperature should also be maintained. Preoperative medication should be administered judiciously to avoid depression of ventilation. Regional anesthesia may be preferred over general anesthesia, although compensatory vasoconstriction and decreased arterial oxygen partial pressures in the unblocked area may predispose patients to infarction.

G. Thalassemia

DEFINITION

Certain inherited disorders resulting in a person's inability to synthesize structurally normal hemoglobin.

INCIDENCE AND PREVALENCE

β-Thalassemia major usually affects Greek and Italian children.

ETIOLOGY

Patients have a genetic inability to synthesize structurally normal hemoglobin. β-Thalassemia major reflects an inability to form the β chains of hemoglobin. As a result, adult hemoglobin A is not formed, and anemia develops during the first year of life, as fetal hemoglobin disappears. β-Thalassemia minor reflects a heterozygote state that results in mild anemia. α-Thalassemia results from the lack of production of α chains of adult hemoglobin. The homozygous form of α-thalassemia is incompatible with life, resulting in intrauterine demise or early neonatal death.

LABORATORY RESULTS

Check the complete blood count preoperatively, based on need and the patient's underlying condition.

CLINICAL MANIFESTATIONS

β-Thalassemia major is associated with jaundice, hepatosplenomegaly, and susceptibility to infection. Death can result from cardiac hemochromatosis. Supraventricular cardiac dysrhythmias and congestive heart failure are common. Hemothorax and spinal cord compression may occur secondary to massive extramedullary hematopoiesis and destruction of vertebral bodies. Overgrowth of the maxillae can make visualization of the glottis difficult during direct laryngoscopy for tracheal intubation.

In β-thalassemia minor, a relatively normal RBC count distinguishes anemia caused by thalassemia minor from iron-deficiency anemia. Finally, the homozygous form of α-thalassemia is incompatible with life; the heterozygous presentation usually results in mild hypochromic and microcytic anemia.

TREATMENT

Treatment varies depending on variant form. β-Thalassemia major can be treated with hydroxyurea. Occasionally, bone marrow transplantation may be recommended in these patients, and a splenectomy may be necessary if hypersplenism leads to pancytopenia. For α-thalassemia, blood transfusion is occasionally necessary.

ANESTHETIC CONSIDERATIONS

Check the patient's complete blood count preoperatively.

HEPATIC SYSTEM

A. Cirrhosis/Portal Hypertension

DEFINITION

Cirrhosis/portal hypertension is a chronic disease process that destroys the hepatic parenchyma and replaces it with collagen. This distorts the liver's normal architecture and leads to obstruction of portal venous flow and subsequent portal hypertension as well as impairment of physiologic functions of the liver. Other complications include variceal hemorrhage secondary to the portal hypertension, intractable fluid retention in the form of ascites and the hepatorenal syndrome, and hepatic encephalopathy or coma.

ETIOLOGY

The most common cause of cirrhosis in the United States is alcohol abuse (Laennec's cirrhosis). Other causes include chronic active hepatitis (postnecrotic cirrhosis), chronic biliary inflammation or obstruction (biliary cirrhosis), chronic right-sided congestive heart failure (cardiac cirrhosis), hemochromatosis, and Wilson's disease.

DIAGNOSTIC AND LABORATORY RESULTS

Laboratory changes in the presence of portal hypertension include a hematocrit of 30% to 35%, hyponatremia resulting from increased secretion of antidiuretic hormone, blood urea nitrogen greater than 20 mg/dL, and elevated plasma bilirubin, transaminases, and alkaline phosphatase concentrations.

CLINICAL MANIFESTATIONS
Gastrointestinal

Portal hypertension leads to the formation of ascites, esophageal varices, hemorrhoids, and gastrointestinal bleeding. Peptic ulcer disease is twice as common in patients with cirrhosis and may result in further hemorrhage. Patients develop anorexia and lose skeletal muscle mass. Gastric emptying is often slow, warranting premedication (cimetidine, metoclopramide) and a rapid sequence induction.

Circulatory

A hyperdynamic circulation characterized by an increased cardiac output is attributed to increased vascular volume, decreased blood viscosity secondary to anemia, and generalized peripheral vasodilation. Cardiomyopathy can manifest as congestive heart failure. Palmar erythema and spider angiomas over the face, upper back, and arms are prominent. Hepatomegaly occurs with or without splenomegaly and ascites.

Pulmonary

Hyperventilation commonly results in primary respiratory alkalosis. Arterial hypoxemia develops because of right-to-left shunting (up to 40% of cardiac output). Elevation of the diaphragm from ascites reduces functional residual capacity and predisposes patients to atelectasis.

Renal

Decreased renal perfusion, enhanced proximal and distal sodium reabsorption, impaired free water clearance, hyponatremia, and hypokalemia are common. The hepatorenal syndrome may develop in these patients following gastrointestinal bleeding, aggressive diuresis, sepsis, or major surgery. This syndrome is characterized by progressive oliguria, azotemia, intractable ascites, and a high mortality rate unless liver transplantation is undertaken.

Hematologic

Anemia, thrombocytopenia, and leukopenia may be present. Coagulopathies result from decreased hepatic synthesis of coagulation factors (all except factor VIII and fibrinogen are affected), and reduced or impaired platelet function. Enhanced fibrinolysis resulting from decreased clearance of activators of the fibrinolytic system may also contribute to the coagulopathy.

Metabolic

Hypoalbuminemia, hyperaldosteronism, and hypoglycemia may be present.

Central Nervous System

Hepatic encephalopathy as well as coma may be manifested. Mental obtundation, asterixis (flapping motion of the hands), and fetor hepaticus (musty, sweet breath odor) are evident. Elevated intracranial pressure may require prompt treatment and continuous intraoperative monitoring.

TREATMENT

Treatment is supportive until liver transplantation can be undertaken. Variceal bleeding involves replacement of blood loss, vasopressin infusion (0.1 to 0.9 units/min intravenously), balloon tamponade (Sengstaken-Blakemore tube), endoscopic sclerosis, or the transjugular intrahepatic portosystemic shunt/stent procedure to stop the bleeding. If bleeding does not stop or recurs, emergency surgical procedures such as shunts (portocaval or splenorenal), esophageal transection, or gastric devascularization may be needed. Coagulopathies should be corrected by replacing clotting factors with fresh-frozen plasma or cryoprecipitate. Platelet transfusions should be performed preoperatively for counts less than 100,000 mm³. Preservation of renal function involves avoiding aggressive diuresis while correcting acute intravascular fluid deficits with colloid infusions.

ANESTHETIC CONSIDERATIONS

The dosage of muscle relaxants should be reduced, depending on hepatic elimination (e.g., pancuronium, vecuronium) because of reduced plasma clearance. Cisatracurium may be the relaxant of choice. The duration of action of succinylcholine may be prolonged as a result of reduced levels of pseudocholinesterase. Half-lives of opioids may be prolonged, leading to prolonged respiratory depression. Regional anesthesia may be used in patients without thrombocytopenia or coagulopathy if hypotension is avoided (perfusion to the liver becomes highly dependent on hepatic arterial blood flow). Following removal of large amounts of ascitic fluid, colloid fluid replacement may be necessary to prevent hypotension. Whole blood may be preferable to packed red blood cells when replacing blood loss. Coagulation factors and platelet deficiencies should be corrected with fresh-frozen plasma and platelet transfusions, respectively. Citrate toxicity can occur in these patients because of impaired metabolism of the citrate anticoagulant in blood products. Intravenous calcium should be given to reverse the negative inotropic effects of a reduction in serum ionized calcium levels.

B. Hepatic Failure

DEFINITION

Hepatic failure occurs when massive necrosis of liver cells results in the development of a life-threatening loss of functional capacity that exceeds 80% to 90%. Hepatic failure can result from acute or chronic liver disease.

INCIDENCE

The major causes of hepatic failure in the United States are related to the effects of viral hepatitis or drug-related liver injury. Each year, an estimated 2000 cases of hepatic failure in the United States are related to viral hepatitis. This accounts for 1% of all deaths and 6% of all liver-related deaths.

ETIOLOGY

Following is a categoric list of the potential causes of hepatic failure.

Viral
Hepatitis A, B, C, D, E viruses
Herpes simplex virus
Cytomegalovirus
Adenovirus
Epstein-Barr virus
Varicella zoster virus
Dengue fever virus
Rift Valley fever virus

Toxic Damage
Isoniazid
Phenytoin
Halothane
Methyldopa
Tetracycline
Valproic acid
Nicotinic acid
Carbon tetrachloride
Phosphorus
Pesticides
Ethyl alcohol

Metabolic
Wilson's disease
Acute fatty liver of pregnancy
Reye's syndrome
Sickle cell disease
Galactosemia

Other
Autoimmune hepatitis
Amanita phalloides (mushroom) poisoning
Acetaminophen
Budd-Chiari syndrome
Veno-occlusive disease
Hyperthermia
Partial hepatectomy
Jejunoileal bypass

DIAGNOSTIC AND LABORATORY FINDINGS

Most proteins associated with the promotion or inhibition of coagulation are synthesized in the liver. When one is reviewing laboratory data, special attention should be given to coagulation studies, liver function studies, complete blood count, electrolytes, glucose, blood urea nitrogen, and creatinine.

A 12-lead electrocardiogram should be performed to rule out any possible cardiac arrhythmias related to acidemia, electrolyte abnormalities, or hypoxemia associated with hepatic failure. The patient with liver failure is at risk for the development of acid-base derangements. Respiratory alkalosis may result from hyperventilation related to an abnormality of central regulation. Respiratory acidosis may be caused by endotoxins, increased intracranial pressure, or pulmonary sequelae, which depress respiratory centers. Metabolic acidosis is also possible, related to substantial tissue damage and decreased clearance of lactic acid by the failing liver.

The hypoxemia associated with liver failure can be attributed to aspiration, atelectasis, infection, hypoventilation, or their combinations. Results of chest x-ray studies should be obtained to rule out evidence of pulmonary edema or adult respiratory distress syndrome. Listed in the following table is a guide to laboratory results in liver failure.

Laboratory Results in Liver Failure

Laboratory Study	Normal	Liver Failure
White blood cell count	3.5–10.6 cells/mm^3	Decreased
Hemoglobin	11.5–15.1 g/dL	Decreased
Hematocrit	34.4%–44.2%	Decreased
Platelet count	150–450/mm^3	Decreased
Prothrombin time	11–14 sec	Increased
Partial thromboplastin time	20–37 sec	Increased
Bilirubin	Plasma: 0.3–1.1 mg/dL Indirect: 0.2–0.7 mg/dL Direct: <0.5 mg/dL	Increased: jaundice seen with plasma bilirubin levels >3 mg/dL
Serum glutamic-oxaloacetic transaminase (aspartate aminotransferase)	10–40 units/L	Increased
Serum glutamic-pyruvic transaminase (alanine aminotransferase*)	5–35 units/L	Increased
Lactate dehydrogenase (LD-5*)	5.3%–13.4%	Increased
Alkaline phosphatase	87–250 units/L	Normal; used to differentiate biliary obstruction

*Specific for liver damage.

Laboratory Results in Liver Failure—cont'd

Laboratory Study	Normal	Liver Failure
Albumin	3.3–4.5 g/dL	Decreased; levels <2.5 g/dL are precarious
Ammonia	<50 g/dL	Increased ammonia converted to urea by the normal liver
Blood urea nitrogen	7–20 mg/dL	Normal or decreased by impaired excretion of sodium and retention of water; increased in hepatorenal syndrome
Creatinine	0.6–1.3 mg/dL	Increased in hepatorenal syndrome
Sodium	135–145 mEq/L	Usually decreased; increased sodium may result after the administration of lactulose or if replacement of free water is inadequate
Potassium	3.6–5 mEq/L	Decreased; related to the secondary effects of hyperaldosteronism, vomiting, diuretic use, or inadequate replacement; increased potassium may result from the use of blood products
Magnesium	1.6–3 mEq/L	Decreased
Calcium	8.8–10.4 mg/dL	Decreased
Phosphorus	2.5–4.5 mg/dL	Decreased
Glucose	70–110 mg/dL	Decreased; related to impaired gluconeogenesis and decreased insulin clearance

CLINICAL MANIFESTATIONS

No matter the exact cause of the patient's liver failure, it inevitably affects the entire physiologic makeup. Physical examination is important for the approximation of liver and spleen size, evidence of bleeding abnormalities, identification of extravascular fluid shifts, and any other organ dysfunction. Listed in the following table are common clinical features of hepatic failure and their associated causes.

Clinical Features of Hepatic Failure and Associated Causes

Clinical Feature	Cause
Anemia	Iron, vitamin B_{12}, or folate deficiency; hypersplenism; bone marrow suppression
Ascites	Portal hypertension; hypoalbuminemia; sodium and water retention
Fetor hepaticus (pungent sour odor detected in exhaled breath)	Inability to metabolize methionine
Gynecomastia	Increased circulating estrogen
Hepatic encephalopathy (hepatic coma)	Inability to metabolize ammonia; increased cerebral sensitivity to toxins; hypoglycemia
Hepatorenal syndrome	Decreased renal blood flow, particularly to the cortex; vasoconstriction; decreased glomerular filtration rate; renal retention of sodium
Increased bleeding tendencies, nosebleeds, gingival bleeding, menstrual bleeding, easy bruising	Anemia; thrombocytopenia; decreased production of clotting factors; decreased adherence of circulating platelets
Increased risk of infection	Endotracheal intubation with impaired cough reflex; intravenous catheters; central lines; urinary catheters; leukopenia; decreased neutrophil adherence; complement deficiencies
Increased skin pigmentation	Increased activity of melanocyte-stimulating hormone
Jaundice	Increased circulating bilirubin
Leukopenia	Hypersplenism; bone marrow suppression
Palmar erythema	Increased circulating estrogen
Pectoral and axillary alopecia	Increased circulating estrogen
Peripheral edema	Hypoalbuminemia; failure of the liver to inactivate aldosterone and antidiuretic hormone, with subsequent sodium and water retention
Spider angiomas, "nevi"	Increased circulating estrogen
Testicular atrophy	Increased circulating estrogen
Thrombocytopenia	Hypersplenism; bone marrow suppression
Weight loss and muscle wasting	Nausea and vomiting; anorexia; impaired gluconeogenesis; impaired insulin functioning; hypoproteinemia

TREATMENT

Management of the patient with liver failure should include admission to the intensive care unit. The health care team should be on constant guard for complications associated with liver failure, such as sepsis, cerebral edema, hypoglycemia, and electrolyte and bleeding abnormalities. Liver failure associated with acetaminophen poisoning or mushroom poisoning should be identified immediately, because antidotes are available for both. Patients not responsive to conventional treatment should be considered for liver transplantation as early as possible, before they are excluded by the development of infection or encephalopathic brain damage.

General treatment modalities for the patient with liver failure include the following:

- Antibiotic prophylaxis
- Urinary catheter
- Central venous pulmonary catheter
- Histamine-2 (H_2) antagonist or sucralfate
- Blood glucose checks every 1 to 2 hours
- Aspiration precautions
- Periodic assessment of neurologic status (Neurologic status may rapidly deteriorate because of increasing ammonia levels or increasing intracranial pressure)
- Prevention of sepsis
- Monitoring of renal function and fluid status
- Monitoring of fluid volume
- Increase gastric pH and decrease risk of gastrointestinal bleeding
- Prevention of hypoglycemia and guide administration of intravenous dextrose
- Prevention of aspiration pneumonia and adult respiratory distress syndrome
- Early nutritional supplementation: prevention of nutrition-related complications

ANESTHETIC CONSIDERATIONS

Only surgery to correct life-threatening conditions should be performed on the patient with liver failure. The patient's condition should be optimized before the surgical procedure. A normally "minor" procedure can become a major catastrophe in the patient with liver failure.

Premedication must be considered, taking into account the severity of the patient's disease process, the presence of altered consciousness, and the liver's diminished ability to metabolize pharmacologic agents. If the patient is thought to have a full stomach, antacids and H_2 antagonists may be administered.

Monitoring should conform to the established standards of care. The size and number of intravenous catheters should be individualized. Most cases involving liver failure require the use of an arterial line, a central venous pressure or pulmonary artery catheter, and a urinary drainage catheter to monitor the patient's fluid status.

The use of local anesthesia with sedation or regional anesthesia should be considered whenever possible. Coagulopathies must first be ruled out, and the surgical procedure itself must be considered. Patients may be considered to have a full stomach, especially in the presence of ascites. In this case, a rapid-sequence induction is standard. The choice of induction agent and dosage administered should reflect the liver's diminished ability to metabolize pharmacologic agents and the patient's increased volume of distribution.

Both nondepolarizing and depolarizing muscle relaxants may be administered. Dosages may need to be individualized according to the patient's initial response. A peripheral nerve stimulator aids the practitioner in gauging the patient's response and adjusting subsequent doses. The breakdown of succinylcholine remains relatively normal despite advanced disease states. Muscle relaxants metabolized by the liver (e.g., vecuronium) should be avoided. *Cis*-atracurium may be the muscle relaxant of choice because of its unique metabolic properties, which do not involve either the liver or the kidneys. If *cis*-atracurium is unavailable, any other nondepolarizing muscle relaxant may be used, taking into account the patient's specific organ involvement and the drug's metabolic properties.

Isoflurane and desflurane are the inhalational agents of choice. Enflurane may also be considered, but the practitioner must consider the neurologic status of the patient. Halothane is contraindicated in patients with liver disease. Nitrous oxide may be safely instituted according to the nature of the surgical procedure and as long as a high fraction of inspired oxygen is not required.

The use of opioids must take into account a prolonged half-life and decreased clearance. Because fentanyl does not decrease hepatic blood flow, it is often the opioid of choice for the patient with liver failure.

The patient with liver failure is at risk for major blood loss with any invasive procedure. Blood products should be available, and all losses should be replaced accordingly.

PROGNOSIS

In the United States, mortality rates from liver disease have increased since the 1960s. Overall, the mortality rate from hepatic failure is 70% to 95%. Liver transplantation should be considered when conventional medical management fails; such consideration should take place early, before infection or encephalopathic brain damage renders the potential candidate ineligible for the procedure. One-year patient survival rates after liver transplantation are 63% to 78%.

C. Hepatitis

DEFINITION

Hepatitis is an inflammatory disease of hepatocytes that may be either acute or chronic (lasting more than 6 months) and can progress to cell necrosis and eventual hepatic failure.

ETIOLOGY

Some of the causes of acute and chronic hepatitis include viral infections and drug-induced toxicity. The organisms responsible for viral hepatitis include hepatitis A virus, hepatitis B virus, hepatitis C virus (formerly non-A, non-B virus), Epstein-Barr virus, cytomegalovirus, and herpes simplex virus. Hepatitis A, or infectious hepatitis, is transmitted by the fecal-oral route or by ingestion of food contaminated with sewage. Hepatitis types B and C are transmitted percutaneously and by contact with body fluids. Hepatitis B, or serum hepatitis, is the most common type of viral hepatitis and may also be transmitted by nonparenteral routes (oral-to-oral and sexual). Drug-induced hepatitis may result from dose-dependent toxicity of a drug (or drug metabolite), from an idiosyncratic drug reaction, or from a combination of both. Halothane has been associated with hepatic dysfunction with repeat administration at short intervals in adults.

DIAGNOSTIC AND LABORATORY RESULTS

Laboratory evaluation should include blood urea nitrogen, serum electrolytes, serum creatinine, glucose, transaminases, bilirubin, alkaline phosphatase, albumin, prothrombin time, platelet count, and hepatitis B surface antigen. Concentrations of plasma transaminase enzymes are elevated 7 to 14 days before the onset of jaundice and begin to decline shortly after jaundice is clinically evident. Severe hepatitis is suggested by a plasma albumin concentration of less than 2.5 g/dL or a markedly prolonged prothrombin time unresponsive to vitamin K therapy. The presence of hepatitis B surface antigen in plasma indicates the potential for infectivity, and persistence for longer than 6 months in the absence of antibodies indicates that the patient is a chronic carrier and is potentially infective to others.

CLINICAL MANIFESTATIONS

Symptoms of viral hepatitis include jaundice, dark urine, fatigue, anorexia, nausea, fever, and abdominal discomfort. Mild anemia and lymphocytosis also occur. Hypomagnesemia may be present in patients with chronic alcoholism and can predispose to arrhythmias.

TREATMENT

Dehydration and electrolyte abnormalities should be corrected. Vitamin K or fresh-frozen plasma is used to correct coagulopathies. Bacterial infections should be treated, and neomycin, lactulose, or both should be used to decrease plasma ammonia levels. Factors that may aggravate hepatic encephalopathy should be avoided. Orthotopic liver transplantation may be considered in selected patients.

ANESTHETIC CONSIDERATIONS

Coagulopathy should be corrected with fresh-frozen plasma. Premedication with sedatives should be avoided. Barbiturates, opioids, and some muscle relaxants may have prolonged effects because of altered hepatic metabolism. Response to succinylcholine may also be prolonged because of depression of pseudocholinesterase. Factors known to reduce hepatic blood flow, such as hypotension, excessive sympathetic activation, and high mean airway pressures during controlled ventilation, should be avoided. Hypoglycemia can be prevented by administering exogenous glucose. Blood should be administered at a controlled rate to minimize the likelihood of citrate intoxication. Patients with alcoholism may develop cross-tolerance to both intravenous and volatile anesthetics.

MUSCULOSKELETAL SYSTEM

A. Arthritis

DEFINITION

Osteoarthritis (OA) is a degenerative disease affecting the articular surface of the joints, most commonly the hip and knees. Rheumatoid arthritis (RA) is an immune-mediated joint destruction characterized by chronic and progressive inflammation of synovial membranes. Unlike OA, RA is associated with systemic involvement and is usually symmetric.

INCIDENCE AND PREVALENCE

The incidence of RA is approximately 1% worldwide. It predominately affects women between the ages of 30 and 50 years.

ETIOLOGY

OA is usually caused by repetitive joint trauma. It is commonly associated with advancing age or morbid obesity. The etiology of RA is unknown.

LABORATORY RESULTS

Rheumatoid factor is the antibody that is present in most patients with RA.

CLINICAL MANIFESTATIONS

Patients with OA experience pain with motion. Spinal involvement usually includes the lower cervical and lower lumbar areas.

Swelling, pain, limited mobility, and morning stiffness of the joints occur with RA. Cervical spine involvement is frequent, although the thoracic, lumbar, and sacral spine is rarely affected. The heart may be involved, including pericardial thickening, effusion, pericarditis, myocarditis, arteritis involving the coronary arteries, cardiac valve fibrosis, and rheumatoid nodules in the conduction system. In addition, dilation of the aortic root may result in aortic regurgitation. Pleural effusion is the most common pulmonary manifestation of RA. Restrictive lung changes may result from costochondral involvement.

TREATMENT

Nonsteroidal antiinflammatory drugs (NSAIDs) are often used for pain management in both OA and RA. Corticosteroids are often used for the management of inflammation associated with RA. Gold salts or cytotoxic drugs may be used with severe RA that is difficult to control with NSAIDs and steroids. Reconstructive joint surgery is indicated to relieve pain and improve joint function.

ANESTHETIC CONSIDERATIONS

Joint deformities related to RA may make intravenous access difficult. Careful preoperative evaluation for cardiac and pulmonary disease is imperative because the joint effects of arthritis often prohibit exercise testing. Effects of medications such as NSAIDs and corticosteroids should be considered.

Careful neck positioning is important because of the high frequency of cervical spine involvement with both OA and RA. In addition, atlantoaxial subluxation may occur with severe RA. This carries a risk of protrusion of the odontoid process into the foramen magnum during intubation, thus compromising blood flow and compressing the spinal cord or brain stem. Atlantoaxial subluxation may be asymptomatic, so lateral radiographs are imperative in patients with severe RA. Atlantoaxial instability greater than 5 mm necessitates awake fiberoptic intubation with neck stabilization. Tempomandibular joint involvement may also complicate intubation by limiting jaw mobility. Cricoarytenoid arthritis may cause narrowing of the glottic opening, as evidenced by hoarseness or inspiratory stridor. In this case, a smaller endotracheal tube is warranted. Postextubation airway obstruction is also a risk.

B. Malignant Hyperthermia

DEFINITION

Malignant hyperthermia (MH) is an uncommon, life-threatening, hyper-metabolic disorder of skeletal muscle triggered in susceptible individuals by potent inhalation agents, including sevoflurane, desflurane, isoflurane, and halothane, and the depolarizing muscle relaxant succinylcholine.

INCIDENCE AND PREVALENCE

About 52% of cases occur in patients under age 15 years, with a mean age of 18.3 years. The exact incidence of MH is unknown, but the rate of occurrence has been estimated to be 1 in 50,000 in adults and 1 in 15,000 in children. High-incidence areas in the United States include Wisconsin, West Virginia, and Michigan. A genetic component seems to be related to the incidence of MH. MH has been found to be associated with other muscle disorders, such as Duchenne muscular dystrophy.

PATHOPHYSIOLOGY

Although the cause of MH is not yet known with certainty, it is generally agreed that it is an inherited disorder of skeletal muscle in which a defect in calcium regulation is expressed by exposure to triggering anesthetic agents; intracellular hypercalcemia results. The ryanodine receptor modulates calcium release from channels in the sarcoplasmic reticulum, and much attention has been focused on this receptor as a site of the MH defect. There is no evidence for a primary defect in cardiac or smooth muscle cells.

MH is initiated when specific triggering agents induce increased concentrations of calcium in the muscle cells of MH-susceptible (MHS) patients. Actomyosin cross-bridging, sustained muscle contraction, and rigidity result. Energy-dependent reuptake mechanisms attempt to remove excess calcium from the muscle cells, increasing muscle metabolism twofold to threefold. The accelerated cellular processes increase oxygen consumption, augment carbon dioxide (CO_2) and heat production, deplete adenosine triphosphate (ATP) stores, and generate lactic acid. Acidosis, hyperthermia, and ATP depletion cause sarcolemma destruction, producing a marked egress of potassium, myoglobin, and creatine kinase to the extracellular fluid. The precise cause of MH is not well understood; however, it is thought that a defect in calcium metabolism in the sarcoplasm leads to high concentrations. The high concentration of calcium allows for sustained muscle contraction. Accelerated metabolism associated with the sustained contractions is accompanied by acidosis and heat production. There is depletion of ATP, acidosis, cell membrane destruction, and cell death.

LABORATORY RESULTS

The most accurate and commonly accepted test available for determining MH susceptibility is the caffeine halothane contracture test (CHCT). This test involves taking a biopsy of skeletal muscle from the patient's thigh and measuring its contractile response to caffeine, halothane, or both. Normal muscle contracts in response to caffeine or halothane, but this response is augmented in the patient with MH. The test is available at eight medical centers in North America, and because it must be completed within hours after muscle biopsy, the patient must travel to the testing site. The test has a sensitivity of 92% and a specificity of 78%. Patients who have survived an unequivocal episode of MH are considered MHS patients. The CHCT is indicated for family members of an MHS patient or for patients who have had a previous suspicious but undiagnosed reaction to anesthesia.

CLINICAL MANSIFESTATIONS

There is a spectrum or continuum of severity, ranging from an insidious onset with mild complications to an explosive response with pronounced rigidity, temperature rise, arrhythmias, and death. Although MH may present in several ways, a typical MH episode begins while the patient is under general anesthesia with a volatile anesthetic. Succinylcholine administration may or may not precede the MH episode. The onset of MH symptoms may occur immediately after induction of anesthesia or several hours into the surgical procedure. Succinylcholine appears to accelerate the onset and increase the severity of the MH episode. The presentation of MH may follow a dose-dependent response, with lower concentrations of volatile anesthetics resulting in a more protracted onset of hypermetabolic symptoms. Rarely, MH occurs in the recovery room, usually within 1 hour after general anesthesia.

The clinical features of MH reflect increased intracellular muscle calcium concentration and the greatly increased body metabolism (see later). Common signs of MH include tachycardia, tachypnea, skin mottling, cyanosis, and total body or jaw muscle rigidity. Muscle rigidity is clinically apparent in 75% of cases. The most sensitive indicator of MH is an unanticipated increase in end-tidal CO_2 ($ETCO_2$) levels out of proportion to minute ventilation. The increased $ETCO_2$ may be abrupt, or it may rise gradually over the course of the anesthetic. Hyperthermia, which may climb at a rate of 1° to 2° C every 5 minutes and may exceed 43.3° C (110° F), is often a late but confirming sign of MH.

Clinical Events and Laboratory Findings During Malignant Hyperthermia

Clinical events

- Unexplained, sudden rise in $ETCO_2$
- Unexplained tachycardia, tachypnea, labile blood pressure, or arrhythmias
- Masseter muscle or generalized muscle rigidity
- Unanticipated respiratory or metabolic acidosis
- Rising patient temperature
- Cola-colored urine (myoglobinuria)
- Mottled, cyanotic skin, decreased oxygen saturation

Laboratory findings consistent with malignant hyperthermia

- Arterial blood gases: partial pressure of CO_2 greater than 60 mm Hg, base excess more negative than −8 mEq/L, pH lower than 7.25
- Potassium ion greater than 6 mEq/L
- Creatine kinase (CK) greater than 10,000 units/L after anesthetic without succinylcholine
- Serum myoglobin greater than 170 mg/L
- Urine myoglobin greater than 60 mg/L

The combination of acidosis, hyperkalemia, and hyperthermia leads to cardiac irritability, labile blood pressure, and arrhythmias that can rapidly progress to cardiac arrest. Laboratory findings mirror the muscle breakdown and include myoglobinuria and increased serum potassium and CK values. CK levels peak 12 to 24 hours after the onset of MH. Myoglobin appears in the plasma within minutes of the muscle injury response. Arterial and venous blood gas analysis reveals decreased oxygen tension and mixed metabolic and respiratory acidosis. Late complications may include cerebral edema, myoglobinuric renal failure, consumptive coagulopathy, hepatic dysfunction, and pulmonary edema.

The variable time course and the nonspecific clinical features and laboratory findings can make the diagnosis of MH difficult. Insufficient anesthetic depth, hypoxia, neuroleptic malignant syndrome, thyrotoxicosis, pheochromocytoma, and sepsis can share several characteristics with MH and make the clinical picture ambiguous and the differential diagnosis challenging to even the most experienced practitioner.

Manifestations That Mimic Malignant Hyperthermia: Signs and Symptoms

- Tachycardia
- Hypoxia
- Hypercarbia
- Hypovolemia
- Insufficient anesthetic depth
- Anticholinergics, sympathomimetics, cocaine
- Pheochromocytoma
- Hyperpyrexia
- Heat stroke
- Blood transfusion reaction
- Infection
- Drug reaction
- Neuroleptic malignant syndrome, serotonin syndrome

- Hypermetabolic states (sepsis, thyroid storm, pheochromocytoma)
- Tachypnea, hypercapnia
- Congestive heart failure, pulmonary edema
- Intraperitoneal CO_2 insufflation
- Airway obstruction, pneumothorax
- Excess dead space, low minute volume
- Masseter muscle rigidity
- Insufficient neuromuscular blockade
- Temporomandibular joint syndrome
- Myotonia

ANESTHETIC CONSIDERATIONS

Patients who are MHS may be otherwise healthy and completely unaware of their risk until exposed to a triggering anesthetic. Furthermore, not everyone who has the MH gene develops an MH episode on each exposure to triggering anesthetics. It is estimated that about 21% of MHS patients have at least one uneventful anesthetic before having an MH episode. Although MH susceptibility cannot be ruled out by history alone, every surgical patient should be questioned about the following:

- Family or personal history of muscle disorders
- Family history of unexpected intraoperative complications or deaths
- Family or personal history of muscle rigidity/stiffness or high fever under anesthesia
- Personal history of dark or cola-colored urine following surgery

Because MH is considered an inherited disorder, all members of a family in which MH has occurred must be considered MHS unless proven otherwise. Moreover, the absence of a positive family history does not preclude MH susceptibility.

Certain disorders should alert the anesthetist to an increased possibility of MH susceptibility. A clear genetic association between MH and the inherited myopathy central core disease has been demonstrated. Case reports have also linked MH to Duchenne and Becker muscular dystrophies and forms of periodic paralysis and myotonia. MH triggering agents should not be administered to patients with these disorders. This caveat is especially consequential in patients undergoing outpatient procedures who will have limited postoperative observation and same-day discharge.

CK levels are imprecise and nonspecific as a diagnostic test for MH. Stress, fever, prior exercise, and cocaine and alcohol ingestion have been implicated as causal factors, but it is debated whether these factors cause, exacerbate, or have no affect on clinical MH triggering.

A detailed anesthesia history is imperative. If the patient or family has a history of MH, all triggering agents should be avoided. The anesthesia machine vaporizers should be removed, and the circuit and CO_2 absorber canisters should be changed. The machine should be flushed with oxygen (10 L/min) for 10 to 20 minutes before surgery. The patient should be well sedated. Consider administering dantrium preoperatively (do not use phenothiazine). If MH is diagnosed, patient and family counseling and education will be necessary.

Anesthesia for the Patient Susceptible to Malignant Hyperthermia

Standard intraoperative monitoring for the MHS surgical patient includes blood pressure, electrocardiography, pulse oximetry, capnography, and continuous measurement of core body temperature (nasopharyngeal, distal esophageal, tympanic, or pulmonary artery). A cooling water mattress should be placed under the MHS patient at the start of the procedure. Inconsistent reports of emotional stress or anxiety predisposing a patient to MH have led to recommendations that anxiolytic agents be included in the premedication.

If the surgical site permits, a regional or local anesthetic technique is preferable for the MHS patient. Local anesthetics (both amide and ester) are nontriggering drugs. Nontriggering general anesthetics can also be administered safely in concert with close monitoring of appropriate vital functions. The list of "nontriggering" anesthetic agents is comprehensive enough to meet most anesthetic requirements. The volatile inhalation anesthetics and succinylcholine are MH triggers and should not be administered to the MHS patient. Potassium salts can depolarize the muscle membrane and are considered unsafe for the MHS patient.

Triggering and Nontriggering Agents
Triggering agents
- All volatile inhalation anesthetics (halothane, desflurane, isoflurane, sevoflurane)
- Succinylcholine
- Potassium salts

Nontriggering agents
- Local anesthetics
- Opioids
- Nitrous oxide
- Barbiturates, propofol, ketamine, etomidate
- Benzodiazepines
- Nondepolarizing skeletal muscle relaxants (vecuronium, atracurium, *cis*-atracurium, pancuronium, mivacurium, rocuronium, doxacurium, pipecuronium)
- Digoxin, tricyclic antidepressants, magnesium
- Anticholinesterase agents
- Anticholinergic agents

Not all drugs have been thoroughly screened as potential MH triggers, but it is clear that most prescription and nonprescription drugs are safe, including antibiotics, antihypertensive agents, and drugs used in the treatment of gastrointestinal disorders. Keys to successful perioperative outcome include the following:

- Avoidance of MH-triggering medications
- Preparation of an anesthesia machine by changing the soda lime and breathing circuits, removing or inactivating vaporizers, and flushing with oxygen or air at 10 L/min for at least 20 minutes or 10 minutes if the fresh gas hose is also replaced
- Assiduous perioperative observation for the signs of MH, including continuous intraoperative monitoring of the patient's $ETCO_2$ concentration, arterial oxygen saturation, and central temperature

• A full appreciation of a preestablished treatment protocol by all perioperative medical personnel

A machine to manufacture ice or the ready availability of ice and the ability to crush it, and a refrigerator containing at least 3000 mL of cold intravenous solution, should be available. Because early arterial blood gas analysis is an integral part of MH diagnosis and treatment, some MH experts recommend that every facility where MH-triggering agents are administered have ready access to blood gas analysis.

Ambulatory surgery can be safely performed in most MHS patients, provided appropriate monitoring is employed and an adequate supply of dantrolene is available. Outpatient surgical cases for the MHS patient are best scheduled early in the day to allow for adequate recovery and at least 4 hours of observation time after surgery. As with any ambulatory procedure, patient selection for outpatient surgery should be individualized. Patients known or suspected of having MH should be assessed well before their date of outpatient surgery, so anesthesia records and MH testing center reports (if available) can be collected to corroborate the history. Some experts recommend conservative management with overnight hospital admission for patients who have survived a previous fulminant or severe MH episode or when dantrolene prophylaxis is used.

All locations where general anesthesia is administered should contain a fully stocked MH cart with drugs and supplies, including 36 vials of dantrolene. Because minutes count in an MH emergency, a dantrolene supply should never be shared with a nearby facility, but rather it should be kept in or very close to the operating room so that it is available immediately if MH occurs.

TREATMENT

Enhanced patient monitoring, earlier diagnosis and treatment, and the introduction of dantrolene are responsible for the dramatic decrease in mortality from nearly 80% in the mid-1980s to less than 10% today. Clearly, the nurse anesthetist plays a critical role in the early recognition and treatment of MH.

Dantrolene is a unique muscle relaxant that works by reducing the release of calcium from skeletal muscle sarcoplasmic reticulum, thus counteracting the abnormal intracellular calcium levels accompanying MH. It does not work at the neuromuscular junction as do standard neuromuscular blocking drugs. At clinical concentrations, dantrolene does not render the muscle totally flaccid and without tone, but it may cause significant muscle weakness and respiratory insufficiency, especially in patients with preexisting muscle disease.

Dantrolene pretreatment for the MHS surgical patient is no longer routine, but it may be used prophylactically in specific surgical patients who cannot tolerate hypermetabolic states (e.g., the MHS patient with severe cardiac or cerebrovascular disease) or myoglobinuria (e.g., the MHS patient with renal disease). A single intravenous dose (2.5 mg/kg) immediately before induction is recommended. Dantrolene should not be used with calcium channel blockers because the combination may induce life-threatening hyperkalemia and myocardial depression.

The Malignant Hyperthermia Association of the United States provides an "Emergency Therapy for MH" poster that should be posted in every surgical site. The following treatment sequence is recommended for an acute MH episode:

- Call for help and alert the surgeon to conclude the procedure promptly.
- Discontinue the volatile anesthetic and succinylcholine.
- Hyperventilate with 100% oxygen at high flows (at least 10 L/min) to improve tissue oxygenation and eliminate CO_2.
- Administer 2.5 mg/kg dantrolene intravenous bolus and repeat as necessary until symptoms abate. Occasionally, a total dose greater than 10 mg/kg may be needed.
- Dysrhythmias will usually respond to treatment of acidosis or hyperkalemia. Treat persistent or life-threatening arrhythmias with standard antiarrhythmic agents (avoid calcium channel blockers).
- If fever is present, initiate cooling by lavage (orogastric, bladder, open cavities), administration of chilled intravenous normal saline and surface cooling (hypothermia blanket; ice packs to the groin, axillae, and neck).
- Determine arterial blood gases, serum electrolytes, and blood glucose every 15 minutes until the syndrome stabilizes. Correct metabolic acidosis with sodium bicarbonate. Baseline values for coagulation studies, CK, myoglobin, and liver enzymes should be established.
- Treat hyperkalemia with hyperventilation, bicarbonate, and intravenous insulin and glucose (10 units regular insulin in 50 mL 50% glucose) titrated to potassium level. Life-threatening hyperkalemia may be cautiously treated with calcium administration.
- Maintain urine output greater than 2 mL/kg/hour by hydration and mannitol (300 mg/kg) and/or furosemide (0.5 to 1 mg/kg). Large losses of intravascular volume should be anticipated. Consider central venous or pulmonary artery hemodynamic monitoring.

Dantrolene must be reconstituted with sterile water, and its poor water solubility makes it very time consuming to mix and administer the requisite doses. During an MH emergency, the full-time efforts of additional medical personnel should be enlisted. Documentation of an MH episode should include patient responses, personnel involved, medications, interventions, and patient outcomes.

The Malignant Hyperthermia Association of the United States MH hotline consultant may be contacted for expert medical advice. The MH event should be reported to the North American Malignant Hyperthermia Registry.

Postoperative Care

The patient who has experienced an acute MH episode should be observed in an intensive care unit for at least 24 hours. Recrudescence of an intra-operative episode occurs in 25% of cases. Dantrolene treatment is continued for a minimum of 24 hours after control of the episode.

For the MHS patient who has undergone an uneventful surgical course, close observation and assiduous monitoring should continue into the postanesthesia care unit. MH can first become manifest in the recovery room after uneventful surgery and anesthesia. Most MHS patients undergoing outpatient surgery may be discharged on the day of surgery, but each case should be individualized.

C. Muscular Dystrophy

DEFINITION

Muscular dystrophy is a heterogeneous set of diseases that includes fascio-scapulohumeral dystrophy, limb-girdle dystrophy, Becker muscular dystrophy, Duchenne muscular dystrophy (DMD), and others. DMD, also known as *pseudohypertrophic muscular dystrophy*, is the most common and most severe form.

ETIOLOGY

DMD is an inherited, sex-linked recessive disease. The disease presents in early childhood between 2 and 6 years of age. It is clinically evident in boys and has an incidence of 1 in 3500 live male births. Girls and women are generally unaffected but are carriers of the disorder. Mental retardation, of varying degrees, occurs in about 30% of patients with DMD. Death often occurs in late adolescence or early adulthood and is usually caused by respiratory failure.

CLINICAL MANIFESTATIONS

Patients with DMD experience an infiltration of fibrous and fatty tissue into the muscle, followed by a progressive and painless degeneration and necrosis of muscle fibers. Muscle weakness ends with muscle destruction.

DMD is characterized by an unremitting weakness and a steady deterioration of the proximal muscle groups of the pelvis and shoulders. The child exhibits a clumsy, waddling gait and falls frequently. Weakness of the pelvic girdle leads to the classic finding of Gower's sign, in which patients use their hands to climb up their legs to arise from the floor. A steady deterioration of muscle strength forces most of these boys to be wheelchair bound by the age of 8 to 12 years.

Skeletal muscle atrophy is usually preceded by fat and fibrous tissue infiltration, resulting in pseudohypertrophy. The infiltrative process is most apparent in the calf muscles, which become particularly enlarged.

Degeneration of respiratory muscles occurs and leads to a restrictive type of ventilatory impairment. Unopposed action by healthy, nondystrophic axial muscles predisposes these patients to kyphoscoliosis, which further decreases the pulmonary reserve. Decreasing muscle strength also results in ineffective cough, impaired swallowing, and inability to mobilize secretions.

More progressive forms of the disease affect not only skeletal muscle but also smooth muscle of the alimentary tract and cardiac muscle. Alimentary tract involvement can lead to intestinal hypomotility, delayed gastric emptying, and gastric dilation.

Myocardial involvement occurs in almost all patients with progressive disease. Myocardial disease includes fibrotic changes localized primarily to the left ventricle. Echocardiography can effectively evaluate left ventricular function in patients with DMD. Clinical symptoms of heart failure do not usually appear unless the patient is severely stressed or until advanced stages of the disease.

Electrocardiographic changes characteristic of preclinical cardiomyopathy include a large or polyphasic R wave in lead V_1, deep Q waves in the lateral precordial leads (V_4 through V_6), premature beats (atrial and ventricular), and labile sinus or atrial tachycardia.

Although often severe, the compromised cardiac and respiratory conditions may be masked by the limited activity imposed by the patient's skeletal myopathy. Added stress, such as that produced by surgery and anesthesia, may suddenly increase cardiorespiratory demand and uncover the weakened cardiac and respiratory states.

LABORATORY RESULTS

Laboratory findings include a serum creatine kinase level that is 30 to 300 times normal, even early in the disease, reflecting skeletal muscle necrosis and the increased permeability of skeletal muscle membranes. Creatine kinase concentration is elevated in approximately 70% of female carriers. Skeletal muscle biopsy early in the course of the disease may demonstrate necrosis and phagocytosis of muscle fibers.

ANESTHETIC CONSIDERATIONS

Patients with DMD are susceptible to untoward anesthesia-related complications. When possible, local or regional anesthesia should be considered.

Generalized muscle weakness, especially in the advanced stages of muscular dystrophy, makes these patients exquisitely sensitive to the respiratory depressant properties of opioids, sedatives, and general anesthetic agents. Preoperative sedation should be minimal, and the smallest possible amounts of anesthetic agents should be used.

Preoperative and postoperative respiratory therapy can help to maximize the patient's pulmonary condition. In patients with more advanced disease, arterial blood gas determinations and preoperative pulmonary function studies may elucidate the extent of respiratory involvement and the amount of respiratory reserve. A forced vital capacity of less than 35% of that predicted indicates a risk for postoperative pulmonary complications.

The effects of nondepolarizing muscle relaxants must be scrupulously monitored. There is increased muscle relaxant sensitivity, and recovery may be prolonged by three to six times in patients with DMD. Short-acting nondepolarizing muscle relaxants that are carefully titrated with the use of a nerve stimulator are recommended.

Assiduous attention to respiratory function must be continued into the postoperative period. Delayed pulmonary insufficiency, as late as 36 hours after surgery, has been reported. At least 24 hours of observation should be instituted after the patient undergoes anesthesia.

Their decreased cardiac reserve makes these patients sensitive to the myocardial depressant effects of general anesthetic agents, sedatives, and narcotics. Cardiac arrests associated with inhalation anesthetics have been reported. A carefully titrated intravenous "balanced" technique may help to provide a smoother cardiovascular course. Ketamine has been used successfully for anesthesia during diagnostic muscle biopsy in patients with DMD. Judicious administration of intravenous fluids is warranted. The sudden occurrence of tachycardia during anesthesia may herald heart failure.

The potential for delayed gastric emptying, in addition to the presence of weak laryngeal reflexes, dictates that the anesthesia plan of care include measures for guarding against aspiration of stomach contents. Gastrokinetic agents and the prophylactic use of a nasogastric tube are recommended to avoid gastric dilation.

Succinylcholine and the potent inhalational agents should not be used in patients with muscular dystrophy because the altered sarcolemma can lead to rhabdomyolysis with their administration. The resultant massive breakdown of muscle fibers produces a profound hyperkalemia that requires extensive and tenacious treatment with hyperventilation, calcium chloride, sodium bicarbonate, and glucose and insulin. Several cases of ventricular fibrillation or cardiac arrest occurring during anesthetic induction have been associated with succinylcholine or potent inhalational agent administration. Additionally, DMD is included among the myopathies that may be associated with malignant hyperthermia (MH). The anesthetist should avoid MH-triggering agents and should vigilantly observe for signs and symptoms of MH when these children undergo surgery. Dantrolene and other treatment modalities for MH should be readily available.

D. Myasthenic Syndrome

DEFINITION

Lambert-Eaton myasthenic syndrome (LEMS) is a rare autoimmune disease that classically occurs in patients with malignant disease, particularly small cell carcinoma of the bronchi. In one third to one half of patients, however, no evidence of carcinoma is present. Most patients with myasthenic syndrome are men between the ages of 50 and 70 years.

CLINICAL MANIFESTATIONS

The basic defect associated with LEMS appears to be an autoantibody-mediated derangement in presynaptic calcium channels leading to a reduction in calcium-mediated exocytosis of acetylcholine (ACh) at neuromuscular and autonomic nerve terminals. The decreased release of ACh quanta from the cholinergic nerve endings produces a reduced postjunctional response. Unlike in myasthenia gravis, the number and the quality of postjunctional ACh receptors remain unaltered, and the end-plate sensitivity is normal. The neuromuscular junction abnormality of LEMS resembles that of magnesium intoxication or botulism poisoning, in which the release of presynaptic ACh is attenuated. Clinical manifestations include skeletal muscle weakness in patients with small cell carcinoma of the lung.

ETIOLOGY

Myasthenic syndrome is an autoimmune disease in which immunoglobulin G antibodies are produced in response to presynaptic calcium channels.

TREATMENT

Anticholinesterase drugs that are effective in treating myasthenia gravis are *not* effective in patients with this syndrome. 4-Aminopyridine, which stimulates the presynaptic release of ACh, may improve skeletal muscle strength.

ANESTHETIC CONSIDERATIONS

Muscle weakness, fatigue, hyporeflexia, and proximal limb muscle aches are the dominant features of LEMS. The diaphragm and other respiratory muscles are also involved. Autonomic nervous system dysfunction is often present and is manifested as impaired gastric motility, orthostatic hypotension, and urinary retention.

Patients with LEMS experience a brief increase in muscle strength with voluntary contraction, distinguishing it from myasthenia gravis. Tetanic stimulation results in a progressive augmentation in muscle strength as the frequency of the stimulation is increased. Posttetanic potentiation is also enhanced.

There is no cure for LEMS. Treatment is aimed at improving muscle strength and reversing autonomic deficits. 3,4-Diaminopyridine is used in some patients to improve muscle strength. It acts presynaptically to promote calcium influx and to increase the number of ACh quanta that are liberated by a single nerve action potential. Anticholinesterase agents, plasmapheresis, corticosteroids, intravenous immunoglobulin,[107] and immunosuppressive drugs provide improvement for some patients with LEMS. Patients being treated with aminopyridine derivatives should have their medication continued into the preoperative period.[30]

An index of suspicion for LEMS should be maintained in patients undergoing surgery who have suspected or diagnosed carcinoma of the lung. Patients with LEMS are extremely sensitive to the relaxant effects of both depolarizing and nondepolarizing muscle relaxants. Inhalational anesthetics alone may provide adequate relaxation, but if muscle relaxants are required, their dosages should be reduced, and the neuromuscular blockade should be closely monitored.[108] Neuromuscular reversal with an anticholinesterase agent may be used. Prolonged ventilatory assistance may be required postoperatively.

E. Kyphoscoliosis

DEFINITION

Kyphoscoliosis is a deformity of the costovertebral skeletal structures that is characterized by anterior flexion (kyphosis) and lateral curvature (scoliosis) of the vertebral column.

ETIOLOGY

The incidence of idiopathic kyphoscoliosis is about 4 in 1000. The disease seems to have a familial predisposition, with girls and women being affected about four times more often than boys and men.

A vertebral column curve of greater than 40 degrees is considered severe and is most likely associated with physiologic alterations in cardiopulmonary function. Restrictive lung disease and pulmonary hypertension progressing to cor pulmonale are the principal causes of mortality in patients with kyphoscoliosis. As the scoliotic curve worsens, more lung tissue is compressed, resulting in decreased vital capacity and dyspnea with mild exertion. Work of breathing is increased by abnormal mechanical properties of the thorax and by increased airway resistance resulting from small lung volumes. The alveolar-to-arteriolar difference for oxygen is increased. The arterial carbon dioxide pressure is usually normal, but relatively minor insults such as bacterial or viral upper respiratory tract infections may result in acute respiratory failure. A poor cough reflex contributes to frequent pulmonary infections. Pulmonary hypertension reflects increased pulmonary vascular resistance resulting from compression of lung vasculature by the curve in the spine and the pulmonary vascular response to arterial hypoxemia.

ANESTHETIC CONSIDERATIONS

Anesthetic management of these patients should begin with a thorough preoperative assessment of the physiologic derangements produced by the skeletal deformity. Pulmonary function tests, specifically vital capacity and forced expiratory volume in 1 second, reflect the magnitude of restrictive lung disease. Arterial blood gases are helpful in detecting unrecognized arterial hypoxemia or acidosis that could be contributing to pulmonary hypertension. These patients may enter the preoperative period with pneumonia resulting from chronic aspiration of gastric fluid. Any reversible components of pulmonary dysfunction, such as infections or bronchospasm, should be corrected before elective surgery is performed. Preoperative medication should be administered judiciously because of the narrow margin of safety in these patients (decreased ventilatory reserve) and the adverse effects on the pulmonary vascular resistance that would occur with respiratory acidosis from hypoventilation. Intraoperatively, controlled ventilation facilitates adequate arterial oxygenation and elimination of carbon dioxide. Nitrous oxide should be used with caution because it may increase pulmonary vascular resistance. Arterial oxygen saturation should be monitored continuously to ensure adequacy of oxygenation/ventilation. Central venous pressure measurements may provide an early warning of increased pulmonary vascular resistance produced by nitrous oxide. It has been suggested that these patients have an increased incidence of malignant hyperthermia, so vigilant monitoring of end-tidal carbon dioxide and temperature is recommended.

RENAL SYSTEM

A. Acute Renal Failure

DEFINITION

Acute renal failure is a rapid deterioration in renal function that results in retention of nitrogenous waste products (azotemia).

ETIOLOGY

Azotemia can be divided into prerenal, renal, and postrenal types, depending on its causes. Prerenal azotemia results from an acute decrease in renal perfusion. Renal azotemia is usually the result of intrinsic renal disease, renal ischemia, or nephrotoxins. Postrenal azotemia is the result of urinary tract obstruction or disruption. Up to 50% of cases are caused by ischemia and nephrotoxins following major trauma or surgery. This is also called *acute tubular necrosis*. Potential toxins include aminoglycosides, x-ray contrast dyes, and (in some patients) nonsteroidal antiinflammatory drugs. Other factors predisposing to acute renal failure include preexisting renal impairment, advanced age, atherosclerotic vascular disease, diabetes, and dehydration.

LABORATORY RESULTS

Acute renal failure is thought of as either oliguric (urinary volume less than 400 mL/day) or anuric (urinary volume less than 100 mL/day). However, nonoliguric acute renal failure (urine volume greater than 400 mL/day) may now account for up to 50% of cases. These patients have a lower urine sodium concentration than do oliguric patients. Moreover, they appear to have a lower complication rate and require shorter hospitalization. Creatinine clearance is the best predictor of early acute tubular necrosis and the best laboratory value for distinguishing between acute tubular necrosis and prerenal azotemia.

CLINICAL MANIFESTATIONS

Please refer to the later discussion of chronic renal failure.

TREATMENT

Standard treatment includes restriction of fluids, sodium, potassium, and protein intake. Dialysis may be employed to treat or prevent uremic complications. Peritoneal dialysis and hemodialysis can be equally effective, yet elevation and immobilization of the diaphragm associated with continuous peritoneal dialysis may predispose patients to respiratory complications. Standard hemodialysis may also be replaced by continuous arteriovenous or venovenous hemofiltration, which may be better tolerated in critically ill patients.

ANESTHETIC CONSIDERATIONS

Please refer to the later discussion of chronic renal failure. Fenoldopam (direct dopamine-1 receptor agonist) infusion of 0.1 to 0.3 mcg/kg/min, to increase renal perfusion and, potentially, urine output, may be of benefit.

PROGNOSIS

Sepsis remains the most common cause of death in patients with acute renal failure. Urinary function improves over the course of several weeks but may not return to normal for up to 1 year.

B. Chronic Renal Failure

DEFINITION

Chronic renal failure is characterized by a progressive decrease in the number of functioning nephrons that leads to an irreversible reduction in the glomerular filtration rate.

ETIOLOGY

Common diseases that lead to chronic renal failure are chronic glomerulo-nephritis, diabetic nephropathy, hypertensive nephrosclerosis, and polycystic renal disease.

LABORATORY RESULTS

The chest x-ray study should be examined for possible fluid overload (be aware of when the patient last underwent dialysis) or pulmonary edema. Electrolytes, complete blood count, and coagulation factors should be checked, because all may be affected.

CLINICAL MANIFESTATIONS
Metabolic

Hyperkalemia, hyperphosphatemia, hypocalcemia, hypermagnesemia, hyperuricemia, and hypoalbuminemia are possible. Water and sodium retention results in extracellular fluid overload and hyponatremia. Failure to excrete nonvolatile acids causes a high anion gap and metabolic acidosis. Chronic renal failure interferes with normal excretion of hydrogen ions by the kidneys and results in metabolic acidosis. Treatment of the acidosis may include hemodialysis or intravenous administration of sodium bicarbonate.

Hematologic

Anemia is present because of decreased erythropoietin production, decreased red cell production, and decreased cell survival. Anemia and metabolic acidosis result in a rightward shift of the oxyhemoglobin dissociation curve. Both platelet function and white cell function are impaired in patients with renal failure. This is clinically manifested as a prolonged bleeding time and increased susceptibility to infection. Patients who have recently undergone hemodialysis may also have residual anticoagulant effects from heparin. Observe the prothrombin time and partial thrombo-plastin time, especially if regional anesthesia is being considered.

Cardiovascular

Cardiac output is increased to maintain oxygen delivery. Sodium retention and abnormalities in the renin-angiotensin system result in systemic arterial hypertension. Left ventricular hypertrophy is common. Extracellular fluid overload, along with the increased demands of anemia and hypertension, predispose these patients to cardiomegaly and congestive heart failure. Arrhythmias may result from metabolic abnormalities. Hypovolemia may develop if too much fluid is removed with dialysis.

Pulmonary

Chronic renal failure interferes with normal excretion of hydrogen ions by the kidneys and results in metabolic acidosis. Treatment of the acidosis may include hemodialysis or intravenous administration of sodium bicarbonate. Pulmonary edema may result from an increase in permeability of the alveolar-capillary membrane with the appearance of "butterfly wings" on chest x-ray studies.

Endocrine

Diabetes mellitus is common because of peripheral resistance to insulin. Secondary hyperparathyroidism resulting from chronic hypocalcemia leads to osteodystrophy and vulnerability to pathologic fractures.

Gastrointestinal

Anorexia, nausea, vomiting, and ileus are associated with azotemia. Gastric fluid volume and acidity are increased. These changes, combined with delayed gastric emptying related to autonomic neuropathy, predispose these patients to pulmonary aspiration.

Neurologic

Asterixis, lethargy, confusion, seizures, and coma are manifestations of uremic encephalopathy. Autonomic and peripheral neuropathies are common. Peripheral neuropathies are typically sensory and involve the distal lower extremities. The median and common peroneal nerves are most often affected.

TREATMENT

Treatment may include intermittent hemodialysis using an arteriovenous fistula or continuous peritoneal dialysis through an implanted catheter. Renal transplantation may become necessary.

ANESTHETIC CONSIDERATIONS

Monitoring

Avoid measuring blood pressure in an arm with an arteriovenous fistula. Consider invasive monitoring, especially for procedures involving major fluid shifts. Intraarterial monitoring is indicated for patients with poorly controlled hypertension.

Premedication

Aspiration prophylaxis with a histamine-2 blocker, a nonparticulate antacid (sodium citrate [Bicitra]), and metoclopramide may be indicated.

Induction

Rapid sequence induction with cricoid pressure is indicated for patients with nausea, vomiting, or gastrointestinal bleeding. Reduced protein binding of drugs results in more unbound drug to act at receptor sites. Succinylcholine should be avoided in patients with a serum potassium level greater than 5 mEq/L. Atracurium, mivacurium, and *cis*-atracurium are the muscle relaxants of choice. Expect a prolonged response to the other nondepolarizing muscle relaxants.

Maintenance

Agents that reduce cardiac output (principal compensatory mechanism for anemia) should be avoided. Isoflurane and desflurane are the preferred volatile agents because they have the least effect on cardiac output. Use of meperidine may result in accumulation of the metabolite normeperidine. Morphine and its effects may be prolonged. If regional anesthesia is considered, the adequacy of coagulation should be confirmed, and the presence of uremic neuropathies should be excluded. The duration of action of local anesthetics may be shortened because of elevated tissue blood flow secondary to increased cardiac output. Ventilation of the lungs should maintain normocapnia and reduce the effects of positive-pressure ventilation on cardiac output. Hypoventilation, which results in respiratory acidosis, should also be avoided. However, hyperventilation causing respiratory alkalosis shifts the oxyhemoglobin dissociation curve to the left and reduces tissue oxygen availability.

Fluid Management

The use of lactated Ringer's injection should be avoided in hyperkalemic patients when large volumes of fluid may be required because of the potassium concentration of 4 mEq/L. Consider colloid earlier versus traditional crystalloid fluid replacement to increase intravascular volume and to promote renal perfusion and less interstitial fluid leakage (i.e., pulmonary edema reduction).

C. Urolithiasis

DEFINITION

Urolithiasis, or "kidney stones," refers to the presence of calculi, typically composed of calcium oxalate. These calculi result from hypercalciuria or hyperoxaluria. Other types of stones include magnesium ammonium phosphate, calcium phosphate, and uric acid.

ETIOLOGY

Causes of hypercalcemia and hypercalciuria are primarily hyperparathyroidism, vitamin D intoxication, malignancies, and sarcoidosis. Small bowel bypass is associated with hyperoxaluria. Alterations in urine pH and the presence of metabolic disturbances can also result in formation of renal stones, which differ in composition from the typical oxalate variety.

TREATMENT

Extracorporeal shock wave lithotripsy is a noninvasive treatment of renal stones. It transmits shock waves through water and focuses them on the stone by biplanar fluoroscopy. For patients with arrhythmias, shock waves can be delivered during the heart's refractory period (approximately 20 milliseconds after R wave) to avoid initiating further cardiac arrhythmias. Patients with artificial cardiac pacemakers risk pacemaker dysfunction with this form of therapy. Percutaneous nephrostomy can also be performed for removal of stone, obstruction, or biopsy. A needle is passed into the renal collecting duct, a catheter can be placed over the needle, and the kidney is drained. Anesthetic options include local anesthesia with sedation, regional anesthesia, and general anesthesia.

ANESTHETIC CONSIDERATIONS

General anesthesia, intravenous sedation, or regional anesthesia, including epidural and intercostal nerve blocks with local infiltration, may be used to provide analgesia during lithotripsy. Regardless of the anesthetic regimen, the patient must remain still because movement (including excessive diaphragmatic excursion) can move the stone from the wave focus. The sitting position may be associated with peripheral pooling of blood, especially with the use of regional anesthesia and resultant vasodilatation. Immersion in water increases hydrostatic pressures on the abdomen and thorax, which can displace blood into the central circulation. This increase in central venous pressure may result in acute congestive heart failure in patients with limited cardiac reserve. The hydrostatic forces on the thorax likewise result in decreases in chest wall compliance and functional residual capacity. This may produce ventilation/perfusion mismatches. Water in the immersion tub should be kept warm, to avoid hypothermia. An alternative option to an immersion tank is a lithotripsy table. Extracorporeal shock wave lithotripsy is contraindicated in patients with abdominal aortic aneurysms, spinal cord tumors, or orthopedic implants in the lumbar region. Parturients, obese patients, and patients with coagulopathies are also not good candidates for this procedure.

A. Adult Respiratory Distress Syndrome

DEFINITION

Adult respiratory distress syndrome (ARDS) is characterized by arterial hypoxemia associated with acute lung injury. It is characterized by diffuse alveolar damage and noncardiogenic pulmonary edema. ARDS can lead to acute respiratory failure and death. Acute respiratory failure is often synonymous with acute (formerly adult) respiratory distress syndrome. Common features include the following: a history of a preceding noxious event that served as a trigger for the subsequent development of ARDS, an interval from hours to days of relatively normal lung function following the insult, and the rapid onset and progression over several hours of dyspnea, severe hypoxia, diffuse bilateral pulmonary infiltration, and stiffening and noncompliance of the lungs.

INCIDENCE AND PREVALENCE

Approximately 150,000 to 200,000 new cases of ARDS are diagnosed yearly in the United States. ARDS is precipitated by numerous conditions and frequently affects young people who were previously in excellent health.

Risk factors for the development of ARDS appear to be additive. The incidence of occurrence is 25% with the presence of one risk factor, 42% with the presence of two, and 85% with the presence of three. The mortality rate for ARDS remains high, ranging from 50% to 70%. However, the mortality rate often exceeds 90% when gram-negative septic shock precedes ARDS development.

ETIOLOGY

Events and risk factors associated with the development of ARDS include the following: (1) shock (septic, cardiogenic, or hypovolemic), (2) trauma, (3) pulmonary infection (e.g., with *Pneumocystis carinii* or *Escherichia coli*), (4) disease states that result in the release of inflammatory mediators (e.g., extrapulmonary infections, disseminated intravascular coagulation, anaphylaxis, coronary bypass grafting, and transfusion reactions), (5) exposure to various agents (e.g., narcotics, barbiturates, or oxygen), (6) diseases of the central nervous system, (7) aspiration (e.g., of gastric contents, or as in drowning), and (8) metabolic events (e.g., pancreatitis and uremia). Alveolar damage may occur directly, as a result of aspiration, pneumonia, pulmonary contusions, and inhalation injuries. The damage may also result from indirect lung injury in response to sepsis, trauma, shock, activation of complement, multiple blood transfusions, and cardiopulmonary bypass.

The diffuse alveolar damage results in an increase in capillary alveolar permeability leading to increased lung water and high concentrations of proteins in the lung parenchyma and alveoli. This leads to pulmonary edema, inactivation of surfactant, impaired gas exchange, and decreased lung compliance. As the syndrome progresses, collagen formation leads to progressive obliteration of alveoli, respiratory bronchioli, and interstitium, resulting in a decreased ventilation/perfusion ratio, arterial hypoxemia, and right ventricular failure.

LABORATORY RESULTS

The chest x-ray study may initially be clear or may exhibit bilateral diffuse infiltrates. Later, infiltrates will become extensive and progress to complete opacification. In early stages, arterial blood gases may show hyperventilation-induced respiratory alkalosis and mild hypoxemia that improves with the administration of supplemental oxygen. In the later stages of ARDS, hypoxemia is not improved by oxygen administration, and hypercarbia develops because of increased dead-space ventilation.

CLINICAL MANIFESTATIONS

Classically, patients with ARDS are dyspneic, hypoxic, and hypovolemic and often require intubation and mechanical ventilation. In late stages, metabolic acidosis, hypotension, decreased cardiac output, and death may occur. The clinical presentation of ARDS resembles that of pulmonary edema and aspiration pneumonitis. Findings on histologic examination are similar to those of aspiration pneumonitis, except fibrosis of lung is more pronounced. Recovery of lung function is unpredictable. Milder cases resolve quickly, whereas others progress to fibrosis and death.

TREATMENT

Early recognition and treatment with supportive therapy and prevention of complications afford the best chance of recovery from ARDS. Maintenance of tissue oxygenation and replacement of lost intravascular fluids are the main goals of therapy. Preservation of end-organ perfusion is of utmost importance. Treatment is supportive and includes correction of hypoxia, preload and afterload reduction, and inotropic support as indicated.

Therapy may include oxygen administration, intravascular fluid management, and mechanical ventilation with the use of positive end-expiratory pressure (PEEP), inspiratory hold, or reverse inspiratory/expiratory ratio. Medications that may be used include steroids, diuretics, inhaled β-adrenergic agonists, and cardiac drugs such as digitalis and inotropes. Extracorporeal membrane oxygenation is sometimes used in the most severe cases, but it is associated with complications and has not been shown to improve survival. Because lung infections (e.g., *P. carinii* pneumonia) mimic ARDS, antibiotic therapy often is initiated before the cause of respiratory failure is known.

ANESTHETIC MANAGEMENT

Anesthetic preparation includes evaluation of the patient's respiratory, cardiac, and renal status. Ventilator settings should be noted, and special attention should be devoted to peak inspiratory pressures and PEEP levels. If the anesthesia ventilator cannot accommodate these settings, then arrangements must be made to bring the patient's ventilator into the operating room. The nature of lung sounds and amount of secretions should be noted. The presence of excess secretions should alert the anesthetist to the potential risk of airway obstruction. The degree of barotrauma from prolonged mechanical ventilation with high levels of PEEP can be assessed by the presence of chest tubes and subcutaneous emphysema secondary to pneumothorax. The effectiveness of therapy with bronchodilators should be assessed because the use of these drugs may be initiated preoperatively and continued intraoperatively if effective. An arterial line should be placed preoperatively and arterial blood gas analysis performed. If possible, lactic acid values should be determined.

Volume status should be evaluated closely because patients with ARDS often are hypovolemic. Invasive monitoring through central venous lines and pulmonary artery catheters often is available, and cardiac filling pressures along with cardiac output values should be assessed. Patients requiring inotropic support may arrive for surgery with infusions of dopamine or dobutamine. For all procedures, renal function should be monitored with a bladder catheter. Antibiotic therapy should be continued intraoperatively, and steroid preparations should be considered if patients were receiving these medications preoperatively.

Because patients with ARDS often are hemodynamically unstable, careful titration of anesthetic agents and adjunct agents is necessary. Owing to the multisystemic involvement characteristic of ARDS, drug metabolism and elimination should be carefully considered. An altered volume of distribution and rate of drug metabolism, as well as altered liver and kidney function, require more gradual and decreased dosing of benzodiazepines, narcotics, muscle relaxants, induction agents, and inhalation agents. The use of nitrous oxide is rarely possible because of high fractional inspired oxygen requirements.

Transport should be carefully planned so that complications are minimized and safe arrival in the intensive care unit is ensured. Patients should undergo pulse oximetry, electrocardiography, and blood pressure transport monitoring (by arterial line or noninvasively) before departure from the operating room. Breath sounds should be continually assessed with a precordial stethoscope. A full tank of oxygen and PEEP adaptor valves should be available for transport. The potential need for emergency medications and a defibrillator should be considered. If the patient's ventilator needs to be returned to the intensive care unit, plans should be made so that it arrives there before the patient does. Finally, if possible, another member of the anesthesia team should accompany the patient during transport. Regional anesthesia may be acceptable, if it is not contraindicated by hemodynamic instability, coagulopathy, or sepsis.

B. Aspiration Pneumonia

DEFINITION

Pulmonary aspiration has two components: gastric contents escape from the stomach into the pharynx and then enter the lungs. This situation results from preexisting disease, airway manipulation, and the inevitable compromise in protective reflexes that accompanies the anesthetic process. Aspirates are commonly categorized as contaminated, acidic, particulate, and nonparticulate. Pneumonia is an acute infection of the lung parenchyma caused by bacteria or viruses.

INCIDENCE AND PREVALENCE

Fewer than half of all aspirations lead to pneumonia. Pneumonia occurs most often in patients suffering pulmonary ingestion of virulent material or who are immunocompromised. Ingestion of highly acidic or particulate aspirate may cause severe respiratory damage without an infectious component. Patients who initially show no signs of infection, however, may develop pneumonia over the long term because of the severity of the lung injury and prolonged respiratory support.

ETIOLOGY

Aspiration usually occurs when normal protective reflexes (swallowing, coughing, and gagging) fail, although vomiting and gastroesophageal reflux are common clinical events. Reflex responses to aspiration are automatically blunted with depression of consciousness. The most common setting for depression of reflex protection occurs during anesthesia induction and emergence.

Three aspiration syndromes have been identified: chemical pneumonitis (Mendelson's syndrome), mechanical obstruction, and bacterial infection. Characteristics of Mendelson's syndrome include the triphasic sequence of immediate respiratory distress combined with bronchospasm, cyanosis, tachycardia, and dyspnea followed by partial recovery and a final phase of gradual return of function. This acute chemical pneumonitis is caused by the irritative action of hydrochloric acid, which is quite damaging to the lungs.

PATHOPHYSIOLOGY

The pathophysiology of aspiration pneumonia often is characterized according to the pH, volume, and type of gastric material aspirated. It has long been believed that gastric fluid volume greater than 0.4 mL/kg (25 mL/70 kg) and a pH lower than 2.5 are significant indicators of risk for aspiration sequelae. It has been suggested that the focus be shifted away from gastric fluid volume and pH toward patient characteristics, condition, and anesthetic practices that place the patient at risk for pulmonary aspiration.

When aspiration is severe, damage to the entire alveolocapillary barrier, including the basement membranes and capillary endothelial cells, may occur. Damage to these structures causes an increase in the permeability of the pulmonary blood vessels, followed by a profound capillary leak syndrome. Hypoxia occurs secondary to a shunting effect. Initially, the arterial carbon dioxide tension tends to be low because of hyperventilation from hypoxic drive and the mechanical and irritative stimuli to the large airways and parenchyma. Hypercarbia associated with hypoventilation occurs from either acute or chronic lung obstruction and is a negative prognostic sign.

CLINICAL MANIFESTATIONS

Arterial hypoxemia, the hallmark sign of aspiration pneumonia, may not be suspected until after surgery, when unanticipated instability occurs in an otherwise healthy patient. Signs to alert the anesthetist include tachypnea, dyspnea, tachycardia, hypertension, and late cyanosis.

Diagnosis may be difficult to establish unless the aspiration is witnessed or gastric contents are visualized directly in the airway or suctioned from an endotracheal tube. Arterial blood gas analysis and chest radiography are needed for evaluation. Infiltrates in perihilar and basilar regions along with pulmonary edema are most common findings on radiography; however, aspiration pneumonitis may not be revealed for up to 6 to 12 hours after insult. Determination of tracheal aspirate pH, once advocated, has proved to be an inaccurate means of detection owing to the neutralization of secretions by mucus.

TREATMENT

When the use of general anesthesia is unavoidable, minimizing the risk of aspiration can be accomplished by pharmacologic prophylaxis and/or use of rapid sequence intubation and awake extubation.

Pharmacologic prophylaxis for aspiration has been common practice for many years. Much of the concern arose from the finding that large volumes of acidic gastric contents, if aspirated, caused lung damage and increased the risk of serious morbidity and mortality. Agents such as gastrokinetics, histamine blockers, anticholinergics, antacids, proton pump inhibitors, and antiemetics are all used alone or in various combinations to raise gastric pH and to lower volume. Evidence does not support the practice of routine preoperative administration of these gastric-related agents. Use of these agents in patients believed to exhibit risk factors should be continued.

The administration of clear nonparticulate antacids such as sodium citrate has been shown to be clinically effective in increasing the pH of gastric contents. Desired onset of action occurs within 15 minutes, and duration of action is 1 to 3 hours. Intravenous administration of the histamine-2 (H_2)-receptor blockers cimetidine, ranitidine, and famotidine, 45 to 60 minutes before surgery, can raise gastric pH. Metoclopramide stimulates gastric emptying, increases lower esophageal pressure, and acts as an antiemetic. When this agent is used in combination with H_2-receptor blockers or antacids, the resultant reduction in gastric volume and acidity may be helpful in reducing the risk of aspiration.

ANESTHETIC CONSIDERATIONS

If intubation is not expected to be difficult, a rapid sequence induction (rather than awake endotracheal intubation) is indicated. If awake or rapid sequence intubation is indicated for decreasing the risk of aspiration, awake extubation is needed. Premature extubation before the patient is fully awake, manifests reflexes, and can follow commands may place him or her at risk of aspiration and laryngospasm.

If vomiting or aspiration occurs during induction, immediate treatment includes tilting of the patient's head downward or to the side, rapid suctioning of the mouth and pharynx, and intubation. The outcome is related to the amount and type of aspirate. Patients should be observed for the following symptoms: a new cough or a wheeze, a decrease in oxygen saturation as measured by pulse oximetry greater than or equal to 10% of preoperative levels while breathing room air, or radiographic evidence of pulmonary aspiration. For patients who experience more severe aspirations, endotracheal intubation should be performed quickly and the cuff inflated so that further aspiration is prevented. Before 100% oxygen is administered and positive-pressure ventilation is initiated, the endotracheal tube should be suctioned. This measure has been advocated to avoid pushing aspirated material further down the tracheobronchial tree. A nasogastric tube should be placed for emptying of the stomach. If aspiration is severe, surgery may be postponed. Arterial blood gas analysis should be performed for determination of the extent of hypoxia. Early application of positive end-expiratory pressure is recommended for improving pulmonary function. Bronchoscopy should be reserved for those patients who are suspected of having aspirated solid material. Pulmonary lavage is not recommended unless conducting airways are obstructed. The use of steroids is controversial, and the routine use of antibiotics is not recommended.

C. Asthma

DEFINITION

Asthma is a respiratory condition that encompasses periodic attacks of bronchospasm associated with dyspnea, cough, and wheezing. Its hallmark is airway hyperreactivity in response to many stimuli, such as airborne substances (pollens, animal dander, chemicals), medications (aspirin, nonsteroidal antiinflammatory drugs), exercise, emotional excitement, and viral infections. Many factors (e.g., autonomic, endocrine, infectious, and immunologic) play a role in this disorder. Bronchospastic episodes are typically short-lived and reversible, and patients respond to therapy with complete recovery between episodes.

INCIDENCE AND PREVALENCE

Up to 14 to 15 million persons are afflicted with asthma in the United States. It is the most common chronic disease of childhood, affecting an estimated 4.8 million children. Asthma results in approximately 5000 deaths in the United States each year. Boys and men are affected twice as often as girls and women.

ETIOLOGY

Asthma is a heterogeneous clinical syndrome characterized by episodic hyperresponsive airways, interspersed with symptom-free periods. Airway inflammation and nonspecific hyperirritability of the tracheobronchial tree are now recognized as central to the pathogenesis. Environmental factors such as dust, cold, fumes, animal dander, pollen, chemicals, or stress (emotional or physical) can precipitate a bronchospastic episode. An overreactive parasympathetic nervous system allows the release of mediators causing the bronchiolar hyperreactivity. Immunoglobulin E (IgE) plays a role. An antigen that binds to IgE on mast cells causes degranulation. Bronchoconstriction is the result of subsequent release of the following: histamine; bradykinin; leukotrienes C, D, and E; platelet-activating factor; prostaglandins E_2, $F_{2\alpha}$, and D_2. Serotonin, a potent bronchoconstrictor, may also play a role. Vagal afferents in the bronchial tree are sensitive to these stimuli and to noxious stimuli, such as cold air, inhaled irritants, and instrumentation. Reflex vagal activation results in bronchoconstriction. Airway obstruction develops as airway passages constrict and become edematous (producing mucus); this inevitably leads to inspiratory and expiratory resistance to air flow. Hyperinflation distal to airway obstruction, altered pulmonary mechanics, and an increase in the work of breathing occur secondary to impaired expiration. Respiratory alkalosis occurs as a result of the alteration in the ventilation/perfusion (V/Q) relationships. Resultant hypoxemia occurs without hypercapnia and hyperventilation. Worsening obstruction invariably leads to hypercapnia and respiratory acidosis.

LABORATORY RESULTS

The chest x-ray study is normal in more than 75% of patients with asthma. A chest radiograph may exhibit hyperinflation with flattening of the diaphragm as well as other causes and complications of asthma (e.g., pulmonary edema, pneumonia, or pulmonary hypertension). Arterial blood gases in the early phase of an asthma attack reveal mild hypoxemia, hypocarbia, and respiratory alkalosis. As the attack intensifies, hypoxemia worsens, and hypercarbia and respiratory acidosis develop. Pulmonary function tests show a decrease in forced expiratory volume in 1 second. Residual volume, functional residual capacity, and total lung compliance are increased as a result of an increase in volume of the gas trapped beyond closed airways, and lung deflation is less because of airway obstruction. The electrocardiogram may show right ventricular strain (ST-segment changes, right-axis deviation, right bundle branch block, or right atrial or ventricular compromise). Eosinophilia (more than 275/mm^3) is common in patients with active IgE-mediated bronchial asthma. An increasing total eosinophil count often signals the acceleration of bronchial asthma before the patients experience symptoms.

CLINICAL MANIFESTATIONS

During remission, patients are asymptomatic (i.e., pulmonary function is normal). Key hallmarks of asthma in the awake patient include wheezing, dyspnea, cough (productive or nonproductive; frequently at night or early morning), labored respirations with accessory muscle use, tachypnea, chest tightness, prolonged expiratory phase of respiration, and fatigue. Typically, most attacks are short-lived, lasting minutes to hours. The asthmatic episode produces not only airflow obstruction, but also gas exchange abnormalities. The resulting low ventilation/perfusion (V/Q) state produces arterial oxygen desaturation. Hypoxemia is common, and carbon dioxide elimination is relatively well preserved until V/Q abnormalities are severe. Chronic asthma eventually leads to irreversible lung destruction, loss of lung elasticity, pulmonary hypertension, and lung hyperinflation.

In the anesthetized patient, manifestations of the asthmatic episode are wheezing, mucus hypersecretion, high inspiratory pressures, a blunted expiratory carbon dioxide waveform, and hypoxemia (see the following table).

Clinical Asthma Classification and Associated Pharmacotherapy

	Clinical Characteristics before Therapy	Pharmacologic Treatment*
Step 1 Mild intermittent asthma	Signs and symptoms up to twice per week Generally asymptomatic with normal peak flows between exacerbations Exacerbations brief, although intensity may vary Nighttime symptoms occur up to twice per month FEV_1 or PEFR ≥80% of predicted value	Short-acting bronchodilator, as needed: inhaled β_2-agonists are the first-line selection
Step 2 Mild persistent asthma	Signs and symptoms more than twice per week but less than once per day Exacerbations may affect activity Nighttime symptoms occur more than twice per month FEV_1 or PEFR ≥80% of predicted value	Long-term antiinflammatory medication: inhaled corticosteroid (low dose) Cromolyn or nedocromil, particularly in children Sustained-release theophylline is an alternative Zafirlukast or zileuton may be considered for patients ≥12 years old
Step 3 Moderate persistent asthma	Daily symptoms Daily use of short-acting β_2-agonist Exacerbations that affect activity occur at least twice a week and may last for days Nighttime symptoms occur more than once per week FEV_1 or PEFR 60%–80% of predicted value	Long-term control medications: medium-dose inhaled corticosteroids or low- to medium-dose inhaled corticosteroids plus long-acting bronchodilator (inhaled or oral β_2-agonist, sustained-release theophylline), especially for nocturnal symptoms
Step 4 Severe persistent asthma	Continuous signs and symptoms, frequently exacerbated Frequent nighttime symptoms Limited physical activity FEV_1 or PEFR ≤60% of predicted value	High-dose inhaled corticosteroids Long-acting bronchodilators, as indicated in step 3 Systemic corticosteroids (e.g., prednisone)

*For all severity steps, β_2-agonists are used for quick relief of acute symptoms.
FEV$_1$, Forced expiratory volume in 1 second; *PEFR,* peak expiratory flow rate.

TREATMENT

Treatment includes β_2-adrenergic agonists (albuterol, isoproterenol [Isuprel], metaproterenol [Alupent]), methylxanthines (theophylline) glucocorticoids (by metered-dose inhaler or intravenously), anticholinergics (ipratropium [Atrovent]), and mast cell stabilizing agents. All except the last may be used for short- or long-term treatment (see the following table).

Drug Therapy for Asthma

Drug Group	Specific Agent	Dose
Antiinflammatory drugs, cortico-steroids, mast cell–inhibiting agents	Hydrocortisone, intravenous	4 mg/kg bolus followed by infusion of 0.5 mg/kg/hr
	Methylprednisolone, intravenous	0.8 mg/kg bolus followed by infusion of 0.1 mg/kg/hr
	Beclomethasone dipropionate (Beclovent, Vanceril) (MDI)	42 mcg/puff; two puffs four times/day or four puffs twice/day
	Budesonide (Pulmicort Turbuhaler)	One–two inhalations twice/day
	Flunisolide (AeroBid) by MDI	250 mcg/puff; two–four puffs twice/day
	Fluticasone propionate (Flovent)	44 mcg/puff; two–four puffs twice/day
	Triamcinolone (Azmacort) by MDI	100 mcg/puff; two puffs three–four times/day or four puffs twice/day
	Cromolyn sodium (Intal) by MDI	100 mcg/puff; two–four puffs twice/day; two–four puffs four times/day
	Nedocromil (Tilade)	1.75 mg/puff; two puffs q6h
Bronchodilators, β₂-selective adrenergic drugs	Albuterol (Proventil, Ventolin) by MDI	90 mcg/puff; two puffs q4–6h (nebulized solution, 2.5 mg q1–4h)
	Bitolterol mesylate (Tornalate) by MDI	370 mcg/puff; two–three puffs q4–6h (nebulized solution, 1.5–3.5 mg q4–6h)
	Salmeterol xinafoate (Serevent) by MDI	21 mcg/puff; two puffs q12h
	Pirbuterol (Maxair)	200 mcg/puff; two puffs q4–6h
	Terbutaline (Brethine, Bricanyl) subcutaneous	0.25 mg (may repeat once after 15–30 min; maximum dose, 0.5 mg in 4 hr)
	Levalbuterol (Sepracor)	0.63 mg q6–8h nebulized PRN
Antimuscarinics	Ipratropium bromide (Atrovent)	18 mcg/puff; two puffs four times/day maximum, 12 puffs in 24 hr
Methylxanthine	Theophylline (Theo-Dur and others)	Extended-release capsules or tablets, 300–600 mg/day. Intravenous: 5–6 mg/kg loading; 0.9–1 mg/kg maintenance via slow infusion
Leukotriene modifiers	Montelukast (Singulair)	10-mg tablets once/day
	Zafirlukast (Accolate)	20-mg tablets twice/day
	Zileuton (Zyflo)	600-mg tablets twice/day
Anti-immuno-globulin E antibody	Omalizumab (Xolair)	150–300 mg every 4 wk to 225–375 mg every 2 wk subcutaneous injection

MDI, Metered-dose inhaler; PRN, as needed.

ANESTHETIC CONSIDERATIONS

A complete preoperative evaluation should be performed and should include history of the disease and current status, auscultation of lung sounds, and prescribed medication. Active wheezing may predispose the patient to a life-threatening event in the perioperative period. Therapeutic levels of theophylline, bronchodilating inhalers, and, in some cases, glucocorticoids should be verified. Preoperative administration of these drugs is advocated following recommended dosing guidelines. Sedatives (e.g., benzodiazepines) are desirable, especially for those whose disease has an emotional component, but these drugs should be administered carefully to avoid respiratory depression and apnea. Use care when opioids are administered, especially those associated with histamine release, which may lead to bronchospasm.

The onset of an asthmatic episode may occur abruptly in surgical patients. Airway manipulation, acute exposure to allergens, or the stress of surgery can provoke wheezing in a patient who was previously asymptomatic. The patient should be deeply anesthetized before intubation with propofol or one of the barbiturates. The barbiturates may cause histamine release; however, higher doses blunt this problem. Intravenous lidocaine given approximately 3 minutes before laryngoscopy and intubation may help to blunt untoward airway responses.

All volatile agents possess bronchodilating properties; however, isoflurane and desflurane can also cause airway irritation. When muscle relaxation is required, those drugs that have a potential to release histamine (e.g., atracurium) should be used with caution.

Intraoperative bronchospasm may be detected by noting changes in lung sounds, rising airway pressures, and difficulty in ventilation. If intraoperative bronchospasm occurs, inhaled bronchodilators, subcutaneous terbutaline, aminophylline, and/or volatile agents may be used for treatment.

Reversal agents (i.e., anticholinesterase combined with anticholinergics) are typically administered together to reverse the effects of nondepolarizing muscle relaxants. Anticholinesterase drugs may themselves precipitate bronchospasm. To prevent the likelihood of this occurrence, it has been suggested that the anticholinergic drug be given before the anticholinesterase agent (i.e., given separately). "Deep" extubation to decrease the likelihood of bronchospasm on emergence has been recommended for those not at risk of aspiration. Risk reduction strategies are listed in the following table.

Risk Reduction Strategies for Anesthetizing Asthmatic Patients

Preoperative
Encourage cessation of cigarette smoking for at least 8 weeks.
Aggressively treat airflow obstruction.
Administer antibiotics and delay surgery if respiratory infection is present.
Begin patient education regarding lung-expansion maneuvers.

Intraoperative
Limit duration of surgery to less than 3 hours.
Use regional anesthesia when possible.
Avoid the use of long acting neuromuscular blocking agents.
Use laparoscopic procedures when possible.
Substitute less ambitious procedure for upper abdominal or thoracic surgery when possible.

Postoperative
Encourage deep-breathing exercises or incentive spirometry.
Use continuous positive airway pressure.
Use intercostal nerve blocks and local anesthesia infiltration of incisional area for pain when appropriate.

D. Chronic Obstructive Pulmonary Disease

DEFINITION

Chronic obstructive pulmonary disease (COPD) is a term used to describe a variety of airway-related disease processes, such as emphysema, asthma, chronic bronchitis, bronchiectasis, and cystic fibrosis. These conditions cause an increase in resistance to flow of gases in the airway that often results in acute and chronic disease states that are reversible or irreversible. Chronic bronchitis and emphysema are the most common causes of COPD.

INCIDENCE AND PREVALENCE

COPD affects an estimated 15 to 20 million Americans and is the fifth leading cause of death in the United States. Chronic bronchitis and emphysema are the most common causes of COPD.

ETIOLOGY

The primary predisposing factor is a history of cigarette smoking. COPD results from progressive airflow obstruction as reflected by a decreased forced expiratory volume in 1 second (FEV_1). The decrease of FEV_1 is related to a decrease in the intrinsic size of the bronchial lumina, an increase in the collapsibility of bronchial walls, and a decrease in the elastic recoil of the lungs. Exacerbations may be precipitated by infection, congestive heart failure, oxygen therapy that blunts hypoxic drive, and pulmonary thromboembolism. The stages, characteristics, and recommended treatments for COPD are listed in the table on p. 145.

LABORATORY RESULTS

Chest x-ray studies often show hyperinflation and diaphragmatic flattening, right ventricular hypertrophy, a dilated proximal pulmonary artery, and attenuated pulmonary vasculature in the presence of associated pulmonary vascular disease. Pulmonary function tests show a decreased FEV_1/forced vital capacity ratio less than 75% of predicted values. Emphysematous patients have increased respiratory volume and total lung compliance but decreased diffusing capacity for cardiac output. The partial pressures of both oxygen (PaO_2) and carbon dioxide ($PaCO_2$) are generally not affected until the later stages of COPD. The electrocardiogram may exhibit right ventricular hypertrophy when right-sided heart failure is present. With the chronic respiratory acidosis that often accompanies COPD, $PaCO_2$ is elevated, and pH is low or normal. Acute exacerbations often result in an elevated $PaCO_2$ and an acidic pH. Hematocrit may be elevated in both acute and chronic disease states.

CLINICAL MANIFESTATIONS

Patient History

Chronic bronchitis is often manifested by a chronic productive cough, exertional dyspnea, and wheezing. Clinically, it is defined as the presence of a productive cough for more than 3 months over more than 3 successive years. Emphysema is primarily manifested by exertional dyspnea that is progressive, with or without a productive cough or wheezing.

Physical Examination

Patients with COPD often have an increased anteroposterior chest diameter ("barrel chest"), hyperresonance to percussion, and wheezing or rhonchi on

Therapy at Each Stage of Chronic Obstructive Pulmonary Disease

Stage	Character	Recommended Treatment
All		Avoidance of risk factors Influenza vaccination
0: At risk	Chronic symptoms (cough, sputum) Exposure to risk factors Normal spirometry	
I: Mild COPD	FEV_1/FVC <70% FEV_1 >80% predicted With or without symptoms	Short-acting bronchodilator when needed
II: Moderate COPD	IIA FEV_1/FVC <70% 50% < FEV_1 <80% predicted With or without symptoms	Regular treatment with one or more bronchodilators Rehabilitation Inhaled glucocorticosteroids if significant symptoms and lung function response
	IIB FEV_1/FVC <70% 30% ≤ FEV_1 >50% predicted With or without symptoms	Regular treatment with one or more bronchodilators Rehabilitation Inhaled glucocorticosteroids if significant symptoms and lung function response or if repeated exacerbations
III: Severe COPD	FEV_1/FVC <70% FEV_1 <30% predicted or presence of respiratory failure or right heart failure	Regular treatment with one or more bronchodilators Inhaled glucocorticosteroids if significant symptoms and lung function response or if repeated exacerbations Treatment of complications Rehabilitation Long-term oxygen therapy if respiratory failure Consider surgical treatments

COPD, Chronic obstructive pulmonary disease; *FEV₁*, forced expiratory volume in 1 second; *FVC*, forced vital capacity.

auscultation of the chest. Accessory muscles for breathing are used; these patients have a prolonged expiratory phase of respiration and use "pursed lip" breathing; clubbing of the fingers also may occur. The clinical features of the various types of COPD are listed in the following table.

Differential Diagnosis of Chronic Obstructive Pulmonary Disease

Diagnosis	Suggestive Features*
Chronic obstructive pulmonary disease	Onset in midlife; symptoms slowly progressive; long smoking history; dyspnea during exercise; largely irreversible airflow limitation
Asthma	Onset early in life (often childhood); symptoms vary from day to day; symptoms at night/early morning; allergy, rhinitis, or eczema also present; family history of asthma; largely reversible airflow limitation
Congestive heart failure	Fine basilar crackles on auscultation; chest x-ray study shows dilated heart, pulmonary edema; pulmonary function tests indicate volume restriction, not airflow limitation
Bronchiectasis	Large volumes of purulent sputum; commonly associated with bacterial infection; coarse crackles on auscultation; chest x-ray study or computed tomography shows bronchial dilation, bronchial wall thickening.
Tuberculosis	Onset at all ages; chest x-ray study shows lung infiltrate or nodular lesions; microbiologic confirmation; high local prevalence of tuberculosis
Obliterative bronchiolitis	Onset in younger age, nonsmokers; may have history of rheumatoid arthritis or fume exposure; computed tomography on expiration shows hypodense areas
Diffuse panbronchiolitis	Most patients male and nonsmokers; almost all have chronic sinusitis; chest x-ray study and high-resolution computed tomography show diffuse small centrilobular nodular opacities and hyperinflation

*These features tend to be characteristic of the respective diseases, but do not occur in every case. For example, a person who has never smoked may develop chronic obstructive pulmonary disease (especially in the developing world, where other risk factors may be more important than cigarette smoking); asthma may develop in adult and even elderly patients.

TREATMENT

Conservative management includes low-flow oxygen by nasal cannula or Venturi mask, bronchodilators, β_2-adrenergic agonists, ipratropium bromide, theophylline, and antiinflammatory agents (e.g., cromolyn sodium and adrenocortical steroids). Aggressive therapy includes subcutaneous injection of epinephrine or terbutaline sulfate, inhaled bronchodilators, aminophylline, adrenocortical steroids, and intubation and mechanical ventilation in cases not responsive to other therapies. The commonly used bronchodilator drugs are listed in the following table.

Commonly Used Bronchodilator Drugs

Drug	Metered-dose Inhaler (mcg)	Nebulizer (mg)	Oral (mg)	Duration of Action (hr)
β_2-Agonists				
Fenoterol	100–200	0.5–2	—	4–6
Salbutamol (albuterol)+	100–200	2.5–5	4	4–6
Terbutaline	250–500	5.10	5	4–6
Formoterol	12–24	—	—	12+
Salmeterol	50–100	—	—	12+
Anticholinergics				
Ipratropium	40–80	0.25–0.5	—	6–8
Tiotropium (Spiriva)	18 (dry powder)			24–72
Methylxanthines				
Aminophylline (SR)	—	—	225–450	Variable, ≤24
Theophylline (SR)	—	—	100–400	Variable, ≤24

ANESTHETIC CONSIDERATIONS

Preoperatively, patients should be optimally prepared before elective procedures. Assessment of recent changes in dyspnea, sputum, and wheezing should be addressed. Patients with FEV_1 less than 50% (1.2 to 1.5 L) usually have dyspnea on exertion. Those with FEV_1 less than 25% (less than 1 L) typically have dyspnea with minimal activity. Both general anesthesia and regional anesthesia have proved acceptable, but these patients are susceptible to postoperative respiratory failure. When sedation is given, as during a regional technique, great care should be taken because these patients are extremely sensitive to the respiratory depressant effects of these drugs. Blockade above a sensory level of T6 may decrease expiratory reserve volume, so there is an ineffective cough and thus poor clearance of secretions.

With general anesthesia, patients who are at high risk have an increased likelihood of postoperative ventilation, and this should be discussed with both the patient and the surgeon. The clinician should attempt to avoid cold, dry inspired gases. Volatile agents may produce bronchodilation. Nitrous oxide can cause enlargement and rupture of pulmonary bullae, leading to pneumothorax. Opioids may be used but can be associated with preoperative and postoperative ventilatory depression. Controlled ventilation with high tidal volume (10 to 15 mL/kg) and slow inspiratory rates optimizes PaO_2, minimizes airflow turbulence, and optimizes V/Q matching. During spontaneous ventilation with volatile agents, a greater degree of respiratory depression can be seen in patients with COPD. Perioperative arterial blood gases should be monitored.

E. Cor Pulmonale

DEFINITION

The term *cor pulmonale* or pulmonary heart disease is used loosely to describe three broad groups of patients that exhibit pulmonary hypertension resulting in progressive right ventricular hypertrophy, dilation, and eventual cardiac decompensation. This condition arises from the following: disorders that affect ventilatory drive or musculoskeletal respiratory mechanics; pulmonary airway, infiltrative, fibrotic, or vascular diseases; and diseases that are primarily cardiac but affect the pulmonary circulation and the lungs.

INCIDENCE AND PREVALENCE

In patients older than 50 years of age, cor pulmonale is the third most common cardiac disorder (after ischemic heart disease and hypertensive cardiac disease). The male-to-female ratio of incidence of the disease is 5:1; 10% to 30% of patients admitted to the hospital with coronary heart failure exhibit cor pulmonale.

The pulmonary disease responsible for the increased pulmonary vascular resistance (PVR) determines prognosis. In patients with chronic obstructive pulmonary disease (COPD) in whom alveolar oxygen tension can be maintained at near-normal levels, the prognosis is favorable. However, cor pulmonale associated with hypoxic lung disease is associated with a 70% rate of mortality within 5 years after onset of associated peripheral edema. Prognosis is poor for those patients in whom cor pulmonale is the result of gradual obstruction of pulmonary vessels by intrinsic pulmonary vascular disease or pulmonary fibrosis. These anatomic changes cause irreversible alterations in the pulmonary vasculature, resulting in fixed elevations of PVR.

ETIOLOGY

COPD is associated with the functional loss of pulmonary capillaries and the subsequent arterial hypoxemia; these events initiate pulmonary vasoconstriction, which is the leading cause of chronic cor pulmonale. The World Health Organization has proposed a classification of conditions associated with cor pulmonale. Diseases associated with hypoxic pulmonary vasoconstriction include the following: COPD, bronchiectasis, chronic mountain sickness, cystic fibrosis, idiopathic alveolar hypoventilation, obesity-related hypoventilation syndrome, neuromuscular disease, kyphoscoliosis, pleuropulmonary fibrosis, and upper airway obstruction. Diseases that produce obstruction or obliteration of the pulmonary vasculature include the following: pulmonary embolism, pulmonary fibrosis, pulmonary lymphangitic carcinomatosis, idiopathic pulmonary hypertension (PH), progressive systemic sclerosis, sarcoidosis, intravenous drug abuse, pulmonary vasculitis, and pulmonary veno-occlusive disease.

PATHOPHYSIOLOGY

Sustained pulmonary vasoconstriction produces hypertrophy of the smooth muscle in the tunica media and an irreversible increase in the PVR. In the presence of chronically elevated pulmonary capillary pressure, the lungs are increasingly resistant to pulmonary edema because lymph vessels expand and their ability to carry fluid away from the interstitial spaces increases. The lymphatic pumping action creates a suction effect, which results in negative pleural pressure. The rate with which right ventricular dysfunction develops depends on the magnitude of pressure increase in the pulmonary circulation and on the rapidity with which this increase occurs. When PH occurs gradually, as it does in COPD, right ventricular compensation occurs; congestive heart failure rarely occurs before mean pulmonary artery pressure (PAP) exceeds 50 mm Hg.

Patients with COPD have larger-than-normal increases in PAP when they execute maneuvers that increase pulmonary blood flow (e.g., exercise, even if resting hemodynamic status is normal). Derangements in intrapulmonary gas exchange are the major factors involved in the hemodynamic changes. Alveolar hypoxia appears to mediate locally the vasoconstriction of precapillary pulmonary vessels, and acidosis and hypercarbia potentiate this effect.

The compensatory mechanism for pressure overload on the right ventricle involves enhancement of contractility and an increase in preload, which result in an increase in right ventricular end-diastolic volume. In response to chronic pressure overload imposed by PH, right ventricular hypertrophy occurs. Right ventricular hypertrophy is characterized by increased firmness of the myocardium and increased thickness of its wall, most prominently in the pulmonary outflow tract. The papillary muscles and the trabeculae carneae may be twice as thick as normal. The thickness of individual muscle fibers also is greater than normal and may approximate that of left ventricular myofibers.

LABORATORY RESULTS

Chest x-ray study reveals evidence of COPD, right ventricular hypertrophy, dilation of the main pulmonary artery, and decreased markings of peripheral pulmonary vasculature. The electrocardiogram may reveal signs of right atrial enlargement (peaked P waves in the limb leads) and/or right ventricular hypertrophy (R greater than S in V_1, right-axis deviation), atrial fibrillation, or right bundle branch block (rSR' in V_1). Pulmonary function tests generally exhibit those changes consistent with the primary pulmonary disease.

CLINICAL MANIFESTATIONS

Clinical manifestations of cor pulmonale often are nonspecific and are obscured by coexisting COPD. Right-sided heart catheterization usually is required for diagnosis. Cardiac catheterization combined with pulmonary angiography provides the most definitive information on the degree of PH, cardiac reserve, and the effects of pulmonary vasodilator treatment.

Symptoms of cor pulmonale are retrosternal pain, cough, dyspnea on exertion, weakness, fatigue, early exhaustion, and hemoptysis. Occasionally, hoarseness secondary to left recurrent laryngeal nerve compression by the enlarged pulmonary artery is present. Syncope on effort may occur, reflecting the inability of the right ventricular stroke volume to increase in the presence of a fixed elevation of PVR. Physical signs of cor pulmonale include the following: elevation of jugular venous pressure, cardiac heave or thrust along the left sternal border and S_3 gallop, presence of an S_4 secondary to significant right ventricular hypertrophy, a widely split S_2, possible murmur of pulmonic and tricuspid insufficiency, hepatomegaly, ascites, and lower extremity edema (late signs).

TREATMENT

The goals of treatment are decreasing the workload of the right ventricle, reducing PVR, preventing increases in PAP, and avoiding major hemodynamic changes. Improvement of gas exchange is the primary focus of treatment in patients with COPD and cor pulmonale. Treatment includes supplemental administration of oxygen to maintain a PaO_2 greater than 60 mm Hg or an arterial oxygen saturation greater than 90%. Oxygen is the only vasodilator with a selective effect on pulmonary vessels whose use does not entail a risk of worsening hypoxemia. (See the listing of vasodilators in the table in the discussion of PH). A heart-lung transplantation may ultimately be needed when cor pulmonale progresses despite the provision of maximal medical therapy.

ANESTHESIA MANAGEMENT

In general, preoperative preparation for the patient with cor pulmonale includes the following: elimination and control of acute or chronic pulmonary infections, reversal of bronchospasm, improvement in clearance of secretions, expansion of collapsed or poorly ventilated alveoli, and adequate hydration. Regional anesthesia technique may be appropriate as long as a high sensory level of anesthesia is not required, because any decrease in systemic vascular resistance in the presence of a fixed PVR may produce undesirable degrees of systemic hypotension. Volatile agents decrease PVR. Nitrous oxide has been shown to increase PVR in patients with primary PH. Intravenous agents, with the exception of ketamine, appear to have little effect on PVR. During all stages of anesthesia, manipulations that increase PAP must be avoided. The following key principles should be followed:

- Keep the patient well oxygenated.
- Avoid acidosis.
- Avoid the use of exogenous and endogenous vasoconstrictors.
- Avoid presenting stimuli that increase sympathetic tone.
- Avoid hypothermia.

F. Cystic Fibrosis

DEFINITION

Cystic fibrosis is the most common life-shortening autosomal recessive disorder.

INCIDENCE AND PREVALENCE

Cystic fibrosis affects an estimated 30,000 persons in the United States, with 1000 new cases per year. Most are diagnosed between the ages of 3 months and 6 years, but 8% are not diagnosed until after 18 years. One in 31 Americans is an asymptomatic carrier of the defective gene. More than 80% of those born with cystic fibrosis are born to parents with no prior history of the disease.

ETIOLOGY

Cystic fibrosis is caused by a mutation of a gene on chromosome 7. The result is defective chloride ion transport in epithelial cells in the lungs, pancreas, liver, gastrointestinal tract, and reproductive organs. This decrease in chloride transport results in a decrease of sodium and water transport. This results in dehydrated, viscous secretions that can cause obstruction, destruction, and scarring of exocrine glands.

LABORATORY RESULTS

Because cystic fibrosis is an expiratory airflow obstructive disease, most pulmonary function test results will be abnormal. The white blood cell count may be elevated because of frequent pulmonary infections.

CLINICAL MANIFESTATIONS

Pancreatic insufficiency, meconium ileus at birth, diabetes mellitus, azospermia, and obstructive hepatobiliary tract disease (cirrhosis and portal hypertension) are often present. The primary causes of morbidity and mortality are bronchiectasis and chronic obstructive pulmonary disease (COPD). Typically, a cough, chronic purulent sputum production, and exertional dyspnea will be seen.

TREATMENT

Treatment is similar to that for bronchiectasis and focuses on alleviation of symptoms (mobilization and clearance of lower airway secretions and treatment of pulmonary infections) and correcting organ dysfunction (pancreatic enzyme replacement). Treatment of secretions is usually done by chest physical therapy with postural drainage. Bronchodilator therapy may also be instituted. Antibiotics are often given to relieve the increased secretions from pulmonary infections. If no pathogens are seen, bronchoscopy to remove lower airway secretions may be indicated if there is no response to common antibiotics.

ANESTHETIC CONSIDERATIONS

Management is based on the same principles as in patients with COPD and bronchiectasis. Elective procedures are delayed until optimal pulmonary function is ensured by controlling infections and removing secretions from the airways. Vitamin K may be given if liver function is poor or if absorption of fat-soluble vitamins is poor in the gastrointestinal tract. Preoperative sedation is probably unnecessary because of possible respiratory depression. Maintenance of anesthesia with a volatile agent and oxygen can decrease airway resistance by decreasing the bronchial smooth muscle tone. Volatile agents are also helpful in decreasing the responsiveness of hyperreactive airways. Humidified gases are also important to decrease the viscosity of secretions. Frequent suctioning is also necessary.

G. Pneumothorax and Hemothorax

DEFINITION

Pneumothorax is the presence of air or gas in the pleural space. Hemothorax is the presence of blood in the pleural space.

INCIDENCE AND PREVALENCE

Spontaneous pneumothorax occurs unexpectedly in healthy persons, most often in men 20 to 40 years of age. Secondary pneumothorax and hemo-pneumothorax are generally the result of trauma.

ETIOLOGY AND TREATMENT
Pneumothorax

Pneumothorax can be subdivided into three categories, depending on whether air has direct access to the pleural cavity. In *simple pneumothorax,* no communication exists with the atmosphere. Additionally, no shift of the mediastinum or hemidiaphragm results from the accumulation of air in the intrapleural space. The severity of pneumothoraces is graded on the basis of the degree of collapse: collapse of 15% or less is small; collapse of 15% to 60% is moderate; and collapse of greater than 60% is large. Treatment of simple pneumothorax is determined by the size and cause of injury and may include catheter aspiration or tube thoracostomy; close observation of the patient with simple pneumothorax is essential.

In *communicating pneumothorax,* air in the pleural cavity exchanges with atmospheric air through a defect in the chest wall. Because the exchange of air through the site of injury may often be heard, this entity is commonly known as a "sucking chest wound." Communicating pneumothorax represents a severe ventilatory disturbance because the affected lung collapses on inspiration and expands slightly on expiration. The exchange of air in and out of the wound results in a large functional dead space and a decrease in the efficacy of ventilation. The wound should be covered with an occlusive dressing immediately. Development of tension pneumothorax is possible (see next section). The injury should never be packed during inspiration because the negative pressure could suck the dressing into the chest cavity. Treatment measures include administration of supplemental oxygen, tube thoracostomy, and intubation; mechanical ventilation may be indicated.

Tension pneumothorax develops when air progressively accumulates under pressure within the pleural cavity. If the pressure becomes too great, the mediastinum shifts to the opposite hemithorax, and this causes compression of the contralateral lung and great vessels. Subsequently, venous return is decreased, and air enters the pleural space but cannot exit. Respiratory and cardiac disturbances ensue, exhibited by a decrease in cardiac output, a decrease in blood pressure, an increase in central venous pressure, and a shunting of blood to nonventilated areas. The hallmark signs of tension pneumothorax are hypotension, hypoxemia, tachycardia, increased central venous pressure, and increased airway pressure. Other findings include absence of breath sounds on the affected side, asymmetric chest wall movement, tracheal shift, displacement of the cardiac impulse, and hyperresonance to percussion in the affected hemithorax. In addition, the patient may exhibit extreme anxiety.

Tension pneumothorax is potentially lethal; therefore, immediate treatment is essential. Decompression of the chest can be performed with the insertion of a 16- or 18-gauge angiocatheter into the second or third interspace anteriorly or the fourth or fifth interspace laterally. A rush of air is heard when decompression occurs. The angiocatheter must be covered if the sucking of more air into the pleura is to be prevented.

Hemothorax

Hemothorax is the accumulation of blood in the pleural cavity. It usually is a result of trauma, but other causes include the rupture of small blood vessels in the presence of inflammation, pneumonia, tuberculosis, or erosion by tumors. The treatment of hemothorax consists of airway management as necessary, restoration of circulating blood volume, and evacuation of the accumulated blood. Thoracostomy may be indicated if the initial bleeding rate is greater than 20 mL/kg per hour. If bleeding subsides but its rate remains greater than 7 mL/kg per hour, if chest radiographic findings worsen, or if hypotension persists after initial blood replacement and decompression, thoracostomy is indicated.

PATHOGENESIS

Different presentations may be distinguished, according to the mechanism of injury, as described in the following sections.

Spontaneous

Pneumothorax usually is caused by rupture of alveoli near the pleural surface of the lung after a forceful sneeze or cough. This mechanism is most common in persons with a long, narrow chest and in those with emphysema.

Traumatic

Hemothorax, pneumothorax, and flail chest may occur after blunt chest trauma; however, they most frequently occur after rib fracture. Hemopneumothorax also may occur with penetrating injury.

Iatrogenic

Hemothorax and pneumothorax may occur after any of the following:

- Subclavian central line insertion (incidence, 2% to 16%)
- Supraclavicular block to the brachial plexus (incidence, 1%; hemothorax and pneumothorax can be complications of interscalene block but are rare with intercostal block)
- Barotrauma (from overdistention of the alveoli by positive end-expiratory pressure [PEEP]; an abrupt deterioration of alveolar oxygen tension and cardiovascular function during PEEP administration should arouse suspicion of pulmonary barotrauma, especially pneumothorax)
- Exposure to high airway pressures (e.g., during mechanical ventilation)
- Other surgical procedures (e.g., mediastinoscopy, radical neck dissection, mastectomy, or nephrectomy)

LABORATORY RESULTS

Chest x-ray study usually shows subcutaneous emphysema, pneumomediastinum, and pneumopericardium. Free fluid, as with hemothorax, may be best seen on a cross-table lateral film.

ANESTHETIC CONSIDERATIONS

Pneumothorax or hemothorax can significantly interfere with oxygenation and ventilation. Decreased cardiac output, as with tension pneumothorax, can exacerbate intrapulmonary shunting. Cyanosis indicates both cardiac and pulmonary involvement. Nitrous oxide can quickly expand the size of a pneumothorax if a chest tube is not in place. Nitrous oxide is acceptable for use if the chest tube is patent and functioning. A closed pneumothorax is a contraindication to the administration of nitrous oxide. Decreased pulmonary compliance (increased pulmonary inspiratory pressure) during administration of anesthesia to patients with a history of chest trauma may reflect the expansion of an unrecognized pneumothorax.

In the case of ventilator-related pneumothorax, mortality is significantly reduced if a chest tube is placed in less than 30 minutes. Development of tension pneumothorax during general anesthesia is manifested by sudden hypotension, loss of pulmonary compliance, or decreased ventilating volume. Patients with significant trauma may require fluid resuscitation and cardiovascular support. Agents chosen should have minimal cardiac depressant effects.

H. Pulmonary Edema

DEFINITION

Pulmonary edema is the accumulation of excess fluid in the interstitial and air-filled spaces of the lung. The mechanisms responsible for its development include an increase in hydrostatic pressure within the pulmonary capillary system, an increase in the permeability of the alveolocapillary membrane, and a decrease in intravascular colloid oncotic pressure. Pulmonary edema is classified as being either cardiogenic (high pressure, hydrostatic) or noncardiogenic (increased permeability).

TYPES

Cardiogenic Pulmonary Edema

Some type of left-sided heart incompetence or failure initiates cardiogenic pulmonary edema. *Left ventricular failure* implies that there is a decrease in left ventricular contractility, which ultimately leads to a reduction in both stroke volume and cardiac output. Incomplete left ventricular emptying elevates left ventricular end-diastolic volume, which, in turn, elevates left ventricular end-diastolic pressure. Increased left ventricular end-diastolic pressure is "reflected back," causing elevation of the left atrial, pulmonary venous, and pulmonary capillary pressures. When pulmonary capillary pressure reaches levels of 20 to 25 mm Hg (normal range, 10 to 16 mm Hg), the rate of fluid transudation often exceeds lymphatic drainage capacity, and alveolar flooding occurs.

Coronary artery disease, hypertension, cardiomyopathies, mitral regurgitation, and mitral stenosis are a few of the cardiac conditions that may increase pulmonary intravascular hydrostatic pressure and predispose a patient to the development of pulmonary edema. Several noncardiac problems, including pulmonary veno-occlusive disease, fibrosing mediastinitis, head trauma, cerebrovascular accident, exposure to high altitudes, and overhydration, are additional causes.

Noncardiogenic Pulmonary Edema

Noncardiogenic pulmonary edema is associated with an increase in endothelial permeability caused by an insult that disrupts the barrier function of the blood-tissue interface. Noncardiogenic pulmonary edema is associated with the leakage of both fluid and protein from the vascular space. Because this respiratory membrane disruption cannot be easily or directly measured, noncardiogenic pulmonary edema is said to exist when suspicious chest radiographic evidence coexists with insufficient hemodynamic basis. The presence of pulmonary wedge pressure less than 12 mm Hg and the absence of a significant history of cardiac disease generally suffice for exclusion of a hemodynamic mechanism.

Although many disorders are associated with noncardiogenic pulmonary edema, the most commonly encountered cause is systemic sepsis that leads to adult respiratory distress syndrome. Other clinical conditions associated with noncardiogenic pulmonary edema include the aspiration syndromes, inhalation of toxic fumes and gases, and embolization phenomenon.

Pulmonary edema is nearly always associated with some type of preexisting disease state or insult. If a patient with pulmonary edema presents with a prior history of congestive heart failure, hypertension, or ischemic heart disease, then the presence of cardiogenic pulmonary edema can be assumed. In addition to systemic sepsis, anaphylaxis, pancreatitis, disseminated intravascular coagulation, trauma, multiple transfusions, and near-drowning can all result in noncardiogenic pulmonary edema.

Neurogenic Pulmonary Edema

Neurogenic pulmonary edema begins with a massive outpouring of sympathetic nervous system stimulation triggered by central nervous system insult. This centrally mediated central nervous system overactivity typically occurs in the hypothalamic area. Excessive sympathetic activation induces remarkable hemodynamic alterations, primarily systemic and pulmonary vasoconstriction. The left ventricle fails because of the inordinate pressure work imposed by the systemic hypertension, and pulmonary blood volume increases because of the functional imbalance between the failing left ventricle and the normal right ventricle. Although this sequence seems to parallel that of hemodynamic pulmonary edema, a permeability component exists, as evidenced by the high protein concentration found in the pulmonary secretions of these patients.

Uremic Pulmonary Edema

Uremic pulmonary edema is seen in those patients with renal insufficiency or failure. Overhydration and expansion of the circulating blood volume lead to increases in pulmonary capillary pressures. Again, a "leaky" component exists because of the metabolic abnormalities associated with uremia. Reducing the circulating blood volume of these patients by hemodialysis promotes the resolution of this type of pulmonary edema.

High Altitude–Related Pulmonary Edema

High altitude–related pulmonary edema may occur in the absence of left ventricular failure whenever someone overexerts himself or herself before acclimating to a high altitude. The pathogenesis of this form of pulmonary edema is unclear but may be the result of intense hypoxic pulmonary arterial vasoconstriction or massive sympathetic discharge triggered by cerebral hypoxia.

Pulmonary Edema Caused by Upper Airway Obstruction

Pulmonary edema resulting from upper airway obstruction is caused by the prolonged, forced inspiratory effort against an obstructed upper airway. The most common cause of this type of pulmonary edema in adults is laryngospasm following extubation and general anesthesia. In children, pulmonary edema following obstruction caused by croup, epiglottitis, and laryngospasm also is well documented. Vigorous inspiration against obstruction creates high negative intrathoracic, transpleural, and alveolar pressures that enlarge the pulmonary vascular volume and subsequently the interstitial fluid volume. The capacity of the lymphatics becomes overwhelmed, and interstitial fluid transudes into the pulmonary alveoli. Hypoxia causes a massive sympathetic discharge that results in systemic vasoconstriction and a translocation of fluid from the systemic circulation to the already expanding pulmonary vascular and interstitial spaces. Hypoxia also increases pulmonary capillary pressures. Because hypoxia alters myocardial activity, left atrial function and left ventricular function are reduced.

During obstruction, vigorous inspiratory efforts are unsuccessful because of the airway obstruction. Unsuccessful expiration produces an increase in intrathoracic and alveolar pressures. Intrinsic positive end-expiratory pressure (PEEP) also is produced during this stage. Relief of the obstruction results in cessation of intrinsic PEEP.

The consequence of these events is the sudden massive transudation of fluid from the pulmonary interstitium into the alveoli, which results in pulmonary edema. The severity of pulmonary edema is determined by the extent of prior alveolar and capillary damage and the immensity of hemodynamic and cardiovascular alterations.

RISK FACTORS

Not all those who experience acute airway obstruction develop pulmonary edema, and no specific risk factors for its occurrence have been identified. Factors that may predispose to its formation following obstruction include youth, male gender, long periods of obstruction, overzealous perioperative fluid administration, and the presence of preexisting cardiac and pulmonary disease.

CLINICAL MANIFESTATIONS

Physical examination reveals an increased work of breathing. As water accumulates, the lungs become heavy and noncompliant, and a decrease in functional residual capacity occurs. This increase in the volume of extravascular lung fluid provides a potent stimulus for surrounding interstitial stretch receptors (J-receptors), whose activation results in tachypnea. Tachypnea is not relieved by the administration of oxygen and the return of arterial oxygen tension (PaO_2) to normal. Intercostal retractions and use of accessory muscles are apparent on physical examination. Signs of sympathetic stress stimulation such as hypertension, diaphoresis, and tachycardia often are noted. The expectoration of pink, frothy sputum signals that alveoli have been flooded.

The detection of basilar crackles on auscultation is the traditional hallmark of early pulmonary edema. In reality, by the time these crackles become audible, excess water has already flooded the alveoli and has overflowed into the terminal bronchioles. It is in the bronchioles, not in the alveoli, that the crackles of pulmonary edema are generated. The earliest and most often disregarded clinical sign is rapid, shallow breathing.

In cardiogenic pulmonary edema, heart size may be increased. High central venous pressures, an S_3 or S_4 gallop, and jugular venous distention often are observed. Chest radiography is still the most reliable and expedient tool for early detection of pulmonary edema. In cardiogenic pulmonary edema, the cardiac silhouette may appear abnormal or enlarged; in noncardiogenic pulmonary edema, it can be enlarged or remain normal. Interstitial edema can be observed before the alveoli flood and the onset of clinical signs occurs. Pleural effusions are common, and a "whited-out" or "butterfly" appearance may be noted.

Arterial blood gas analysis reveals hypoxemia secondary to ventilation/perfusion (V/Q) abnormalities. When right-to-left shunting is great, the PaO_2 can be affected by any change in the central venous oxygen content. Increases in oxygen consumption or decreases in cardiac output further reduce the PaO_2. The arterial carbon dioxide tension ($PaCO_2$) may be low, normal, or elevated. The initial hypocarbia is related to tachypnea and high minute volumes; at later stages, hypercarbia is frequently secondary to muscle fatigue and exhaustion. Changes in pH usually reflect changes in $PaCO_2$, but metabolic and V/Q or lactic acidosis may occur from tissue oxygen deficiency, low cardiac output, or sepsis.

TREATMENT AND ANESTHETIC CONSIDERATIONS

Treatment includes prompt recognition of the condition, the securing of a patent airway, supportive therapy with oxygenation, and the administration of diuretics. Although the onset of pulmonary edema after laryngospasm usually is immediate, cases have been reported of the occurrence of pulmonary edema several hours after laryngospasm. Therefore, it is recommended that patients who develop laryngospasm be observed postoperatively longer than the typical 60 to 90 minutes. The diagnosis of pulmonary edema and its differentiation into cardiogenic and noncardiac categories require the taking of a detailed medical history, physical examination, chest radiography, and arterial blood gas analysis.

Pulmonary edema is considered a medical emergency, and immediate intervention is required for treating the underlying disease, supporting other failing organ systems, and optimizing oxygen delivery. Oxygen should be administered by nasal cannula, face mask, or endotracheal tube. If oxygenation does not improve with the administration of high fractions of inspired oxygen, positive-pressure ventilation with either PEEP or continuous positive airway pressure must be initiated. Institution of positive-pressure mechanical ventilation in patients with acute pulmonary edema usually results in a prompt increase in oxygenation and, in some cases, in cardiac output. Improvement occurs because of superior inflation and V/Q matching.

Pharmacologic therapy includes the use of vasodilators, inotropes, steroids, and diuretics. Morphine sulfate has been used in the treatment of cardiogenic pulmonary edema because of its venodilatory and preload-reducing properties. Nitroprusside is a very effective preload and afterload reducer. By reducing systemic blood pressure, nitroprusside decreases the afterload on the left ventricle; this may result in better cardiac function, with a subsequent lowering of left atrial pressures. Inotropic agents such as dopamine or dobutamine improve myocardial contractility and lower cardiac filling pressures. In patients with chronic congestive heart failure and pulmonary congestion, digitalis augments contractility and promotes decreases in left atrial and ventricular filling pressures.

Fluid balance is managed with both fluid restriction and diuresis. This therapy helps achieve a "negative" fluid balance in hydrostatic pulmonary edema. Potent diuretics such as furosemide not only lower left atrial filling pressure by decreasing systemic venous tone but also induce diuresis of the expanded extravascular volume.

The type of fluid, whether crystalloid or colloid, that should be used in the presence of pulmonary edema remains controversial. Regardless of type used, it is generally agreed that fluid administration proceeds slowly.

I. Pulmonary Embolism

DEFINITION

Pulmonary embolism (PE) is an occlusion of the pulmonary vascular bed by an embolus. It may result from blood clots, fat, tissue fragments, tumor cells, air, amniotic fluid, or foreign objects.

INCIDENCE AND PREVALENCE

PE is responsible for approximately 50,000 deaths per year. It is the most common cause of acute pulmonary disease in hospitalized patients. It is the third most common cause of cardiovascular death after myocardial infarction and stroke. PEs originate from deep vein thrombosis (DVT) of the iliofemoral vessels in about 90% of patients, and the clinical course depends on the size of the clot. Evidence suggests that at least 5 million episodes of DVT occur annually in the United States, with about 10% leading to PE. Of those exhibiting PE, about 10% are fatal.

ETIOLOGY

PE is primarily the result of venous stasis, alterations or abnormalities in the blood vessel wall, and hypercoagulation. Most of these emboli arise from thromboses in vessels of the pelvis or lower extremities. The emboli can result in massive occlusion or blockage of a major branch of the pulmonary circulation, embolus with infarction of a portion of lung tissue, embolus without infarction (i.e., not severe enough to cause permanent lung injury), or multiple PEs, either chronic or recurrent. The pattern of occurrence and the severity determine the degree of hypoxic vasoconstriction, pulmonary edema, atelectasis, vagal stimulation, and release of neurohumoral substances such as histamine. PEs may also cause systemic hypotension, pulmonary hypertension (PH), decreased cardiac output, and shock.

DVT at proximal sites is more likely to cause symptoms. Three major factors promote the formation of venous thrombi: stasis of blood flow, venous injury, and hypercoagulation states. Other less common causes of PE include air, tumor, bone, fat, catheter fragments, and amniotic fluid. Fillers used in illicit drug preparations by intravenous drug abusers also may cause PE. Of particular concern to anesthesia providers are air emboli caused by the opening of venous structures during surgery or by disconnected intravenous lines.

LABORATORY RESULTS

Pulmonary angiography is the gold standard as a definitive diagnostic tool. Chest x-ray study may be normal or may show only subtle changes. A ventilation/perfusion scan may reveal an embolus if a perfusion defect exists in an area of normal ventilation. In the patient with PE, arterial blood gas (ABG) analysis generally reveals hypoxemia and increased differences between alveolar and arterial carbon dioxide tension (P_ACO_2 and $PaCO_2$), which result from ventilation of unperfused alveoli. Massive PE is associated with severe hypoxemia and hypocapnia. An initial difference between P_ACO_2 and end-tidal carbon dioxide tension ($PETCO_2$) is common early during the embolic event.

Echocardiographic and electrocardiographic (ECG) signs are noted in the following table.

Electrocardiographic and Echocardiographic Signs of Pulmonary Embolism

Method	Signs
Electrocardiography	Incomplete or complete right bundle branch block
	S in leads I and aV_L >15 mm
	Transition zone shift to V_5
	QS in leads III and aV_F but not in lead II
	QRS axis >90 degrees or indeterminate axis
	Low limb lead voltage
	T-wave inversion in leads III and aV_F or in leads V_1 to V_4
Echocardiography	Direct visualization of thrombus (rare)
	Right ventricular dilatation
	Right ventricular hypokinesis (with sparing of the apex)
	Abnormal interventricular septal motion
	Tricuspid valve regurgitation
	Pulmonary artery dilatation
	Lack of decreased inspiratory collapse of inferior vena cava

Imaging and laboratory tests available for diagnosis, and their advantages and disadvantages, are listed in the following table.

Advantages and Disadvantages of Diagnostic Tests For Suspected Pulmonary Embolism

Diagnostic Test	Advantages	Disadvantages
Plasma D-dimer enzyme-linked immunosorbent assay	A normal result makes PE exceedingly unlikely	Level is elevated in many systemic illnesses that mimic PE; unless a rapid assay is available, the turnaround time will be long
Electrocardiography	Universally available; may indicate acute cor pulmonale	Acute cor pulmonale on electrocardiography is not specific for PE; not a sensitive test
Impedance plethysmography	Portable, inexpensive, easy to use	Inaccurate, with failure to detect major non-obstructive proximal DVT
Chest radiography	Usually has minor abnormalities but occasionally pathognomonic; may suggest alternative diagnoses; may guide workup toward chest computed tomography rather than lung scan	Not specific

DVT, Deep venous thrombosis; *PE,* pulmonary embolism.

Continued

Advantages and Disadvantages of Diagnostic Tests For Suspected Pulmonary Embolism—cont'd

Diagnostic Test	Advantages	Disadvantages
Venous ultrasonography	Excellent for detecting symptomatic proximal DVT; surrogate for PE	Cannot image iliac vein thrombosis; imaging of calf is operator dependent; DVT may have embolized completely, resulting in a normal result
Nuclear venography	Image pelvic and calf veins; differentiate acute versus chronic DVT	Limited experience with this test
Contrast venography	Used to be gold standard; excellent for calf veins	Can cause chemical phlebitis; uncomfortable; costly; may fail to diagnose massive DVT because veins are filled with thrombus and cannot be opacified
Lung scanning	Standard initial imaging test for PE; high-probability scans are reliable for detecting PE; normal/near-normal scans are reliable for precluding PE	Most scans are neither high probability nor normal/near-normal; ventilation scans are falling out of favor; most test results are equivocal
Chest computed tomography	Excellent for PE in the proximal pulmonary arterial tree	Insensitive for important but distal PE
Magnetic resonance imaging	Excellent for anatomy and cardiac function	In preliminary use; not widely available; experience very limited
Echocardiography	Excellent for identifying right ventricular dilatation and dysfunction that is not obvious clinically, thus providing an early warning of potentially adverse outcome	Not specific; many patients with PE have normal echocardio-grams; the test cannot reliably differentiate causes of right ventricular dysfunction
Pulmonary angiography	Considered the gold standard for diagnosis	Invasive, costly, uncomfortable

DVT, Deep venous thrombosis; *PE,* pulmonary embolism.

CLINICAL MANIFESTATIONS

The patient's clinical presentation depends largely on the size of the embolus. Signs and symptoms of PE vary, and the differential diagnosis according to size of emboli may be difficult. Dyspnea of sudden onset appears to be the only common historical complaint. Hypoxia is a constant feature of PE, possibly owing to intrapulmonary shunting. Several clinical features can be associated with emboli of varying sizes.

Small emboli frequently go unrecognized; uncommonly, however, multiple small emboli can produce extensive obstruction of the pulmonary capillary bed, possibly causing PH and cardiac failure. Generally, however, small thromboemboli are incorporated into the arterial wall and have little effect on either parenchyma or the circulation. Patients may complain of dyspnea on exertion that may lead to syncope; sometimes, a right ventricular "heave" or a split second heart sound can be detected on examination. For the patient with chronic embolization, medical therapy with anticoagulant, thrombolytic, or vasodilating drugs does not alter the prognosis.

Patients with medium-sized emboli may present with pleuritic pain accompanied by dyspnea, a slight fever, and a productive cough yielding blood-streaked sputum. These patients usually are tachycardic. A small pleural effusion may develop and may mimic the appearance of pneumonia.

Massive emboli can produce sudden cardiac collapse. Preceding symptoms range from pallor, shock, and central chest pain to sudden loss of consciousness. In patients with cardiac collapse, the pulse becomes rapid and weak, blood pressure decreases, neck veins become engorged, and cardiogenic shock may be present or impending. In addition, a decrease in $PETCO_2$ and an increase in $PACO_2$ occur, with the difference between the values for these two indices increasing as conditions worsen. If a pulmonary artery catheter is in place, pulmonary artery pressures are observed to increase rapidly; the ECG may also begin to show right ventricular strain. The prognosis for these patients is very poor.

The most common clinical signs are dyspnea, respiratory rate greater than 20/min, heart rate greater than 100 beats/min, chest pain, cough, syncope, and hemoptysis.

TREATMENT

Aggressive efforts at prevention have been successful in reducing the incidence of DVT in surgical patients. Some suggested preventive measures are noted in the next table. Treatment mainly is aimed at preventing further embolism and at providing ventilatory support. Use of graded compression stockings, intermittent pneumatic compression, administration of various anticoagulants and thrombolytics, and ambulation are typical measures for preventing embolus formation. PE is a mechanical disease caused by acute pulmonary obstruction in a previously healthy patient.

Prevention of Venous Thromboembolism

Condition	Strategy
Total hip or knee replacement; hip or pelvis fracture	Warfarin (Coumadin) (target INR, 2–2.5) × 4–6 wk
	Low-molecular-weight heparin (e.g., enoxaparin [Lovenox], 30 mg subcutaneously twice daily)
	IPC ± warfarin (Coumadin)
Gynecologic cancer surgery	Warfarin (Coumadin) (target INR, 2–2.5) ± IPC
	Unfractionated heparin, 5000 units q8h ± IPC
	Dalteparin (Fragmin) 2500 units once daily ± IPC
	Enoxaparin 40 mg subcutaneously once daily
Urologic surgery	Warfarin (Coumadin) (target INR, 2–2.5) ± IPC
Thoracic surgery	IPC *plus* unfractionated heparin, 5000 units q8h

INR, International Normalized Ratio; *IPC,* intermittent pneumatic compression.

Continued

Prevention of Venous Thromboembolism—cont'd

Condition	Strategy
High-risk general surgery (e.g., prior VTE, current cancer, or obesity)	IPC *or* GCS *plus* unfractionated heparin 5000 units q8h
General, gynecologic, or urologic surgery (without prior VTE) for noncancerous conditions	GCS *plus* unfractionated heparin 5000 units q12h Dalteparin 2500 units subcutaneously once daily Enoxaparin 40 mg subcutaneously once daily IPC alone
Neurosurgery, eye surgery, or other surgery when prophylactic anticoagulation is contraindicated	GCS ± IPC
Medical conditions	GCS ± heparin 5000 U q-12h IPC alone Enoxaparin (Lovenox) 40 mg subcutaneously once daily
Orthopedic surgery	Enoxaparin 30 mg twice daily Enoxaparin 40 mg once daily* Dalteparin 5000 units once daily* Danaparoid 750 units twice daily* Warfarin (target INR, 2–3) GCS plus IPC
General surgery	Enoxaparin 40 mg daily Dalteparin 2500 or 5000 units once daily GCS plus IPC
Pregnancy	Enoxaparin 40 mg daily Dalteparin 5000 units daily
Medical patients	Enoxaparin 40 mg daily GCS plus IPC

*Approved only for total hip replacement prophylaxis.
GCS, Graduated compression stockings; *INR*, International Normalized Ratio; *IPC*, intermittent pneumatic compression; *VTE*, venous thromboembolism.

Guidelines for the Treatment of Pulmonary Embolism

- Treat DVT or pulmonary thromboembolism with therapeutic levels of unfractionated intravenous heparin, adjusted subcutaneous heparin, or low-molecular-weight heparin for at least 5 days and overlap with oral anticoagulation for at least 4 to 5 days. Consider a longer course of heparin for massive pulmonary thromboembolism or severe iliofemoral DVT.
- For most patients, heparin and oral anticoagulation can be started together and heparin can be discontinued on day 5 or 6 if the International Normalized Ratio (INR) has been therapeutic for 2 consecutive days.
- Continue oral anticoagulant therapy for a least 3 months with a target INR of 2.5 (range, 2 to 3).
- Patients with reversible or time-limited risk factors can be treated for 3 to 6 months. Patients with a first episode of idiopathic DVT should be treated for at least 6 months. Patients with recurrent venous thrombosis

or a continuing risk factor such as cancer, inhibitor deficiency states, or antiphospholipid antibody syndrome should be treated indefinitely.

- Isolated calf vein DVT should be treated with anticoagulation for at least 3 months.
- The use of thrombolytic agents continues to be highly individualized, and clinicians should have some latitude in using these agents. Patients with hemodynamically unstable pulmonary thromboembolism or massive iliofemoral thrombosis are the best candidates.
- Inferior vena caval filter placement is recommended when there is a contraindication to or failure of anticoagulation, for chronic recurrent embolism with PH, and with concurrent performance of surgical pulmonary embolectomy or pulmonary endarterectomy.

Surgery

Surgical intervention often is indicated for patients who are unresponsive to other measures. The most common surgical procedure for patients with PE is placement of an umbrella filter, which traps thromboemboli. It is estimated that 30,000 to 40,000 patients receive such filters annually in the United States. The filter is placed in the inferior vena cava under fluoroscopic guidance, usually below the renal veins at the level of the L2-3 intervertebral space. Suprarenal placement is required when a thrombus directly involves the renal veins or has propagated above the level of the renal veins.

The presence of an infrarenal filter in a pregnant woman may place her and her fetus at risk because of the possibility that the filter will come into contact with the gravid uterus. Suprarenal placement prevents this risk.

Thromboendarterectomy is the treatment of choice for chronic large-vessel thromboembolic PH. Desired results include decreased pulmonary vascular resistance (PVR), improved cardiac output, restoration of exercise tolerance, and resolution of hypoxemia. Improvements in right ventricular function and hemodynamics may be prompt, whereas gas exchange improvements occur over weeks to months. Although the role of pulmonary embolectomy remains controversial, in the few patients who do not benefit from optimal medical therapy, it remains an acceptable procedure.

ANESTHESIA MANAGEMENT

Anesthesia for patients at risk for PE is aimed at supporting vital organ function and minimizing anesthetic-induced myocardial depression. The use of a high fraction of inspired oxygen (FiO_2) aids in preventing pulmonary vasoconstriction, and the monitoring of pulmonary artery pressure helps the anesthesia provider to optimize right-sided heart function and to assess the effects of anesthetic management on PVR. Many anesthesia providers choose not to place pulmonary artery catheters because of concerns about the possibility that these catheters dislodge clots in the right side of the heart.

Intravenous fluid infusion must be adjusted so right ventricular stroke volume is optimized in the presence of marked increase in afterload. A continuous catecholamine infusion may be needed to enhance cardiac contractility.

Induction is often performed with etomidate or ketamine (for maintenance of hemodynamic stability), but ketamine must be titrated judiciously because it may increase PVR.

The use of nitrous oxide is generally believed to be acceptable. However, this may not be possible with the use of a high FiO_2. Use of nitrous oxide should be discontinued if PVR increases. Obviously, the use of nitrous oxide is contraindicated in patients with venous air embolism. Patients with moderate to severe PE often are experiencing acute right-sided heart failure. Cardiac function can be optimized by the use of minimally depressing cardiac agents such as narcotics.

Persistent severe hypotension, such as that accompanying massive PE, may necessitate the use of a cardiotonic agent. The goal is preservation of perfusion to the brain and heart until cardiopulmonary bypass is started and surgical removal of the clot is attempted. Heparin should be readily available, and when needed, it should be administered into a central line while blood aspiration is verified before and after injection. Reports of operative mortality during pulmonary embolectomy range from 11% to 55%, with much higher rates among patients suffering cardiac arrest.

Detection of Pulmonary Embolism during Anesthesia

In the intubated patient under general anesthesia, combinations of the symptoms may occur. A decreasing $PETCO_2$ and tachycardia usually are the first symptoms seen in PE. These can be followed by a decrease in arterial oxygen saturation and the generation of ABG values that indicate unexplained arterial hypoxemia. Increased pulmonary artery and central venous pressures can be seen in combination with a decrease in systolic and diastolic blood pressures. Bronchospasm may occur. Finally, ECG changes indicating right-axis deviation, incomplete or complete right bundle branch block, or peaked T waves may be observed in the presence or absence of an accompanying systolic ejection murmur.

Intraoperative Management

Several measures can be taken to support the anesthetized patient with suspected PE. First and most important, an airway must be established by intubation if the patient is not already intubated. Second, delivery of the anesthetic agent must be discontinued, and administration of 100% O_2 must be initiated. Next, the circulatory system should be supported with the infusion of intravenous fluids or blood (or both) as needed, and the use of sympathomimetics (e.g., dobutamine or dopamine) initiated, if necessary. Dysrhythmias should be treated with intravenous administration of lidocaine, and the patient should receive positive end-expiratory pressure for optimization of oxygen transport across the alveolar membrane.

Pulmonary embolectomy may be necessary. Severe hemodynamic difficulty should be anticipated, and resuscitative efforts should be continued. Patients with PE are extremely sensitive to any anesthetic agent and likely require femoral bypass under local anesthesia with partial cardiopulmonary bypass before induction. Again, it is critical to have heparin ready to infuse into a central line (if available). Depending on the insult to the right ventricle, pulmonary vasodilation and catecholamine infusions may be indicated. Simultaneous left atrial and right atrial pressure monitoring is helpful.

Patients with PE present particular management challenges in their postoperative course, including reperfusion edema, persistent hypoxemia, pericardial effusion, psychiatric disorders, and pulmonary blood flow steal. The areas of the lung to which pulmonary artery flow has been restored are subject to development of reperfusion pulmonary edema, presumably as a manifestation of oxidant- and protease-mediated acute lung injury.

Other possible causes are extracorporeal circulation, anticoagulation, and an increase in perfusion pressure in a previously obstructed pulmonary artery.

Complications include immediate pulmonary hemorrhage and respiratory disturbance, and death may occur. This syndrome may develop 3 to 5 days after surgery. After pulmonary thromboendarterectomy for relief of chronic thromboembolic PH, perfusion lung scans frequently reveal new perfusion defects in segments served by undissected pulmonary arteries. This phenomenon has been labeled *pulmonary blood flow steal* and is believed to be caused by postoperative redistribution of regional PVR and not by rethrombosis or embolism.

J. Pulmonary Hypertension

DEFINITION

Pulmonary arterial hypertension (PH) exists if the mean level of pulmonary artery pressure (PAP) increases by 5 to 10 mm Hg or if pulmonary artery systolic pressure exceeds 30 mm Hg and mean PAP exceeds 20 mm Hg. PH usually represents an advanced stage of a large number of cardiovascular diseases. The mortality rate associated with PH is high.

INCIDENCE AND PREVALENCE

PH may be (1) primary or idiopathic (unexplained) or (2) secondary to an associated condition. In young adults, the female-to-male incidence of primary PH (PPH) is 4:1; this incidence is similar to that in older groups of men and women. PPH is a rare disorder, and its true incidence is unknown; however, it is found on autopsy in 1% of patients in whom cor pulmonale had been diagnosed.

ETIOLOGY

PH may be caused by many associated conditions, including pulmonary venous hypertension caused by left atrial outflow obstruction or pulmonary venous occlusive disease and pulmonary arterial hypertension caused by hyperdynamic circulation (e.g., secondary to burns or sepsis), vasoconstriction, viscosity, obstruction, and reactive vascular disease. PPH is characterized by a rapidly progressive course with a 79% mortality rate within 5 years of clinical diagnosis. The degree of increase in pressure in the pulmonary circulation has an important influence on the patient's life expectancy. Resistant PH has long been identified as a major cause of early death. Prognosis is largely determined by right ventricular integrity.

PATHOPHYSIOLOGY

PH is characterized by an increase in vascular tone and by the growth and proliferation of pulmonary vascular smooth muscle. Initial reversible vasoconstriction may progress to muscle hypertrophy and irreversible degeneration.

Pulmonary vasoconstriction appears to occur in some (but not all) patients with PH. Some investigators speculate that the disease progresses from vasoconstriction to fixed obstruction of the pulmonary vascular bed. Pathologic changes associated with a fixed resistance are the presence of intimal sclerosis, plexiform (resembling a plexus or network) lesions, and the obliteration of as many as 90% or more of the small vessels within the lung. Other reported abnormalities include impairment of endothelium-dependent vasodilation.

CLINICAL FEATURES AND DIAGNOSIS

PH may be either acute or chronic. In almost all patients with PH, dyspnea and exercise intolerance usually are the first complaints. Patients also may present with angina. PH may be associated with chest pain and electrocardiographic (ECG) changes typical of myocardial infarction even in the absence of coronary artery disease. Some clinicians propose that the source of the chest pain is (1) an increase in right ventricular myocardial oxygen demand secondary to an increase in wall stress or (2) a decrease in coronary blood flow because of a decrease in flow in the arteries supplying the right ventricle during systole.

Right atrial hypertrophy or right ventricular hypertrophy (or both) may be evident on ECG. Chest radiography may demonstrate an enlarged pulmonary artery. Cardiac catheterization combined with pulmonary angiography is most informative in assessing PH, cardiac reserve, and the effects of pulmonary vasodilator therapy. Vasodilator therapy is attempted when a vasoconstrictor component is identified. Vasodilator challenge may be performed with cardiac catheterization using a rapid and effective pulmonary vasodilator such as nitroglycerin, isoproterenol, nifedipine, prostaglandin E_1, prostacyclin, prostaglandin E_2, hydralazine, nitroprusside, or adenosine for evaluation of the reversibility of PH. Frequently, open lung biopsy is performed for assessment of the histopathologic composition of small pulmonary arteries. Noninvasive evaluation includes Doppler echocardiography for measuring the velocity of tricuspid regurgitation (which correlates well with invasive PAP measurements) and pulmonic peak flow velocity.

LABORATORY RESULTS

Diagnosis is confirmed with cardiac catheterization when other possible causes have been excluded. Chest x-ray studies may show an enlarged border of the right side of the heart. ECG may reveal signs of right ventricular hypertrophy (i.e., R greater than S in V_1).

CLINICAL MANIFESTATIONS

Signs and symptoms are often masked by primary pulmonary or cardiovascular disease. PH may not be evidenced until PAP equals systemic pressure. Resting PAP generally does not rise until the effective cross-sectional area of the vascular bed is decreased by 50% or more. Patients may complain of fatigue, chest discomfort, and dyspnea, especially with exertion, and tachypnea.

ANESTHETIC CONSIDERATIONS

Attempts to alleviate PH disease states have had varied success. Vasodilator agents are used most commonly and may be helpful in patients with reversible vasoconstriction. A list of vasodilators used in PH is provided in the next table. Possible beneficial effects of pulmonary arterial dilation are preservation of lung function, prevention of right ventricle deterioration, and, one hopes, improved survival.

The principal objectives during anesthesia in patients with PH are prevention of increases in PH and avoidance of major hemodynamic changes. Considerations that apply to the care of patients with cor pulmonale also apply to patients with PH. Information regarding PH and intravenous induction agents is lacking; however, most agents have either little effect on pulmonary vascular resistance (PVR) or decrease it. Ketamine, which causes an increase in PVR, may be the exception (see the following table).

Drug Treatment Options for Patients with Pulmonary Hypertension

Drug or Drug Class	Rationale	Potentially Responsive Types of Pulmonary Hypertension	Limitations
Anticoagulants	Reduce risk of pulmonary thromboembolism	Primary and that secondary to acute pulmonary thromboembolism, chronic pulmonary thromboembolism, and anorectic drugs	For primary hypertension, concomitant vasodilator treatment also required
Vasodilators			
Calcium antagonists	Inhibit influx of calcium into smooth muscle cells with elevated vasomotor tone Preferentially act on pulmonary vasculature	Primary and that secondary to connective tissue vascular disease and COPD	Initial treatment in specialized centers recommended to avoid severe adverse outcomes such as negative inotropic effects
Epoprostenol (Flolan) Prostacyclin	May replace deficiencies in endogenous prostacyclin Also inhibits smooth muscle proliferation and platelet aggregation	Primary, persistent pulmonary hypertension of the neonate, and that secondary to ARDS, crises after heart surgery in infants, and connective tissue disease in adults	Peripheral adverse effects occur when administered by continuous intravenous infusion
Nitric oxide	Interferes with endogenous vasoconstrictor mechanisms	Primary, persistent pulmonary hypertension of the neonate, and that secondary to corrective cardiac surgery in children, lung or lung/heart transplant surgery in adults, and COPD	Potential adverse effects include increased bleeding times, negative inotropic effects and formation of potentially toxic products (i.e., nitrogen dioxide, methemoglobin)

Continued

Drug Treatment Options for Patients with Pulmonary Hypertension—cont'd

Drug or Drug Class	Rationale	Potentially Responsive Types of Pulmonary Hypertension	Limitations
Alprostadil (prostaglandin E₁)	Interferes with endogenous vasoconstrictor mechanisms	Secondary to ARDS	Impaired pulmonary metabolism may result in systemic hypotension
Bosentan (Tracleer)	Oral endothelin receptor antagonist	Severe pulmonary hypertension	Hepatotoxicity
Treprostinil (Remodulin)	Prostacyclin analogue	Primary pulmonary hypertension; class II–IV	Given by continuous infusion via wearable infusion pump
Inhibitors of Vasoconstriction			
α-Adrenoceptor antagonists	Inhibit the formation of the vasoconstrictor angiotensin II	Persistent pulmonary hypertension of the neonate (especially preterm infants) and that secondary to COPD	Can cause severe systemic adverse effects
Angiotensin converting enzyme inhibitors	Inhibit the formation of the vasoconstrictor angiotensin II	Secondary to connective tissue disease, high altitude, and congestive heart failure	Prolonged treatment required to obtain an effect

ARDS, Adult respiratory distress syndrome; *COPD*, chronic obstructive pulmonary disease.

Reversible coexisting disease should be corrected preoperatively, and baseline arterial blood gases should be obtained. Preoperative sedation may depress ventilation. Anticholinergics may depress mucociliary activity and impair clearance of secretions. Bronchospasm and increases in pulmonary and systemic pressures may be avoided during intubation if the depth of anesthesia is adequate. Regional anesthesia may be appropriate for patients not requiring high sensory levels of blockade. Nitrous oxide may increase PVR when high doses of opioids are given. Monitoring requirements depend on the severity of disease and type of surgery.

K. Restrictive Pulmonary Diseases

DEFINITION

Restrictive pulmonary disease is defined as any condition that interferes with normal lung expansion during inspiration. Typically, it includes disorders that increase the inward elastic recoil of the lungs or chest wall. Consequently, the alteration in pulmonary dynamics results in decreases in lung volumes and capacities and in lung or chest wall compliance. Some restrictive diseases produce ventilation abnormalities and ventilation/perfusion mismatching, whereas others lead to impairment of diffusion. The forced expiratory volume in 1 second (FEV_1) and the forced vital capacity (FVC) are both decreased owing to a reduction in total lung capacity (TLC) or a decrease in chest wall compliance or muscle strength. However, the FEV_1/FVC ratio is normal or elevated.

INCIDENCE AND PREVALENCE

Statistics vary according to the acute intrinsic, chronic intrinsic, or chronic extrinsic nature of the restrictive disease.

ETIOLOGY

Impairment-producing restrictive pulmonary diseases can be classified as (1) acute intrinsic, (2) chronic intrinsic, or (3) chronic extrinsic. *Acute intrinsic disorders* are primarily caused by the abnormal movement of intravascular fluid into the interstitium of the lung and alveoli secondary to the increase in pulmonary vascular pressures occurring with left ventricular failure, fluid overload, or an increase in pulmonary capillary permeability. Examples of acute intrinsic disorders include pulmonary edema, aspiration pneumonia, and acute respiratory distress syndrome.

Chronic intrinsic diseases are characterized by pulmonary fibrosis. Conditions producing fibrosis of the lung include idiopathic pulmonary fibrosis, radiation injury, cytotoxic and noncytotoxic drug exposure, oxygen toxicity, autoimmune diseases, and sarcoidosis.

Chronic extrinsic diseases can be defined as disorders inhibiting the normal lung excursion. They include flail chest, pneumothorax, atelectasis, and pleural effusions. They also include conditions that interfere with chest wall expansion, such as ascites, obesity, pregnancy, and skeletal and neuromuscular disorders.

CLINICAL MANIFESTATIONS

Clinical manifestations depend on the disorder but may include tachypnea, dyspnea, cough, bronchospasm, pulmonary vascular vasoconstriction, pulmonary hypertension, cor pulmonale, and arterial hypoxemia. The pulmonary function tests reveal decreased vital capacity with normal expiratory flow rates.

TREATMENT
Treatment also depends on the specific restrictive disorder and may include oxygen therapy, bronchodilators, corticosteroids, and mechanical ventilation with positive end-expiratory pressure.

ANESTHETIC CONSIDERATIONS
- Restrictive pulmonary disease does not dictate drug choices for induction and maintenance of general anesthesia.
- Drugs should be selected and administered to avoid postoperative ventilatory depression.
- Regional anesthesia may be acceptable, but sensory levels of blockade above T10 may impair respiratory muscle function.
- Controlled ventilation may maximize oxygenation and ventilation.
- Poorly compliant lungs may require high inspiratory pressures.
- Postoperative mechanical ventilation may be necessary.
- Extubation should be done only when patients clearly meet the criteria.
- Decreased lung volumes may impair cough and interfere with postoperative secretion removal.

L. Severe Acute Respiratory Syndrome

DEFINITION
Severe acute respiratory syndrome (SARS) is a viral respiratory illness.

INCIDENCE AND PREVALENCE
SARS was first reported in Asia in February, 2003, and spread to North America, South America, and Europe in the following months. By late July, 2003, the illness was considered contained. A total of 8437 people became infected, and 813 died during the outbreak.

ETIOLOGY
SARS is caused by a previously unrecognized coronavirus, called SARS-associated coronavirus (SARS-CoV). The virus is spread by person-to-person contact through respiratory droplets. It is unknown whether SARS-CoV is spread through other routes (i.e., airborne spread).

LABORATORY RESULTS
A reverse transcription polymerase chain reaction test can detect SARS-CoV in blood, stool, and nasal secretions. In addition, the blood can be tested for SARS-CoV antibodies. Viral cultures can also be used to detect SARS-CoV. Arterial blood gases may reveal hypoxia, and with severe respiratory distress, hypercarbia and acidosis may be evident. Chest x-ray study may show evidence of pneumonia.

CLINICAL MANIFESTATIONS
Initial manifestations include the following: fever (temperature higher than 38° C), which may be associated with chills; headache, body aches, and

generalized discomfort. Diarrhea may also occur. Two to 7 days following onset, a dry, nonproductive cough occurs and may progress to hypoxia. Pneumonia also commonly develops.

It is believed that people infected with SARS are infectious only while they have symptoms. The most infectious period is during the second week of illness.

TREATMENT

Primary treatment includes supportive measures. Face masks should be worn by infected persons. Antibiotics have not shown effectiveness in the treatment of SARS, although they may be used initially until pneumonia is excluded. Ribavirin has also been used, but its effectiveness has not been proved.

ANESTHETIC CONSIDERATIONS

The U.S. Centers for Disease and Prevention recommends that all nonessential staff, including students, should not partake in care of the patient with SARS. Hand washing after all patient contact is imperative, and alcohol-based skin disinfectants can be used if there is no obvious organic material contamination.

A patient with SARS should remain in airborne isolation. If negative pressure isolation is not available, recirculation of the room air should be avoided, and entry and exit should be minimized. All equipment should be disposable or disinfected with a broad-spectrum disinfectant after use. Personal protective equipment should be worn by all care providers. The arms, torso, eyes, nose, mouth, and all exposed skin should be covered. Providers should be fit-tested for disposable particulate respirators (i.e., N-95, N-99, or N-100). Powered air purifying respirators are also appropriate. Disposable masks should not be reused.

To minimize the spread of SARS, it is suggested that aerosol-generating procedures (administration of aerosolized medications, bronchoscopy, airway suctioning, endotracheal intubation, positive-pressure ventilation by face mask) be limited to those deemed medically necessary. Therefore, local anesthesia with intravenous sedation or regional anesthesia, when appropriate, should be considered in the patient with SARS. If not contraindicated, intubation should be completed during a deep plane of anesthesia, to minimize coughing and subsequent spread of the virus.

M. Tuberculosis

DEFINITION

Tuberculosis is a chronic granulomatous disease that is spread primarily by aerosol transmission.

INCIDENCE AND PREVALENCE

In the past and before specific antimicrobial therapy, tuberculosis was a significant cause of death and disability in North America. It currently affects approximately 28,000 persons in North America. The elderly, debilitated, malnourished, and those immunosuppressed and living in crowded conditions are most often affected.

ETIOLOGY

Tuberculosis is caused by the acid-fast bacillus *Mycobacterium tuberculosis.* Once inspired, the bacilli multiply, causing nonspecific pneumonitis.

Some bacilli migrate to the lymph nodes, encounter lymphocytes, and precipitate the immune response. Phagocytes engulf colonies of bacilli in the lung, isolate them, and form granulomatous tubercules. Infected tissues inside the tubercles create caseation necrosis (a cheeselike material). Isolation of the bacilli is completed by formation of scar tissue around the tubercle. After approximately 10 days, the immune response is complete, and further bacilli multiplication is prevented. After isolation of bacilli and development of immunity, tuberculosis can remain dormant for life. Reactivation may occur if live bacilli escape into bronchi or in states of decreased immunity. Patients with laryngeal tuberculosis or lung cavitation have the highest infectivity rate.

LABORATORY RESULTS

Diagnosis is made by positive tuberculin skin (purified protein derivative) testing, chest x-ray study, and positive sputum culture. A positive skin test alone may indicate only exposure to the tuberculin bacteria and is not by itself evidence of active disease. Chest x-ray findings consistent with tuberculosis in the presence of acquired immunodeficiency syndrome (AIDS) may be atypical.

CLINICAL MANIFESTATIONS

Many patients are asymptomatic. Common manifestations include low-grade fever, fatigue, weight loss, anorexia, lethargy, and a worsening cough (i.e., purulent sputum). Some patients occasionally develop pleural effusions, meningitis, bone or joint disease, genitourinary abscesses, or peritonitis. Chest pain, dyspnea, and hemoptysis are not common.

TREATMENT

Drugs of choice for treatment include isoniazid, rifampin, streptomycin, and ethambutol.

ANESTHETIC CONSIDERATIONS

Patients are placed in respiratory isolation until such time/therapy that they are no longer transmitters of the disease. Whenever possible, disposable equipment (i.e., filters and anesthesia circuits) should be used. Nondisposable equipment must be thoroughly sterilized. Postpone elective surgery in actively infected persons until adequate chemotherapy has been administered (usually 3 weeks of treatment) and verified by a negative sputum sample. Consider the implications of organ dysfunction that may be secondary to the disease or its treatment. Although the disease most commonly affects the pulmonary system, chemotherapeutic agents used for treatment may lead to organ toxicity (i.e., liver, kidneys, or peripheral nervous system).

OTHER CONDITIONS

A. Anaphylaxis

DEFINITION

Anaphylaxis is a life-threatening response that a sensitized person develops within minutes after administration of a specific antigen.

INCIDENCE AND PREVALENCE

The estimated incidence of anaphylactic reaction during anesthesia is estimated at 1 in 5000 to 1 in 25,000 anesthetic administrations.

ETIOLOGY

Prior exposure to an antigen causes the production of antigen-specific immunoglobulin E (IgE) antibodies, causing host sensitization. Anaphylaxis occurs after subsequent exposure to the antigen and is mediated by a type I hypersensitivity reaction. Mediators include histamine, leukotrienes, prostaglandins, eosinophil chemotactic factor, neutrophil chemotactic factor, and platelet-activating factor.

LABORATORY RESULTS

Laboratory tests to determine susceptibility to anaphylactic reactions include intradermal skin testing, leukocyte or basophil degranulation testing (histamine release test), and radioallergosorbent testing. Serum levels of IgE, tryptase, and histamine are elevated immediately following an anaphylactic reaction.

CLINICAL MANIFESTATIONS

Anaphylaxis is manifested by respiratory distress, often followed by vascular collapse or by shock without respiratory difficulty. There may be upper or lower airway obstruction or both. Hoarseness, stridor, or wheezing may be evident. Cutaneous manifestations include pruritus, urticaria, and angioedema. Angioedema can result in mechanical obstruction of the epiglottis and larynx. Gastrointestinal manifestations include nausea, vomiting, crampy abdominal pain, and diarrhea. Loss of up to 50% of intravascular blood volume from capillary leakage and vasodilation may result in hypotension and cardiovascular collapse. Myocardial ischemia may be evident as a result of coronary hypoperfusion and hypoxemia. The onset is generally within seconds to minutes after introduction of the antigen. However, anaphylactic reactions to latex exposure can be delayed for more than an hour after exposure.

TREATMENT

When anaphylactic reactions are suspected, the probable drug or causative agent should be discontinued. One hundred percent oxygen should be administered, and endotracheal intubation may be indicated to maintain oxygenation. Epinephrine, 0.01 to 0.5 mg intravenously, subcutaneously, or intramuscularly, should be given. The route and dose of epinephrine should be determined based on the severity of the reaction. The dose of epinephrine may be doubled and repeated every 1 to 3 minutes until symptoms are controlled. Intravenous fluids including crystalloids and colloids should be infused rapidly; up to 4 L may be required to restore intravascular volume. Additional vasopressors should be used as needed to treat hypotension. Diphenhydramine, 50 to 100 mg intravenously, may help to attenuate the symptoms; however, there is no evidence that antihistamine administration is effective in treating anaphylaxis. Inhaled β_2-agonists, such as albuterol, are beneficial for the treatment of bronchospasm. Hydrocortisone, up to 200 mg intravenously, or methylprednisolone, 1 to 2 mg/kg intravenously, may also be given; the beneficial effects of steroids seem to be related to inhibition of production of leukotrienes and prostaglandins.

ANESTHETIC CONSIDERATIONS

Anesthetic considerations include prompt recognition and treatment of anaphylactic reactions. Key initial signs of anaphylaxis in patients under general anesthesia include hypotension, bronchospasm, and urticaria; patients at risk should be closely monitored for these signs.

B. Difficult Airway

DEFINITION

A difficult airway presents the challenge of a "can't intubate, can't ventilate" scenario requiring the prompt initiation of various airway management strategies. Failure to acknowledge that the patient cannot be intubated or ventilated and reluctance to accept that the endotracheal tube is in the esophagus contribute to adverse outcomes. These include brain injury, death, cardiopulmonary arrest, unnecessary tracheotomy, airway trauma, and damage to teeth. Continued attempts at intubation and exertion of unnecessary force can cause bleeding and edema of the mucous membranes. Ventilation can become progressively more difficult, leading to morbidity from hypoxemia and hypercarbia.

AIRWAY ASSESSMENT

A complete airway assessment and physical examination should be done in the preoperative period. This assessment includes evaluation of multiple patient physical characteristics to identify potential airway problems indicative of the difficult airway. Criteria that can be assessed to identify potentially difficult airways include measurement of interincisor distance, thyromental distance, head and neck extension, Mallampati classification, body weight, and a past history of difficult airway. Evaluation of the length of upper incisors, visibility of the uvula, shape of the palate, compliance of the mandibular space, and length and thickness of the neck provides further assessment. The most prominent factors that are predictive of a difficult airway are obesity, decreased head and neck movement, decreased jaw movement, receding mandible, and buck teeth. In determining the probability of a difficult airway, there is no ideal method that is highly sensitive and specific, with minimal false-positive or false-negative reports. In an attempt to standardize the physical examination, it is recommended that all tests be completed with the patient in the sitting position with ead in full extension, mouth opened wide, tongue extruded, and with phonation. The history should focus on prior airway management problems, acute or chronic diseases, and syndromes associated with difficult airways.

During the airway physical examination, notation of findings that may indicate a difficult airway are integrated into the proposed airway management. Normally, the interincisor distance should be at least 4 cm, with less than 3 cm indicative of potential problem. If the mouth is narrow, it may be difficult to get the 2-cm flange of the laryngoscope blade and the endotracheal tube into the mouth while maintaining good visualization of the vocal cords. The thyromental distance is measured from the thyroid notch to the inner border of the mandible with the head extended. A thyromental distance less than 6 cm or three ordinary fingerbreaths is associated with a higher incidence of difficult intubation. The full range of flexion and extension of the neck varies from 90 to 165 degrees, decreasing approximately 20% between ages 16 and 75 years. The atlanto-occipital joint is capable of extending up to 35 degrees and provides the highest degree of mobility in the neck. When extension is reduced to 23 degrees, visualization may become difficult. Patients should be able to touch the tip of the chin to their chest.

The Mallampati classification is an indirect method of relating the size of the base of the tongue to the oral cavity. It is based on the theory that the tongue is singularly the largest obstacle to direct visualization of the glottis.

INCIDENCE AND PREVALENCE

The incidence of Mallampati grades III and IV laryngoscopic views varies throughout the literature. Variability in observation, years of experience, and definitions of airway categories cause differences in reporting statistics. Approximately 15% to 18% of patients have a grade III view requiring multiple intubation attempts. Approximately 1% to 4% have a grade IV view, and approximately 0.0001% to 0.02% fit into the "cannot intubate, cannot ventilate" category.

Difficult direct laryngoscopy occurs in 1.5% to 8.5% of general anesthetic administrations, and difficult intubation occurs with a similar incidence. Failed intubation occurs in 0.13% to 0.3% of general anesthetic administrations.

ANESTHETIC CONSIDERATIONS

The Difficult Airway Algorithm established the standardized approach to the management of the anticipated or unanticipated difficult airway (see Appendix V). The airway algorithm provides guidelines to manage difficult face mask–ventilation, difficult laryngoscopy, difficult tracheal intubation and failed intubation. An organized plan should be initiated when a difficult airway is encountered.

All departments have a dedicated difficult airway cart or box that must be readily available and well stocked. This cart should be checked on a routine basis to determine whether the materials are all available and working. Devices and techniques used for difficult intubation and ventilation may include different laryngoscopes blades, fiberoptic scope, the light wand, Bullard scope, laryngeal mask airway, intubating stylet, retrograde intubation kit, Eschmann stylet, transtracheal jet ventilation, and Combitube. A commercial kit is available for retrograde intubation, or the practitioner can choose to insert either a "J-wire" or #2 Mersiline suture through a cricothyrotomy and pass the device into the oropharynx. Adjunct airway equipment should be routinely used in nonemergency or practice situations to increase familiarity with the equipment and to facilitate ease of use in emergency situations (see the following box).

Components of a Cart for Difficult Airway Management

Airways (oral and nasal): various sizes
Tongue blades
Flexible stylets
Endotracheal tubes (cuffed and uncuffed): 2.5, 3, 3.5, 4, 4.5, 5, 5.5, 6, 7, 8 (two of each size)
Miller laryngoscope blades: sizes 0, 1, 2, 3, 4
MacIntosh laryngoscope blades: sizes 2, 3, 4
Laryngoscope handles: regular and stubby
Extra laryngoscope batteries and bulbs
Magill forceps
Syringes: 3, 5, 10, and 20 mL (three to four of each size)
Angiocatheters: 14-, 16-, 18-, 20-gauge (three each)
Lidocaine (Xylocaine) jelly 2%
Surgilube
Salem sump: 16 and 18 French
Suction catheters: 10, 12, 14 French
Nebulizer
Atomizer
Oxygen mask
Nasal cannula
Oxygen with 15-L/min regulator

Alternate Airway Devices
Laryngeal mask airways: sizes 3, 4, 5
Intubating laryngeal mask airway
Combitube
Lighted stylet (Trachlite) (two)
Eschmann stylet
Tube exchanger: small, medium, large
Ventilating stylet
Needle cricothyrotomy set
Retrograde intubation set
Melker percutaneous dilational cricothyrotomy set
Transtracheal jet ventilator
Ambu bag
Bullard or Upsher scope
Intubating bronchoscope
Tongue clamp
Light source
Endoscopy mask
Ovassapian intubating airway
Lidocaine: 4% topical, 2% for injection

Preparation

The patient with a potentially difficult airway should be optimally positioned. Pillows and blankets should be built up under the head and shoulders to afford the optimal "sniffing" position. This also provides more space for introduction of the laryngoscope blade into the mouth. Locating and marking the cricoid cartilage or cricothyroid ligament enable the assistant who is performing cricoid pressure to find the correct position easily and to identify landmarks should a surgical airway be needed.

Preoxygenation is an essential component in patients with a difficult airway, to delay arterial desaturation during subsequent apnea. It increases the oxygen content and eliminates much of the nitrogen (79% of room air) from the functional residual capacity (FRC). Adequate preoxygenation should include having the patient breathe at normal tidal volumes for 3 to 5 minutes with a fresh gas flow of no less than 5 L and a tight mask fit. This is easily accomplished by applying the face mask as soon as the patient arrives in the operating room, before application of other monitors. If time is limited, "fast-track" preoxygenation in which the patient takes four vital capacity breaths in 30 seconds can be used before induction of anesthesia. This will not completely denitrogenate the blood but is useful in an emergency situation.

Alternative anesthetic management options exist if a difficult airway is anticipated, including use of monitored anesthesia care and regional anesthesia. The selection of monitored anesthesia care or regional anesthesia does not obviate the need to plan for management of the difficult airway. Failure of the regional block or complications resulting from placement may require emergency intubation under less than desirable conditions. It is not recommended that regional anesthesia be used for conditions in which the patient is unwilling to cooperate, the surgery cannot be quickly terminated, or access to the airway is lost.

C. Geriatrics

DEFINITION

Geriatrics is the branch of medicine that deals with the physiologic effects of aging and the diagnosis and treatment of persons who are 65 years of age or older. In the year 2000, as children of the "baby boom" entered their sixth decade, nearly 50 million Americans were older than 70 years of age and made up 13% of the general population.

ETIOLOGY

Human organ function shows a linear decline with age. The rate constant for this decline is slightly less than 1% per year of the functional capacity present at age 30 years. As a consequence, a 70-year-old geriatric patient may have a 40% decrease in the function of any specific organ compared with that present at the age of 30 years.

CLINICAL MANIFESTATIONS

Clinical manifestations include an increased prevalence of age-related, concomitant disease (hypertension, renal disease, atherosclerosis, myocardial infarction, chronic obstructive pulmonary disease, cardiomegaly, diabetes, liver disease, congestive heart failure, angina, cerebrovascular

Common Age-Related Anatomic and Physiologic Changes

General Changes
- Decreased organ function
- Increased body fat
- Decreased blood volume
- Loss of protective reflexes
- Decreased ability to retain body heat
- Decreased lean body mass
- Decreased skin elasticity
- Collagen loss
- Decreased intracellular water

Cardiovascular Changes
- Impaired pump function
- Prolonged circulation time
- Myocardial fiber atrophy
- Hypertension
- Impaired cardiac adrenergic receptor quality
- Increased peripheral vascular resistance
- Decreased cardiac output
- Decreased organ perfusion
- Left ventricular hypertrophy
- Coronary artery disease

Pulmonary Changes
- Increased lung compliance
- Decreased forced expiratory volume
- Increased closing volume
- Decreased resting arterial oxygen tension
- Increased alveolar-arterial difference
- Ventilation/perfusion mismatch
- Decreased functional residual capacity
- Decreased total lung capacity

Central Nervous System Changes
- Decreased activity
- Decreased oxygen consumption
- Reduced number of functioning receptors
- Reduced production of neurotransmitters
- Neuron loss
- Decreased cerebral blood flow

Renal Changes
- Decreased renal blood flow
- Decreased urine concentrating ability
- Decreased ability to conserve water
- Decreased elimination of drugs
- Decreased glomerular filtration rate

Hepatobiliary Changes
- Decreased hepatic blood flow
- Decreased plasma drug clearance

Endocrine Changes
- Decreased pancreatic function
- Increased incidence of diabetes
- Decreased tolerance to glucose load

accident). The commonly age related anatomic and physiologic changes that occur are listed in the box on p. 178.

ANESTHETIC CONSIDERATIONS

The choice of anesthetic technique should be based on the changes in organ system function in the patient, the pharmacokinetic and pharmaco-dynamic effects anticipated, the surgical requirements, and the needs and predisposition of the patient. As a rule, the geriatric patient is likely to be predisposed to hypotension as a result of reduced activity of the sympathetic nervous system and decreased intravascular volume. Decreased cardiac output and delayed drug clearance are likely to prolong the onset of drug effects and prolong the duration of action (see the following table).

Age-Related Changes and Pharmacokinetics

Change	Effect
Contracted vascular volume	High initial plasma concentration
Decreased protein binding	Increased availability of free drug
Increased total body lipid storage sites	Prolonged action of lipid-soluble drugs
Decreased renal and hepatic blood flow	Prolonged action of drugs dependent on kidney and liver elimination

Regional, general, and monitored anesthesia care techniques are appropriate selections for the geriatric patient. Each technique has its cor-responding cadre of supporters. No conclusive study has demonstrated the superiority of any one specific anesthetic technique. With regional and local techniques, maintenance of consciousness during the surgical procedure may be associated with less confusion during the postoperative period. However, general anesthesia, with endotracheal intubation, may be advan-tageous for promoting bronchopulmonary toilet and facilitating surgical conditions. A progressive decrease in the reactivity of protective airway reflexes, such as coughing and swallowing, can be expected with age. Because elderly patients often are edentulous, a sealed fit with the anesthetic face mask may be difficult. These factors may increase the likelihood of regurgitation of gastric contents, with aspiration of vomitus into the lungs. The changes that accompany cervical arthritis and osteoarthritis, limiting extension and flexion of the neck, often make endotracheal intubation difficult.

It appears likely that the patient's preoperative health status and events during the course of the anesthetic that precipitate such physiologic changes as hypotension, hypoxia, hypercarbia, and hypertension do more to affect patient outcome than does anesthetic technique.

Great care must be taken to prevent trauma to skin and bony promi-nences when the geriatric patient is positioned for surgery on the operating table. Collagen loss and decreased elasticity of tissue make the skin more sensitive to damage from tape, monitoring devices, and contact with hard table surfaces. Additionally, any invasive procedure, including insertion of intravenous, spinal, and epidural catheters, should be accomplished with the goal of protecting the integrity of the skin.

PART I   Common Diseases

D. Glaucoma/Open Globe

DEFINITION AND ETIOLOGY

In glaucoma, intraocular pressure (IOP) is increased, resulting in impaired capillary flow to the optic nerve. If the condition is left untreated, loss of sight may result.

Types of Glaucoma

- *Open-angle glaucoma:* This is characterized by elevated IOP with anatomically open anterior chamber. Sclerosed trabecular tissue impairs aqueous filtration and drainage. Treatment: miosis and trabecular stretching should be produced medically (eyedrops, epinephrine, timolol).
- *Closed-angle glaucoma:* The peripheral iris moves in direct contact with the posterior corneal surface, mechanically obstructing aqueous flow. This is caused by a narrow angle between the iris and posterior cornea and produces swelling of the crystalline lens.
- *Congenital glaucoma* is associated with some eye diseases (retinopathy of prematurity, aniridia, mesodermal dysgenesis syndrome). Surgical goniotomy or trabeculotomy should be performed to route aqueous flow into Schlemm's canal. Cyclocryotherapy decreases aqueous formation by destroying the ciliary body by freezing tissue with a probe.

Open Globe

This condition usually follows traumatic injury.

DIAGNOSTIC AND LABORATORY FINDINGS

Normal IOP is 10 to 25 mm Hg; abnormal IOP is greater than 25 mm Hg. Pressure becomes atmospheric when the globe is opened. Any sudden rise in IOP at this time may lead to prolapse of the iris and lens, extrusion of the vitreous humor, and loss of vision. Coagulation studies should be evaluated before retrobulbar block is instituted.

CLINICAL MANIFESTATIONS

The clinical manifestations of acute glaucoma are a dilated, irregular pupil and pain in and around the eye.

TREATMENT

IOP is increased by the following: external pressure on the eye, including venous congestion associated with coughing, vomiting, or the prone position; scleral rigidity, which is increased in aged persons; and changes in the intraocular structure or fluids. Pilocarpine hydrochloride decreases resistance to improve drainage of aqueous humor. Acetazolamide reduces the rate at which aqueous humor is formed.

ANESTHETIC CONSIDERATIONS

Drug therapy should be continued to maintain miosis. Anticholinergic drugs are acceptable in preoperative medication. Increases of IOP, hypercarbia, and central venous pressure should be avoided. Succinylcholine causes transient increases in IOP. Rapid sequence induction generally is acceptable for patients with open globe and a full stomach. Awake intubations are not desirable because they may contribute to increases in IOP. Techniques and drugs associated with decreasing IOP include volatile anesthetics, intravenous anesthetics, hypocarbia, hypothermia, mannitol, glycerin, nondepolarizing muscle relaxants, and timolol. General anesthesia or retrobulbar blocks are acceptable for eye surgery. General anesthesia is typically used for open globe repair.

Drug interactions must also be considered. Echothiophate prolongs the effect of succinylcholine. Timolol may result in bradycardia. Etomidate may induce myoclonus.

ANESTHETIC GOALS FOR OPHTHALMIC SURGERY

The goals for ophthalmic surgery are akinesia, profound analgesia, minimal bleeding, avoidance of the oculocardiac reflex, control of IOP, awareness of drug interactions, and smooth induction and emergence without vomiting or coughing/bucking.

E. Latex Allergy

DEFINITION

Latex allergy means having an allergic reaction when exposed to a latex protein allergen. It is a systemic allergic reaction to natural rubber. The diagnosis of latex allergy is based on the identification of persons with latex-specific immunoglobulin E (IgE) and symptoms consistent with IgE-mediated reactions to latex-containing devices. Materials that aerosolize or contact the skin, mucosa, respiratory and vascular system are likely to cause reactions. *Latex sensitivity* means testing positive for specific immunologic changes related to exposure to latex. Having a sensitivity does not necessarily mean that the person will experience any clinical symptoms when exposed to the allergen. The presence of specific latex IgE antibodies only demonstrates that sensitization has occurred and does not indicate when someone will have a reaction or the severity of a potential reaction. The most commonly used latex products causing reactions are balloons, condoms, and gloves.

INCIDENCE AND PREVALENCE

In the general population, the prevalence rate is reported as 1% to 7.6%. The prevalence among health care workers has been reported in a range from 0.9% to 30%. High-risk populations include persons with occupational exposure (health care workers, rubber industry workers, hair stylists), atopy (rhinitis, eczema, and asthma), spina bifida and congenital genitourinary abnormalities, and other conditions that require multiple surgical procedures. In addition to these risk groups, persons who have certain food allergies may have a coexisting latex allergy. Foods with possible cross-sensitivity with latex allergy include banana, avoado, chestnut, kiwi, apricot, papaya, and passion fruit.

ETIOLOGY

Latex allergy is an IgE-mediated immunologic response. The most significant factors that contribute to latex sensitivity include the frequency and duration of exposure to latex as well as the specific amount of available protein content of the product.

LABORATORY RESULTS

Diagnostic tests for latex allergy include skin testing, serum immunoassays, and challenge studies. Skin prick testing has been the gold standard for diagnosis of latex allergy and is the most sensitive means of detecting IgE antibody. In vitro immunoassays are tests used to measure the IgE responses in the serum of latex-allergic persons. Latex-IgE binding proteins vary in size and appear different in various risk groups, a feature that accounts for some of the variations in testing results. Three tests are currently approved by the U.S. Food and Drug Administration for use: AlaSTAT (American Diagnostics Corporation), CAPS (Pharmacia), and Hycor (Labcor).

CLINICAL MANIFESTATIONS

In health care workers, most clinical reactions are caused by skin contact, mucosal exposure, or inhalation to latex allergens. Repeated exposures to latex can precipitate escalating severity in symptomatic reactions. Clinical manifestations associated with latex allergy include contact dermatitis (irritant and allergic), rhinitis and asthma, and anaphylaxis.

TREATMENT

Treatment of latex reactions depends on their severity. If there is a high suspicion of a severe reaction, histamine-1 (H_1)- and H_2-receptor antagonists and corticosteroids are considered. This pretreatment is not routine practice. For mild reactions, the aforementioned medications are usually sufficient. Severe anaphylactic-type reactions may require epinephrine administration and respiratory and cardiovascular support. The best treatment is prevention of contact in susceptible patient populations.

ANESTHETIC CONSIDERATIONS

Intraoperative management is characterized by a latex-free environment. Nonlatex gloves are used by all personnel who may be in contact with patients, especially their mucous membranes. Medications should not be withdrawn from multidose bottles with latex caps or injected through latex ports on intravenous delivery tubing. Adhesive tape, intravenous and bladder catheters, drains, anesthesia delivery tubing, ventilator bellows, endotracheal tubes, laryngeal mask airways, nasogastric tubes, blood pressure cuffs, pulse oximeter probes, electrocardiogram pads, and syringes are selected on the basis of being latex free. Despite these precautions, it can never be guaranteed that allergic reactions to latex will not occur. The American Association of Nurse Anesthetists Latex Allergy Protocol is listed in Appendix III.

F. Malnutrition

DEFINITION

Malnutrition, or nutritional failure, is associated with protein depletion in the presence of adequate calories or with combined protein-calorie deficiency. Protein-calorie depletion is a frequent finding in surgical patients and in the critically ill.

INCIDENCE AND PREVALENCE

Critically ill patients experience negative caloric intake because of the hypermetabolic state produced by their illness. Trauma, fever, sepsis, and wound healing result in a drastically increased metabolism.

ETIOLOGY

Basic energy requirements are an intake of 1500 to 2000 calories/day. An increase in body temperature of 1° C increases daily caloric requirements by 15%. Multiple fractures increase in energy needs by 25%. Major burns cause the greatest increase in energy requirements, 100%. In addition, patients with large tumors may also have their energy requirements greatly increased.

LABORATORY RESULTS

The lack of a specific test for protein-calorie malnutrition often makes diagnosis difficult. The best single index of malnutrition is evidence of weight loss from the patient's normal level of weight. Plasma albumin levels lower than 3 g/dL and transferrin levels less than 200 mg/dL have also been used to diagnose malnutrition. Nitrogen balance, which requires the careful collection of all drainage and excretions over 24 hours, may be used to evaluate nutritional status. Nitrogen balance provides an estimate of net protein degradation or synthesis.

CLINICAL MANIFESTATIONS

Protein depletion affects the protein content of all organs. The liver and gastrointestinal tract are rapidly depleted; the brain is affected less than other organs. If protein depletion is severe, the gastrointestinal system will be unable to tolerate or digest food because protein is needed to produce digestive enzymes. Skeletal muscle is most affected and may lose as much as 70% of its protein. Patients with malnutrition are at increased risk of infections and complications in the postoperative period.

TREATMENT

The steps in planning a nutritional regimen are first to identify the need for intervention, then to determine the route of delivery, and finally to adjust the amounts of macronutrients and micronutrients the patient requires.

ANESTHETIC CONSIDERATIONS

Enteral and parenteral are the two routes of choice. At times, these two routes are combined. Enteral supplements can be sipped or administered through a nasogastric feeding tube or gastrostomy tube. If the gastrointestinal tract is nonfunctional, intravenous (parenteral) nutrition is instituted. Isotonic solutions can be delivered through peripheral veins. However, if the solution is hypertonic because of a greater caloric need, a central line should be used.

Patients receiving exogenous nutritional support are prone to deficits or an overabundance of certain electrolytes. Careful evaluation of laboratory values preoperatively as well as of any function tests performed is imperative. Parenteral nutrition has the greatest potential for complications. Hypoglycemia and hyperglycemia are common. Increased carbon dioxide resulting from metabolism of large amounts of glucose may hinder early extubation postoperatively. Patients with compromised cardiac function are at risk of congestive heart failure related to fluid overload. Electrolyte abnormalities include hypokalemia, hypomagnesemia, hypocalcemia, and hypophosphatemia. If parenteral nutrition is continued intraoperatively, infusions of other fluids should be minimized. Malnutrition is a clinical finding that must be partially corrected preoperatively. Therapy must be maintained.

G. Obesity

DEFINITION
Obesity is a complex multifactorial chronic disease that develops from an interaction of genotype and the environment. Overweight is defined as a body mass index (BMI) of 25 to 29 kg/m^2 and obesity as a BMI of 30 kg/m^2.
BMI can be calculated by:

- BMI = Weight (in kilograms)/Height (in meters)^2
- BMI = [Body weight (in pounds)/Height (in inches)^2] × 703

Classification of Overweight and Obesity by Body Mass Index

	Obesity Class	Body Mass Index (kg/m^2)	Risk of Disease
Underweight		<18.5	Increased
Normal		18.5–24.9	Normal
Overweight		25–29.9	Increased
Obesity	I	30–34.9	High
	II	35–39.9	Very high
	III	>40	Extremely high

INCIDENCE AND PREVALENCE
Obesity is a disease that affects more than one third of the adult American population. It is the second leading cause of preventable death in the United States. The number of overweight and obese adults has continued to increase since the mid-1990s. It is estimated that 64.5% of U.S. adults (about 127 million) are either overweight or obese. Demographically, obesity has dramatically increased among civilian, black, white, and Hispanic populations of both sexes and all ages. Obesity in children and adolescents has also increased significantly since the mid-1990s. In the United States, 30% of this population is overweight and 15% is obese.

ETIOLOGY
Obesity is a complex and multifactorial disease. Body size is dependent on genetic and environmental factors. Genetic predisposition, believed to be a primary factor in the development of obesity, explains only 40% of the variance in body mass. The significant increase in the prevalence of obesity has resulted from environmental factors that increase food intake and reduce physical activity. Other factors such as socialization, age, sex, race, and economic status affect its progression. In the United States, food consumption has risen as a result of the supersizing of portions and the availability of fast food and snacks with high fat content. Physical activity has been reduced as a result of modernization (television and computers), sedentary life-style, and work activities. Cultural and life-style variations play an important role in the development of obesity.

LABORATORY RESULTS
Findings include hypercholesterolemia, hypertriglyceridemia, and altered pulmonary function test results. Baseline arterial blood gases, chest x-ray studies, electrocardiograms, and echocardiograms are used for diagnosis.

CLINICAL MANIFESTATIONS

Manifestations include increased cardiac output, blood volume, oxygen consumption, minute ventilation, work of breathing, and carbon dioxide production, as listed in the next box. Obesity is associated with an increase in the incidence of more than 30 medical conditions. The risk of cardiovascular disease, certain cancers, diabetes, and disease overall is linearly related to weight gain. Type 2 diabetes, coronary heart disease, hypertension, and hypercholesterolemia are prominent conditions in overweight and obese patients. With increasing weight gain and increased adiposity, glucose tolerance deteriorates, blood pressure rises, and the lipid profile becomes more atherogenic. Hormonal and nonhormonal mechanisms contribute to the greater risk of breast, gastrointestinal, endometrial, and renal cell cancers. Psychologic health risks often stem from social ostracism, discrimination, and impaired ability to participate fully in activities of daily living. The physiologic changes associated with obesity are listed in the following box.

Physiologic Changes Occurring with Obesity

Cardiovascular Changes
- Increased cardiac output
- Increased blood volume
- Hypertension
- Pulmonary hypertension
- Ventricular hypertrophy
- Congestive heart failure

Respiratory Changes
- Increased oxygen consumption
- Increased carbon dioxide production
- Increased work of breathing
- Increased minute ventilation
- Decreased chest wall compliance
- Decreased lung volumes (including functional residual capacity), restrictive pattern
- Arterial hypoxemia
- Obstructive sleep apnea
- Obesity hypoventilation syndrome

Metabolic Changes
- Increased metabolic rate
- Diabetes mellitus due to insulin resistance

Gastrointestinal Changes
- Fatty liver infiltration
- Elevated intraabdominal pressure (gastroesophageal reflux disease, hiatal hernia)
- Increased gastric volume
- Increased gastric acidity

Other Changes
- Osteoarthritis

TREATMENT

A multimodal approach in the treatment of obesity includes dietary intervention, increased exercise, behavior modification, drug therapy, and surgery. Weight loss programs are individualized to each patient based on the degree of obesity and coexisting conditions. Drug therapy is initiated in patients with a BMI greater than 30 kg/m² or a BMI between 27 and 29.9 kg/m² with a coexisting medical condition. Pharmacologic management includes the administration of anorexiant drugs that affect the monoamine oxidase system. Through interactions with norepinephrine, dopamine, and serotonin, anorexiant agents affect satiation (level of fullness) or satiety (level of hunger after eating) or both. The most commonly used anorexiant drug is sibutramine hydrochloride (Meridia). Gastrointestinal lipase inhibitors such as Orlistat (Xenical) have been used to block the absorption of dietary fat. Overweight and obese patients may self-prescribe "natural" herbs and plant concoctions such as *ma huang* or diet teas that contain ephedra and unknown quantities of other stimulants.

Surgical approaches designed to treat obesity can be classified as malabsorptive or restrictive. Malabsorptive procedures, which include jejunoileal bypass and biliopancreatic bypass, are rarely used at the present time. Restrictive procedures include the vertical banded gastroplasy† (VBG) and gastric banding, including adjustable gastric banding (AGB). Roux-en-Y gastric bypass (RYGB) combines gastric restriction with a minimal degree of malabsorption. VBG, AGB, and RYGB can all be performed laparoscopically. RYGB, the most commonly performed bariatric procedure in the United States, involves anastomosing the proximal gastric pouch to a segment of the proximal jejunum and bypassing most of the stomach and the entire duodenum. It is the most effective bariatric procedure to produce short-term and long-term weight loss in severely obese patients. Advances in laparascopic surgery have significantly improved surgical procedure times, morbidity, and mortality related to bariatric surgery.

PHARMACOLOGIC CONSIDERATIONS

Obesity is associated with significant alterations in body composition and function that can alter the pharmacodynamics and pharmacokinetics of drugs. Alterations in the volume of distribution are related to the following factors: size of the fat organ, increased blood volume, increased cardiac output, increased total body weight, and alterations in protein binding and lipophilicity of the drug. Highly lipophilic drugs have an increased volume of distribution in obese persons compared with persons of normal weight. The increased volume of distribution requires higher doses of lipophilic drugs to produce the required pharmacologic effect and prolongs the elimination of certain drugs such as thiopental (Pentothal) and benzodiazepines. Factors such as protein binding and end-organ clearance affect volume of distribution.

There is no relationship for some highly lipophilic drugs (digoxin, remifentanil, and procainamide) between their solubility and distribution in obese patients. Dosing by ideal body weight is appropriate for these drugs. Drugs with weak or moderate lipophilicity are usually dosed based on ideal body weight or lean body mass. Recommendations for dosing commonly used anesthetics are listed in the following table.

Dosing Guidelines for Intravenous Anesthetics

Anesthetic Agent	Dosing	Guidelines
Midazolam (Versed)	TBW	Increased central V_d; increase initial dose to achieve therapeutic effect, prolonged sedation
Thiopental	TBW	Increased V_d; increase initial dose, prolonged time to awakening
Propofol	TBW: Initial and infusion	Increased V_d; increase initial dose, high affinity for fat, high hepatic extraction
Fentanyl	TBW	Increased V_d; increased elimination half-time
Sufentanil	TBW	Increased V_d; increased elimination half-time
Remifentanil	IBW	Consider age and lean body mass
cis-Atracurium	TBW	No difference normal weight
Vecuronium	IBW	Increased V_d; impaired hepatic clearance; prolonged duration of action
Rocuronium	IBW	Faster onset and similar duration of action
Succinylcholine	TBW	Increased plasma pseudo-cholinesterase activity; increase dose

IBW, Ideal body weight; *TBW*, total body weight; V_d, volume of distribution.

Elimination of drugs in obese individuals is normal or increased in phase I reactions (oxidation, reduction, and hydrolysis) and increased in phase II reactions (metabolism). Renal clearance is increased by the augmented renal blood flow and glomerular filtration rate.

ANESTHETIC CONSIDERATIONS

No demonstrable difference in emergence from inhalation versus narcotic technique has been discerned in obese patients. The use of short-acting water-soluble anesthetics facilitates smooth anesthetic induction, maintenance, and emergence from anesthesia. Objectives for maintenance of anesthesia in obese patients include the following: strict maintenance of airway, adequate skeletal muscle relaxation, optimum oxygenation, avoidance of the residual effects of muscle relaxants, provision of appropriate intraoperative and postoperative tidal volume, and effective postoperative analgesia. Depending on the patient's condition, these can be achieved by either general or regional anesthesia regimens. An epidural anesthetic with concomitant "light" general anesthesia is frequently chosen. A light general anesthetic can facilitate management of the airway, ventilation, and the patient's level of consciousness while the epidural anesthetic provides surgical analgesia and anesthesia. Combining these techniques accomplishes all the objectives. The epidural catheter can be used for postoperative analgesic administration. This will enhance earlier resumption of deep breathing and coughing maneuvers.

Airway Evaluation

A thorough airway evaluation is warranted to determine the optimal airway management technique in overweight and obese patients. Most practitioners use evaluation of multiple patient physical characteristics to identify potential airway problems indicative of the unanticipated difficult airway. These include measurement of interincisor distance, thyromental distance, head and neck extension, Mallampati classification, body weight, and a past history of difficult airway. Evaluation of the length of upper incisors, visibility of the uvula, shape of the palate, compliance of the mandibular space, and length and thickness of the neck provides further assessment. Increasing neck circumference and Mallampati's classification higher than grade III have been identified as the two most important factors in morbidly obese patients.

Anatomic aberrations of the upper airway induced by severe obesity include reduced temporomandibular and atlanto-occipital joint movement. Unsatisfactory mouth opening, presence of neck or arm pain, or inability to place the head and neck into "sniffing position" may indicate the need for awake fiberoptic intubation. Extreme airway narrowing, in conjunction with shortened mandibular-hyoid distance (less than three fingerbreadths) can complicate mask ventilation and intubation. Presence of a short, thick neck, pendulous breasts, hypertrophied tonsils and adenoids, and beards can contribute to a difficult airway. Marginal room air pulse oximeter saturations, abnormal arterial blood gases, and previous history of complicated airway management also indicate a potentially difficult intubation, which occurs in at least 13% of severely obese patients.

Aspiration Prophylaxis

Of significance to the airway in the anesthetized obese patient is the increased risk of regurgitation (passive and active) and subsequent pulmonary aspiration. Obese persons have greater volumes and more acidic gastric fluid than persons of normal weight. Gastroesophageal reflux and hiatus hernia, which are more prevalent in obese patients, also predispose them to esophagitis and pulmonary aspiration. Other conditions that cause delayed gastric emptying, such as diabetes mellitus or traumatic injury, further increase the risk of aspiration. For these reasons, the obese patient is considered to have a "full stomach," even if the prescribed nothing-by-mouth (NPO) intake restriction has been followed. Debate and controversy exist as to the relative risk of aspiration in obesity; most practitioners use techniques to attenuate this complication.

Timely preinduction administration of histamine-2– and dopamine-receptor antagonists coupled with oral administration of nonparticulate antacids decreases morbidity resulting from pulmonary aspiration and Mendelson's syndrome. Head-up positioning of the patient, with application of the Sellick maneuver during rapid sequence induction, limits the volume of vomitus that enters the trachea if regurgitation occurs. Nasogastric or orogastric suctioning before emergence further reduces the amount of fluid available for aspiration.

Intubation

The obese patient should be positioned with the head elevated (reverse Trendelenberg's position) on the operating room table. This position facilitates patient comfort, reduces gastric reflux, provides easier mask ventilation, improves respiratory mechanics, and helps to maintain functional residual capacity. The reduced functional residual capacity in obese patients contributes to the rapid desaturation that occurs with induction of general anesthesia. To attenuate the desaturation and to maximize oxygen content in the lungs, patients are preoxygenated with 100% mask oxygen for at least 3 to 5 minutes. The patient's head, neck, and shoulders should be carefully moved into "sniffing position" by using pillows, "doughnuts," or foam head supports.

Some practitioners advocate the use of an "awake look" to visualize the difficulty of the airway. Careful administration of sedative drugs, application of topical anesthesia to the oropharyngeal structures, and transtracheal and superior laryngeal nerve blocks are performed. Nasal oxygen is used as a supplement during awake laryngoscopy. If epiglottic and laryngeal architecture is easily visualized, successful asleep intubation can be done. If the airway structures cannot be visualized, an intubating laryngeal mask airway or awake fiberoptic intubation should be performed. The surgeon and another skilled anesthesia provider must also be in attendance during the induction. Muscle hypotonus in the floor of the mouth, followed by rapid occurrence of soft tissue obstruction and hypoxia, requires one person to support the mask and airway while another person bag ventilates the patient. In the case of inability to ventilate or intubate, the American Society of Anesthesiologists' difficult airway algorithm should be followed (see Appendix V).

Volume Replacement

The normal adult percentage of total body water is 60% to 65%. In the severely obese patient, it is reduced to 40%. Therefore, calculation of estimated blood volume should be 45 to 55 mL/kg actual body weight rather than the 70 mL/kg apportioned to the nonobese adult. Use of reduced parameters for volume replacement and avoidance of rapid rehydration lessen cardiopulmonary compromise. Fluid management is guided by blood pressure, heart rate, and urine output measurements. Volume expanders, such as hetastarch (Hespan), should not be administered at greater than recommended volumes per kilogram of ideal body weight (20 mL/kg). Dilutional coagulopathy, factor VIII inhibition, and decreased platelet aggregability can result from excessive administration. Albumin 5% and 25% should be used as indicated to support circulatory volume and oncotic pressure. When replacing blood loss with crystalloid, the 3:1 ratio (3 mL of crystalloid to 1 mL of blood loss) is applicable to the severely obese patient.

Intraoperative Positioning

Surgical positioning of morbidly obese patients necessitates extra precautions to prevent nerve, integumentary, and cardiorespiratory compromise. The type of surgery, combined with inordinate stretching or compression of nerve plexus, and prolonged immobility cause local tissue ischemia and damage that begins at the cellular level. Hypothermia, hypotension, table positioning, and the hydraulic pressure effect that the adipose patient places on orthopedic or cardiopulmonary structures potentiate impairment.

Regional Anesthesia

Regional anesthesia can be used as the primary anesthetic technique in selected cases or as an accompaniment to postoperative pain and mobility management. Difficulties are frequently encountered, however, in the severely obese patient. Anatomic landmarks used to guide conduction blockade are not easily visualized or palpable.

Extubation

The risk of airway obstruction following extubation is increased in the obese patient. A decision to extubate depends on evaluation of the ease of mask ventilation and tracheal intubation, the length and type of surgery, and presence of preexisting medical conditions, including obstructive sleep apnea. Criteria for extubation include the following: an awake patient; tidal volume and respiratory rate at preoperative levels; sustained head lift or leg lift for at least 5 seconds; strong, constant hand grip, effective cough; adequate vital capacity of at least 15 mL/kg; and inspiratory force of at least 25 to 30 cm H_2O negative. Patients must be placed with their head up or in a sitting position. If doubt exists about the ability of the patient to breathe adequately, the endotracheal tube is left in place. Extubation over an airway exchange catheter or through a fiberoptic bronchoscope may be performed.

H. Scleroderma

DEFINITION

Widespread, symmetric lesions that cause induration of the skin and are followed by atrophy and pigmentation changes characterize scleroderma. It is a systemic disease that affects muscles, bones, heart, and lungs. Intestinal and pulmonary changes also occur. Lung volumes, vital capacity, compliance, and dead space all decrease. The respiratory rate increases, and diffusion capacity is impaired. Pulmonary hypertension can occur.

ANESTHETIC CONSIDERATIONS

Tightening of the skin around the neck may limit mobility and mouth opening. Alternate methods to secure the airway (e.g., fiberoptic intubation) should be considered. Baseline pulmonary function tests and arterial blood gases may assist in optimizing these patients preoperatively, intraoperatively, and postoperatively. Postoperative ventilatory assistance may be needed. Be alert for vasospastic phenomena following induction of anesthesia: these should be treated with a plasma expander. Regional anesthesia is acceptable. Core temperature must be maintained. Gastrointestinal pretreatment (e.g., histamine blockers, metoclopramide) may be necessary because of poor gastric emptying.

I. Systemic Lupus Erythematosus

DEFINITION

Systemic lupus erythematosus (SLE) is a chronic inflammatory disorder of connective tissues that affects multiple organ systems with periods of remissions and exacerbations.

INCIDENCE AND PREVALENCE

SLE occurs 8 to 15 times more often in women than in men and affects approximately 75 people in 1,000,000 every year. It occurs most often in Asians and in blacks. Exacerbations are more common in spring and summer and during stresses such as infection, pregnancy, and surgery.

ETIOLOGY

The origin of SLE is unknown. One theory is that it is an antibody-antigen autoimmune response. Another theory deals with predisposing factors that promote susceptibility to SLE. These factors include stressors such as infection, exposure to ultraviolet light, immunizations, and pregnancy. A third theory suggests that drugs such as procainamide, hydralazine, penicillin, anticonvulsants, oral contraceptives, and sulfa drugs may trigger SLE.

LABORATORY RESULTS

Complete blood count with differential may reveal anemia, a decreased white blood cell count, and a decreased platelet count. Specific tests for SLE include antinuclear antibodies, anti-DNA, and lupus erythematosus cell tests; urine analysis may reveal both red and white blood cells. Chest x-ray examination may reveal pulmonary involvement, and electrocardiography may show conduction abnormalities.

CLINICAL MANIFESTATIONS

Clinical manifestations of SLE include arthritis of the upper and lower extremities as well as avascular necrosis of the femur. Systemically, SLE affects major organ systems (heart, lungs, kidneys, liver, neuromuscular system, skin). Pericarditis, myocarditis, tachycardia, arrhythmias, and congestive heart failure may develop. Left ventricular dysfunction and endocarditis have also been associated with SLE. About 50% of patients with SLE develop such cardiopulmonary abnormalities. Pneumonia, pleural effusions, cough, dyspnea, and hypoxemia are common. Glomerulonephritis and oliguric renal failure may result. Some patients develop lupoid hepatitis, which may be fatal. They may also incur intestinal ischemia. The neuromuscular system may be affected by myopathies. Psychologic changes include schizophrenia and deterioration of the intellect. The skin may exhibit the typical lesion associated with SLE; this "butterfly rash" appears over the nose and is erythematous. Alopecia may also be seen clinically.

TREATMENT

The usual treatment of SLE includes antiinflammatory therapy with aspirin. Corticosteroids are often used to suppress adverse renal and cardiovascular system changes. For patients who do not respond well to steroids, immunosuppressive agents may be used. Antimalarial drugs, in small doses, have been found to be effective in treating arthritis and skin lesions.

ANESTHETIC CONSIDERATIONS

Anesthesia management is based on medications used to treat the disorder as well as the organ involvement. Care must be taken in positioning the patient to avoid hyperextension of the neck. These patients may be difficult to intubate because of their inflammatory changes, and they frequently have restrictive lung disease and therefore may be difficult to ventilate. Rapid rates with smaller tidal volumes may be helpful. Overall, a thorough preoperative evaluation should be performed to establish organ system involvement.

Cutaneous lesions on the nose and mouth may make mask fit difficult. Cricoarytenoid arthritis rarely occurs. Patients with advanced disease may be debilitated, and chest x-ray findings, complete blood cell count, and electrolytes should be checked. Anemia and thrombocytopenic purpura have been identified. The partial thromboplastin time may be falsely elevated because antibodies of SLE react with phospholipids used to determine partial thromboplastin time. If renal dysfunction is advanced, drugs dependent on renal elimination should be avoided. If the patient is currently receiving steroids or has taken them within 6 months, a steroid bolus should be used.

CARDIOVASCULAR SYSTEM

Management of anesthesia for cardiac surgery requires a thorough understanding of normal and altered cardiac physiology, knowledge of the pharmacology of anesthetic, vasoactive, and cardiac drugs, and an understanding of the physiologic alterations associated with cardiopulmonary bypass and the specific surgical procedures.

A. Cardiac Tamponade and Constrictive Pericarditis

1. **Pathophysiology**
   a) A large pericardial effusion, which can develop slowly, may cause few or no symptoms. A small and rapidly forming effusion may lead to cardiac tamponade.
   b) Right ventricular pressure waveforms are unchanged during tamponade but show a dip and a prominent y descent in constrictive pericarditis.
   c) Severity of the condition is determined by the degree of tachycardia, hypotension, and filling pressures.
2. **Anesthetic considerations**
   a) Primary goals are to avoid decreases in myocardial contractility, peripheral vascular resistance, and heart rate.
   b) Pericardiocentesis in patients with tamponade may be advisable before induction.
   c) Induction agents include etomidate and ketamine. A dopamine infusion during induction and the preparation phase is helpful.
   d) Transesophageal and transvenous pacing modalities should be readily available.
   e) In severely compromised patients, an awake intubation and having the patient prepared and draped before induction is advisable.

B. Coronary Artery Disease

The rate of coronary artery disease (CAD) has rapidly progressed to make it the predominant cause of death for patients in their 40s and 50s. There are upwards of 519,000 adult coronary artery surgical procedures yearly, and this number represents 80% of all adult heart operations performed in the United States.

1. **Risk factors**
   a) Age: Increased risk with increased age
   b) Gender: Men at greater risk than women
   c) Genetic predisposition
   d) Obesity

e) Hyperlipidemia: High levels of low-density and intermediate-density lipoproteins associated with atherosclerosis
f) Hypertension: Increased risk with high blood pressure, especially diastolic
g) Smoking: Risk of those who smoke one pack per day 70- to 200-fold that of nonsmokers
h) Diabetes mellitus: Increases risk of myocardial infarction twofold

2. **Myocardial oxygen supply and demand**
Management of patients with CAD requires controlling the factors determining myocardial oxygen demand and optimizing oxygen delivery to the heart. When myocardial demand exceeds supply, ischemia develops.

a) Determinants of oxygen demand
   (1) Myocardial wall tension: According to the Law of Laplace, wall tension is directly proportional to the chamber's distending pressure and internal radius and is indirectly proportional to wall thickness.
       (a) Preload: This refers to left ventricular end-diastolic (LVED) volume, which determines the end-diastolic fiber length and, in turn, profoundly affects myocardial performance.
       (b) Afterload: This refers to the force distributed by the ventricular wall during ejection, usually equated with the ventricular pressure during ejection and varies with time; it is an impedance to ventricular ejection.
       (c) Goal: Lowering the end-diastolic volume will decrease wall tension and therefore decrease myocardial oxygen demand. (Nitroglycerin, morphine, and nitroprusside [Nipride] all accomplish this goal.)
   (2) Contractility
       (a) This is the ability of the myocardium to develop force; it is not dependent on the load of the heart. In the normal heart, sympathetic stimulation and inotropes increase myocardial contractility and oxygen demand.
       (b) Goal: If wall tension is constant and contractility is decreased, oxygen demand will decrease. (Calcium channel blockers, β-blockers, and volatile agents decrease myocardial oxygen demand.)
   (3) Heart Rate
       (a) Oxygen demand increases as the number of contractions per minute increases.
       (b) Goal: Avoid tachyarrythmias. (β-Blockers decrease heart rate.)

b) Determinants of oxygen supply
   (1) Coronary blood flow: This is directly related to the perfusion pressure across the coronary vascular bed and is inversely related to total coronary resistance.
       (a) Coronary perfusion pressure: This is the difference between aortic diastolic pressure and the LVED pressure (LVEDP).
       (b) Total coronary resistance: This consists of the basal resistance during diastole and the compressive resistance during systole.
       (c) Goal: A low LVEDP is ideal for improving perfusion because of the higher pressure gradient.

(d) Heart rate: Coronary arteries fill during the diastolic phase of the cardiac cycle; increased heart rates decrease coronary filling time.

(e) Arterial oxygen content (CaO_2): Maintaining the blood's oxygen-carrying capacity is vital to perfusion of vital organs, including the heart. Variables affecting CaO_2 include the hemoglobin level and oxygen saturation (see the following equation).

$$CaO_2 = (SaO_2)(Hgb)(1.34) + (PaO_2)(0.003)$$

3. **Coronary artery bypass grafting**
   a) Methods have been devised to promote coronary blood flow because it has been determined that thrombosis causes the development of myocardial infarction. Some of these methods involve shunting collateral pericardial blood to epicardial arteries and implantation of the internal mammary artery as meant without ligating side branches. Saphenous veins can also be anastomosed to the epicardial coronary arteries. The technique of coronary artery bypass grafting involves bypass of a narrowed or occluded epicardial coronary greater than 1 mm in diameter with a small-diameter conduit distal to the narrowed segment. The proximal arterial inflow source is the ascending aorta.
   b) The surgeon approaches the heart through a median sternotomy, and the patient is supported on full coronary artery bypass. The most common strategy used is for all distal (epicardial) anastomoses to be performed during a period of aortic cross-clamping and cardiac arrest. Myocardial protection is achieved by hypothermia and occasional reperfusion through anterograde or retrograde cardioplegia. Cardiac standstill and a bloodless field are mandatory for these small-diameter anastomoses to be constructed with an obstruction to flow in minimal amount of time.
   c) The cross-clamp is removed, and the heart is allowed to resume beating. A partially occluding aortic cross-clamp can be applied to allow for

PART II **Common Procedures**

Improving Myocardial Oxygen Supply-Demand Balance

1. Decrease myocardial oxygen demand
   a. Decrease wall tension by decreasing chamber size with venous and arterial vasodilators.
   b. Decrease contractility with calcium channel antagonists, β-blockers, or volatile agents. (Use caution in patients with compromised left ventricular function.)
   c. Slow heart rate with β-blockers and anesthetics.
2. Increase oxygen supply
   a. Decrease heart rate to 50 to 60 beats/min to maximize coronary filling time during diastole.
   b. Increase coronary perfusion pressure by increasing aortic diastolic pressure and decreasing left ventricular end-diastolic pressure. (Often a combination of phenylephrine [Neo-Synephrine] and nitroglycerin will achieve these goals.)
   c. Maximize oxygen-carrying capacity with supplemental oxygen and red blood cells to correct anemia.

the construction of the proximal aortic anastomoses. After an adequate period of resuscitation, the patient is weaned from cardiopulmonary bypass (CPB). Decannulation is performed, heparin is reversed, and the chest is closed.

d) Typical target arteries requiring CPB include the distal right coronary artery and its major terminal branch, the posterior descending artery. Typical target arteries on the left include the left anterior descending artery with its diagonal and septal branches. This coronary artery courses in the posterior atrioventricular groove and is not easily accessible for bypass. Therefore, this procedure is usually performed to its obtuse marginal or posterolateral branches.

e) The choice of the vein graft depends on its availability and durability. The internal mammary artery appears to have superior long-term performance with patency rates of 90% after 10 years. Conversely, the saphenous vein graft has a 50% patency rate at 10 years.

f) The usual preoperative diagnosis of these patients is CAD with class 3 or 4 angina. This type of angina occurs with minimal exertion or at rest.

4. **Selection of anesthesia**

a) Goal: The goal in anesthesia selection is to decrease myocardial oxygen requirements and prevent myocardial ischemia.

b) The selection of drugs is influenced by the extent of preexisting myocardial dysfunction and the pharmacologic properties of the specific agents.

c) Opioids lack myocardial depressant effects and are useful in patients with severe myocardial dysfunction.

(1) In critically ill patients, fentanyl (50 to 100 mcg/kg) or sufentanil (5 to 20 mcg/kg) may be used as the sole anesthetic.

(2) In patients with good left ventricular function, opioids may be inadequate in suppressing sympathetic nervous system activity, requiring the addition of volatile anesthetics and sedative/hypnotics.

d) Inhalation agents

(1) Advantages: These include dose dependency, easy reversibility, and reliable suppression of sympathetic nervous system responses to surgical stress and CPB.

(2) Disadvantages: These are myocardial depression and systemic hypotension.

(3) Combinations of opioids and volatile agents produce the advantages of each and minimize undesirable side effects.

(4) Isoflurane is a coronary vasodilator, although effects are clinically insignificant in doses less than 1 minimum alveolar concentration.

e) Sedative/hypnotics: Thiopental, propofol, ketamine, and etomidate may be useful as co-induction agents in particular situations. Of these drugs, etomidate causes the least amount of myocardial depression.

f) Muscle relaxants

(1) The best drugs are those with minimal cardiovascular effects (e.g., vecuronium, cisatracurium, rocuronium).

(2) A "priming dose" will help to counteract chest wall rigidity that is often encountered with narcotic induction.

(3) Succinylcholine may cause bradycardia but can be used in modified rapid sequence inductions for patients with reflux or a full stomach.

(4) Pancuronium can be used to produce a graded increase in heart rate when desirable.

C. Cardiopulmonary Bypass

1. **Extracorporeal circuit (ECC):** To proceed with all but the least invasive procedures involving surgery on the heart, an ECC must be used. The ECC is also called the "heart-lung machine," named for the cardiovascular function it must support during open heart surgery and cardiopulmonary bypass (CPB).

2. **Goals of the ECC:** The primary goals of the ECC are vascular transport, oxygenation, physiologic homeostasis, hemodynamic control, thermoregulation, and organ system preservation.

3. **ECC components:** The ECC consists of an oxygenator (membrane or bubble), venous reservoir, cardiotomy reservoir, circuit tubing, filters (arterial, prebypass, cardiotomy), tubing connectors, and cannulas (arterial, venous, and cardioplegic).

4. **Prime**
   a) Before bypass, the ECC is filled with fluid to eliminate air and to coat the surface of the membrane oxygenator, filters, and system tubing with the constituents of the prime solution. Establishment of an air-free circuit is essential for unimpaired fluid volume transport and prevention of air embolism.
   b) Most circuits require at least 2000 mL of a solution such as Normosol, Plasmalyte A, or Isolyte S with pH and electrolytes closely matching the composition of whole blood. Added to this base are heparin, sodium bicarbonate, mannitol, hetastarch, albumin, and possibly corticosteroids or antihyperfibrinolytic agents. The result is priming volumes in excess of 2000 mL, which, when transfused to the patient at the onset of CPB, can equate to a hemodilutional bolus of 30% to 50% of the patient's circulating blood volume.

5. **Safety mechanisms:** These mechanisms function to alert the operator to low venous operating reserve, high arterial pressures, disconnection from air supply, and introduction of air embolus into the arterial line.

6. **Cardioplegia delivery system:** This provides and maintains hypothermic and pharmacologic arrest of the heart during revascularization.

7. **Ultrafiltration and red blood cell–sequestering devices:** These devices may be incorporated into the ECC to counteract hemodilution by removing excess volume through dialysis or centrifugal separation of fluid and plasma components from the circulating blood volume.

8. **Cardiac output control:** Cardiac output is controlled by a pump delivery system (centrifugal or rollerhead) that maintains patient blood flow and perfusion pressure in accordance with physiologic state and requirements.

9. **Pulmonary control:** For control of pulmonary function, an oxygenator and blender are used to maintain appropriate oxygen saturation levels and respiratory acid-base homeostasis.

10. **Temperature regulation:** Core thermal regulation is maintained by a heater/cooler system that propels fluid housed separately in a compartment parallel to the blood pathway.

11. **Vascular transport**
    a) Vascular access at sites on the right side of the heart (atrial/venous) and the left side of the heart (aortic/arterial) are necessary for the shunting of deoxygenated blood away from the patient, to the heart-lung machine, and back to the aorta as propelled arterialized blood.

PART II **Common Procedures**

b) Isolation of the heart and lungs from systemic blood flow is accomplished by right atrial or vena caval cannulation with subsequent diversion of venous blood returning to the heart into a venous reservoir situated at a level below the patient's heart to facilitate gravity exsanguination.

c) Blood from the reservoir is propelled to the oxygenator, where it becomes arterialized. A heat exchanger mounted on the oxygenator provides for thermal control of blood temperature.

d) Oxygenated blood passes through an arterial filter and an arterial gas monitoring device.

e) Aortic cannula placement is distal to the sinus of Valsalva and proximal to the brachiocephalic artery.

f) Cardiac index and mean arterial pressure are maintained according to metabolic requirements and surgical demand.

12. **Myocardial protection techniques**

a) Rapid cardioplegia-induced cardiac arrest, decompression of the ventricles, and hypothermia are the underlying concerns for myocardial protection during CPB.

b) The severity of preexisting ischemia determines the magnitude of injury associated with reperfusion. The duration of aortic cross-clamping time, collateral coronary blood supply, frequency of cardioplegia delivery, and composition of cardioplegia are factors influencing the extent of reperfusion injury.

c) Intermittent doses of cold crystalloid cardioplegia help to maintain cardiac arrest, hypothermia, and pH to counteract edema, to wash out metabolites, and to provide oxygen substrate for aerobic metabolism.

(1) Maintenance doses are delivered in an antegrade fashion through the aortic root at intervals corresponding to completion of individual distal graft anastomoses.

(2) Retrograde delivery of cardioplegia through the coronary sinus in the right atrium may be used in the presence of severe cardiovascular disease, emergency revascularization for recent or ongoing myocardial infarction, or high-grade stenosis, in which antegrade delivery may prove ineffective in protecting myocardium distal to the lesion.

D. Pacemakers

1. **Indications**

a) Sick sinus syndrome, second-degree block type 2, and third-degree heart block are indications for pacemakers.

b) Heart blocks

(1) Atrioventricular block including complete heart block and type 2 second-degree block are pacemaker indications.

(2) Fascicular block including symptomatic bifascicular block and trifascicular block are pacemaker indications.

c) Temporary pacemakers are indicated for same reasons as permanent pacemakers. They may serve as a bridge until permanent pacing is available or until the cardiac condition stabilizes, such as after coronary artery bypass grafting.

2. **Preoperative evaluation**

a) Assess the patient's current cardiac status and symptoms.

b) Determine the original reason for the pacemaker.

c) Determine the type of pacemaker and the settings.

d) Determine the location of the generator. Usually, it is located in the upper chest, but occasionally it may be located in the abdomen.

e) Pacemaker wires may become easily dislodged in the first 6 weeks after placement. Central line placement may need to be done under fluoroscopy to avoid lead disruption.

3. **Intraoperative management**

Although most pacemakers now are resistant to electromagnetic interference (EMI) from the use of electrocautery, it can occasionally occur. The pacemaker output may be inhibited or the pacemaker may be reset to a preset pacing mode (DOO or VOO).

a) If EMI occurs, a doughnut magnet can be applied directly over the pacemaker, which will cause it to convert to the magnet or a committed mode. Most pacemakers will automatically convert to an asynchronous mode when prolonged EMI is detected, so the magnet intervention is rarely needed.

b) Heart rate should be monitored with a precordial or esophageal stethoscope, pulse oximeter, or arterial line or by palpating the pulse during electrocautery.

c) Postoperatively, pacemaker function is not routinely checked unless interference was detected or the surgical procedure involved primary insertion or generator change.

4. **Pacemaker insertion**

a) Insertion sites can be the subclavian vein or through the cephalic vein in the deltopectoral groove.

b) Leads are placed through the subclavian vein, through the tricuspid valve into the right atrium, or dual chamber leads may be placed with one in the right atrium and one in the right ventricle.

c) Anesthetic requirements are usually local anesthesia administered by the surgeon and intravenous sedation.

d) Common complications during placement are dysrhythmias.

e) Less common potential complications include pneumothorax, dislodging of electrodes, and cardiac tamponade.

5. **Pacemaker types (definitions and nomenclature)**

a) Unipolar pacing involves a negative electrode in the atrium or ventricle and a positive ground far from the heart. These are rarely used and are more prone to interference from electrocautery and other devices such as microwaves.

b) Bipolar pacing involves placement of both electrodes in the chamber being paced or sensed.

c) Asynchronous generators simply provide electrical impulses without sensing.

d) Synchronous generators have both pulse-sensing and generating circuits.

e) A five-letter code describes the functions and settings of the pacemaker (see the following table).

f) The two most common types of pacemakers are VVI and DDD, with the last two letters frequently omitted.

6. **Automatic internal cardiac defibrillator**

Internal cardiac defibrillators (ICDs) are used in populations that are at high risk of sudden death from cardiac tachydysrhythmias.

a) ICD consists of two defibrillating electrodes or patches and separate electrodes that are used for pacing and sensing. The patches are placed

PART II   Common Procedures

Chamber Paced	Chamber Sensed	Response to Sensing	Program-mability	Antitachy-arrhythmia Function
O = none	O = none	O = none	O = none	O = none
A = atrium	A = atrium	T = triggered	P = simple	P = pacing
V = ventricle	V = ventricle	I = inhibited	M = multipro-grammable	S = shock
D = dual (atrium and ventricle)	D = dual (atrium and ventricle)	D = dual (triggered and inhibited)	C = communi-cating	D = dual (pacing and shock)
			R = rate modulation	

near the pericardium. The generator is implanted in either the abdomen or chest wall.

b) All ICDs are extremely sensitive to EMI used in electrocautery. EMI is detected as ventricular fibrillation by the device and will deliver a shock to the patient.

c) Magnet application will cause the device to suspend detection, but it will not interfere with the pacing function. Intraoperatively, if ventricular fibrillation occurs, the magnet can simply be removed, and the device can deliver a shock, usually within 10 seconds. External defibrillators should always be readily available in case of failure.

d) The ICD can be turned off manually for the duration of the operation before the patient is taken into the operating room, and it can be turned back on in the postanesthesia care unit. Personnel trained in the use of an external cardiac defibrillator should be readily available while the device is turned off.

e) If only bipolar cautery is used, the device can usually remain on.

E. Valvular Heart Disease

1. **Aortic stenosis**
   Disease of the aortic valve may present as aortic valvular stenosis, insufficiency, or a combination of both. Valvular disease is usually caused by rheumatic disease, but it may also occur secondary to calcific degeneration in elderly patients. Endocarditis and a congenitally bicuspid valve account for most of the remainder. It is rarely possible to repair the aortic valve; therefore, most conditions require valve replacement.

   a) Pathophysiology: Chronic obstruction to left ventricular (LV) ejection results in concentric LV hypertrophy and myocardium that is highly susceptible to ischemia (even in the absence of coronary artery disease). Stenosis is severe when the valve area is less than 0.6 cm^2 and the pressure gradient is greater than 70 torr.

   b) Hemodynamic goals: LV filling is dependent on atrial contractions, heart rate, and normal intravascular volume. Decreases in systemic vascular resistance (SVR) are dangerous because of the fixed ventricular ejection; decreased SVR results in decreased blood pressure (BP), coronary perfusion pressures, and resultant ischemia.

   c) Dysrhythmias should be aggressively treated. Because the ventricle is stiff, atrial contraction is critical for ventricular filling and stroke volume.

d) Anesthetic considerations
  (1) Induction
    (a) Usually a high-dose narcotic technique is used: fentanyl, etomidate, and a muscle relaxant.
    (b) Avoid anesthetic agents that reduce vascular tone. Vasopressors should be available for induction.
    (c) Maintain intravascular volume and sinus rhythm.
    (d) Avoid increased heart rate; avoid decreased SVR and BP.
    (e) External cardiac massage is not effective in these patients. Ventricular tachycardia and fibrillation are usually fatal.
  (2) Maintenance: Use a high-dose narcotic, a low-dose volatile agent, oxygen, and air.
  (3) After bypass
    (a) The patient may have higher filling pressures because of the noncompliant ventricle. Inotropic support is commonly required.
    (b) The patient may be hyperdynamic or require vasodilators for hypertension.

2. **Aortic regurgitation**
  a) Pathophysiology
    (1) The incompetent aortic valve results in a decrease in forward LV stroke volume because part of the ejected LV volume regurgitates back into the LV from the aorta, resulting in chronic volume overload of the left ventricle and eccentric hypertrophy.
    (2) Aortic regurgitation causes a decrease in aortic diastolic BP and decreased coronary artery perfusion pressures resulting in subendocardial ischemia and angina (even in the absence of coronary artery disease).
    (3) The magnitude of regurgitation is dependent on the duration of flow and the pressure gradient across the valve. Regurgitation can be reduced by increasing heart rate and decreasing SVR.
    (4) In chronic aortic regurgitation, as end-diastolic volume increases, stroke volume increases so that the ejection fraction is well maintained until LV failure occurs. When failure occurs, cardiac output decreases, end-diastolic volume increases, and pulmonary edema results.
    (5) In acute aortic regurgitation, the sudden increase in LV volume without ventricular hypertrophy results in sudden cardiac failure.
  b) Anesthetic considerations
    (1) Maintenance of adequate ventricular volume in the presence of mild vasodilation and increases in heart rate is most likely to optimize forward LV stroke volume.
    (2) Avoid increases in SVR and BP; avoid decreases in heart rate.

3. **Mitral stenosis**
  a) Pathophysiology
    (1) Increased left atrial pressure and volume overload occur as a result of the narrowed mitral orifice. Persistent increases in the left atrial pressure are reflected back through the pulmonary circulation, leading to right ventricular hypertrophy and failure, tricuspid regurgitation, and perivascular edema in the lungs.
    (2) The left atrial enlargement predisposes the patient to formation of thrombi and systemic emboli, especially with the development of atrial fibrillation.
  b) Anesthetic considerations

(1) Tachycardia results in inadequate LV filling and concomitant hypotension. Continued preoperative administration of digitalis and β-antagonists, the selection of anesthetics with a minimal propensity to increase heart rate, and achievement of an anesthetic depth sufficient to suppress sympathetic nervous system responses are recommended.

(2) Administer induction agents slowly to avoid drug-induced reductions in SVR and resultant hypotension in the presence of a fixed LV stroke volume. Avoid ketamine because of the increase in heart rate associated with this drug.

(3) Preoxygenation and brief laryngoscopy reduce the potential for hypoxia, hypercarbia, and acidosis. (These potentiate pulmonary vasoconstriction, which will potentiate right-sided heart failure.)

(4) Avoid increases in heart rate; avoid decreases in myocardial contractility, SVR, and BP.

4. Mitral regurgitation
a) Pathophysiology

(1) Chronic volume overload of the left atrium occurs, resulting in a decreased LV stroke volume because of part of the stroke volume's regurgitating through the incompetent valve. The increase in left atrial pressure results in elevated pulmonary pressures and right-sided heart failure. LV hypertrophy results to compensate for the decreased cardiac output.

(2) The amount of regurgitation depends on the size of the valve orifice, the heart rate, and the pressure gradient across the valve.

(3) Mild increases in heart rate improve LV stroke volume. Bradycardia results in acute volume overload of the left atrium.

(4) The pressure gradient across the valve is determined by the compliance of the LV and the impedance to LV ejection into the aorta. Reducing SVR can improve forward flow.

b) Anesthetic considerations

(1) Select agents that promote vasodilation and increase the heart rate.

(2) Avoid myocardial depression, which will decrease cardiac output.

(3) Barbiturates, benzodiazepines, etomidate, and succinylcholine are good choices.

(4) Maintain normocarbia and oxygen saturation to prevent increases in pulmonary hypertension associated with pulmonary vasoconstriction.

F. Cardiac Surgery Plan of Care

1. Patient assessment
a) Cardiac evaluation

(1) Hypertension, heart disease (coronary artery disease [CAD], angina, myocardial infarction [MI], congestive heart failure [CHF], smoking, chronic obstructive pulmonary disease [COPD], carotid artery stenosis, transient ischemic attack/cardiovascular accident [TIA/CVA]) diabetes, renal disease, age greater than 70 years, male sex

(2) Electrocardiogram (ECG), previous history of MI, angina, causes, symptoms, treatment, laboratory tests performed (abnormalities always indicate increased perioperative risks)

(3) Cardiac catheterization report:

(a) Degree of vessel occlusion; presence of collateral vessels

(b) Chamber pressures; pulmonary artery (PA) pressures

(c) Left ventricular (LV) function:

Good LV Function:	**Poor LV Function:**
History	History
Angina	Multiple MI
Hypertension/obesity	Symptoms of CHF
No signs of CHF	Cardiac catheterization
Cardiac catheterization	EF less than 40%
Ejection fraction (EF) greater than 50%	LVEDP greater than 18 mm Hg
LV end-diastolic pressure (LVEDP) less than 12 mm Hg	Multiple areas of dyskinesia
	Decreased cardiac output
Normal cardiac output (CO)	

(4) Chest radiography (heart size, pulmonary vascular flow), exercise tolerance test (dysrhythmias, ischemic threshold, location of ischemia, ventricular dysfunction), induced ischemia, arrhythmias, and hemodynamic changes (ambulatory)

(5) ECG (Holter 12 to 48 hours, with symptoms diary; dysrhythmias, ST-segment depression)

(6) Echocardiography (EF, valvular function, congenital defects, segmental wall motion)

(7) Pharmacologic stress perfusion imaging (dipyridamole thallium scan). A vasodilator (dipyridamole) is administered to cause maximal dilation of coronary arteries. Vessels with fixed stenoses will not dilate, allowing less perfusion agent to reach the myocardium.

(8) Dobutamine echocardiography. Abnormally contracting muscle segments seen on resting echocardiography are classified as ischemic or infarcted; this is a good test for patients taking theophylline or caffeine or with COPD.

b) Pulmonary evaluation

(1) Asthma, emphysema, smoking history (to decrease carboxyhemoglobin and nicotine tachycardia, quit at least 2 days preoperatively)

(2) Pulmonary function tests with increased operative risk:

(a) Forced vital capacity (FVC) less than 50% predicted

(b) Forced expiratory volume in 1 second (FEV_1) less than 2 L

(c) FEV_1/FVC ratio less than 50%

(d) Arterial carbon dioxide pressure ($PaCO_2$) greater than 45 mm Hg on room air

(3) Assess lung sounds; relieve bronchospasm with β_2-adrenergic agents (terbutaline sulfate, albuterol), phosphodiesterase inhibitors (aminophylline), parasympatholytics (atropine), steroids, and mast cell stabilizers (cromolyn sodium).

(4) Chest radiography

c) Neurologic evaluation: Carotid stenosis, TIA/CVA

d) Renal evaluation: Chronic end-stage renal diagnosis

e) Laboratory tests: Arterial blood gases, electrolytes, complete blood count, platelet count, coagulation tests, activated clotting time (ACT), type and cross-match with blood available (2 units packed red blood cells [PRBCs] in room for redos)

f) Medications: Aspirin, digoxin, β-blockers

2. **Room preparation**

a) Monitors: Five-lead ECG, arterial line/central venous pressure/PA transducers, CO setup, zero all lines

b) Two units of PRBCs in room and ensure availability of platelets for redos

c) Oxygen (O_2) tank and Ambu bag for transport to the surgical intensive care unit (SICU)

d) Transesophageal echocardiography (TEE) in room for valves (TEE permits on-line evaluation of regional wall motion and global ventricular function)

e) Cordis kit and Swan-Ganz catheter; lidocaine, 10 mg/mL; arterial line setup and 10-mL flush; intravenous materials, sterile gloves, and gown

f) Drips
   (1) Nitroglycerin
   (2) Sodium nitroprusside
   (3) Phenylephrine (Neo-Synephrine)
   (4) Epinephrine
   (5) Dobutamine
   (6) Dopamine
   (7) Levophed
   (8) Amrinone

3. **Patient preparation**
   a) Assess airway, heart, and lung sounds. Review history.
   b) Check laboratory values: Note potassium, resting blood sugar (RBS), hematocrit and hemoglobin, blood urea nitrogen, creatinine.
   c) Verify that blood is available. Keep 2 to 4 units in the operating room for redos.
   d) Assess sedation needs and supply O_2 through a nasal cannula.
      (1) Good LV function: heavy premedication
      (2) Poor LV function: light premedication
   e) Place two large-bore peripheral intravenous tubes.
   f) Start an arterial line. (If radial artery harvest is planned, do not use that site; if use of the left internal mammary artery is planned, use the right side).
   g) Check allergies and give antibiotic as ordered.
   h) Radial artery grafts: Diltiazem (Cardizem) and heparin are used preoperatively.
      (1) Diltiazem (Cardizem) 0.1 mg/kg/hour to decrease spasm of artery with manipulation
      (2) Heparin at 1000 units/hour
   i) Redos: Aprotinin may be given preoperatively.
      (1) Test dose: 1 mL (1.4 mg); given preoperatively; observation for anaphylaxis for 10 minutes
      (2) Loading dose: 100 mL over 20 minutes (140 mg); cannot be given until the Swan catheter is in place
      (3) Pump prime: 200 mL (280 mg); given by perfusionist
      (4) Continuous infusion: 50 mL/hour (35 mg/hour); discontinued at the end of the case
      (5) Rationale: Used for repeat coronary bypass surgery or when transfusions are unavailable or unacceptable (e.g., in Jehovah's Witnesses). During CPB, levels of plasminogen activator are markedly enhanced, and platelets are activated directly. Aprotinin is a proteinase inhibitor that inhibits the fibrinolytic activity while preserving platelet adhesion function; it is considered an antifibrinolytic agent, and its mechanism of action is unknown.

(6) Pharmacokinetics: Eliminated by the kidneys, half-life of 2 hours (reason for continuous infusion)
(7) Adverse reactions:
    (a) Anaphylaxis (increased risk with repeat exposure)
    (b) Kidney dysfunction/failure
(8) Drug interactions: Many (reason for central line with no other drips); ACT standard on bypass less than 400 seconds; ACT with aprotinin used less than 600 seconds
(9) Other considerations with redos:
    (a) Have blood in the room at start of the case in case of cutting through great vessels or old grafts with sternotomy.
    (b) Be ready for emergency during CPB (femoral-femoral bypass); have heparin drawn up, and have rapid infuser and resuscitation measures ready.
    (c) Keep lungs inflated with sternotomy for redos.

4. Perioperative management
  a) Induction
    (1) Goals: Minimal hemodynamic effects, reliable loss of consciousness, and sufficient depth of anesthesia to prevent vasopressor response to intubation are the goals.
    (2) The choice of drugs and speed of induction are based on the patient's underlying LV function.
      (a) Poor LV function requires slow narcotic/relaxant technique.
      (b) Good LV function permits narcotic/relaxant/thiopental (Pentothal) induction with use of an inhalation agent.
    (3) Administer 100% O_2 via mask; avoid using nitrous oxide if possible.
    (4) A muscle relaxant priming dose, 1 mL, helps to decrease chest wall rigidity, whereas the vagolytic effect of pancuronium bromide offsets the bradycardia of sufentanil citrate.
    (5) Give a benzodiazepine: Lorazepam, 2 to 4 mg; midazolam, 2 to 5 mg.
    (6) Have nitroglycerin, phenylephrine (Neo-Synephrine), and atropine ready.
    (7) Use lidocaine (1 to 1.5 mg/kg) to decrease the sympathetic nervous system response to laryngoscopy.
    (8) High-dose narcotic technique: Opioids alone are associated with minimal or no cardiac depression. Fentanyl versus sufentanil: Data are conflicting.
      (a) Fentanyl: Dose: 20 to 100 mcg/kg (usually 1 mL/kg)
        Onset: 1 to 2 minutes
        Depth of anesthesia (DOA): 30 to 60 minutes
        Half-life: 3 to 4 hours
        Better choice than sufentanil in very compromised patients
      (b) Sufentanil: Dose: 5 to 20 mcg/kg
        Onset: 1 to 3 minutes.
        DOA: 20 to 45 minutes.
        Half-life: 2.5 hours (from smaller volume of distribution than fentanyl)

Special considerations with sufentanil: Analgesia is more profound than with fentanyl. It suppresses the catecholamine response 10 times more than fentanyl (better for a more robust person). The vagolytic effects greater than those of fentanyl, thus patients become bradycardic. It has some sedative qualities and hypnosis (unlike fentanyl). The incidence of skeletal muscle rigidity is increased.

(c) Sequence: Usually give $\frac{1}{10}$ muscle relaxant dose before opioid administration because of chest wall rigidity related to high-dose opioid. Slowly administer the opioid dose until the patient loses consciousness. Treat hypotension with intravenous fluid and then small doses of phenylephrine, 25 to 50 mcg intravenously.

(d) Treat bradycardia with atropine, 0.2 to 0.4 mg intravenously.

(e) If the patient remains conscious after a full opioid dose, give a benzodiazepine.

(9) Muscle relaxant:

   (a) Avoid those that cause release of histamine (atracurium, *d*-tubocurarine, mivacurium [Mivacron])

   (b) Best choices: Rocuronium [Zemuron], vecuronium [Norcuron], pancuronium [Pavulon].

   (c) Vecuronium [Norcuron] may precipitate severe bradycardia when combined with a high-dose opioid.

(10) Aortic and mitral valve stenosis anesthesia goals: Avoid SVR decrease and tachycardia (keep heart rate at 60 beats/min).

(11) Aortic and mitral valve regurgitation anesthesia goals: Avoid SVR increase and bradycardia (keep heart rate at 90 beats/min).

(12) While waiting for full muscle relaxation, the saphenous veins may be drained by elevation of the legs, and the Foley catheter with thermistor may be inserted.

(13) Laryngoscopy, intubation: Note the patient's response; confirm endotracheal tube placement.

(14) Check and pad pressure points (ulnar nerves, radial nerves, occiput, and heels).

   (a) Ischemia secondary to compression and compounded by decreases in temperature and perfusion pressure on CPB may cause peripheral neuropathy or damage to soft tissues.

   (b) Brachial plexus injury can occur if the arms are hyperextended or if chest retraction is excessive.

   (c) Ulnar nerve injury can occur from compression of the olecranon against the metal edge of the operating room table. Provide adequate padding under the olecranon.

   (d) Radial nerve injury can occur from compression of the upper arm against the ether screen or the support post of the retractor used in internal mammary artery dissection. Provide adequate padding of the arm.

   (e) Finger injury can occur secondary to pressure when members of the operating room team lean against the table. Position the patient with the hands next to the body in a neutral position and away from the edge of the table.

   (f) Occipital alopecia can occur 3 weeks after the operation secondary to ischemia of the scalp. Provide adequate padding of the head, reposition the head frequently during the procedure.

   (g) Heel of foot ischemia and tissue necrosis can occur. The heels should be well padded.

(15) Postinduction: ether screen, TEE if valve involvement is present, obtain postinduction cardiac output, draw laboratory test samples (arterial blood gases, ACT, potassium, RBS, hematocrit), and give antibiotics.

5. **Prebypass**
   a) High levels of patient stimulation occur at the following times: induction/intubation, incision, sternal split and spread, sympathetic nerve dissection, and cardiotomy. Maintain adequate levels of anesthesia to avoid increasing catecholamine levels (treat with an additional narcotic as necessary), which can precipitate hypertension, ischemia, and heart failure. Treat hypertension with nitroglycerin or sodium nitroprusside.
   b) Low levels of stimulation occur before the incision and during mammary dissection and CPB cannulation. Deep levels of anesthesia may cause hypotension, bradycardia, and ischemia.
   c) Skin incision: Supplement the narcotic as needed to avoid tachycardia and breakthrough hypertension.
   d) Sternotomy: Supplement the narcotic as needed and keep the patient paralyzed. The lungs must be deflated during sternal sawing by disconnecting the exhalation limb and providing adequate muscle relaxation (redos need not deflate lungs; decrease tidal volume and increase respiratory rate because a different saw is used and it is a slower process). Confirm equal inflation of lungs after the chest is open. This is the most common period for awareness and recall. (Redo heart procedures must have aminocaproic acid infusing and 2 units of PRBCs checked and ready in the room because vein grafts, right atrium, right ventricle, or great vessels may be cut or torn. The femoral vein should be identified and prepared by the team).
   e) Harvesting the left internal mammary artery/right internal mammary artery and/or saphenous vein: Decrease tidal volume and increase respiratory rate while the surgeon is dissecting the mammary artery. The chest is retracted to one side, with the table up and rotated away from surgeon. Keep the BP up to prevent vasospasm, which leads to ischemia. The surgeon sprays nitroglycerin or sodium nitroprusside over the vessel to prevent vasospasm (watch for a decreasing BP and maintain normotensive state).
   f) Pericardiotomy: Ensure adequate DOA. Observe wall motion and myocardial contractility. A pericardial sling is made before heparinization and cannulation. This provides a dam for the cardioplegia solution and iced normal saline slush. The sling can also serve to lift the heart. After the pericardium is opened, the postganglionic sympathetic nerves are dissected from the aorta to allow insertion of aortic cannula. This is a period of high-level stimulation because of sympathetic discharge with nerve manipulation. Attenuate with β-blockers and vasodilators.
   g) Heparinization: Activate antithrombin III (stops blood clotting during CPB).
      (1) The onset is immediate; duration, metabolism is by heparinases in the liver.
      (2) Aspirate back on the central line to ensure venous access.
      (3) The dose is 3 mg/kg (300 units/kg), (10,000 units/kg [1 mg = 100 units]).
      (4) Give before aortic cannulation. The surgeon can also administer heparin directly into the heart. (This decreases viscosity; watch for decreased BP and a reflex increase in heart rate.)
      (5) Check the ACT 3 minutes after heparin is given. It must be greater than 400 seconds before initiation of CPB (normal ACT, 70 to 110 seconds). Keep the surgeon aware of all ACTs.

(6) If ACT is not adequate, then one third of original dose should be given (if necessary, up to three times until the original dose is doubled). Check the ACT every 5 minutes until it is greater than 400 seconds. If a double dose is given and the ACT is still low, consider heparin resistance or low antithrombin III. Replace antithrombin III with fresh-frozen plasma.

h) Aortic cannulation: This is done first to provide access for rapid infusion if urgently required. Keep systolic BP at 100 mm Hg to avoid blood spray or aortic dissection. The cannula is placed in the ascending aorta proximal to the innominate artery and distal to the sites of the saphenous vein graft, if used. Pay attention to perfusionist and surgeon communication about cannula pressure readings. Complications include entering innominate, carotid, or subclavian arteries, embolism, dysrhythmias, and aortic dissection.

i) Venous cannulation: This is placed in the right atrium (through the appendage). It can result in hypotension from volume depletion or mechanical compression, especially if the inferior vena cava is cannulated. Dysrhythmias, mainly atrial, can result from surgical manipulation. Purse-string sutures are used to keep the cannulas in place and to close the incision after the cannulas are removed. CPB can be started immediately if the patient is hemodynamically unstable.

j) LV vent: Even though venous return is bypassed from the right ventricle, 2% to 5% of the CO is drained into the LV from bronchial, thebesian, and pleural veins. An LV sump prevents overdistention of the LV, which may cause postpump failure.

6. **Cardiopulmonary bypass**

CPB sustains systemic blood flow, oxygenation, and ventilation during periods when the heart and lungs are arrested.

a) Ensure an adequate level of muscle relaxation and amnesia. The surgeon notifies the perfusionist to go on CPB (record time and maintain mean arterial pressure [MAP] at 50 to 70 mm Hg to maintain coronary perfusion before cross-clamping; treat with phenylephrine [Neo-Synephrine]).

b) When pulmonary blood flow ceases, stop ventilation; disconnect the exhalation limb of the circuit to deflate the lung (increases surgeon visibility); and turn off the vent, gas analyzer, and pulse oximeter. Continue O_2 flow at 2 L/min.

c) Hypotension is associated with CPB because of the 2 L of prime solution, which causes hemodilution, decreases blood viscosity, dilutes circulating catecholamines, and contains no O_2; thus, hypoxic vasodilation occurs.

d) Patient assessment occurs 30 to 60 seconds after initiation of CPB.
   (1) Check the pupils. Examine the conjuctiva for chemosis and reassess pupil size and for unilateral dilation, which may indicate arterial inflow into the innominate artery (unilateral carotid perfusion).
   (2) Examine the face for color, symmetry, temperature, and edema.
   (3) Check the carotid pulses, which should feel like trills because of nonpulsatile flow.
   (4) Examine the heart for distention and contractility.
   (5) Examine the pump lines for arterial-venous color difference.

e) Hypothermia
   (1) The patient is cooled to 28° to 32° C, which decreases the O_2 demands of tissues and allows for lower CPB flows. This shifts

cerebral autoregulation to the left to 25 to 125 mm Hg. Each 1° C decrease in temperature leads to an 8% decrease in metabolic rate. A 10° C decrease in temperature leads to a decrease in metabolism by half. CO_2 and O_2 are more soluble; thus expect lower $PaCO_2$ on arterial blood gas testing.

    (2) Iced saline around heart cools it to 8° to 15° C.

    (3) Watch for ventricular fibrillation, which causes increased utilization of O_2 and requires immediate cardioplegia to arrest the heart.

f) Cardioplegia

The goal is to obtain a motionless heart and a clean, dry, operative field.

    (1) The aorta is cross-clamped. (Record time of CPB on/off and cross-clamp on/off.) Pay attention to perfusionist and surgeon communication in regard to "flow up/flow down" accompanying clamping and unclamping. The effects of aortic cross-clamping are as follows:

        (a) Cessation of coronary perfusion: This stops the blood from the coronary sinus from flooding the operative field.

        (b) If the aortic valve is incompetent, this prevents blood from regurgitating through the valve and flooding the field.

        (c) As the heart becomes hypoxic, it relaxes and can be manipulated more easily.

        (d) If there is any question of air entering the beating heart, the clamp will prevent air from reaching the brain.

    (2) Cardioplegia is the application of a cold solution (4° C) high in potassium (20 to 40 mEq/L) that produces electromechanical quiescence. It arrests the heart in diastole and produces energy conservation. (If it is arrested in systole, as seen with calcium, tetany results).

        (a) This solution causes the myocardial cells to depolarize; contraction occurs, calcium enters the cells, the myocardium relaxes, but membrane repolarization is prevented.

        (b) Four parts blood for one part of cardioplegic solution. Components of the cardioplegia solution may include potassium, sodium, calcium, magnesium, mannitol, and/or albumin, nitroglycerin (coronary dilator), bicarbonate (HCO_3; buffer), calcium channel blockers, propranolol HCl, glucose (cellular energy), hemoglobin (O_2 carrying), and lidocaine or procaine (membrane stabilization).

        (c) Repeat application of solution every 20 to 30 minutes, or if the heart temperature is greater than 18° C, to maintain hypothermia, prevent lactic acid accumulation, and deliver some minimal available O_2.

g) Keep MAP between 30 and 60 mm Hg. Patients with carotid stenosis may require higher pressures. Cerebral perfusion pressure equals MAP. LVEDP = 0. Pulmonary artery pressures should be less than 15 mm Hg; central venous pressure should be less than 5 mm Hg.

h) Potassium can cause systemic hyperkalemia. Treat with 10 units of regular insulin intravenously, 50 g of glucose, hyperventilation, HCO_3, calcium, and furosemide.

i) Ventricular fibrillation usually occurs twice during CPB: during cooling and during warming. Inform the surgeon.

j) Urine output should be maintained at more than 1 mL/kg (notify the surgeon if it is less). Large outputs of 300 to 1000 mL/hour can be seen if mannitol is used in the priming solution. Low urine outputs can be attributed to absent pulsatile flow, hypothermia, and decreased renal blood flow; increased catecholamines cause release of antidiuretic hormone. Treat low urine outputs with mannitol, furosemide, adequate perfusion, and renal-dose dopamine.

  k) Hemodynamics during CPB

    (1) Maintain MAP between 30 and 70 mm Hg with a venous saturation greater than 60%. If cerebral circulation is impaired, keep MAP at 60 mm Hg. Low MAP causes decreased peripheral perfusion. High MAP damages blood components, increases the blood in the operative field, and increases warmed blood to the heart. Treat low SVR with phenylephrine (Neo-Synephrine) and high SVR with nitroglycerin or sodium nitroprusside.

    (2) Reasons for decreased venous saturation: increased O_2 consumption with light anesthesia, low CPB flows, decreased O_2 delivery from oxygenator, or decreased O_2 carrying capacity of hemoglobin secondary to hemodilution.

  l) Physiologic response to CPB

    (1) Platelets: Clumping and degranulation occur after contact with nonendothelial surfaces. This leads to a reduction in numbers and inhibits adhesiveness and aggregation.

    (2) Proteins: Denaturation of oncotic and carrier proteins (albumin, lipoproteins, and gamma globulin) occurs. This leads to increased viscosity, clumping of red blood cells, and fat embolism. Amplification of "humoral system" proteins occurs. Factor XII stimulation of coagulation and fibrinolytic cascade is present. Complement system activation releases kallikrein and bradykinin, a generalized inflammatory response that increases capillary permeability. Enzymatic function is altered.

    (3) Blood: Red blood cells become stiffer and less distensible, which leads to lysis and hemoglobinuria and then impaired renal tubular function. Leukocyte damage and activation lead to degranulation. Complement activation causes pulmonary sequestration of neutrophils resulting in an inflammatory response and lung injury.

    (4) Endocrine: Elevated epinephrine levels during hypothermia cause peripheral vasoconstriction and impair release of insulin (hyperglycemia and release of free fatty acids). Norepinephrine levels rise early during CPB in patients and lead to postoperative hypertension. Renin and aldosterone levels are increased, promoting sodium retention and potassium excretion. Increased vasopressin produces increases in sodium and water diuresis. Angiotensin elevation leads to vasoconstriction.

    (5) Hemodilution reduces requirements for homologous blood transfusion, reduces blood viscosity and improves tissue perfusion, and counteracts the negative effects of hypothermia on tissue perfusion (vasoconstriction and impaired O_2 release from hemoglobin). It dilutes coagulation factors and platelets, contributing to coagulopathy. It also may increase interstitial edema.

    (6) Hypothermia reduces tissue metabolism and O_2 consumption. It improves myocardial protection, provides end-organ (brain, kidney) protection in case of low-flow negative effects, decreases intraoperative awareness, and increases SVR. It shifts the oxyhemoglobin curve to the left, impairing tissue O_2 release. This effect is offset by increased O_2 solubility at lower temperatures and lower metabolic demand. It contributes to decreased platelets and platelet function.

(7) Renal: The renin-angiotensin-aldosterone system alterations promote increased renal vascular resistance and sodium and water retention and lead to decreased renal blood flow, glomerular filtration rate, and tubular function. Hemodilution protects kidneys by increasing cortical plasma flow. Hemoglobinuria may result from long CPB runs (greater than 4 hours).

(8) Liver/intestines: Jaundice may occur in up to 23% of patients following CPB. Mucosal ischemia may result from splanchnic vasoconstriction induced by elevated angiotensin, as well as from microembolism of platelets and leukocytes.

(9) Changes in cerebral autoregulation from 50 to 100 mm Hg to lower values occur, as do embolic phenomena from fat, thrombi, platelets, foreign substances, and air embolism. It is important to keep blood glucose levels between 100 and 200 mg/dL to prevent cerebral ischemic episodes.

(10) Pulmonary: The lungs inactivate catecholamines under normal circumstances. This lack of degradation during CPB may contribute to increased catecholamines seen during CPB and may contribute to high peripheral vascular resistance. The lungs have a high affinity for narcotics, especially fentanyl. One may see decreased pulmonary blood flow after CPB because of embolism (ventilation-perfusion mismatch and edema), as well as localized vasoconstriction from elevated catecholamines.

m) Potential bypass catastrophes

(1) Aortic dissection (cannula placed within arterial wall during cannulation): The cannula should always be transduced; ensure that the pulsation correlates with the arterial line. Treatment is repositioning of the aortic cannula by surgeon.

(2) Carotid or innominate artery hyperperfusion: Reposition the catheter.

(3) Stone heart.

(4) Reversed cannulation: Blood is drained from the aorta, causing hypotension, and is infused into the vena cava at high pressures. Execute gas embolism protocol.

(5) Massive gas embolism (from oxygenator reservoir vortexing or clotting, opened beating heart, or a leak or kink in the lines): Vigilance is the prevention. Treatment includes the following:

(a) Stop CPB and place the patient in Trendelenburg's position.

(b) Remove the aortic cannula, vent air from cannulation site, and institute retrograde superior vena cava perfusion for 2 to 4 minutes.

(c) Perform carotid compression to allow purging of air from the vertebral arteries.

(d) When no additional air can be expelled, resume anterograde CPB, maintaining hypothermia for 40 to 50 minutes. (Lower temperatures increase gas solubility and help reabsorption of gas bubbles.)

(e) Express coronary air by massaging and needle aspiration. Induce hypertension because hydrostatic pressure shrinks bubbles and "pushes" them through the vessels.

(f) Administer steroids and wean from CPB. Ventilate the patient with 100% O_2 for at least 6 hours to maximize the blood-alveolar gradient for elimination of nitrogen. Hyperbaric chambers may accelerate the reabsorption of residual bubbles.

PART II **Common Procedures**

7. Rewarming

a) Rewarming is sensed as hyperthermia by the hypothalamus. Awareness is possible. Supplemental doses of pancuronium, lorazepam, and sufentanil may be required. Watch for the return of electrical activity of the heart (treat ventricular fibrillation with lidocaine and defibrillation). Consider a lidocaine drip if ventricular fibrillation is refractory.

b) Check TRIPLE

(1) T = temperature (Increase the operating room temperature. The patient is rewarmed to a core temperature of 37° C 20 minutes before termination of CPB. When the temperature rises close to 32° C, the SVR and MAP may decrease [treat with phenylephrine]. Rewarming accelerates metabolism of drugs given.)

(2) R = rate and rhythm (For adequate cardiac output, the patient requires sinus rhythm with a heart rate of 70 to 100 beats/min. Use a pacer, atropine, or cardioversion, if needed.)

(3) I = inhalation (FiO_2 equals 100%. Reexpand the lungs with two to four breaths at 30 to 40 cm H_2O to resolve atelectasis. Observe the field to ensure that you are not affecting the grafts. Resume mechanical ventilation.)

(4) P = pressure (Support as needed. High BP places stress on new grafts; low BP can cause ischemia.)

(5) L = laboratory test results (Check test results: prothrombin time, partial thromboplastin time, ACT, fibrinogen, Sonoclot, arterial blood gases, hematocrit, electrolytes, glucose. If potassium is trending less than 4 mEq/L at separation, supplement.)

(6) E = everything else (Level the table, zero all lines.)

c) Unclamping of the aorta: Observe the heart for volume, rate, and contractility. The perfusionist may give or take 50 to 100 mL increments of blood. Monitor filling pressures, distention, or hypotension as indicators that the heart cannot handle the volume. Consider treatment with calcium chloride, epinephrine, or dobutamine for support.

8. Discontinuing CPB

a) Flow is decreased by 50%; the heart is visually inspected for distention of chambers and wall motion abnormalities. Observe ECG for dysrhythmias. Most patients fall into one of four groups listed in the table below when CPB is being discontinued.

b) Ensure adequate hemodynamic parameters; use inotropes and pressors as needed. Pulmonary capillary wedge pressure is a poor indicator of left atrial function after CPB.

	Group I: Vigorous	Group II: Hypovolemic	Group III: Pump Failure	Group IV: Hyperdynamic
Filling pressure	Low	Low	Normal or high	Low
Blood pressure	Normal	Low	Low or normal	Low
Cardiac output	Normal	Low	Low	High
Systemic vascular resistance	Normal	High	High	Low
Treatment	None	Volume	Inotrope afterload reduction, intraaortic balloon pump	Vasoconstrictor

c) The venous line is removed first.

d) Protamine is administered, 1 mg per 1 mg of heparin. Calcium chloride, 500 to 1000 mg, is mixed with protamine to counteract depressed contractility, decreased pH, decreased calcium levels. (Extreme Caution: This may lead to stone heart in a digitalized patient.)

   (1) Protamine is a base that combines with acidic heparin to form a stable salt and inactivates the anticoagulant effect.

   (2) Administer slowly, over 5 to 10 minutes, into a peripheral venous site. Notify the surgeon when one half is administered so that pump suckers can be turned off to prevent coagulation in the pump. Observe for hypotension and increased pulmonary artery pressure.

   (3) Reactions can include histamine release, anaphylactic/ anaphylactoid reactions (immunoglobulin E–mediated venodilation, decreased cardiac filling, and decreased SVR), and pulmonary vasoconstriction (increased airway pressures). The risk of allergic reactions is increased in patients allergic to fish, in patients who have been treated with protamine-containing insulin, or in the presence of antiprotamine antibodies in serum of infertile or vasectomized men. Treat the reaction with diphenhydramine and/or epinephrine, 0.1 to 0.3 mg.

e) Check hemoglobin, hematocrit, potassium, ACT, and arterial blood gases. Begin infusing cardiotomy blood because the patient will require volume. The ACT goal is to return to the patient's preoperative level. A hematocrit of 25% or less may be acceptable without transfusion. The patient will slowly hemoconcentrate.

f) The aortic line is removed, chest tubes are inserted, hemostasis is obtained, and the incision is closed. Chest closure causes a transient increase in intramediastinal pressure, which may depress systemic venous return.

g) Check the CO when the sternal wires closed and the patient is stabilized.

h) Transport to the SICU when the patient is hemodynamically stable. Take a Lifepak, Ambu bag with O_2 tank, Omni-Flow, and tabletop drugs. Ventilation settings: respiratory rate, 8 to 12 breaths/min (for $PaCO_2$ of 35 to 45 mm Hg); FiO_2, 100%; tidal volumes, 10 mL/kg; positive end-expiratory pressure, 5 cm H_2O.

9. **Postoperative complications**

   a) Hypokalemia

   b) MI and acute graft closure

   c) Ischemia

   d) Tamponade

   e) Hemorrhage

   f) Prosthetic valve failure

10. **"Mini" coronary artery bypass graft procedures**

   a) This refers to those coronary artery bypass graft procedures done off CPB with a hemisternotomy.

   b) Prepare the heart for ischemia by reducing myocardial O_2 demand with β-blockers and calcium channel blockers while increasing O_2 supply with nitroglycerin infusion.

   c) Coronary anastomosis is facilitated by inducing bradycardia with adenosine, β-blockers, and calcium channel blockers.

   (1) Usually, these patients have healthier hearts and can tolerate the slow heart rate.

(2) Adenosine will induce a sinus pause lasting 10 to 20 seconds and will decrease BP.

(3) Pacing wires should be in place.

d) After anastomosis: Discontinue β-blockers, continue nitroglycerin, continue calcium channel blockers to decrease vasospasm, and vigorously treat LV dysfunction and/or arrhythmias.

e) Heparin dose requirements are half of those required for traditional coronary artery bypass grafting (150 units/kg); no Amicar is given.

f) Less narcotic and benzodiazepine required.

g) Left radial arterial line; the right arterial system will be used for angiography.

G. Supplemental Information

1. Hemodynamic variables: Calculations and normal values

Variable	Calculation	Normal Values
Cardiac index (CI)	CO/BSA	2.5 to 4 L/min/m^2
Stroke volume (SV)	CO/HR	60 to 90 mL/beat
Stroke index (SI)	SV/BSA	40 to 60 mL/beat/m^2
Mean arterial pressure (MAP)	2(DBP) + SBP/3	80 to 120 mm Hg
Systemic vascular resistance (SVR)	MAP − CVP/CO × 80	1200 to 1500 dynes/cm/sec^{-5}
Pulmonary vascular resistance (PVR)	PAP − PWP/CO × 80	100 to 300 dynes/cm/sec^{-5}
Ejection fraction (EF)	SV/EDV	65%
Cardiac output (CO)	SV × HR	5 to 6 L/min

BSA, Body surface area; *DBP,* diastolic blood pressure; *EDV,* end-diastolic volume; *HR,* heart rate; *PAP,* pulmonary artery pressure; *PWP,* pulmonary capillary wedge pressure; *SBP,* systolic blood pressure.

2. Commonly used drugs

Commonly Used Drugs

Agent	Dosage	Onset	Duration	Action
Nitroprusside	0.5 to 10 mcg/kg/min	30 to 60 sec	1 to 5 min	Direct arterial and venous vascular smooth muscle relaxation
Nitroglycerin	5 to 100 mcg/min	1 min	3 to 5 min	Direct venous dilation
Esmolol	0.5 mg/kg over 1 min	1 min	12 to 20 min	Direct β$_1$-antagonist
Labetalol	2.5 to 20 mg	1 to 2 min	4 to 8 hr	Direct α$_1$-, β$_1$-, and β$_2$-antagonist
Propranolol	0.2 to 3 mg	1 to 2 min	4 to 8 hr	Direct β$_1$-antagonist

Continued

Commonly Used Drugs—cont'd

Agent	Dosage	Onset	Duration	Action
Hydralazine	2.5 to 20 mg	5 to 20 min	4 to 8 hr	Direct vascular smooth muscle relaxation
Nifedipine	10 mg	5 to 10 min	4 hr	Direct vascular smooth muscle relaxation
Epinephrine	1 to 4 mcg/min	30 to 60 sec	1 to 5 min	Direct α_1-, α_2-, β_1-, and β_2-agonist
Ephedrine	2.5 to 10 mg	30 to 60 sec	1 to 5 min	Mixed α_1-, α_2-, β_1-, and β_2-agonist
Aminocaproic acid	10 g loading; 1 g/hr	30 to 60 sec	3 to 5 hr	Coagulant
Protamine	1 mg per mg heparin	30 to 60 sec	2 hr	Heparin antagonist
Phenylephrine	10 to 200 mcg/min	30 to 60 sec	15 to 30 min	Pure α
Norepinephrine	2 to 20 mcg/min	30 to 60 sec	10 min	α_2-agonist, β_2-agonist

GASTROINTESTINAL SYSTEM

A. Adrenalectomy

1. **Introduction**
   a) Adrenalectomy is a procedure in which the adrenal glands are removed by open dissection or laparoscopic approach. The left adrenal gland is exposed by manipulating the spleen and pancreas. The right adrenal gland is exposed by retracting the liver cephalad. Adrenal veins are exposed and ligated before removal.
   b) Pathophysiology: The procedure is performed for medullary or cortical tumors, Cushing's syndrome resulting from adrenal calcium or hyperplasia, pituitary hypersecretion, pheochromocytoma, hypercortisolism, primary hyperaldosteronism, and adenocarcinoma (see the discussion of pheochromocytoma, Cushing's disease, and hyperaldosteronism in Section III of Part 1).

2. **Preoperative assessment**
   This includes differentiating the underlying pathophysiologic features.
   a) History and physical examination
      (1) Cardiac: Assess for volume status, hypertension, dysrhythmias, orthostatic hypotension, myocardial infarction, and congestive heart failure.
      (2) Respiratory: Cushing's syndrome may cause truncal obesity and a buffalo hump.
      (3) Neurologic: Assess for headache, mood changes, psychosis, muscular wasting, and anxiety.
      (4) Renal: Assess for sodium retention and potassium excretion, glucose intolerance from excess steroids, and renal hypertension.
      (5) Gastrointestinal: Assess for obesity and muscle wasting. The patient may need rapid sequence induction and aspiration prophylaxis.
      (6) Endocrine: Assess for underlying pathologic changes in hormones.
   b) Patient preparation
      (1) Laboratory tests: These are as indicated by the patient's condition
      (2) Diagnostic tests: These are as indicated by the patient's condition. Computed tomography or magnetic resonance imaging may be useful.
      (3) Medications: Consider the need for a steroid preparation; hydrocortisone dose: 100 mg every 8 hours.

3. **Room preparation**
   a) Monitoring equipment: This is standard, with a central line and an arterial line as indicated.
   b) Additional equipment: Positioning devices: The patient may be supine or in a nephrectomy or prone jackknife position. Careful padding is needed for patients with Cushing's syndrome because of their easy bruising, thin skin, and osteopenia.

c) Drugs
  (1) Continuous infusions: Intravenous fluids: Large fluid loss is possible. Use isotonic crystalloid at 10 mL/kg per hour.
  (2) Blood: Estimated blood loss is 200 to 300 mL but can be significant. Type and cross-match are needed.
  (3) Tabletop: This is standard. Have atropine available for unopposed parasympathetic response, lidocaine for ventricular arrhythmias (hypokalemia), and syringes of a vasoactive agent (ephedrine) available.
4. **Perioperative management and anesthetic technique**
  a) Induction: Select the appropriate induction agent based on the patient's medical condition. Use a nondepolarizer if rapid sequence induction is not used. Consider decreased muscle mass.
  b) Maintenance: This includes the use of volatile agent, opiates, and a muscle relaxant. Epidural anesthesia can improve surgical exposure by contracting the bowel.
  c) Emergence: The patient may be hemodynamically labile and may have large third-space fluid accumulation. Consider postoperative ventilation.
5. **Postoperative complications**
  Complications include hypoadrenocorticism after tumor resection, hypoglycemia, pneumothorax, and hypertension. Continue steroid therapy after the procedure.

B. Anal Fistulotomy/Fistulectomy

1. **Introduction**
  Most perianal fistulas arise as a result of infection within the anal glands located at the dentate line (cryptoglandular fistula). Fistulas may also arise as the result of trauma, Crohn's disease, inflammatory processes within the peritoneal cavity, neoplasms, or radiation therapy. The ultimate treatment is determined by the cause and the anatomic course of the fistula and can include fistulotomy and fistulectomy. The primary goal is palliation, specifically to drain abscesses and prevent their recurrence. This is often accomplished by placing a Silastic seton (a ligature placed around the sphincter muscles) around the fistula tract and leaving it in place indefinitely. In the absence of active Crohn's disease in the rectum, attempts at fistula cure may be undertaken.
2. **Preoperative assessment**
  a) History and physical examination
    (1) Respiratory: A careful evaluation of respiratory status is important. If the patient has significant respiratory disease, the lithotomy position is better tolerated than the prone or jackknife positions.
    (2) Musculoskeletal: Pain is likely at the surgical site and should be considered when positioning the patient for anesthetic induction. (If the patient has pain while sitting, regional anesthesia should be performed with the patient in the lateral decubitus position.)
    (3) Hematologic: If regional anesthesia is planned and the patient is taking acetylsalicylic acids, nonsteroidal antiinflammatory drugs, or dipyridamole, check the platelet count and bleeding time.
  b) Patient preparation
    (1) Laboratory tests: As indicated per history and physical examination
    (2) Diagnostic tests: As indicated per history and physical examination
    (3) Medication: Standard premedication

3. **Room preparation**
   a) Monitoring equipment: Standard
   b) Drugs
      (1) Standard emergency drugs
      (2) Standard tabletop
      (3) Intravenous fluids: 18-gauge line, normal saline/lactated Ringer's at 5 to 8 mL/kg per hour
4. **Anesthetic technique**
   General anesthesia, local anesthesia with sedation, and spinal or epidural techniques may be used.
5. **Perioperative management**
   a) Induction: Standard. Procedures done with the patient in the jackknife position may require endotracheal intubation for airway control if a regional technique is not performed.
   b) Maintenance
      (1) Standard
      (2) Position: Use chest support or bolster to optimize ventilation in the jackknife position; take care in positioning the patient's extremities and genitals after turning the patient into the jackknife position. Avoid pressure on the eyes and ears after turning the patient. Avoid stretching the brachial plexus. Limit abduction to 90 degrees.
   c) Emergence: No special considerations are needed. The patient is extubated awake and after return of airway reflexes.
6. **Postoperative implications**
   a) Lithotomy position possibly leading to damage to the peroneal nerve, which can lead to foot drop.
   b) Urinary retention
   c) Poor wound healing
   d) Atelectasis

C. Appendectomy

1. **Introduction**
   Appendectomy is performed for acute appendicitis, and a laparoscopic approach is most commonly used.
2. **Preoperative assessment and patient preparation**
   a) History and physical examination
      (1) Gastrointestinal: Patients point to localized pain at McBurney's point, which is midway between the iliac crest and umbilicus; rebound tenderness, muscle rigidity, and abdominal guarding are noted.
      (2) Pregnancy: Alder's sign is used to differentiate between uterine and appendiceal pain. The pain is localized with the patient supine. The patient then lies on her left side. If the area of pain shifts to the left, it is presumed to be uterine.
   b) Diagnostic tests
      (1) The white blood cell count is elevated, with a shift to the left: 10,000 to 16,000 mm^3; 75% neutrophils.
      (2) Urinalysis shows a small number of erythrocytes and leukocytes.
      (3) Computed tomography and abdominal films are used.
      (4) Other laboratory tests include electrolytes, glucose, hemoglobin, and hematocrit. Perform tests as indicated from the history and physical examination.

c) Preoperative medication and intravenous therapy
   (1) An antibiotic is given for enteric gram-negative bacilli, anaerobic bacteria.
   (2) A single 18-gauge intravenous catheter is used because the patient is dehydrated from fever, anorexia, and vomiting.

3. Room preparation
   a) Monitoring equipment
      (1) Standard
      (2) Fetal heart tone monitoring with pregnancy
   b) Pharmacologic agents
      (1) Standard
      (2) For fetal safety, must avoid teratogenic anesthetic during the first trimester
   c) Position
      (1) Supine
      (2) Left uterine displacement with pregnancy

4. Anesthetic technique
   a) Regional block: Analgesia to level T6 to T8
   b) General anesthesia: Endotracheal intubation required

5. Perioperative management
   a) Induction
      (1) Use general anesthesia with rapid sequence induction because patients may have a nasogastric tube or are considered to have a full stomach (emergency).
      (2) In the pregnant patient, special care should be taken to prevent aspiration pneumonitis.
   b) Maintenance
      (1) No specific indications exist.
      (2) Muscle relaxation is necessary.
   c) Emergence: Awake extubation secondary to rapid sequence induction

6. Postoperative implications
   None are reported.

D. Cholecystectomy

1. Introduction

Surgery of the upper abdomen is used in the treatment of gallstones and other diseases of the gallbladder. Open cholecystectomy is performed in patients with adhesions, previous surgical procedures, infection, or major medical problems. The mortality rate for elective cholecystectomy is less than 0.5%. In patients older than 70 years of age, the mortality rate rises to 2% to 3%, mostly because of preexisting cardiopulmonary disease.

2. Preoperative assessment
   a) History and physical examination
      (1) Standard
      (2) Gastrointestinal assessment: Pain is localized in the right subcostal region. The patient may experience referred pain in the back at the shoulder level. Anorexia, nausea, and vomiting are common. Infection and fever are rare.
   b) Diagnostic tests: These are as indicated by the patient's history and medical condition.

    c) Preoperative medication and intravenous therapy
      (1) Use an antimicrobial to prevent bacteremia.
      (2) Narcotics must be used with caution to minimize potential spasm in the biliary tract and sphincter of Oddi.
      (3) Use a single, large-bore (18-gauge) intravenous tube with fluid replacement.
      (4) Use prophylactic antiemetics and aspiration prophylaxis.

3. Room preparation
    a) Monitoring equipment: Standard
    b) Pharmacologic agents
      (1) Standard
      (2) Caution advised with use of narcotic agents because of potential changes in biliary pressure
    c) Position: Supine

4. Anesthetic technique
General endotracheal anesthesia with muscle relaxation is used.

5. Perioperative management
    a) Induction: Rapid sequence induction with oral endotracheal intubation if the patient is considered to have a full stomach
    b) Maintenance
      (1) No specific requirements
      (2) Muscle relaxation per abdominal surgery
      (3) Antiemetic administration
    c) Emergence: Awake extubation after airway reflexes are adequate

6. Postoperative implications
    a) Retraction in the right upper quadrant during surgery can lead to atelectasis in the right lower lobe; postoperative pain and splinting may lead to impaired ventilation.
    b) Right intercostal nerve blocks improve postoperative pain management.
    c) Use patient-controlled analgesia for pain management.

E. Colectomy

1. Introduction
Colectomy is performed most commonly for adenocarcinomas and diverticulosis. Other indications include penetrating trauma, ulcerative colitis, volvulus, and inflammatory bowel disease.

2. Preoperative assessment and patient preparation
    a) History and physical examination: Assess hydration status, nutritional level, and electrolyte state.
    b) Diagnostic tests: These are as indicated by the patient's condition
    c) Preoperative medication and intravenous therapy
      (1) Patients may be receiving steroid therapy or immunosuppressant drugs.
      (2) Bowel preparation is usually indicated with electrolyte preparations.
      (3) Expect fluid shifts requiring moderate to large fluid resuscitation. Two large-bore intravenous access tubes are indicated.

3. Room preparation
    a) Monitoring equipment: Standard with warming modalities
    b) Pharmacologic agents: Standard
    c) Position: Supine, with arms extended

4. **Anesthetic technique**
   a) Epidural (T2 to T4 level) with "light" general anesthetic
   b) General anesthesia with oral endotracheal tube (most common)
5. **Perioperative management**
   a) Induction: Consider the possibility of a full stomach; rapid sequence induction may be indicated.
   b) Maintenance
      (1) Muscle relaxation is required.
      (2) Closely monitor fluid and hydration status and blood loss.
      (3) Avoid nitrous oxide, which may cause bowel distention.
   c) Emergence: This involves awake extubation after rapid sequence induction or placement of a nasogastric tube.
6. **Postoperative implications**
   a) Pain and splinting may lead to hypoventilation and decreased postoperative ventilation.
   b) Control pain with epidural or patient-controlled analgesia.

F. Colonoscopy

1. **Introduction**
   Colonoscopy is used to examine the colon and rectum to diagnose inflammatory bowel disease, including ulcerative colitis and granulomatous colitis. Polyps can be removed through the colonoscope. The colonoscope is also helpful in diagnosing or locating the source of gastrointestinal bleeding; a biopsy of lesions suspected to be malignant may be performed.
2. **Preoperative assessment and patient preparation**
   a) History and physical examination: Assess the patient's hydration status, nutritional level, and electrolyte state.
   b) Diagnostic tests: These are as indicated by the patient's condition
   c) Preoperative medication and intravenous therapy
      (1) Patients may be receiving steroid therapy or immunosuppressants.
      (2) Bowel preparation is required for visualization of the mucosa. Use colon electrolyte lavage preparations (Colyte, GoLYTELY).
      (3) One 18-gauge intravenous tube is used; adequate fluid replacement is ensured.
      (4) The patient is lightly sedated with midazolam because the procedure lasts less than 30 minutes and is an outpatient procedure.
3. **Room preparation**
   a) Monitoring equipment: Standard
   b) Pharmacologic agents
      (1) Standard
      (2) Glucagon
   c) Position: Left lateral decubitus; position changes sometimes required to aid advancement of the scope at the descending sigmoid colon junction and splenic fixture
4. **Anesthetic technique**
   a) Monitored anesthesia care
   b) Intravenous sedation: Midazolam (Versed), fentanyl, or propofol in sedative doses
5. **Perioperative management**
   a) Induction: Oxygenation of the patient with the use of nasal cannula or a face mask

PART II **Common Procedures**

b) Maintenance: No specific indications

c) Emergence: No specific indications

6. **Postoperative implications**

Complications of the procedure include perforation of the bowel, abdominal pain and distention, rectal bleeding, fever, and mucopurulent drainage.

G. Esophageal Resection

1. **Introduction**

Esophagectomy is commonly performed for malignant disease of the middle and lower thirds of the esophagus. It may also be indicated for Barrett's esophagus (peptic ulcer of the lower esophagus) and for peptic strictures that do not respond to dilation. Lesions in the lower third are usually approached through a left thoracoabdominal incision, whereas middle-third lesions are best approached by the abdomen and right side of the chest. Resections of the esophagogastric junction for malignant disease are best performed through a left thoracoabdominal approach in which a portion of the proximal stomach is removed along with a celiac node dissection.

Total esophagectomy may be done through an abdominal and right thoracotomy approach with colonic interposition and anastomosis in the neck. Either the right or the left side of the colon can be mobilized for interposition. Both depend on the middle colic artery and the marginal artery of the colon for their vascular supply.

2. **Preoperative assessment**

a) History and physical examination

(1) Cardiovascular: The patient may be hypovolemic and malnourished from dysphagia or anorexia. Chemotherapeutic drugs (daunorubicin, doxorubicin [Adriamycin]) may cause cardiomyopathy. Chronic alcohol abuse may also produce toxic cardiomyopathy.

(2) Respiratory: A history of gastric reflux suggests the possibility of recurrent aspiration pneumonia, decreased pulmonary reserve, and increased risk of regurgitation and aspiration during anesthetic induction. If a thoracic approach is planned, the patient should be evaluated to ensure that one-lung ventilation can be tolerated.

(a) Chemotherapeutic drugs (bleomycin) may cause pulmonary toxicity that may be made worse by high concentrations of oxygen. Many patients with esophageal cancer have a long history of smoking, with consequent respiratory impairment.

(b) Pulmonary function tests and arterial blood gases can be helpful in predicting the likelihood of perioperative pulmonary complications and whether the patient may require postoperative mechanical ventilation. Patients with baseline hypoxemia/hypercarbia on room air arterial blood gases have a higher likelihood of postoperative complications and a greater need for postoperative ventilatory support. Severe restrictive or obstructive lung disease will also increase the chance of pulmonary morbidity in the perioperative period.

b) Patient preparation

(1) Laboratory tests: Type and cross-match packed red blood cells, electrolytes, glucose, blood urea nitrogen, creatinine, bilirubin,

transaminase, alkaline phosphatase, albumin, complete blood count, and platelet count. Prothrombin time, partial thromboplastin time, urinalysis, arterial blood gases, and other tests are as indicated by the patient's history and physical examination.

(2) Diagnostic tests: Chest radiographs, electrocardiography, pulmonary function tests, and other tests are as indicated by the patient's history and physical examination. If congestive heart failure or cardiomyopathy is suspected, consider cardiac or medical consultations.

(3) Medications: For premedication, consider aspiration prophylaxis.

3. Room preparation
a) Monitoring equipment
   (1) Standard monitoring equipment
   (2) Arterial line and central venous pressure or pulmonary arterial catheter as indicated
b) Additional equipment: Patient warming device
c) Drugs
   (1) Standard emergency drugs
   (2) Standard tabletop
   (3) Intravenous fluids: 14- to 16-gauge (two) normal saline or lactated Ringer's solution at 8 to 12 mL/kg per hour; fluid warmer
   (4) Blood loss possibly significant; blood immediately available

4. Anesthetic technique
General endotracheal anesthesia with or without epidural anesthetic for postoperative analgesia is administered. If the thoracic or abdominothoracic approach is used, placement of a double-lumen tube is indicated, because one-lung anesthesia provides excellent surgical exposure. If the patient is clinically hypovolemic, restore intravascular volume before induction and carefully titrate the induction dose of sedative/hypnotic agents.

5. Perioperative management
a) Induction
   (1) Patients with esophageal disease are often at risk for pulmonary aspiration; therefore, rapid sequence induction is indicated.
   (2) If a difficult airway is anticipated, awake intubation can be done using a fiberoptic bronchoscope.
b) Maintenance
   (1) Standard maintenance uses a narcotic and/or inhalation agent. Avoid nitrous oxide.
   (2) A combined technique with general and epidural anesthesia may be used. If epidural opiates are used for postoperative analgesia, a loading dose should be administered at least 1 hour before the conclusion of surgery.
   (3) Position: The patient is supine, with checked and padded pressure points. Avoid stretching the brachial plexus. Limit abduction to 90 degrees. If the lateral decubitus position is used, an axillary roll and arm holder are needed. Check pressure points, including ears, eyes, and genitals. Check radial pulses to ensure correct placement of the axillary roll (a misplaced axillary roll will compromise distal pulses). Problems that can arise include brachial plexus injuries and damage to soft tissues, ears, eyes, and genitals from malpositioning.
c) Emergence
   The decision to extubate at the end of surgery depends on the patient's underlying cardiopulmonary status and the extent of the

PART II **Common Procedures**

surgical procedure. The patient should be hemodynamically stable, warm, alert, cooperative, and fully reversed from any muscle relaxants before extubation. With patients who require postoperative ventilation, the double-lumen tube should be changed to a single-lumen endotracheal tube before transport to the postanesthesia intensive care unit. Weaning from mechanical ventilation should begin when the patient is awake and cooperative, is able to protect the airway, and has adequate pulmonary function.

6. **Postoperative implications**
   a) For atelectasis or aspiration, recover the patient in Fowler's position.
   b) Hemorrhage: Check coagulation times; replace factors as necessary.
   c) Pneumothorax/hemothorax: Decreased partial oxygen pressure, increased partial carbon dioxide pressure, wheezing, and coughing are noted; confirm with chest radiograph, and institute chest tube drainage as necessary. In an emergency (tension pneumothorax), use needle aspiration, supportive treatment, oxygen, vasopressors, endotracheal intubation, and positive-pressure ventilation.
   d) Hypoxemia/hypoventilation: This ensures adequate analgesia and supplemental oxygen.
   e) Esophageal anastomotic leak: Begin surgical repair for an esophageal anastomotic leak.
   f) Pain management: Patient-controlled analgesia or epidural analgesia is used; the patient should recover in the intensive care unit or in a hospital ward accustomed to treating the side effects of epidural opiates (respiratory depression, breakthrough pain, nausea, and pruritus).

H. Esophagoscopy/Gastroscopy

1. **Introduction**
   Flexible, diagnostic esophagogastroduodenoscopy, a common procedure in pediatrics, is usually performed with the patient under heavy sedation in an endoscopy suite or special procedure area. Rigid esophagoscopy is usually performed for therapeutic indications, such as removal of a foreign body, dilation of an esophageal stricture, or injection of varices. The procedure is similar for each diagnosis and generally is performed with endotracheal intubation. Foreign body removal is normally a short procedure, whereas dilation and variceal injection can be prolonged and may require multiple insertions or removals of the endoscope. Compression of the trachea distal to the endotracheal tube by the rigid esophagoscope is not uncommon.

2. **Preoperative assessment**
   Esophagoscopy for foreign body removal is usually performed in healthy infants and children, although esophageal lodging of a foreign body can occur in any age group. All these patients should be treated with full-stomach precautions. Esophageal dilation usually is performed in two distinct patient populations: those with prior tracheoesophageal fistula repair and those with prior ingestion of a caustic substance.
   a) History and physical examination
      (1) Cardiovascular: There may be persistent congenital cardiac anomalies in the patient with a tracheoesophageal fistula.
      (2) Respiratory: Patients with prior caustic ingestion may have a history of pulmonary aspiration, with resultant chemical pneumonitis, fibrosis, or both. Prolonged intubation after tracheoesophageal

fistula repair may lead to subglottic stenosis. Check any recent anesthesia records for endotracheal intubation.

b) Patient preparation
  (1) Laboratory tests: Routine laboratory analyses are not required if the patient has no underlying chronic illness.
  (2) Diagnostic tests: These are as indicated by the history and physical examination.
  (3) Medications: For foreign body removal, intravenous access may be necessary before induction. No premedication is used if the patient is less than 1 year old.

3. Room preparation
  a) Monitoring equipment: Standard
  b) Drugs
    (1) Standard emergency drugs
    (2) Standard tabletop
    (3) Intravenous fluids: One 20- to 22-gauge intravenous line with normal saline or lactated Ringer's solution at 4 to 6 mL/kg per hour

4. Anesthetic technique
Use general endotracheal anesthesia. For the pediatric patient, a pediatric circle or a nonrebreather circuit may be used. Room temperature can be maintained at 65° to 70° F as long as the patient is covered.

5. Perioperative management
  a) Induction: Rapid sequence induction is usually appropriate for this patient population, unless the patient is presenting for dilation alone and has no evidence to suggest reflux.
  b) Maintenance
    (1) Maintain anesthesia with a volatile agent, nitrous oxide, and oxygen. Opiates are unnecessary because postprocedural pain is negligible. Maintain neuromuscular blockade. Movement must be avoided, particularly with rigid esophagoscopy.
    (2) Position. The patient is supine, with checked and padded pressure points. Avoid stretching the brachial plexus. Limit abduction to 90 degrees.
    (3) Warming modalities for pediatric patients: Increased room temperature, warming blankets, and a Humidivent are used.
  c) Emergence: Extubate when the patient is fully awake. Do not attempt reversal of neuromuscular blockade until first twitch of train-of-four has returned.

6. Postoperative implications
  a) Pneumothorax: Esophageal perforation is more common with rigid esophagoscopy and will lead to pneumothorax.
  b) Aspiration
  c) Accidental extubation
  d) Stridor secondary to subglottic edema
  e) Postoperative pain is negligible; if the patient reports marked substernal discomfort, suspect esophageal perforation.

I. Gastrostomy

1. Introduction
A gastrostomy involves the placement of a semipermanent tube through the abdominal wall directly into the stomach. These tubes are used

for gastric decompression or for feeding. A percutaneous endoscopic gastrostomy is often performed. Feeding gastrostomy tubes are indicated in patients unable to feed by mouth but able to absorb enteral nutrition, such as patients with advanced malignancy and intestinal obstruction, inadequate oral intake, and neurologic impairment.

2. **Preoperative assessment**

Patients undergoing gastrostomy may have neurologic impairment from conditions such as stroke and head injury. This compromises their ability to handle oral secretions and increases their risk for aspiration.

a) History and physical examination

(1) Cardiac: Patients are likely to be hypovolemic secondary to chronically poor oral intake and malnutrition.

(2) Respiratory: Patients may have difficulty swallowing and inadequate laryngeal reflexes, which places them at high risk for aspiration of gastric contents and associated pneumonitis. Hypoxemia and decreased pulmonary reserve can be present with pulmonary infections.

(3) Neurologic: The patient is often neurologically impaired and debilitated.

(4) Renal: Long-term indwelling urinary catheters increase the risk of infection.

b) Patient preparation

(1) Laboratory tests: These are as indicated by the patient's condition.

(2) Diagnostic tests: These are as indicated by the patient's condition.

(3) Medications: These are standard.

3. **Room preparation**

a) Monitoring equipment: Standard monitoring equipment

b) Drugs: Standard emergency drugs

c) Standard tabletop

d) Intravenous fluids: One 18-gauge intravenous line with normal saline or lactated Ringer's solution at 5 to 8 mL/kg per hour

4. **Anesthetic technique**

Intravenous sedation or monitored anesthesia care with local anesthesia is used.

5. **Perioperative management**

a) Induction

(1) If general anesthesia is planned, use rapid sequence induction with cricoid pressure.

(2) Titrate narcotics (fentanyl) and/or benzodiazepines (midazolam) as indicated.

b) Maintenance

(1) General anesthesia: Standard muscle relaxants may be necessary.

(2) Position: The patient is supine, with checked and padded pressure points.

c) Emergence: Tracheal extubation is performed after the return of protective laryngeal reflexes.

6. **Postoperative implications**

Mild to moderate postoperative pain intensity may be controlled with parenteral narcotics or intercostal blocks. Postoperative complications include aspiration pneumonia, wound infection, and atelectasis.

J. Gastrectomy

1. **Introduction**

Total gastrectomy is usually performed for gastric cancer.

2. **Preoperative assessment and patient preparation**
   a) History and physical examination: Assess fluid and hydration status. The patient may be vomiting or bleeding or may have anorexia.
   b) Diagnostic tests
      (1) Abdominal radiography
      (2) Laboratory tests include complete blood count, electrolytes, blood urea nitrogen, glucose, magnesium, calcium, phosphate, prothrombin time, and partial thromboplastin time. Perform other tests based on history and physical examination.
   c) Preoperative medication and intravenous therapy
      (1) Expect a moderate fluid shift with moderate to large fluid losses. Two large-bore intravenous catheters (14 to 16 gauge) are indicated.
      (2) Antibiotic therapy is indicated.
      (3) Blood transfusions are given.
3. **Room preparation**
   a) Monitoring equipment
      (1) Standard
      (2) Full warming modalities
   b) Pharmacologic agents: Standard
   c) Position: Supine, with arms extended
4. **Anesthetic technique**
   a) Routine general anesthesia
   b) Epidural for intraoperative and/or postoperative management
5. **Perioperative management**
   a) Induction: Most patients are considered to have full stomachs; therefore, rapid sequence induction is indicated.
   b) Maintenance
      (1) Muscle relaxation is required.
      (2) A narcotic and/or inhalation agent is administered.
      (3) Closely monitor hydration status and blood loss.
      (4) Avoid nitrous oxide to minimize gastric or colonic distention.
   c) Emergence: Awake extubation is performed after rapid sequence induction or placement of a nasogastric tube.
6. **Postoperative implications**
   Pain may lead to hypoventilation, reduced cough, splinting, and atelectasis.

K. Hemorrhoidectomy

1. **Introduction**
   Hemorrhoids are masses of vascular tissue found in the anal canal. Internal hemorrhoids are found above the pectinate line, arise from the superior hemorrhoidal venosus plexus, and are covered with mucosa. External hemorrhoids are found below the pectinate line, arise from the inferior hemorrhoidal venosus plexus, and are covered by anoderm and perianal skin. Treatment includes hemorrhoidectomy.
2. **Preoperative assessment and patient preparation**
   a) History and physical examination: Signs include bright red blood on toilet paper or the surface of the stool, iron-deficiency anemia, a prolapsed mass of tissue that protrudes from the anus, and thrombosis (blood clot within the hemorrhoidal vein) causing pain
   b) Diagnostic tests: A complete blood count is indicated
   c) Preoperative medication and intravenous therapy

(1) A narcotic with premedication is considered if the patient experiences pain.

(2) An 18-gauge intravenous tube with minimal fluid replacement is used.

3. **Room preparation**
   a) Monitoring equipment: Standard
   b) Position: Prone or lithotomy
4. **Anesthetic technique**
   a) Regional anesthesia, local anesthesia with sedation, or general anesthesia
   b) Regional blockade: Analgesic to S2 to S5 required
      (1) Hypobaric spinal: Lithotomy position
      (2) Hyperbaric spinal: Flexed prone or knee chest position
   c) General anesthesia: Mask or laryngeal mask airway in lithotomy position (endotracheal intubation necessary for prone position)
5. **Perioperative management**
   a) Induction
      (1) Prone: General anesthesia induction is performed while the patient is on the stretcher.
      (2) Position the patient on the operating table with adequate support and padding of the extremities, head, and neck.
   b) Maintenance: General anesthesia: Adequate planes of anesthesia or muscle relaxants are required to relax the anal sphincter.
   c) Emergence: If the prone position is used and general anesthesia is administered, patients are repositioned onto the stretcher before emergence.
6. **Postoperative implications**
   Bearing down to void will be painful; keep fluids to a minimum.

L. Herniorrhaphy

1. **Introduction**
   Inguinal hernias are defects in the transverse abdominal layer; a direct hernia comes through the posterior wall of the inguinal canal, and an indirect hernia comes through the internal inguinal ring. Femoral hernia is when the hernia sac is exposed as it exits the preperitoneal space through the femoral canal. Incisional hernias can occur after any abdominal incision, but they are most common following midline incisions. Factors leading to herniation are ischemia, wound infection, trauma, and inadequate suturing. Treatment is with herniorrhaphy.

2. **Preoperative assessment**
   Predisposing factors for hernia often include increased abdominal pressure secondary to chronic cough, bladder outlet obstruction, constipation, pregnancy, vomiting, and acute or chronic muscular effort. The patient population may range from premature infants to the elderly, with the possibility of various medical problems.
   a) History and physical examination: These are as indicated by the patient's condition.
      (1) Musculoskeletal: Pain is likely in the area of the hernia; evaluate bony landmarks if regional anesthesia is planned.
      (2) Hematologic: If regional anesthesia is planned, check the patient's coagulation status.

(3) Gastrointestinal: Hernias may become incarcerated, obstructed, or strangulated, requiring emergency surgery. Fluid and electrolyte imbalance should be assessed.

b) Patient preparation

(1) Laboratory tests: Complete blood count, electrolytes, and other tests are as indicated by the history and physical examination.

(2) Diagnostic tests: These are as indicated by the history and physical examination.

(3) If necessary, use standard premedication.

3. **Room preparation**

a) Monitoring equipment: Standard

b) Additional equipment: Regular operating table

c) Drugs

(1) Standard emergency drugs

(2) Standard tabletop

(3) Intravenous fluids: One 18-gauge intravenous line with normal saline or lactated Ringer's solution at 5 to 8 mL/kg per hour

4. **Anesthetic technique**

General, regional, and local anesthesia with sedation are all appropriate. The choice depends on such factors as site of incision, the patient's physical status, and the preference of both patient and surgeon. General anesthesia may be preferred for incisions made above T8. Profound muscle relaxation may be needed for exploration and repair.

5. **Perioperative management**

a) Standard induction: General anesthesia by mask or laryngeal mask airway may be suitable for the patient with a simple chronic hernia. If there is obstruction, incarceration, or strangulation, rapid sequence induction with endotracheal intubation is indicated. General endotracheal anesthesia is indicated in the patient with wound dehiscence.

b) Maintenance

(1) Standard: Muscle relaxants may be necessary to facilitate surgical repair.

(2) Position: The patient is supine, with checked and padded pressure points. Avoid stretching the brachial plexus. Limit abduction to 90 degrees.

c) Emergence: Consider extubating the trachea while the patient is still anesthetized to prevent coughing and straining. Patients who are at risk for pulmonary aspiration and who require awake extubation after rapid sequence induction are not candidates for deep extubation.

6. **Postoperative implications**

a) Wound dehiscence may occur with coughing or straining.

b) Urinary retention: Patients with urinary retention may require intermittent catheterization until urinary function resumes.

c) Pain management: Surgical field block or regional anesthesia should provide sufficient analgesia postoperatively.

M. Laparoscopic Cholecystectomy

1. **Introduction**

Laparoscopic cholecystectomy is a minimally invasive surgical procedure used in the treatment of gallstones and diseases of the gallbladder.

PART II **Common Procedures**

This procedure is performed under the guidance of a laparoscope. More than 90% of cholecystectomies are performed laparoscopically.

2. **Preoperative assessment and patient preparation**
   a) History and physical examination: These are as indicated by the patient's history and medical condition
   b) Diagnostic tests: These are as indicated by the patient's history and medical condition.
   c) Preoperative medication and intravenous therapy
      (1) Preoperative antibiotics are used.
      (2) Narcotics must be used with caution to minimize potential spasm in the biliary tract and sphincter of Oddi.
      (3) Use a single, large-bore (18-gauge) intravenous tube with fluid replacement.
      (4) Use prophylactic antiemetics and aspiration prophylaxis.

3. **Room preparation**
   a) Monitoring equipment: Standard
   b) Pharmacologic agents: Standard
   c) Position
      (1) Supine
      (2) Exposure of the operative site optimized with the reverse Trendelenburg position and by tilting the table to the side

4. **Anesthetic technique:** General endotracheal anesthesia with muscle relaxation

5. **Perioperative management**
   a) Induction: Standard or rapid sequence induction with oral endotracheal intubation
   b) Maintenance
      (1) Muscle relaxation with appropriate reversal is used.
      (2) The peritoneal cavity must be insufflated for surgical exposure. Insufflation with carbon dioxide causes a rise in the carbon dioxide partial pressure unless ventilation is controlled.
      (3) Abdominal insufflation may lead to hypercarbia with inadequate ventilation. Special attention should be paid to possible adjustments in ventilator settings with insufflation.
      (4) Basal measurements should be sufficient to control carbon dioxide partial pressure.
      (5) Insufflation leads to increased intraabdominal pressure. An intraabdominal pressure of 20 to 25 cm H_2O produces increases in cardiac output and central venous pressure secondary to changes in the volume of the venous return of blood. An intraabdominal pressure greater than 30 to 40 cm H_2O may lead to decreased central venous pressure and reduced cardiac output secondary to reduced right ventricular preload. Insufflation to a pressure of approximately 15 mm Hg is routine.
      (6) All maintenance anesthetic drugs may be used. Some surgeons request that nitrous oxide not be used to reduce the risk of bowel expansion, which could hinder surgical exposure.
   c) Emergence: Awake extubation is performed after the patient's airway reflexes are adequate.

6. **Postoperative implications**
   a) Pain management: This approach offers the benefit of reduced postoperative pain secondary to smaller abdominal incisions. Patients may experience shoulder pain from pneumoperitoneum, which is

usually self-limiting. Use patient-controlled analgesia or intravenous narcotics.
b) Postoperative nausea and vomiting: Antiemetic prophylaxis is used.

N. Liver Resection

1. Introduction
Patients presenting for hepatic surgery may have primary or metastatic tumors from gastrointestinal and other sources. Liver function may be entirely normal in these patients. Hepatocellular carcinoma is common in men older than 50 years and is associated with chronic, active hepatitis B and cirrhosis. Although most major liver resections can be performed by a transabdominal approach, some surgeons prefer a thoracoabdominal approach. The liver is transected by blunt dissection using the Cavitron ultrasonic suction aspirator and argon beam laser coagulator.

As the principles and techniques of hepatic surgery have evolved, the overall mortality and morbidity rates have improved considerably. Because the normal liver can regenerate, it is possible to resect the right or left lobe along with segments of the contralateral lobe. In patients with cirrhosis, the regeneration process is limited; thus, uninvolved liver should be preserved.

2. Preoperative assessment
The following preoperative considerations are for patients *without cirrhosis:*
a) History and physical examination: These are as indicated by the patient's history and medical condition.
b) Patient preparation
  (1) Laboratory tests: Complete blood count, coagulation profile, liver function test, albumin, creatinine, blood urea nitrogen, blood sugar, bilirubin, and electrolytes are obtained. Perform other tests as indicated by the history and physical examination.
  (2) Diagnostic tests: Chest radiographs, ultrasonography, computed tomography, and magnetic resonance imaging are used as indicated by the history and physical examination.
  (3) Medications: Standard premedication that accounts for the reduced ability of the liver to metabolize drugs is given. Other preoperative medications include antiemetics.

3. Room preparation
a) Monitoring equipment
  (1) Standard monitoring equipment
  (2) Arterial line and central venous pressure as clinically indicated
b) Additional equipment
  (1) Cell saver
  (2) Possibly a rapid transfusion device
c) Drugs
  (1) Standard emergency drugs
  (2) Standard tabletop
  (3) Intravenous fluids: 14- or 16-gauge intravenous lines (two) with normal saline or lactated Ringer's solution at 10 to 20 mL/kg per hour; fluids warmed

(4) Two units of packed red blood cells should be available. Blood loss can be significant, and massive transfusions may be required. Appropriate blood products also include 2 units of fresh-frozen plasma and 10 units of platelets.

4. **Perioperative management and anesthetic technique**
   a) Induction
      (1) General endotracheal anesthesia with rapid sequence intubation is used.
      (2) Restore intravascular volume before anesthetic induction. If the patient is hemodynamically unstable, consider etomidate (0.2 to 0.4 mg/kg) or ketamine (1 to 3 mg/kg).
   b) Maintenance
      (1) Standard
      (2) Combined epidural and general anesthesia: Be prepared to treat hypotension with fluid and vasopressors. General anesthesia is administered to supplement regional anesthesia and for amnesia.
      (3) Position: The patient is supine, with checked and padded pressure points. Avoid stretching the brachial plexus. Limit abduction to 90 degrees.
   c) Emergence
      (1) For major hepatic resections, the patient will be best cared for in an intensive care unit.
      (2) Consider keeping the patient mechanically ventilated until the patient's condition is hemodynamically stable and ventilatory status is optimized.
      (3) If surgical resection was minimal, the patient can be extubated awake and after reflexes have returned.

5. **Postoperative implications**
   a) Decreased liver function: Patients with normal preoperative liver function may have significant postoperative impairment of liver function secondary to loss of liver mass or surgical trauma.
   b) Pulmonary insufficiency (atelectasis, effusion, and pneumonia): More than 90% of patients will develop some form of respiratory complication.
   c) Hemorrhage
   d) Disseminated intravascular coagulation
   e) Electrolyte imbalance
   f) Hypoglycemia
   g) Hypothermia

O. Liver Transplantation

1. **Introduction**
   Liver transplantation is the treatment of choice for patients with acute and chronic end-stage liver disease. The liver transplant operation can be divided into three stages: (1) hepatectomy; (2) anhepatic phase, which involves the implantation of the liver; and (3) postrevascularization, which involves hemostasis and reconstruction of the hepatic artery and common bile duct. Hepatectomy can be associated with marked blood loss. Contributing factors include severe coagulopathy, severe portal hypertension, previous surgery in the right upper quadrant, renal failure, uncontrolled sepsis, retransplantation, transfusion reaction, venous

bypass–induced fibrinolysis, primary graft nonfunction, and intraoperative vascular complications.

The anhepatic phase may be associated with significant hemodynamic changes. This stage consists of implantation of the liver allograft, with or without venovenous bypass. Benefits of using the venovenous bypass system include improved hemodynamics during the anhepatic phase, decreased blood loss, and possible improvement of perioperative renal function. Complications of using the system include pulmonary embolism, air embolism, brachial plexus injury, and wound seroma/infection.

Before revascularization, the liver must be flushed with a cold solution (i.e., albumin 5%) through the portal vein and out the infrahepatic vena cava. The reperfusion of the liver may be the most critical part of the operation. Patients may experience pulmonary hypertension, followed by right ventricular failure and profound hypotension. The hepatic artery reconstruction is performed after stabilization of the patient following revascularization. The last part involves hemostasis, removal of the gallbladder, and reconstruction of the bile duct.

2. **Preoperative assessment**

Patients requiring liver transplantation often have multiorgan system failure. Because of the emergency nature of the surgery, there may be insufficient time available for customary evaluation and correction of abnormalities.

a) History and physical examination

(1) Cardiovascular: These patients can present with a hyperdynamic state, with increased cardiac output and decreased systemic vascular resistance. Many of these patients present with dysrhythmias, hypertension, pulmonary hypertension, valvular disease, cardiomyopathy (alcoholic disease, hemochromatosis, Wilson's disease), and coronary artery disease.

(2) Respiratory: Patients are often hypoxic because of ascites, pleural effusions, atelectasis, ventilation-perfusion mismatch, and pulmonary arteriovenous shunting. This normally results in tachypnea and respiratory alkalosis. Pulmonary infection is usually a contraindication to surgery. Adult respiratory distress syndrome is usually not.

(3) Hepatic: Hepatitis serology and the cause of hepatic failure should be determined. Albumin is usually low, with consequent low plasma oncotic pressure leading to edema and ascites. The magnitude of action and duration of drugs may be unpredictable, although these patients generally have an increased sensitivity to all drugs, and the drug actions are prolonged.

(4) Neurologic: Patients are often encephalopathic and may be in hepatic coma. In fulminant hepatic failure, increased intracranial pressure is common, accounting for 40% mortality (herniation), and may require prompt treatment (e.g., mannitol, hyperventilation).

(5) Gastrointestinal: Portal hypertension, esophageal varices, and coagulopathies increase the risk of gastrointestinal hemorrhage. Gastric emptying is often delayed.

(6) Renal: Patients are often hypervolemic, hyponatremic, and possibly hypokalemic. Calcium is usually normal. Metabolic alkalosis is often present. Preoperative dialysis should be considered.

(7) Endocrine: Patients are often glucose intolerant or diabetic. Hyperaldosteronism may be present.

(8) Hematologic: Patients are often anemic secondary to blood loss or malabsorption. Coagulation is impaired because of decreased hepatic synthesis function (all factors except VIII and fibrinogen are decreased), abnormal fibrinogen production, impaired platelets, fibrinolysis, and low-grade disseminated intravascular coagulation.

b) Patient preparation

(1) Laboratory tests: Complete blood count, coagulation profile, liver function tests, albumin, creatinine, blood urea nitrogen, blood sugar, bilirubin, and electrolytes are obtained. Perform other tests as indicated by the history and physical examination.

(2) Diagnostic tests: Chest radiographs, pulmonary function tests, electrocardiography, echocardiogram, and cardiac catheterization are obtained.

(3) Medication: Standard premedication and aspiration prophylaxis are used.

3. Room preparation

a) Monitoring equipment

(1) Standard

(2) Arterial line, transesophageal echocardiogram, central venous pressure, or pulmonary artery catheter as indicated

b) Additional equipment

(1) Patient warming devices

(2) Rapid infusion system

(3) Blood warmers

c) Drugs

(1) Standard tabletop

(2) Standard emergency drugs

(3) Intravenous fluids: 14- to 16-gauge catheters (two), often placed in the right antecubital fossa or the left or right internal/ external jugular. The left arm is avoided because the axillary vein is used for vasovenous bypass.

(4) Blood loss can be significant; blood should be immediately available.

4. Anesthetic technique:

General anesthesia is used. These patients are challenging to manage during the various stages of the surgery. Hemodynamic instability, massive blood loss, electrolyte imbalance (hypocalcemia, hyperkalemia), and coagulopathy may occur.

5. Perioperative management

a) Induction

(1) Rapid sequence induction with oral endotracheal tube is used.

(2) One may use a narcotic (fentanyl, 2 to 5 mcg/kg) just before induction.

b) Maintenance

(1) Standard maintenance is with fentanyl, 10 to 50 mcg/kg, and/or an inhalation agent titrated according to individual patient response.

(2) Antibiotics and immunosuppressants are given at the surgeon's request.

(3) Position the patient supine, and pad pressure points. Avoid stretching the brachial plexus greater than 90 degrees.

(4) Reperfusion syndrome (which occurs during the revascularization phase) is characterized by decreased heart rate, hypotension, conduction defects, and decreased systemic vascular resistance while right ventricular pressures increase. The cause is unknown. Cardiac output can be maintained. An increase in serum potassium can lead to cardiac arrest.

6. **Postoperative implications**
   a) Monitoring of hepatic function using laboratory data: Serial liver function tests, prothrombin time, partial thromboplastin time, ammonia levels, lactate, and bile output
   b) Possible complications: Bleeding, portal vein thrombosis, hepatic artery thrombosis, biliary tract leaks, primary nonfunction, rejection, infection, pulmonary complications, electrolyte imbalances, hypertension, alkalosis, renal failure, peptic ulceration, and neurologic complications

P. Pancreatectomy

1. **Introduction**
   Distal pancreatectomy is performed for tumors in the distal half of the pancreas, whereas subtotal pancreatectomy involves resection of the pancreas from the mesenteric vessels distally, leaving the head and uncinate process intact. In about 95% of patients with pancreatic cancer, the cancer is ductal adenocarcinoma, and most of these tumors occur in the head of the pancreas.

   Pancreatic cancer may appear as a localized mass or as a diffuse enlargement of the gland on computed tomography of the abdomen. Biopsy of the lesion is necessary to confirm the diagnosis. Complete surgical resection is the only effective treatment of ductal pancreatic cancer.

2. **Preoperative assessment**
   Patients requiring pancreatic surgery can be divided into four groups: (1) those with acute pancreatitis in whom medical treatment has failed in the past; (2) patients with adenocarcinoma of the pancreas; (3) patients with neuroendocrine-active or -inactive islet cell tumors; and (4) patients suffering from the sequelae of chronic pancreatitis (abscess or pseudocyst).
   a) History and physical examination
      (1) Cardiovascular: Patients with acute pancreatitis may be hypotensive and may require aggressive volume resuscitation with crystalloid and even blood before surgery. Severe electrolyte disturbances may be associated with acute pancreatitis and some hormone-secreting tumors of the pancreas.
      (2) Respiratory: Respiratory compromise such as pleural effusions, atelectasis, and adult respiratory distress syndrome progressing to respiratory failure may occur in up to 50% of patients with acute pancreatitis.
      (3) Gastrointestinal: Jaundice and abdominal pain are common symptoms in this group of patients. The presence of ileus or intestinal obstruction should mandate full-stomach precautions and rapid sequence induction. Electrolyte disturbances are common in acute pancreatitis and may include hypochloremic metabolic alkalosis, decreased calcium and magnesium, and increased glucose. These abnormalities should be corrected preoperatively.
      (4) Endocrine: Many patients with acute pancreatitis may have diabetes secondary to loss of pancreatic tissue. Hormone-secreting tumors of the pancreas are occasionally associated with multiple endocrine neoplasia syndromes. Insulinoma is the most common hormone-secreting tumor of the pancreas and can result in hypoglycemia.

(5) Renal: Patients should be evaluated for renal insufficiency.

(6) Hematologic: Hematocrit may be falsely elevated because of hemo-concentration or hemorrhage. Coagulopathy may be present.

b) Patient preparation

(1) Laboratory tests: Complete blood count, prothrombin time, partial thromboplastin time, platelet count, electrolytes, blood urea nitrogen, creatinine, blood sugar, calcium, magnesium, amylase, and urinalysis, as well as other tests as indicated by the history and physical examination.

(2) Diagnostic tests: Chest radiographs, pulmonary function tests, electrocardiography, and computed tomography of the abdomen, as well as other tests as indicated by the history and physical examination.

(3) Medication: Standard premedication with consideration for aspiration prophylaxis.

3. Room preparation

a) Standard monitoring equipment

b) Arterial line, central venous pressure, transesophageal echocardiography, or pulmonary artery catheter: As clinically indicated

c) Additional equipment: Patient warming devices

d) Drugs

(1) Standard emergency drugs

(2) Standard tabletop

(3) Intravenous fluids: 14- to 16-gauge intravenous lines (two) with normal saline or lactated Ringer's solution at 10 to 20 mL/kg per hour; warmed fluids

(4) Blood loss possibly significant; blood immediately available

4. Perioperative management and anesthetic technique

General endotracheal anesthesia is used; consider an epidural technique for postoperative analgesia.

a) Induction

(1) This is standard, with consideration of rapid sequence intubation as indicated.

(2) Restore intravascular volume before anesthetic induction.

(3) If the patient is hemodynamically unstable, consider etomidate (0.2 to 0.4 mg/kg) or ketamine (1 to 3 mg/kg)

b) Maintenance

(1) Standard maintenance: This involves a narcotic and/or inhalation agent.

(2) Avoid nitrous oxide to minimize bowel distention.

(3) Combined epidural and general anesthesia: Be prepared to treat hypotension with fluid and vasopressors.

(4) Titrate epidural anesthesia as indicated by patient's response.

(5) General anesthesia is administered to supplement regional anesthesia and for amnesia.

(6) Position: The patient is supine, with checked and padded pressure points. Avoid stretching the brachial plexus. Limit abduction to 90 degrees.

c) Emergence

The decision to extubate at the end of the operation depends on the patient's underlying cardiopulmonary status and the extent of the surgical procedure. Patients should be hemodynamically stable, warm, alert, cooperative, and fully reversed from any muscle relaxants before extubation.

5. **Postoperative implications**

Significant third-space and evaporative losses contribute to hypovolemia. Major hemorrhage can occur during dissection of the pancreas from the mesenteric and portal vessels. Total pancreatectomy is associated with brittle diabetes that can be difficult to control. Subtotal resections lead to varying degrees of hyperglycemia. The patient should recover in an intensive care unit or hospital ward accustomed to treating the side effects of epidural opiates.

Tests for postoperative management include electrolytes, calcium, glucose, complete blood count, platelets, and other tests as indicated. Electrolyte disturbances are common in acute pancreatitis and may include hypochloremic metabolic alkalosis, decreased calcium and magnesium, and increased glucose. These abnormalities should be corrected preoperatively.

Q. Pheochromocytoma

1. **Introduction**
   a) Surgical treatment of pheochromocytoma is 90% curative; 10% to 25% of patients have bilateral tumors. Adrenalectomy is possible, depending on tumor location.
   b) Pathophysiology: Pheochromocytomas are highly vascular tumors associated with adrenal medulla chromaffin tissue that secrete mostly norepinephrine but also epinephrine. Tumors usually are in the abdomen (95%) but may be found anywhere that chromaffin tissue arises. They are malignant in 10% of patients. An inherited autosomal dominant trait is involved 5% of the time. These tumors can be associated with multiple endocrine neoplasia syndrome. They are most common in early to middle adulthood. Catecholamine release does not depend on neurogenic control (see the discussion of Pheochromocytoma in Section III of Part 1).

2. **Preoperative assessment**
   a) History and physical examination
      (1) Cardiac: Paroxysmal severe hypertension, dysrhythmia, myocardial infarction, orthostatic hypotension, hypovolemia, catecholamine-induced cardiomyopathy, and decreased sensitivity to catecholamines
      (2) Neurologic: Headache, tremors, sweating, hypertensive retinopathy, and mydriasis
      (3) Renal: Impairment from hypertension
      (4) Gastrointestinal: None
      (5) Endocrine: Hyperglycemia
   b) Patient preparation
      (1) Laboratory tests: As indicated by the patient's condition
      (2) Diagnostic tests
         (a) Electrocardiogram; left ventricular hypertrophy and nonspecific T-wave changes common
         (b) Echocardiogram for left ventricular function
         (c) Chest radiography to assess cardiomegaly
         (d) Magnetic resonance imaging or computed tomography to localize tumors
         (e) Urinary vanillylmandelic acid, norepinephrine, and epinephrine levels usually elevated in a 24-hour collection

(3) Medications: α-Adrenergic blockade is recommended 10 to 14 days before surgery (phenoxybenzamine, 40 to 400 mg/day). β-Blockers are added only after α-blockade to help manage tachy-dysrhythmias that are caused from α-blockade. If β-blockers are begun before α-blockade, unopposed α response is possible.

3. **Room preparation**
   a) Monitoring equipment: Standard, arterial line, central line, and pulmonary arterial catheter as indicated
   b) Additional equipment: Positioning devices; supine, nephrectomy, or prone jackknife position used, depending on whether incision is midline abdominal, bilateral subcostal, curved posterior, or dorsal flank oblique
   c) Drugs
      (1) Continuous infusions: Nitroprusside, phentolamine, and esmolol are indicated for severe hypertension and tachycardia during tumor manipulation. Hypotension after ligation of tumor's venous supply can be treated with phenylephrine, dopamine, and fluids.
      (2) Intravenous fluids: Prehydrate before surgery because the patient is usually intravascularly depleted. Large third-space loss and blood loss is possible; use isotonic fluids at 10 mL/kg per hour.
      (3) Blood: Type and cross-match 2 units of packed red blood cells.
      (4) Tabletop: Have vasoactive drugs available for prompt treatment (lidocaine, nitroglycerin, nitroprusside, esmolol, phenylephrine) of hemodynamic instability.

4. **Perioperative management and anesthetic technique**
   a) Induction: This is slow and controlled, to avoid sympathetic nervous system response to laryngoscopy. One may pretreat with esmolol. Avoid histamine-releasing drugs, ketamine, or vagolytics.
   b) Maintenance: General anesthesia with a narcotic-inhalation combination is used. An epidural combination can also be used; however, avoid using epinephrine in the test dose.
   c) Emergence: Pay careful attention to labile hemodynamics.

5. **Postoperative complications**
   Catecholamine levels normalize in several days. Pneumothorax, hypoglycemia, cardiac dysfunction, and hypoadrenocorticism are possible.

R. Small Bowel Resection

1. **Introduction**
   Small bowel resection is performed for various diseases including intestinal obstruction, small bowel tumors, abdominal trauma, stricture, adhesions, Meckel's diverticulum, Crohn's disease, and infection.

2. **Preoperative assessment and patient preparation**
   a) History and physical examination: Assess fluid and hydration status. The patient may be vomiting or bleeding or may have third-spacing, diarrhea, or dehydration.
   b) Diagnostic tests: These are as indicated by the patient's condition.
   c) Preoperative medication and intravenous therapy
      (1) Patients may be receiving steroid therapy or immunosuppressant drugs.

(2) Expect fluid shifts requiring moderate to large fluid resuscitation. Two large-bore, intravenous access tubes are indicated.

(3) Preoperative hydration is essential.

3. Room preparation
a) Monitoring equipment: Standard with full warming modalities
b) Pharmacologic agents: Standard
c) Position: Supine with arms extended

4. Anesthetic technique
a) Epidural (T2 to T4 level) with a "light" general anesthetic
b) General anesthesia with an endotracheal tube

5. Perioperative management
a) Induction: Most patients are considered to have full stomachs; therefore, rapid sequence induction is indicated.
b) Maintenance
   (1) Muscle relaxation is required.
   (2) Closely monitor hydration status and blood loss.
   (3) Avoid nitrous oxide, which may cause bowel distention.
c) Emergence: Awake extubation is performed after rapid sequence induction or placement of a nasogastric tube.

6. Postoperative implications
a) Pain may lead to hypoventilation, reduced cough, splinting, and atelectasis.
b) Pain control is with epidural or patient-controlled analgesia.

S. Splenectomy

1. Introduction
Patients presenting for splenectomy can be divided into two groups: trauma patients and patients with myeloproliferative disorders and other varieties of hypersplenism. Anesthetic management is individualized based on the individual patient's medical condition. Patients who have received chemotherapy must be assessed for potential organ system complications.

2. Preoperative assessment
a) History and physical examination
   (1) Cardiovascular: Patients with systemic disease may be chronically ill and have decreased cardiovascular reserve. Patients who have received doxorubicin (Adriamycin) may have a dose-dependent cardiotoxicity that can be worsened by radiation therapy. Manifestations include decreased QRS amplitude, congestive heart failure, pleural effusions, and dysrhythmia.
   (2) Respiratory: Patients may have a degree of left lower lobe atelectasis and altered ventilation. If they are treated with bleomycin, pulmonary fibrosis may occur. Methotrexate, busulfan, mitomycin, cytarabine, and other chemotherapeutic agents may cause pulmonary toxicity.
   (3) Neurologic: Patients may have neurologic deficits following chemotherapeutic agents. Vinblastine and cisplatin can cause peripheral neuropathies. Any evidence of neurologic dysfunction should be documented.
   (4) Hematologic: Patients are likely to have splenomegaly secondary to hematologic disease (Hodgkin's disease, leukemia). Cytopenias are common.

(5) Hepatic: Some chemotherapeutic agents (methotrexate, 6-mercaptopurine) may be hepatotoxic. Evaluation of liver function tests should be considered in patients considered at risk.

(6) Renal: Some chemotherapeutic drugs (methotrexate, cisplatin) are nephrotoxic. Patients exposed to such agents may have renal insufficiency.

b) Patient preparation

(1) Laboratory tests: Complete blood count, prothrombin time, partial thromboplastin time, bleeding time, platelet count, electrolytes, blood urea nitrogen, creatinine, urinalysis, and other tests are obtained as indicated by the history and physical examination.

(2) Medication: Standard premedication. Consider aspiration prophylaxis. Administer steroids (25-100 mg hydrocortisone) if the patient has received them as part of a chemotherapeutic or medical treatment.

3. **Room preparation**

a) Monitoring equipment: Standard and others as indicated by the patient's status

b) Additional equipment: Patient warming device

c) Drugs

(1) Standard emergency drugs

(2) Standard tabletop

(3) Intravenous fluids: 16- to 18-gauge intravenous lines (two) with normal saline or lactated Ringer's solution at 10 to 15 mL/kg per hour; warmed fluids

4. **Anesthetic technique**

General endotracheal anesthesia with or without an epidural for postoperative analgesia is used.

5. **Perioperative management**

a) Induction

(1) This is standard, with consideration of rapid sequence intubation as indicated.

(2) Restore intravascular volume before anesthetic induction. If the patient is hemodynamically unstable, consider etomidate or ketamine.

b) Maintenance

(1) Standard regimens are used.

(2) Combined epidural and general anesthesia: See the earlier discussion of Pancreatectomy.

(3) Position: The patient is supine, with checked and padded pressure points. Avoid stretching the brachial plexus. Limit abduction to 90 degrees.

c) Emergence: The decision to extubate at the end of the operation depends on the patient's underlying cardiopulmonary status and the extent of the surgical procedure. Patients should be hemodynamically stable, warm, alert, cooperative, and fully reversed from any muscle relaxants before extubation.

6. **Postoperative implications**

a) Bleeding

b) Atelectasis, usually in the left lower lobe

c) Pain management: Multimodal approach with epidural local anesthetics, patient-controlled analgesia, and/or opiates

T. Whipple's Resection

1. Introduction

Whipple's resection consists of a pancreatoduodenectomy, pancreatoje-junostomy, hepaticojejunostomy, and gastrojejunostomy. On entering the peritoneal cavity, the surgeon determines the resectability of the pancreatic lesion. Contraindications to resection include involvement of mesenteric vessels, infiltration by tumor into the root of the mesentery, extension into the porta hepatis with involvement of hepatic artery, and liver metastasis. If the tumor is deemed resectable, the head of the pancreas is further mobilized. The common duct is transected above the cystic duct entry, and the gallbladder is removed. Once the superior mesenteric vein is freed from the pancreas, the latter is transected with care taken not to injure the splenic vein. The jejunum is transected beyond the ligament of Treitz, and the specimen is removed by severing the vascular connections with the mesenteric vessels. Reconstitution is achieved by anastomosing the distal pancreatic stump, bile duct, and stomach into the jejunum. Drains are placed adjacent to the pancreatic anastomosis. Some surgeons stent the anastomosis until it has healed.

2. Preoperative assessment
a) History and physical examination: See the earlier discussion of Pancreatectomy.
b) Patient preparation
  (1) Laboratory tests: See the earlier discussion of Pancreatectomy.
  (2) Diagnostic tests: See the earlier discussion of Pancreatectomy.
  (3) Medication: See the earlier discussion of Pancreatectomy.

3. Room preparation
See the earlier discussion of Pancreatectomy in this section.

4. Anesthetic technique
General endotracheal anesthesia with an epidural for postoperative analgesia is used. See the earlier discussion of Pancreatectomy.

5. Perioperative management
See the earlier discussion of Pancreatectomy in this section.

6. Postoperative implications
See the earlier discussion of Pancreatectomy in this section.

PART II Common Procedures

GENITOURINARY SYSTEM

A. Cystectomy

1. Introduction

The bladder is usually removed for cancer but may also be removed for severe hemorrhagic or radiation cystitis. In a radical cystectomy for invasive cancer in women, the uterus, fallopian tubes, ovaries, and a portion of the vaginal wall are removed. In men, the ampulla of the vas deferens, prostate, and seminal vesicles are removed. There is also lymph node dissection, and a urinary diversion is created (through the intestine).

2. Preoperative assessment

a) Cardiac/respiratory/neurologic/endocrine: Assessment is routine.

b) Renal: Gross hematuria may be a symptom. Check renal function tests as well as evidence of a urinary tract infection.

c) Gastrointestinal: Patients are at risk for fluid and electrolyte imbalance because of bowel preparation.

3. Patient preparation

a) Laboratory tests: Complete blood count, electrolytes, blood urea nitrogen, creatinine, glucose, prothrombin time, partial thromboplastin time, type and screen for 2 to 4 units, and urinalysis

b) Diagnostic tests: Electrocardiography and chest radiography for most of this patient population

c) Medication: Sedation as needed

4. Room preparation

a) Monitors: Standard, arterial line, and central venous pressure; urine output not measurable during this procedure; two large-bore, reliable intravenous lines available

b) Additional equipment: Epidural insertion and infusion supplies, if using, and warming devices for the patient and fluids

c) Position: Supine

d) Drugs and fluids: 6 to 10 mL/kg per hour of crystalloid for maintenance; 2 to 4 units of blood readily available

5. Perioperative management

Combined general/epidural or general anesthesia with standard induction is used. The patient may be anemic because of hematuria and hypovolemic because of bowel preparation. Attempt to correct these conditions before induction. Maintenance is routine, with special attention paid to fluid calculations and keeping the patient warm. Plan to extubate immediately postoperatively unless the patient is unstable during the procedure or prior respiratory complications prevent early extubation.

6. **Postoperative considerations**
Epidural or patient-controlled analgesia should be planned for preoperative use. Watch the patients for signs of hypovolemia, anemia, or pulmonary edema resulting from fluid shifts intraoperatively.

B. Cystoscopy

1. **Introduction**
Cystoscopy is the use of instrumentation to examine the urinary tract. A cystoscope may be used for diagnostic or therapeutic procedures such as the following: workup of hematuria, stricture, and tumor; removal and manipulation of stones; placement of stents; and follow-up of therapy. Retrograde pyelography and other dye studies may be used. This procedure is usually performed on an outpatient basis.
2. **Preoperative assessment and patient preparation**
   a) History and physical examination: Standard
   b) Diagnostic tests: Standard
   c) Preoperative medication and intravenous therapy
      (1) Prophylactic antibiotics
      (2) 18-gauge intravenous catheter with minimal fluid replacement
3. **Room preparation**
   a) Monitoring equipment: Standard
   b) Pharmacologic agents: Indigo carmine, methylene blue
   c) Position: Lithotomy
4. **Anesthetic technique**
   The technique of choice is regional blockade or general anesthesia.
   a) Intravenous sedation: Midazolam (Versed), fentanyl, or propofol in sedation doses
   b) Regional blockade: Analgesia to T9 required
   c) General anesthesia: Administered by mask or oral endotracheal tube
5. **Preoperative management**
   a) Induction: No specific indications
   b) Maintenance
      (1) Diagnostic dyes may be administered. Use indigo carmine dye (α-sympathomimetic effects) cautiously in patients with hypertension or cardiac ischemia. Methylene blue dye may cause hypertension. Oxygen saturation readings may be altered by dye administration.
      (2) Persistent erection may occur in younger male patients, thus preventing manipulation of the cystoscope. Use deeper anesthesia.
      (3) Water or irrigation solution may be used to distend the bladder. See the discission of transurethral resection of the prostate later in this section.
      (4) Quadriplegic or paraplegic patients may undergo repeated cystoscopies. Autonomic hyperreflexia is possible if the injury is above level T5.
   c) Emergence: No specific indications
6. **Postoperative considerations**
   Postoperative care is standard.

PART II Common Procedures

C. Extracorporeal Shock Wave Lithotripsy

1. Introduction

Extracorporeal shock wave lithotripsy (ESWL) is a noninvasive technique that pulverizes renal stones with shock waves. Disintegrated stones are passed in the urine. Patients with a history of cardiac arrthythmias and those with a pacemaker are at risk of developing arrhythmias induced by the shock waves. Synchronization of the shock waves to the R wave of electrocardiogram decreases the incidence of arrthythmias and serves as the trigger for shock waves; therefore, the procedure length is somewhat heart rate–dependent—usually 30 to 90 minutes.

a) First-generation lithotripters: Patients are placed in a hydraulically operated chairlift device and are submerged from the clavicles down into a tub of water. The impact of the shock waves at the flank entry site is painful, requiring anesthesia.

b) Second-generation lithotripters: Patients are placed on lithotripsy table and are positioned so shock waves generated within an enclosed casing are directed at area of stone. Lower-voltage shock waves are used, and pain is greatly reduced with this method.

2. Preoperative assessment and patient preparation

a) Routine preoperative assessment with laboratory tests based on any abnormalities found in the history and physical examination. Consider cardiac status; many hemodynamic changes are associated with this procedure.

b) Absolute contraindications are pregnancy, abnormal coagulation parameters, an active urinary tract infection, and a urinary tract obstruction distal to the stone that prevents passage of stone fragments.

c) Relative contraindications include aortic aneurysm, spinal tumors, orthopedic implants in the lumbar region, morbid obesity, the presence of an abdominally placed cardiac pacemaker, uncontrolled arrhythmias, and coagulation disorders.

d) Ureteral stent placement before ESWL may be used to move the stone upward in the ureter, where it is amenable to therapy.

e) Adequate intravenous hydration aids in the passage of stone fragments.

f) Prophylactic antibiotics may be given.

3. Room preparation

a) The lithotripsy suite may be located away from the main operating room. All anesthetizing equipment must be available.

b) Plan emergency and resuscitative measures in advance (immersed anesthetized patient).

c) The gas machine and monitor connections must be long enough to extend between the patient in the tank and the anesthesia machine (immersed patient).

d) Position the electrocardiogram electrode on the trunk and cover with transparent dressings. This results in less artifact interference with R-wave triggering of shock waves.

e) To minimize treatment times, atropine may be used to increase the patient's heart rate.
f) Use waterproof dressings to cover intravenous tubes and epidural catheters (immersed patient).
g) Esophageal or precordial stethoscopes are impractical because of shock discharge noise.
h) Have vasopressors and emergency drugs available to treat hemodynamic changes.
i) Monitor the temperature of the patient and the bath. The bath should be kept at 37° C (immersed patient).

4. **Anesthetic technique**
Use local anesthesia with sedation; general or regional anesthesia is usually required.

5. **Perioperative management**
a) Monitored anesthesia care with intravenous analgesia: Usually this is the method of choice with newer-generation lithotripters. Adequate analgesia and sedation are needed to prevent patient movement during treatment.
b) General or regional anesthesia is used with older water bath lithotripters.
c) Regional anesthesia: Analgesia to T4 is required.
d) Epidural anesthesia: This produces a slower onset of sympathetic block with less hypotension; it can be used along with pre-ESWL cystoscopy and stent placement.
e) Spinal anesthesia: This can result in more profound circulatory changes during positioning.
f) General anesthesia
   (1) Intubation is mandatory.
   (2) Stones may move during ventilation of lungs. Use a low tidal volume and increase the respiratory rate.
g) Position
   (1) The patient is supported in a padded metal frame in a "lawnchair position" and is lowered into the water (immersed) or positioned in supine or in a semilateral position with ESWL.
   (2) Allow shock waves to hit the kidneys and disintegrate stones but not to reach the lungs.
h) Considerations in the immersed patient
   (1) Prevent patient movement: The patient may be paralyzed if general anesthesia is used; sedate with regional anesthesia.
   (2) Hemodynamic responses to the procedure vary. Sitting position and warm water cause vasodilation, venous pooling, and decreased cardiac output. Immersion counteracts this; hydrostatic pressure on vessels increases venous return.
   (3) Slowly remove the patient from the tub or profound hypotension may occur.
   (4) Pressure on the chest from immersion decreases vital capacity and functional reserve capacity and causes ventilation-perfusion mismatch.
   (5) Cardiac arrhythmias may occur during immersion or emergence because of rapid changes in hemodynamics and during the procedure from the discharge of shock waves independent of the cardiac cycle.

PART II **Common Procedures**

i) Emergence (immersed patient): Use maintenance anesthesia or sedation until the patient is removed from the tub.

6. **Postoperative implications**
   a) Renal hematoma, especially in patients with preexisting hypertension
   b) Cardiac dysrhythmias: Bradycardia, premature atrial contractions, and premature ventricular contractions (primarily during the procedure)
   c) Hematuria, treated with hydration and diuretics
   d) Ureteral colic, evident as nausea, vomiting, or bradycardia

D. Kidney Transplant

1. **Introduction**
   The primary indication for kidney transplantation is end-stage renal disease resulting from several causes, including chronic pyelonephritis, diabetic glomerulonephropathy, polycystic kidney disease, obstructive uropathy, lupus nephritis, hydronephrosis, hypertension, Alport's syndrome, and renal trauma. Each of these conditions can potentially lead to uremic syndrome in which the patient is unable to regulate composition and volume of body fluids. Fluid overload, acidemia, electrolyte imbalance, and secondary dysfunction in other organ systems ultimately develop. Dialysis is used to manage volume and electrolyte status before transplantation. Sources for kidneys for transplants can be either cadaveric or a living donor. Ischemic time for kidneys is at least 48 hours; therefore, optimization of recipient condition is possible. Timing of donor and recipient procedures is coordinated so ischemic time for the kidney is minimized.

DONOR CONSIDERATIONS

2. **Preoperative assessment and patient preparation**
   a) History and physical examination: Most donors are healthy adults because the presence of significant systemic disease would increase the risk of general anesthesia and of postoperative complications.
      (1) Cadaveric: The importance of rapid procurement is based on whether circulation to the kidney is intact. If circulation fails, specimens must be removed quickly to minimize ischemic time.
      (2) Living donors: These are usually close relatives because unrelated living donations do not produce improved results as compared with cadaveric donations.
   b) Diagnostic tests
      (1) Renal arteriography, used to determine whether the kidney is suitable for renal transplantation
      (2) Intravenous pyelography
      (3) Computed tomography
      (4) Noninvasive studies to detect coronary ischemia if the donor is a man older than 45 years or a woman older than 50 years
      (5) Laboratory tests
         (a) Tests include screening for ABO blood group compatibility and cytomegalovirus titer, cross-matching of the recipient's serum with donor lymphocytes, and human leukocyte antigen tissue typing
         (b) See the discussion later in this section on Nephrectomy.

c) Preoperative medications and intravenous therapy
  (1) The patient should donate several units of autologous blood 2 to 4 weeks before the procedure.
  (2) Starting the night before the procedure, donors are hydrated with crystalloid to promote active diuresis.
  (3) Epidural catheter: Perform a test dose in the preoperative area.
  (4) Administer antibiotics.
  (5) The peripheral intravenous catheter (16- to 18-gauge) is placed in a location where it will be easily accessible once patient is in lateral decubitus position; aggressive hydration is indicated because the patient should be 2 L positive before incision.

3. Room preparation
  a) Monitoring equipment: Standard and Foley catheter
  b) Pharmacologic agents: See the discussion of Nephrectomy later in this section.
  c) Position
    (1) The lateral decubitus position is used, with the kidney bar raised.
    (2) With low calcium levels, skin and nerve damage occur easily.
    (3) Inadequate support of the head may lead to Horner's syndrome postoperatively.
    (4) Evaluate the radial pulse after placement of an axillary roll.
    (5) Respiration is impaired secondary to ventilation-perfusion mismatching, decreased functional reserve capacity, decreased vital capacity, and decreased thoracic compliance.
    (6) Reassess breath sounds after movement; an endotracheal tube may migrate into the mainstem bronchus during positioning.

4. Anesthetic technique
See the discussion later in this section on Radical Prostatectomy.

5. Perioperative management
  a) Induction
    (1) Opioids can be used because only a small amount of the drug is excreted unchanged by the kidneys.
    (2) Cisatracurium and atracurium do not require a functional kidney because they are degraded by Hofmann elimination. (Atracurium is also degraded by ester hydrolysis.) Both are good choices to use for living donors who will be losing 50% of their renal function.
    (3) Vecuronium, rocuronium, or rapacuronium may be used for muscle relaxation.
    (4) Induction of anesthesia and intubation of the trachea can be safely accomplished with intravenous drugs plus a nondepolarizing muscle relaxant.
  b) Maintenance
    (1) Maintain normal end-tidal carbon dioxide levels.
    (2) Maintain urinary output at a minimum of 1 mL/min; diuresis may need to be induced by treatment with mannitol or furosemide.
    (3) A volatile anesthetic is used to control intraoperative hypertension.
    (4) The eleventh rib may be removed: Pneumothorax is a complication; therefore, nitrous oxide is best avoided.
    (5) Heparin is administered systemically before removal of the donor kidney to limit potential for intrarenal clotting. On removal, the kidney is flushed free of blood with cold crystalloid solution and is transplanted immediately.

PART II **Common Procedures**

c) Emergence
  (1) The length of the procedure, large fluid amounts, and the potential for pneumothorax and pulmonary edema make an "awake" extubation an appropriate choice.
  (2) Initiate regional blockade through the epidural catheter for postoperative analgesia before the end of the case because the large flank incision is painful.

6. **Postoperative implications**
  a) Continue to assess volume status and urine output.
  b) Obtain a chest film to rule out pneumothorax or pulmonary edema, which may occur after administration of large volumes of fluid in the flank position.

RECIPIENT CONSIDERATIONS

2. **Preoperative assessment and patient preparation**
  a) History and physical examination: Individualized based on patient's condition
  b) Diagnostic tests (based on underlying pathologic process)
    (1) Intravenous pyelography with nephrotomography: Identify a renal mass.
    (2) Ultrasonography: This differentiates simple cysts from solid tumor.
    (3) Exercise stress testing and coronary angiography: They assess for potential ischemic heart disease in diabetic patients.
    (4) Computed tomography
    (5) Laboratory tests: See the later discussion in this section on Radical Prostatectomy.
  c) Preoperative medications and intravenous therapy
    (1) Discuss the date of last hemodialysis. Dialysis of the recipient should occur within the 24-hour period before scheduled transplantation to correct fluid and electrolyte derangements.
    (2) Epidural catheter (if used): Perform a test dose in the preoperative area.
    (3) Administer antibiotics.
    (4) Use small incremental doses of benzodiazepines to facilitate anxiolysis.
    (5) Have a minimum of two peripheral intravenous catheters (16- to 18-gauge) with moderate fluid replacement. In patients with renal failure, administer hypotonic solutions: 5% dextrose in water or 5% dextrose and 0.45% saline.
      (a) Avoid normal saline: It may increase sodium levels.
      (b) Avoid plasmolyte or lactated Ringer's solution. It may increase potassium levels.
      (c) Restrict fluids and consider using microdrip tubing.
    (6) A noninvasive blood pressure cuff and arterial line are placed on the arm contralateral to the arteriovenous fistula. Transplanted kidneys may not be functional immediately; therefore, it is imperative to protect existing arteriovenous fistulas and other dialysis ports because posttransplantation dialysis may be necessary.
    (7) Steroid replacement: Full replacement doses of glucocorticoids should be considered in patients receiving long-term steroid therapy.
    (8) Aspiration prophylaxis: Patients undergoing dialysis have delayed gastric emptying.
    (9) Blood transfusion: Uremic patients will have hemoglobin levels in the 6 to 8 g/dL range. Chronic anemia leads to compensatory

changes, which promote enhanced oxygen unloading to the tissues. Therefore, transfusion is not mandatory but may aid in increasing allograft survival.

3. **Room preparation**
   a) Monitoring equipment: See the later discussion of Nephrectomy in this section.
   b) Pharmacologic agents
      (1) See the later discussion of Nephrectomy in this section.
      (2) Indigo carmine or methylene blue is administered (intravenously to assess urinary flow).
   c) Position: Supine
4. **Anesthetic technique**
   a) Regional blockade, general anesthesia, or a combination of both is used.
   b) Technique of choice: General anesthesia with endotracheal intubation is used because it allows for adequate ventilation even when surgical retraction for kidney placement impinges on diaphragmatic movement.
   c) Regional blockade: Epidural catheter placement is done preoperatively; spinal techniques are impractical because of the duration of the transplant procedure; caution in patients with coagulopathies is warranted.
   d) General anesthesia: Endotracheal intubation is performed.
   e) Regional blockade with general anesthesia: Smaller doses of each are needed.
5. **Perioperative management**
   a) Induction
      (1) See the later discussion of Nephrectomy in this section.
      (2) Succinylcholine is contraindicated if potassium is elevated.
      (3) Select a nondepolarizing muscle relaxant based on the patient's medical condition.
      (4) Rapid sequence induction and aspiration prophylaxis should be considered because patients undergoing dialysis have delayed gastric emptying.
      (5) Regardless of blood volume status, renal patients may respond to induction of anesthesia as if they are hypovolemic.
   b) Maintenance
      (1) Maintain urinary output; use medications if necessary (i.e., furosemide, mannitol).
      (2) Volatile anesthetic is used to control intraoperative hypertension.
      (3) Nitrous oxide may be omitted to avoid bowel distention, which may limit surgical exposure.
      (4) Promotion of renal perfusion after anastomoses of the kidney vessels can be achieved by maintaining high-normal blood pressures by reducing the depth of anesthesia, fluid bolus, or temporary dopamine infusion.
      (5) The preservation solution most commonly used is the Euro-Collins solution, which contains potassium 115 mEq, sodium 10 mEq, chloride 15 mEq, bicarbonate 10 mEq, dihydrogen phosphate 15 mEq, monohydrogen phosphate 85 mEq, osmolality 375 mOsm, and pH 7.25.
   c) Emergence
      (1) If hypertension occurs on emergence, administer a vasodilator.
      (2) Renal patients are considered at greater risk for aspiration, so an "awake" patient before extubation may be most appropriate.

PART II   **Common Procedures**

(3) Initiate regional blockade through the epidural catheter (if used) for postoperative analgesia before the end of the case or administer opioids incrementally.

6. **Postoperative implications**
   a) Continue to assess volume status because pulmonary edema can develop if urine output is slow to resume.
   b) For patients with renal failure, normeperidine, the major metabolite of meperidine, may accumulate and may result in prolonged depression of ventilation and seizures. Therefore, meperidine should be avoided because transplant recipients are considered to have renal failure until adequate urine output begins.

E. Nephrectomy

1. **Introduction**
   Indications for nephrectomy include calculus, hemorrhage, hydronephrosis, hypertension, neoplasms, renal donation, trauma, and vascular disease. Partial nephrectomy is performed to preserve as much renal function as possible. Surgery of the kidney is usually accomplished through a flank incision.

2. **Preoperative assessment and patient preparation**
   a) History and physical examination: Individualized for the patient's condition
   b) Diagnostic tests
      (1) Intravenous pyelography with nephrotomography: Identify a renal mass.
      (2) Ultrasonography: This differentiates simple cysts from solid tumor.
      (3) Arteriography: This determines whether the kidney is suitable for renal transplantation.
      (4) Computed tomography
      (5) Laboratory tests
         (a) Prothrombin time, partial thromboplastin time, complete blood count, electrolytes, and glucose
         (b) Glomerular filtration rate: Blood urea nitrogen, plasma creatinine, and creatinine clearance
         (c) Renal tubular function: Urine concentration ability, sodium secretion, proteinuria, hematuria urine sediment, and urine volume
   c) Preoperative medications and intravenous therapy
      (1) Identify the date of last hemodialysis
      (2) Epidural catheter: Perform a test dose in the preoperative area.
      (3) Administer antibiotics.
      (4) Use small incremental doses of benzodiazepines to facilitate anxiolysis.
      (5) Have a minimum of two peripheral intravenous tubes (16- to 18-gauge) with moderate fluid replacement.
      (6) In patients with renal failure, administer hypotonic solutions: 5% dextrose in water or 5% dextrose and 0.45% saline.
         (a) Avoid normal saline: It may increase sodium levels.
         (b) Avoid plasmolyte or lactated Ringer's solution: It may increase potassium levels.
         (c) Restrict fluids and consider using microdrip tubing.

3. **Room preparation**
   a) Monitoring equipment

    (1) Standard equipment is used.
    (2) An arterial line and central venous pressure monitoring may be
        necessary to trend volume status, especially if the patient is elderly
        with coexisting medical disease.
    (3) A noninvasive blood pressure cuff should not be placed in an arm
        with an arteriovenous fistula.
  b) Pharmacologic agents
    (1) Dopamine: Low dose (2 to 5 mcg/kg/min) to increase urinary output
    (2) Furosemide (Lasix) and/or mannitol for stimulation of urinary
        output
    (3) Indigo carmine (hypertension resulting from an α-agonist) or
        methylene blue (hypotension and interference with the pulse
        oximeter) administration (intravenously to assess urinary flow)
    (4) Hetastarch (Hespan)/albumin
    (5) Heparin and protamine with donor kidneys
  c) Position
    (1) A lateral decubitus position is used, with the kidney bar raised.
    (2) With low calcium levels, skin and nerve damage occur easily.
    (3) Inadequate support of the head may lead to Horner's
        syndrome (ptosis, enophthalamos, miosis, and anhidrosis)
        postoperatively.
    (4) Evaluate the radial pulse after placement of an axillary roll.
    (5) Respiration is impaired secondary to ventilation-perfusion mis-
        matching, decreased functional reserve capacity, decreased vital
        capacity, and decreased thoracic compliance.
    (6) Reassess breath sounds after movement; an endotracheal tube
        may migrate into the mainstem bronchus during positioning.
4. **Anesthetic technique**
  a) See the discussion of radical prostatectomy later in this section.
  b) Consider rapid sequence induction because renal patients may be
     considered to have a full stomach.
5. **Perioperative management**
  a) Induction
    (1) Opioids can be used because only a small amount of the drug is
        excreted unchanged by the kidneys.
    (2) Succinylcholine is contraindicated if potassium is elevated.
    (3) Cisatracurium does not require a functional kidney because it is
        degraded by Hofmann elimination and is a good choice for mus-
        cle relaxation. Laudanosine is a metabolite and is associated with
        seizures. This is not a concern with short-term perioperative use.
    (4) Mivacurium metabolism is dependent on pseudocholinesterase
        independent of renal and liver function.
    (5) Vecuronium and rocuronium may be used for muscle relaxation.
    (6) Regardless of blood volume status, renal patients may respond to
        induction of anesthesia as if they are hypovolemic.
    (7) Induction of anesthesia and intubation of the trachea can be safely
        accomplished with intravenous drugs plus a nondepolarizing
        muscle relaxant.
    (8) Thiopental (Pentothal) and propofol are both highly protein-
        bound drugs, and this may necessitate a reduced dosage. Propofol
        is exclusively metabolized by the liver and metabolites are inactive.
        Thiopental has a small amount of renal excretion, and its pento-
        barbitone is active.

PART II **Common Procedures**

(9) Ketamine is less protein bound with less than 3% renal excretion.

(10) Etomidate is 75% protein bound and does not require adjustment.

b) Maintenance

    (1) Maintain normal end-tidal carbon dioxide levels.

    (2) If working on a donor nephrectomy, the eleventh rib may be removed; pneumothorax is a complication; therefore, nitrous oxide is best avoided.

    (3) Maintain urinary output; use medications if necessary.

    (4) Volatile anesthetic is used to control intraoperative hypertension.

c) Emergence

    (1) If hypertension occurs on emergence, administer a vasodilator.

    (2) Renal patients are considered to have a full stomach; some practitioners require an "awake" patient before extubation

    (3) Initiate regional blockade through the epidural catheter for postoperative analgesia before the end of the case.

6. **Postoperative implications**

a) Continue to assess volume status.

b) Obtain a chest film. Rule out pulmonary edema or pneumothorax, which may occur after administration of large volumes of fluid in the flank position or from removal of the eleventh rib, respectively.

c) For patients with renal failure, normeperidine, the major metabolite of meperidine, may accumulate and result in prolonged depression of ventilation and seizures.

F. Penile Procedures

1. **Introduction**

Penile procedures are usually performed for three different indications: (1) for the congenital defect hypospadias, which is usually a pediatric procedure; (2) for penectomy or penile resection as a result of penile cancer; and (3) for implants to compensate for impotence. Organic impotence is often secondary to diabetes, hypertension and its treatment, or spinal cord trauma.

2. **Preoperative assessment**

Assessment is individualized, based on the patient's condition.

3. **Patient preparation**

a) Standard preoperative laboratory testing is as indicated.

b) Preoperative medications are individualized.

4. **Room preparation**

a) Monitoring: Standard

b) Position: Supine

c) Drugs and tabletop: Adult/pediatric setup

5. **Anesthesia and perioperative management**

a) For pediatric patients, use an inhaled induction for general anesthetic. Intubation is desired because hypospadias repair generally takes longer than 2 hours.

b) For penectomy or prosthetic insertion, a regional or general anesthetic may be used, depending on the preferences of the patient and the anesthetist and on the medical condition. Muscle relaxation is not required, and blood loss is minimal.

c) Some practitioners will perform a caudal block for pediatric patients just before awakening for postoperative pain control.

6. **Postoperative implications**
Urinary retention is common and may be intensified with the use of a regional anesthetic.

G. Radical Prostatectomy

1. **Introduction**
Open prostatectomy refers to removal of the prostate with or without the prostatic capsule. Several surgical approaches may be used, including suprapubic, transvesical, retropubic, perineal, and transcoccygeal. In suprapubic or transvesical procedures, the prostate is removed through the cavity of the bladder. Retropubic prostatectomy is performed through a low abdominal incision without opening the bladder. The transcoccygeal approach allows maximal surgical access to the posterior lobes of the prostate. Perineal prostatectomy is most often performed for cancer of the prostate when it is confined to the capsule. This procedure may also be done with the assistance of a robot.

2. **Preoperative assessment and patient preparation**
   a) History and physical examination: These are individualized based on the patient's condition; assess for symptoms of metastatic disease.
   b) Diagnostic tests
      (1) Plasma concentration of prostate-specific antigen is increased in prostate cancer.
      (2) Blood urea nitrogen, creatinine, electrolytes, complete blood count, coagulation profile, and type and cross-match are obtained.
      (3) Ultrasonography is used.
   c) Preoperative medication and intravenous therapy
      (1) Bowel preparation will render the patient in a dehydrated state.
      (2) Have a minimum of two peripheral intravenous lines (18- and 16-gauge) with moderate fluid replacement.
      (3) Epidural catheter: Perform a test dose in the preoperative area.
      (4) Administer antibiotics.
      (5) Small incremental doses of benzodiazepines may be given to ease patient preparation.

3. **Room preparation**
   a) Monitoring equipment
      (1) Equipment is standard.
      (2) Arterial line and central venous pressure monitoring may be necessary to trend volume status, especially if the patient is elderly, with coexisting medical diseases. Central venous pressure monitoring may also be indicated for potential of venous air embolism related to positioning of the patient.
      (3) Warming modalities are used.
   b) Pharmacologic agents
      (1) Dopamine, possibly a low dose (2 to 5 mcg/kg/min) to increase urinary output
      (2) Hetastarch (Hespan) and albumin
   c) Position: Supine; the surgeon may request use of kidney rest and for the patient's body to be partially flexed. Expect to need to rotate the patient from side to side for optimal surgical viewing.

4. **Anesthetic technique**
   a) Regional blockade, general anesthesia, or a combination of both

b) Technique of choice: General anesthesia with endotracheal intubation

c) Regional blockade: Epidural catheter placement in preoperative area; analgesia to T6 to T8

d) General anesthesia: Endotracheal intubation

e) Regional blockade with general anesthesia: Smaller doses of each with the combination technique

5. **Perioperative management**
   a) Induction: The patient may be dehydrated and show an exaggerated response to medications.
   b) Maintenance
      (1) Initiate warming modality and use fluid warmers.
      (2) Position
         (a) Radical retropubic: Supine with the operating room table broken in the midline or kidney rest to provide slight hyperextension; a slight Trendelenburg position until the patient's legs are parallel to the floor
         (b) Radical perianal: Exaggerated lithotomy position combined with flexion of the trunk and a Trendelenburg tilt
      (3) The Foley catheter is discontinued during the case, and volume status (blood loss) is difficult to quantify.
      (4) Muscle relaxation is necessary.
   c) Emergence
      (1) Initiate regional blockade through the epidural catheter for postoperative analgesia before the end of the case.
      (2) Base extubation on the patient's general health, amount of blood loss, and overall status after the procedure.
      (3) An awake or deep extubation may be appropriate.

6. **Postoperative implications**
   a) Obtain hemoglobin and hematocrit.
   b) Continue to trend volume status.
   c) For postoperative pain management, consider patient-controlled analgesia, epidural techniques, or a combination of ketorolac and opiates.
   d) Early postoperative complications include deep venous thrombosis, pulmonary embolus, and wound infection.
   e) Late complications include incontinence, impotence, and bladder neck contracture.
   f) Rhabdomyolysis is seen with the extreme lithotomy position and may progress to acute renal failure. Monitor urine output and maintain at more than 0.5 mL/kg/hour.

H. Scrotal Procedures

1. **Introduction**

   Scrotal procedures are considered minor operative procedures and can be performed on an outpatient basis unless there are preexisting medical conditions. In adults, most elective scrotal procedures can be performed under local anesthesia with sedation. The most common procedures include surgery for infertility, hydrocele, undescended testicle, or orchiectomy for cancer.

   The most common emergency scrotal operation is for testicular torsion. These patients will be in acute pain and should be considered to have a full stomach.

2. **Preoperative assessment**
   a) Most patients who present for infertility concerns, hydrocele, and minor procedures are essentially healthy.
   b) Those who present for orchiectomy require careful preoperative evaluation for possible metastasis.
   c) No specific laboratory tests or medications are required except those that are suggested from the preoperative evaluation.
3. **Room preparation**
   a) Monitoring: This is standard.
   b) Position: Supine. The patient's arms usually are out at the sides. The lithotomy position may be requested.
   c) Drugs and tabletop: Sedatives and narcotics. The tabletop should be set up for emergency general anesthesia.
4. **Anesthesia and perioperative management**
   a) The patient may receive local anesthesia with sedation, regional anesthesia, or general anesthesia, depending on condition and the anesthetist's preference.
   b) There are no specific considerations because muscle relaxation is not required, and blood loss is minimal.
5. **Postoperative considerations**
   Pain management may be commenced intraoperatively by the use of narcotics, ketorolac, or both. Some patients, especially if being treated for malignancy, may experience nausea and vomiting.

I. Transurethral Resection of the Prostate

1. **Introduction**
   Transurethral resection of the prostate is the treatment of choice for benign prostate. Resection consists of applying a high-frequency current to a wire loop with fragments of the obstructive tissue removed under direct endoscopic vision. The prostate gland contains a rich plexus of veins (dorsal venous plexus) that can be opened during the surgical procedure. Hemostasis is effected by sealing vessels with the coagulating current. Continuous irrigation with fluids is required to improve visibility through the cystoscope, to distend the prostatic urethra, and to maintain the operative field free of blood and dissected tissue (see table on p. 256).
2. **Preoperative assessment and patient preparation**
   a) History and physical examination: This is an elderly patient population. Assess for coexisting cardiac, pulmonary, and renal diseases. These patients have a 30% to 60% prevalence of both cardiovascular and pulmonary disorders.
   b) Diagnostic tests
      (1) Complete blood count, blood urea nitrogen, creatinine, electrolytes, coagulation profile, and type and screen are obtained.
      (2) Postpone the procedure if serum sodium is 128 mEq/L or less.
   c) Preoperative medication and intravenous therapy
      (1) Use an 18-gauge intravenous catheter with minimal fluid replacement.
      (2) Administer antibiotics.
3. **Room preparation**
   a) Monitoring equipment: Standard
   b) Pharmacologic agents: Standard

Solution	Osmolality (mOsm)	Advantage	Disadvantage
Distilled water	0	Improved visibility	Hemolysis Hemoglobinemia Hemoglobinuria Hyponatremia
Glycine (1.5%)*	200	Decreased chance of transurethral resection syndrome	Transient postoperative visual impairment Hyperammonemia Hyperoxaluria
Sorbitol (3.5%)*	165	Decreased chance of transurethral resection syndrome	Hyperglycemia, possible lactic acidosis Osmotic diuresis
Mannitol (5%)*	275	Isosmolar solution Not metabolized	Osmotic diuresis, possibility of acute intravascular expansion

*Solutes such as sorbitol, mannitol, glycine, and glucose may be added to water to make osmolality similar to that of plasma.

    c) Position: Lithotomy
    d) Warming modalities
4. Anesthetic technique
    a) Regional blockade or general anesthesia: For regional blockade, analgesia to T10 is required. One may consider adding opioids for postoperative analgesia. An awake patient can provide early warning of complications (restlessness, hypervolemia, hyponatremia).
    b) Technique of choice: Spinal anesthesia enables one to assess the manifestations of transurethral resection of the prostate syndrome, which may be masked under general anesthesia (see table on p. 257).
5. Perioperative management
    a) Induction: No specific indications
    b) Maintenance
       (1) Blood loss: This is difficult to assess because the irrigating fluid dilutes the blood. The average loss is about 4 mL/min of resection time.
       (2) Intravascular absorption of irrigating fluid: The open venous sinuses of the prostate bed cause absorption of irrigating fluid. The primary determinants of fluid absorption are as follows:
          (a) Height of irrigation container, recommended no higher than 30 cm above the table at the beginning and 15 cm during the final stages
          (b) Number and size of venous sinuses opened
          (c) Duration of resection
          (d) Venous pressure at the irrigant-blood interface
          (e) Hydrostatic pressure of irrigation solution (see table above)
       (3) Limit resection time to less than 1 hour (10 to 30 mL of fluid is absorbed per minute of resection time), and monitor resection time closely.
       (4) Absorption of large volumes of irrigating fluids results in increased intravascular volume and dilutional hyponatremia with

Symptoms of Transurethral Resection of the Prostate Syndrome

Serum Sodium (mEq/L)	Electrocardiographic Changes	Central Nervous System Changes
120	Possible widening of QRS	Restless, confusion
115	Widened QRS, elevated ST segment	Nausea, somnolence
110	Ventricular tachycardia, ventricular fibrillation	Seizures, coma

early symptoms of hypertension and reflex tachycardia. Symptoms in an awake patient include restlessness, nausea and vomiting, mental confusion, and visual disturbances.

(5) Hypothermia resulting from large volumes of irrigating fluids at room temperature leads to postoperative shivering with dislodging of clots and promotes bleeding. Prevention includes warming irrigation fluids to body temperature and using a convection blanket (see table above).

6. **Treatment of intraoperative complications**
   a) Dilutional hyponatremia
      (1) Terminate or complete the surgical procedure.
      (2) Send blood for serum sodium determination; if the sodium level is more than 120 mEq/L, administer furosemide and limit fluids.
      (3) If the sodium levels is less than 120 mEq/L, administer 3% sodium chloride at a rate of less than 100 mL/hour. Increase the sodium level no more than 12 mEq/L in a 24-hour period. Discontinue the infusion when it is higher than 120 mEq/L.
   b) Bladder perforation
      (1) Suspect perforation of the prostatic capsule if irrigation fluid fails to return.
      (2) Initial symptoms include hypertension and tachycardia, followed by hypotension and bradycardia.
      (3) An awake patient will experience suprapubic fullness and pain in the upper abdomen or referred from the diaphragm to the precordial region or shoulders.
      (4) Prepare for a possible open surgical procedure.
   c) Glycine toxicity: A metabolite of glycine is ammonia. Glycine absorption can produce central nervous system symptoms such as mild depression, confusion, and transient blindness to coma.
7. **Emergence**
   No specific indications exist.
8. **Postoperative considerations**
   a) Hyponatremia may not be suspected until the postoperative period.
   b) Disseminated intravascular coagulation: Prostate cancer cells may release thromboplastin, which can initiate a state of hypercoagulabilty, followed by a state of fibrinolysis. Treatment includes aminocaproic acid (Amicar), 4 to 5 g over the first hour, followed by an infusion of 1 g/hour for 8 hours or until bleeding is controlled. For other treatment options, see the discussion of disseminated intravascular coagulation in Section V of Part 1 for other treatment options.

HEAD AND NECK

A. Dacryocystorhinostomy

1. Introduction

Dacryocystorhinostomy is performed for patients who have chronic tearing or obstruction at the level of the nasolacrimal duct. This procedure restores drainage into the nose from the lacrimal sac. The surgeon injects lidocaine 1% with 1:100,000 epinephrine, bupivacaine (Marcaine) 0.75%, and hyaluronidase (Wydase) in the operative site along the lacrimal crest. An additional injection may be given along the medial orbital wall, anesthetizing the ethmoidal nerve. This will help to anesthetize the nasal mucosa by blocking the ethmoidal nerve. This block may cause a temporary dilated pupil or medial rectus muscle paralysis.

A small incision is made near the medial canthus to allow a subperiosteal dissection to the lacrimal sac. The bone between the lacrimal fossa and middle fossa is broken and cut, making a small canaliculi. The mucosa of the lacrimal sac is anastomosed to the mucosa of the nose. To prevent closure of the newly formed path by scarring, a silicone tube may be placed inside the duct. Muscles and tissues in the area are then closed. The patient is then asked to open the eyelids, and when the proper height is obtained, the incision is closed.

2. Preoperative assessment and patient preparation

a) History and physical examination: This procedure may be done in patients of varying age. The patient's cardiac history should be determined, because epinephrine is to be used for vasoconstriction. Infections in the surgical area should be treated with antibiotics for several days before surgery. Because of the inaccessibility of the anesthesia provider to the head, patients with obstructive sleep apnea should also be identified and anesthesia planned accordingly.

b) Patient preparation
(1) Laboratory tests: As indicated by the history and physical examination
(2) Diagnostic tests: Electrocardiography as indicated by the history and physical examination
(3) Premedication: Standard

3. Room preparation

a) Monitoring equipment is standard.
b) Additional equipment: An end-tidal carbon dioxide sensing nasal cannula may be used to give additional information about ventilation.

c) An extra long circuit should be available because of turning of the table 90 to 180 degrees.

d) Drugs: Standard emergency and standard tabletop agents are used.

e) Intravenous fluids: An age-appropriate intravenous line and fluid are used for pediatric patients. One 18-gauge intravenous line is used for adults with normal saline/lactated Ringer's at 2 mL/kg/hour (blood loss should be minimal because of the use of epinephrine).

4. **Perioperative management and anesthetic technique**
   Most of these procedures can be done with local anesthesia with sedation; very rarely is general anesthesia used. The choice depends on the preferences of the surgeon and the patient.
   a) Induction is routine for general surgery.
   b) For local anesthesia with sedation, short-acting agents are best because these procedures are usually done on an outpatient basis.
   c) Maintenance is routine.
   d) Emergence: For general anesthesia, the patient should be extubated while awake, unless the condition dictates otherwise (i.e., reactive airway disease).

5. **Postoperative implications**
   As stated earlier, there may be some temporary dilation of the pupil or medial rectus paralysis.

B. Laryngectomy

1. **Introduction**
   Most cancers of the upper respiratory tract are squamous cell carcinomas. When the laryngeal musculature or cartilage is invaded, total laryngectomy is performed. Intractable aspiration, with resultant pneumonia that has been unresponsive to other treatments, is another indication for laryngectomy.

   Total laryngectomy involves removal of the vallecula and includes the posterior third of the tongue if necessary. Surgical exposure is from the hyoid bone to the clavicle. A tracheostomy is performed, and an anode tube is placed. The larynx is usually transected just above the hyoid bone. The trachea is brought out to the skin as a tracheostomy without the need for an endotracheal tube or tracheostomy tube as the pharynx is closed.

   Supraglottic laryngectomy leaves the true vocal cords by resection of the larynx from the ventricle to the base of the tongue. Surgical exposure is similar to that for total laryngectomy. The specimen includes the epiglottis, the false vocal cords, the supraglottic lesions, and a portion of the base of the tongue. The thyroid perichondrium is approximated to the base of the tongue along with the strap muscles for closure. A temporary tracheostomy is required.

   Hemilaryngectomy or vertical partial laryngectomy retains the epiglottis but involves removal of a unilateral true and false vocal cord. Surgical exposure is similar to that of supraglottic laryngectomy, and a tracheostomy is required.

   Near-total laryngectomy involves removal of the entire larynx. One arytenoid is used to construct a phonatory shunt for speaking. A permanent or temporary tracheostomy is created, and the procedure may be combined with neck dissection and pharyngectomy with flap reconstruction.

2. **Preoperative assessment**

Most patients are older and have a long history of tobacco and alcohol abuse. Associated medical problems may include chronic obstructive pulmonary disease, hypertension, coronary artery disease, and alcohol withdrawal.

a) History and physical examination: Individualized

(1) Respiratory: Smoking (more than 40 packs/year) is associated with bronchitis, pulmonary emphysema, and chronic obstructive pulmonary disease, which impair respiratory function. Arterial blood gases may reveal carbon dioxide retention and hypoxemia. Pulmonary function tests demonstrate decreased forced expiratory volume, forced vital capacity, and the ratio of forced expiratory volume to forced vital capacity. Preoperative airway assessment is imperative because edema may distort airway anatomy, and tumor and edema may cause airway compromise. Tracheal deviation must be considered. Fibrosis, edema, and scarring from prior radiation therapy may distort the airway as well.

(2) Assess for signs of alcohol withdrawal (altered mental status, tremulousness, and increased sympathetic activity).

(3) Gastrointestinal: Weight loss, malnutrition, dehydration, and electrolyte imbalance can be significant.

(4) Hematologic: Anemias or coagulopathies may be present.

b) Patient preparation

(1) Laboratory tests: Baseline arterial blood gases, electrolytes, hemoglobin, hematocrit, prothrombin time, partial thromboplastin time, and, if indicated from the history and physical examination, hepatic function tests are obtained.

(2) Diagnostic tests: Chest radiography, electrocardiography, pulmonary function testing, echocardiography, and stress tests are as indicated from the history and physical examination. Indirect and direct laryngoscopies preoperatively and review of computed tomography may help in planning intubation.

(3) Medications: Treatment with a long-acting hypnotic, such as chlordiazepoxide or diazepam, as a precaution for delirium tremens can be considered, unless sedation would be contraindicated because of concerns of airway compromise. An intravenous antisialagogue (glycopyrrolate, 0.2 mg) facilitates endoscopy by the surgeon.

3. **Room preparation**

a) Monitoring equipment

(1) Standard monitoring equipment

(2) Foley catheter

(3) Arterial line: Useful for serial laboratory and arterial blood gas studies

(4) Central venous pressure catheter: If indicated by coexisting disease (prefer basilic/cephalic vein)

b) Additional equipment

(1) Regular operating table: May be turned 180 degrees

(2) Extension tubes

(3) Fluid warmer and humidifier

(4) Fiberoptic laryngoscope with anticipated difficult airway or potential for airway obstruction

(5) Tracheostomy under local anesthesia occasionally necessary for severe airway management.

c) Drugs
   (1) Standard emergency drugs
   (2) Standard tabletop
   (3) Intravenous fluids
   (4) Two 16- to 18-gauge or larger intravenous lines with normal saline/lactated Ringer's solution at 3 to 5 mL/kg/hour
   (5) No sudden large blood losses; transfusion usually not necessary
4. **Perioperative management and anesthetic technique**
   General endotracheal anesthesia is used.
   a) Induction: Standard intravenous induction is appropriate with a normal airway. The choice of an induction drug should be based on the patient's medical condition. If airway difficulty is possible, direct laryngoscopy can be performed while the patient is breathing spontaneously, and a muscle relaxant may be administered once the glottis is visualized. In more difficult cases, awake intubation or fiberoptic laryngoscopy may be required.
   b) Maintenance: The patient is in the supine position, with the head elevated 30 degrees; standard maintenance is used, considering the patient's preexisting medical problems. An inhalation agent and supplemental narcotics will benefit patients with reactive airway disease. Use of nondepolarizing muscle relaxants should be discussed with the surgeon because nerve stimulation for facial nerve localization may be performed.
   c) Emergence: Many patients undergo tracheostomy. If no tracheostomy is performed, the amount of airway edema and distortion needs to be discussed with the surgeon before determining extubation. Gradual emergence with stable hemodynamic parameters is an important consideration in the patient with coronary artery disease.
5. **Postoperative implications**
   a) Injury to the facial nerve can cause facial droop. Recurrent laryngeal nerve injury can result in vocal cord dysfunction; diaphragmatic paralysis may result from phrenic nerve injury.
   b) Pneumothorax may occur with low neck dissection.
   c) Airway impingement results from restrictive neck dressings or hematoma development.
   d) Communication difficulties occur following laryngectomy.

C. LeFort Procedures

1. **Introduction**
   a) The usual preoperative diagnosis for patients with maxillary fractures is facial trauma. LeFort fractures are frequently associated with other skull fractures, zygoma fractures, and possible intracranial fractures and thus with cerebrospinal fluid rhinorrhea.
   b) Maxillary fractures are grouped by the LeFort system.
      (1) Type 1: Horizontal fracture separating the teeth and maxillary components from the upper facial structures
      (2) Type 2 (pyramidal): Triangular fracture across the ethmoid and the nose through the intraorbital rims and extending to the entire maxillary structure
      (3) Type 3 (craniofacial dysfunction): Essentially, a fracture in which the cranium and face are dissociate; common coexisting injuries

include cerebral contusions, intracranial hemorrhage, and cervical spine trauma

2. **Preoperative assessment and patient preparation**

The airway is a priority. If the airway cannot be managed, emergency intubation becomes necessary. Avoid blind nasal intubation in patients with cerebrospinal fluid rhinorrhea, periorbital edema, "raccoon's eyes" bruising, or other evidence of nasopharyngeal trauma.

   a) Neurologic: Document any neurologic deficit; intracranial trauma may require invasive monitoring.

   b) Laboratory tests: Hematocrit and any other tests are as indicated by the history and physical examination.

3. **Room preparation**

   a) Monitoring equipment: Standard

   b) Additional equipment: Fiberoptic cart

   c) Drugs

      (1) Standard emergency

      (2) Standard tabletop

   d) Intravenous fluids: one 18-gauge line with normal saline/lactated Ringer's solution at 6 to 8 mL/kg/hour

4. **Perioperative management and anesthetic technique**

General endotracheal anesthesia is used.

   a) Induction: Fiberoptic laryngoscopy should be performed if there is any doubt about the ease of intubation. Patients with mandibular and maxillary (LeFort I and II) fractures should undergo intubation. Patients with nasal, orbital, or zygomatic fractures usually are intubated orally. Consider using anode or right-angled endotracheal tubes. A LeFort type II or III fracture is a relative contraindication for nasal intubation or nasogastric tube placement.

   b) Maintenance

      (1) Muscle relaxation is usually required. Consider the prophylactic use of antiemetics for patients with wired jaws.

      (2) Position: The patient is supine; check and pad pressure points. Avoid stretching the brachial plexus, and limit abduction to 90 degrees. Protect the patient's eyes with ophthalmic ointment.

   c) Emergence: Extubation should be performed when the patient is fully awake in the case of difficult airway or wired jaws. A wire cutter should be available at all times. Verify that throat packing has been removed before extubating. Patients with facial or airway swelling and those involved in multiple trauma may need continued postoperative intubation and ventilation.

5. **Postoperative implications**

   a) For airway obstruction, wire cutters must be available.

   b) Aggressive treatment of nausea and vomiting is important.

   c) Pain management includes narcotics, as well as antiemetics as needed.

   d) Cerebrospinal fluid leak may occur.

D. Maxillofacial Trauma

1. **Introduction**

Two common causes of maxillofacial fractures are fights and gunshot wounds. Because of the forces required to cause facial fractures, other traumas (e.g., subdural hematoma, pneumothorax, cervical spine injury, and intraabdominal bleeding) often occur with these fractures. These patients are at increased risk for aspiration and should be considered as having full stomachs. Therefore, securing of the airway is of utmost importance. Rapid sequence intubation should be done on these patients, provided the nature of their injuries will allow for this. Airway management can be difficult because of soft tissue injury to the tongue or airway. A tracheostomy under local or awake intubation should be strongly considered if any doubt exists about securing the airway. Nasal intubation is usually indicated for mandibular or maxillary fractures, because at the end of the procedure intermaxillary fixation is performed. The surgeon may require monitoring of the facial nerve; if so, muscle relaxants are contraindicated. The surgical approach depends on the type and complexity of the fracture. The approach can vary from reduction for nasal fractures to the Caldwell Luc approach for extensive maxillary bone fractures. Intermaxillary fixation may be required for zygomatic and maxillary fractures. Mandibular fractures are usually reduced and fixed with wires or plates.

2. **Preoperative assessment**
   a) Respiratory/airway management: The extent of fractures is evaluated to determine appropriate airway management. Fractures of the middle face are not usually nasally intubated. Access to the oropharynx may be difficult with mandibular fractures. An urgent tracheostomy is indicated for massive facial trauma.
   b) Neurologic: Thorough documentation of any neurologic deficits and review of computed tomography (CT) scan are needed if head injury is suspected. Meningitis is possible postoperatively.
   c) Musculoskeletal: Careful positioning is imperative, with special consideration for other trauma-related injuries. Cervical spine and CT scans should be reviewed to rule out cervical fracture if suspected.
   d) Laboratory tests: Hematocrit and others are as indicated from the history and physical examination.
   e) Standard premedication is used as for neurologically intact patients.

3. **Room preparation**
   a) Monitoring equipment: Standard; invasive monitoring may be needed for intracranial or other trauma.
   b) Additional equipment: Regular operating table; some surgeons like the table turned 90 or 180 degrees or to have extension tubings available for the circuit.
   c) Drugs
      (1) Standard emergency drugs
      (2) Standard tabletop
      (3) Intravenous fluids: One 16- to 18-gauge intravenous tube (the patient may have significant blood loss with maxillary repairs) is used; normal saline/lactated Ringer's solution is given at 6 to 8 mL/kg/hour for trauma-related injuries or 2 to 4 mL/kg/hour if surgery is elective. If the fracture is trauma related and intracranial injury is suspected, solutions containing dextrose should be avoided, because they can increase cerebral edema.

4. **Perioperative management and anesthetic technique**
   General endotracheal anesthesia is used.
   a) Induction: Awake fiberoptic laryngoscopy should be performed if any doubt exists concerning the ease of intubation. For patients with LeFort (mandibular or maxillary) fractures, nasal intubation is

preferred. Patients with nasal, orbital, or zygomatic fractures are usually orally intubated. Standard induction is appropriate for patients having elective surgery who have normal airways and whose NPO (nothing by mouth) status can be determined. Trauma patients should be considered to have full stomachs, and induction should be performed using a rapid sequence technique. Nasal or oral right-angled endotracheal tubes are used to optimize the surgical field. If these patients arrive at the operating room already intubated, proper endotracheal tube placement should be confirmed.

b) Maintenance: Muscle relaxation is usually required. An antiemetic is helpful for patients who will have their jaws banded or wired together.
  (1) Standard maintenance is used.
  (2) Position: Supine; check and pad all pressure points; abduct the patient's arms less than 90 degrees to avoid overstretching of brachial plexus.

c) Emergence: Suction oropharynx carefully to avoid aspiration. Verify that any packs are removed before emergence. Patients with difficult airways or wired jaws should be fully awake and have protective reflexes before extubation. Wire cutters should be at the bedside at all times. Depending on the amount of trauma and soft tissue swelling, the patient may require extended intubation and ventilation postoperatively.

5. **Postoperative implications**
  a) Because of the possibility of airway obstruction, wire cutters should be available at all times for airway management. A throat pack may be obstructing the airway.
  b) Aggressive treatment of nausea and vomiting is imperative.
  c) Pain management includes intravenous narcotics and antiemetics as needed.

E. Nasal Surgery

1. **Introduction**
Nasal surgery is performed for cosmetic reasons, to restore the caliber of the nasal airway, or sometimes for both reasons. Whether for rhinoplasty, septoplasty, or septorhinoplasty, the nasal cavity can be anesthetized by placing 4% cocaine–soaked pledgets up each nostril for 5 to 10 minutes. To ensure vasoconstriction and minimize bleeding, the site is infiltrated with 1% lidocaine and 1:100,000 epinephrine.

An incision is made in the septum down to the cartilage, and a submucoperichondrial flap is elevated. This may be repeated on the contralateral side. Bone and cartilaginous deformities are resected or weakened either on the face, or they are removed first, shaped, and then replaced. Once the surgeon is satisfied with the resection, the incision is closed with an absorbable suture. In rhinoplasty, depending on the area needing work, the nasal contours can be remodeled by tip remodeling, humps can be reduced; bone osteotomies can be performed to shape the contour of the nose, or combinations thereof. After surgery, both nasal cavities are packed, and external splints may be used.

2. **Preoperative assessment and patient preparation**
Generally, these procedures are elective and can be performed on an outpatient basis. It is important to identify patients with obstructive apnea.

These patients often have chronic airway obstruction, redundant pharyngeal tissues, or both. Such patients, as well as asthmatic patients, should undergo arterial blood gas and pulmonary function testing. Ketorolac and acetylsalicylic acid should be avoided in patients who also have nasal polyps, because they often are hypersensitive to acetylsalicylic acid, a condition that can precipitate bronchospasm.

  a) History and physical examination: Carefully evaluate cardiovascular status because the use of local vasoconstrictors may cause dysrhythmia, coronary artery spasm, hypertension, and seizures.
  b) Patient preparation
    (1) Laboratory tests: As indicated by the history and physical examination
    (2) Diagnostic tests: As indicated by the history and physical examination
    (3) Standard premedication
3. **Room preparation**
  a) Monitoring equipment: Standard
  b) Additional equipment: Regular operating table, turned 90 to 180 degrees; anesthesia circuit extension available
  c) Drugs
    (1) Standard emergency
    (2) Standard tabletop
  d) Intravenous fluids: Two 18-gauge lines with normal saline/lactated Ringer's solution at 4 to 6 mL/kg/hour
4. **Perioperative management and anesthetic technique**
  Use general endotracheal or local anesthesia with sedation; the choice depends on the preferences of the surgeon and the patient, as well as on the acetylsalicylic acid status of the patient.
  a) Induction: Routine. Use of an oral right-angled endotracheal tube is convenient for the surgeon but is not necessary. If a sedation technique is chosen, short-acting agents are best because these procedures are usually minor, and patients are usually sent home.
  b) Maintenance is routine.
  c) Emergence: Counsel patients that the nose will be packed with bandaging and possibly splinted, so mouth breathing will be necessary on awakening.
5. **Postoperative implications**
  a) Elevate the head of the bed.
  b) Nasal packing and swallowed blood may contribute to postoperative nausea and vomiting.
  c) Mild analgesics after discharge are usually sufficient.

F. Ocular Procedures

OPEN EYE

1. **Introduction**
  Intraocular pressure (IOP) is determined by the balance between production and drainage of aqueous humor and by changes in choroidal blood volume. Resistance to outflow of aqueous humor in the trabecular tissue maintains IOP within physiologic range. Normal IOP is 12 to 16 mm Hg in the upright posture and increases by 2 to 3 mm Hg in the supine position.
  When the globe is open, the IOP is equal to ambient pressure. If the volume of choroid and vitreous should increase while the eye is opened,

the vitreous may be lost. Any deformation of the eye by external pressure on the globe will cause an apparent increase in intraocular volume. This discussion is of open eye procedures.

2. **Preoperative assessment and patient preparation**
   a) History and physical examination: Standard; the patient may come in as an emergency with a full stomach; ensure that the patient has no other injuries.
   b) Diagnostic and laboratory tests: These are as indicated by the history and physical examination.
   c) Preoperative medication and intravenous therapy
      (1) Aspiration prophylaxis is used.
      (2) Atropine or glycopyrrolate reduces oral secretions and may inhibit the oculocardiac reflex.
      (3) Avoid narcotic, which may cause nausea and vomiting.
      (4) Sedatives are given in the preoperative hold area and are titrated to effect.
      (5) One 18-gauge intravenous tube with minimal fluid replacement is used.

3. **Room preparation**
   a) Monitoring equipment: Standard
   b) Pharmacologic agents: Standard, lidocaine and atropine
   c) Position: Supine; table may be turned for the surgeon's access

4. **Anesthetic technique and perioperative management**
   General anesthesia with endotracheal intubation because a retrobulbar block causes a transient rise in IOP, which may cause intraocular contents to be expelled.
   a) Induction (general)
      (1) The goal is to avoid increasing IOP.
      (2) When preoxygenating, avoid pressing face mask onto the eyeball.
      (3) Awake intubation is contraindicated because it may cause coughing and bucking.
      (4) Intravenous lidocaine, 1 mg/kg, may eliminate coughing and bucking.
      (5) The use of succinylcholine in open eye globe injuries is controversial. Many practitioners believe that when succinylcholine has been preceded by pretreatment with a nondepolarizing muscle relaxant and a barbiturate for induction, it is a safe combination for rapid sequence induction in the open eye in a patient with a full stomach.
      (6) Induction may be with thiopental plus a large dose of a nondepolarizing muscle relaxant.
      (7) Use of ketamine is contraindicated; it causes a moderate increase in IOP and nystagmus or blepharospasm.
   b) Maintenance
      (1) Inhalation agents cause dose-related decreases in IOP; the degree of IOP reduction is proportional to the depth of anesthesia.
      (2) Oculocardiac reflex
         (a) This is caused by traction on the extraocular muscles (medial rectus), ocular manipulation, or manual pressure on the globe.
         (b) Signs and symptoms are bradycardia and cardiac dysrhythmias.
         (c) Treatment is to stop surgical stimulus, ensure that dysrhythmia is not the result of lack of oxygen (by oxygen saturation confirmation) or ventilation, and administer atropine if needed.

c) Emergence
(1) The goal is smoothness.
(2) Empty the patient's stomach with a nasogastric tube and suction the pharynx while the patient is still paralyzed or deeply anesthetized.
(3) Administer an antiemetic before the end of surgery.
(4) Administer lidocaine, 1 mg/kg, to prevent coughing during emergence.
(5) The trachea should be extubated before the patient has a tendency to cough.

5. **Postoperative implications**
a) Transport the patient to the recovery room with the head up 10 to 20 degrees to facilitate venous drainage from the eye.
b) The patient can be placed on the side with the operative side upward.
c) Shivering and pain can increase IOP and should be prevented.

STRABISMUS REPAIR

1. **Introduction**
Strabismus repairs are performed to correct ocular malalignment. This malalignment may be esotropia (eyes deviate inward) or exotropia (eyes deviate outward). This procedure straightens the eyes cosmetically and allows the patient binocular vision by the lengthening or shortening of individual muscles or pairs of muscles. The specific muscles involved are the horizontal rectus and the oblique muscles.

A forced duction test is performed by the surgeon after induction and intubation by manipulating the sclera of the operative eye to aid the surgical plan. An incision is made through the conjuctiva in the area of the muscle to be manipulated. The muscle is then isolated and sewn back farther on the globe if the muscle tension is to be increased. If the muscle tension needs to be decreased, a segment of the muscle is removed.

2. **Preoperative assessment**
Strabismus repair is the most common ophthalmic surgical procedure performed on children. These children are usually otherwise healthy. There is, however, a higher incidence of strabismus in children with cerebral palsy and myelomeningocele with hydrocephalus. Malignant hyperthermia also is more common with children undergoing strabismus repair.
a) History and physical examination
(1) A careful family history should be obtained preoperatively, including any history of family problems with anesthesia.
(2) Respiratory: For patients with signs and symptoms of an acute respiratory infection, surgery should be postponed because these children are at greater risk for laryngospasm and bronchospasm.
b) Patient preparation
(1) Laboratory tests: These are as indicated by the history and physical examination. Caffeine and halothane contracture tests may be indicated if the patient is believed to be susceptible to malignant hyperthermia.
(2) Diagnostic tests: These are as indicated by the history and physical examination.
(3) Medications: Midazolam, 0.5 to 0.7 mg/kg orally, is given as a premedication.

3. **Room preparation**
a) Monitoring equipment: Standard

b) Additional equipment
   (1) Standard emergency drugs (including lidocaine and atropine)
   (2) Pediatric standard tabletop
   (3) Intravenous fluids: 20- or 22-gauge intravenous tube with normal saline or lactated Ringer's solution at 5 to 10 mL/kg/hour

4. **Perioperative management and anesthetic technique**
   a) Induction: General endotracheal anesthesia is the technique of choice. Nondepolarizing muscle relaxants may be used after the forced duction test is performed by the surgeon. Bradycardia is common owing to the oculocardiac reflex, so atropine is commonly used.
   b) Maintenance: Routine. Watch for signs and symptoms of malignant hyperthermia.
   c) Emergence: Nausea and vomiting are very common.

5. **Postoperative implications**
   Aggressive prophylaxis and treatment of postoperative nausea and vomiting are required. Minimal analgesia is necessary.

INTRAOCULAR PROCEDURES

1. **Introduction**
   Intraocular procedures may refer to vitrectomy, glaucoma drainage, corneal transplant, and open eye injury. These procedures involve entry into the vitreous humor. It is crucial to avoid increases in IOP with all intraocular procedures.
   The most common of these procedures, vitrectomy, is performed by making three openings into the vitreous cavity. One of these openings is used to instill balanced salt solution; another is made for insertion of a fiberoptic light. The third opening is made for the insertion of various instruments used to remove abnormal tissue from the vitreous cavity. Frequently, a gas bubble is introduced during vitrectomy to tamponade retinal tears.

2. **Preoperative assessment**
   a) History and physical examination: Individualized based on patient's history and medical condition
   b) Patient preparation
      (1) Laboratory and diagnostic tests: These are as indicated from the history and physical examination.
      (2) Medications: Midazolam, 1 to 2 mg, may be given intravenously in divided doses as a premedication. The anesthesia provider must be aware that ocular drugs applied topically can have systemic effects. These include hypertension, arrhythmias, nausea and vomiting, agitation, excitement, disorientation, seizures, hypotension, and metabolic acidosis.

3. **Room preparation**
   a) Monitoring equipment is standard.
   b) Additional equipment includes standard emergency drugs, a long breathing circuit (table will be turned), and right-angled endotracheal tubes.
   c) Intravenous fluids: An 18-gauge intravenous line with normal saline or lactated Ringer's solution at 5 to 10 mL/kg/hour is used.
   d) A Hudson hood may be used to provide oxygen to the patient if a regional block with sedation is to be used. Care must be taken if there is any electrocautery, because the hood will create an oxygen-rich environment under the drape.

4. **Perioperative management and anesthetic technique**
   a) These procedures can be done with the patient under general anesthesia or under a regional block (retrobulbar or peribulbar block) with sedation.
   b) General anesthesia with endotracheal intubation is indicated for the following patients: infants; young children; patients with severe claustrophobia; patients unable to cooperate, communicate, or lie flat for long periods; or patients with a history of acute anxiety attacks.
   c) Most adult patients do well with a regional block with sedation, which is the preferred anesthetic technique. If this method of anesthesia is used, it is important to determine the patient's response to sedatives/narcotics before administration of the block. Once the table is turned and the patient is draped, it can be difficult to maintain an airway if necessary. Care must be taken to avoid oversedation. If oversedated, patients tend to be startled when they arouse and may be confused and move about. A short-acting hypnotic (propofol) may be useful immediately before administration of the block. The surgeon does need to have the patient's cooperation during the block, because the surgeon may ask the patient to look from side to side.
   d) General endotracheal tube anesthesia is also appropriate.
      (1) Induction: Standard intravenous induction. Ketamine is not a drug of choice because increased IOP is to be avoided. Care must be taken to avoid pressure on the eyes with the mask. Nondepolarizing muscle relaxants are used for intubation and continued throughout the procedure, titrated to patient response. It is imperative the patient not move during the procedure. All connections in the breathing circuit should be secured.
      (2) Maintenance: Continuous intravenous anesthesia is an option. Another option is the use of inhalational agents. Nitrous oxide may or may not be used. If used, however, and the surgeon performs a gas-fluid exchange, the nitrous oxide should be discontinued 5 to 10 minutes before this exchange. Consider an antiemetic because of the high incidence of postoperative nausea and vomiting.
   e) Emergence: Smooth emergence and extubation are important. Coughing, bucking, and straining should be avoided to prevent increasing the IOP. Consider deep extubation, although care must be taken not to place pressure on the operative eye with the face mask.

5. **Postoperative implications**
   Again, coughing, straining, and bucking should be avoided. The patient may be positioned prone or to one side (as ordered by the surgeon) for correct positioning of the gas bubble. The patient's respiratory status should be ensured before turning the patient postoperatively.

G. Orbital Fractures

1. **Introduction**
   Surgical access to the orbit may be needed to repair orbital fractures. The orbit may be divided into several compartments, including the peripheral surgical space, subperiosteal space, central surgical space, and subtenon space. The approach for orbital wall fractures depends on the location and the pathologic process involved. The common approach to these fractures is the transperiosteal or extraperiosteal approach. A skin

PART II **Common Procedures**

incision is made in the desired quadrant just outside the orbital rim. The periosteum is identified and incised and is then resected from the wall and orbital margin.

2. **Preoperative assessment and patient preparation**
   a) History and physical examination: Patients are usually healthy, aside from the underlying trauma. Evaluation should focus on any coexisting disease and systemic manifestations of the trauma.
   b) Laboratory tests are as indicated by the history and physical examination.
   c) Diagnostic tests are as indicated by the history and physical examination.
   d) Premedication is standard.
3. **Room preparation**
   a) Monitoring equipment: Standard
   b) Additional equipment: Regular operating table, which will be turned 90 to 180 degrees; availability of an anesthesia circuit extension required
   c) Drugs: Standard emergency and standard tabletop
   d) Intravenous fluids: One 18-gauge intravenous line with normal saline/lactated Ringer's solution at 4 to 6 mL/kg/hour
4. **Perioperative management and anesthetic technique**
   a) Use general endotracheal anesthesia.
   b) Induction: Standard; an oral right-angled endotracheal tube may be preferred.
   c) Maintenance: Standard; muscle relaxation is not required.
   d) Position: Supine; check and pad pressure points. The table is turned 90 degrees; have extension tubes or long tubes for an anesthesia circuit. Check the patient's eyes and tape or use ointment (or do both).
   e) Potential complication
      (1) Oculocardiac reflex is triggered by pain, direct pressure on the eye, and pulling on the extrinsic muscle of the eye. It has both trigeminal afferent and vagal efferent pathways. Bradycardia is usual with oculocardiac reflex, although junctional rhythm, atrioventricular block, ventricular premature contractions, ventricular tachycardia, and asystole also occur.
      (2) To treat, tell the surgeon to stop the stimulus, ensure adequate oxygenation and ventilation and administer atropine as needed. Lidocaine infiltration near the eye muscles may help to attenuate the reflex, which is self-limiting (i.e., it will tire itself with repeated manipulations).
5. **Postoperative implications**
   a) For nausea and vomiting, begin prophylactic treatment before the end of the surgical procedure.
   b) For pain management, use parenteral opiates.

H. Parathyroidectomy

1. **Introduction**
   Primary hyperparathyroidism results from excessive secretion of parathyroid hormone from benign parathyroid adenomas (89% of cases), hyperplasia (9%), or parathyroid carcinoma (2%). Symptoms result from accompanying hypercalcemia. Definitive treatment requires

surgical removal of the adenoma or malignant gland. Hyperplasia of all four glands is treated by excision of all parathyroid tissue except half of one gland. Parathyroidectomy may be indicated in some cases of secondary hyperparathyroidism.

2. **Preoperative assessment and patient preparation**
   a) Assess for clinical manifestations of hypercalcemia. Renal, cardiac, and central nervous system abnormalities are associated with chronic hypercalcemia.
   b) Laboratory tests should include a current calcium level. Consider hemoglobin and hematocrit, electrolytes, magnesium, phosphate, blood urea nitrogen, creatinine, electrocardiography, and radiography.
   c) Correct volume status and electrolyte irregularities. Hypercalcemia can cause nausea and vomiting; subsequently, these patients may be markedly dehydrated and anorexic. Hypercalcemia can cause nephrogenic diabetes insipidus, thus inhibiting urine concentration by the kidneys. The resultant polyuria can compound the problem of dehydration.
   d) Elevated calcium levels may be lowered initially with intravenous normal saline and furosemide. Emergency treatment is necessary with levels greater than 15 mg/dL. Treatment includes intravenous phosphates, mithramycin, calcitonin, glucocorticoids, and dialysis.

3. **Room preparation**
   a) A standard tabletop setup is used.
   b) The patient is in the supine position with arms tucked at the side; a small pad may be placed between the shoulder blades to hyperextend the neck. The operating table may be tilted to elevate the head and decrease bleeding.
   c) Consider two large (16-gauge) intravenous lines. The proximity of surgery to vessels of the neck could necessitate aggressive fluid resuscitation if a vessel is accidentally incised. Vigorous fluid therapy is indicated to correct hypervolemia and dilute the hypercalcemia. Volume frequently is contracted.

4. **Perioperative management and anesthetic technique**
   General anesthesia is the usual choice. Rarely is this surgery performed using local anesthesia with sedation.

5. **Considerations**
   a) Avoid hypoventilation because acidosis increases ionized calcium concentrations.
   b) Renal dysfunction coexists; adjust anesthetic techniques accordingly.
   c) Somnolence before induction may decrease anesthetic requirements.
   d) The response to muscle relaxants may be altered. A nerve stimulator is important. The patient may be sensitive to succinylcholine and resistant to a nondepolarizer. Use caution with long-acting muscle relaxants if the surgeon wants to test nerve function.
   e) Osteoporosis predisposes patients to vertebral compression during laryngoscopy and to bone fractures during transport. Position the patient gently to avoid pathologic fractures.
   f) Monitor the electrocardiogram for a short QT interval and a prolonged PR interval.

6. **Postoperative considerations**
   a) Complications include recurrent laryngeal nerve damage, bleeding, and transient or complete hypoparathyroidism.

b) Patients with significant preoperative bone disease may develop decreased calcium (hungry bone syndrome); therefore, monitor serum calcium, magnesium, and phosphorus levels closely.

I. Ptosis Surgery

1. **Introduction**
   If ptosis is severe, the function of the levator palpebrae is poor. Most frequently, ptosis surgery involves shortening or reattaching the muscle at its site of insertion on the superior tarsus. The upper eyelid is marked at the desired height so it matches the opposite eyelid. Local anesthetic is injected by the surgeon. The skin is incised along the upper eyelid crease, and dissection proceeds until the orbicularis oculi is reached. At the medial and lateral ends of the tarsus, scissors incisions are made, and a clamp is placed between the two incisions. The levator muscle is resected as desired, and the eyelid height is evaluated. The skin incision is then closed, with any excess being excised.
2. **Preoperative assessment and patient preparation**
   a) This type of procedure in adults is preferably performed using local anesthesia so the patient can keep the eyes open and the lid position can be adjusted.
   b) History and physical examination are routine.
   c) Patient preparation
      (1) Laboratory tests: As indicated by history and physical examination
      (2) Diagnostic tests: As indicated by history and physical examination
      (3) Premedication: Light sedation as needed
      (4) Intravenous fluids: One 18- or 20-gauge needle with normal saline/lactated Ringer's; keep vein open; blood loss normally minimal
3. **Perioperative management and anesthetic technique**
   a) Patients are kept awake such that they are able to open their eyes to facilitate adjustment of the lids.
   b) Deep sedation is required for only localization; then the patient is kept awake.
4. **Postoperative implications**
   a) Antibiotic steroid ophthalmic ointment is applied to the suture line.
   b) Sometimes, an eye pad is applied or the patient receives iced saline pads in the postanesthesia care unit.

J. Radical Neck Dissection

1. **Introduction**
   Neck dissection is often performed when there is local tumor extension. Radical neck dissection involves complete cervical lymphadenectomy with resection of the sternocleidomastoid muscle, internal jugular vein, and select cranial nerves. Functional neck dissection is complete cervical lymphadenectomy, preserving the sternocleidomastoid muscle, internal jugular vein, and selected cranial nerves. Modified neck dissection is a variation between radical neck dissection and functional neck dissection. Neck dissections are usually combined with resection of the primary lesions, such as those of the tongue, pharynx, and larynx. In composite

resection, radical neck dissection, normally done first, is followed by partial mandibulectomy and possibly partial glossectomy. Tracheostomy is almost always performed with these resections.

Usually, one or two neck incisions, occasionally extending vertically to expose the neck from the mandible to the clavicle, are performed. The accessory nerve (XI), hypoglossal nerve (XII), and lingual nerves are identified and preserved. The sternocleidomastoid muscle, internal jugular vein, and submental triangle may or may not be resected. Drains are placed posteriorly, and the wound is closed in layers.

2. **Preoperative assessment**

Most patients are older and have a long history of tobacco and alcohol abuse. Associated medical problems may include chronic obstructive pulmonary disease, hypertension, coronary artery disease, malnourishment, and alcohol withdrawal.

a) History and physical examination: See the earlier discussion of laryngectomy in this section.

b) Patient preparation: See the earlier discussion of laryngectomy in this section.

3. **Room preparation**

a) Monitoring equipment
   (1) Standard monitoring equipment
   (2) Foley catheter
   (3) Arterial line: Useful for serial laboratory and arterial blood gas studies
   (4) Central venous pressure line: If indicated by coexisting disease (prefer basilic/cephalic vein)

b) Additional equipment
   (1) Regular operating table turned 180 degrees
   (2) Extension tubes
   (3) Fluid warmer and humidifier
   (4) Fiberoptic laryngoscope with anticipated difficult airway or potential for airway obstruction
   (5) Tracheostomy under local anesthesia occasionally necessary for severe airway management.

c) Drugs
   (1) Standard emergency drugs
   (2) Standard tabletop
   (3) Intravenous fluids: two 16- to 18-gauge or larger intravenous lines with normal saline or lactated Ringer's solution at 3 to 5 mL/kg/hour; uncontrolled bleeding of the internal jugular vein at the skull base rare but can result in sudden significant blood losses

4. **Perioperative management and anesthetic technique**

General endotracheal anesthesia is used.

a) Induction: Standard intravenous induction is appropriate with a normal airway. The choice of an induction drug should be based on the patient's medical condition. If airway difficulty is possible, direct laryngoscopy can be performed while the patient is breathing spontaneously, and a muscle relaxant may be administered once the glottis is visualized. In more difficult cases, awake intubation or fiberoptic laryngoscopy may be required.

b) Maintenance: The patient is in the supine position, with the head turned to the opposite side and a pillow placed below the shoulders; standard maintenance is used, considering the patient's preexisting medical problems. An inhalation agent and supplemental narcotics benefit patients with reactive airway disease. Use of nonde-polarizing muscle relaxants should be discussed with the surgeon, because nerve stimulation for cranial nerve XI localization may be done. With right radical neck dissection, a prolonged QT interval on the electrocardiogram can progress to ventricular dysrhythmia and even cardiac arrest. These changes result from interruption of cervical sympathetic outflow to the heart through the right stellate ganglion. The left cardiac sympathetic fibers most likely have different effects on cardiac excitability because prolongation of the QT interval does not occur after left radical neck dissection. Manipulation of the carotid sinus during dissection can result in hypotension and cardiac dysrhythmia. Treatment includes cessation of manipulation and, if necessary, infiltration of surrounding tissues with a local anesthetic or administration of intravenous atropine. Unexplained hypotension or dysrhythmia may indicate venous air embolism through large open neck veins. Treatment is to give 100% oxygen, notify the surgeon, flood the field with normal saline, place the patient's head down, aspirate air through the central venous pressure line, increase venous pressure by positive-pressure ventilation, and administer circulatory support as required.

c) Emergence: Many patients undergo tracheostomy. If no tracheostomy is performed, the amount of airway edema and distortion needs to be discussed with the surgeon before determining extubation. A gradual emergence with stable hemodynamic parameters is an important consideration in the patient with coronary artery disease.

5. **Postoperative implications**
   a) Injury to the facial nerve can cause facial droop. Recurrent laryngeal nerve injury can result in vocal cord dysfunction, and diaphragmatic paralysis may result from phrenic nerve injury.
   b) Painful shoulder syndrome may occur.
   c) Pneumothorax may occur with low neck dissection.
   d) Airway impingement results from restrictive neck dressings or hematoma development.
   e) Communication difficulties occur after laryngectomy.

K. Rhytidectomy/Facelift

1. **Introduction**
   Rhytidectomy is a reconstructive plastic procedure in which the skin of the face is tightened, wrinkles (rhytid-) are removed, and the skin is made to appear firm and smooth. In the preoperative area, the surgeon marks where the planned incisions will be made; before incision, the surgeon will localize the area. Typically, lidocaine 1% with 1:100,000 epinephrine is infiltrated along the incision lines, and lidocaine 0.5% with 1:400,000 epinephrine is infiltrated into the anticipated dissection line.

   The facelift incision begins in the temporal scalp area about 5 cm above the ear and 5 cm behind the hairline, curves down parallel to the hairline toward the superior root, and continues caudally in the natural preauricular skin crease. The dissection will begin in the temporal hair-bearing area; dissection continues through temporoparietal fascia, down to the loose areolar layer. The facial nerve branches enter the facial muscles on their deep surface; dissection during this procedure must be done carefully. The only large sensory nerve that is important is the great auricular nerve. This nerve crosses the surface of the sternocleidomastoid muscle below the caudal edge of the auditory canal and is found posterior to the external jugular.

2. **Preoperative assessment and patient preparation**
   a) History and physical examination
      (1) Most patients are older and have some effects of aging, but the age range may be anywhere from 40 to 70 years. Therefore, cardiovascular status should be evaluated because of the use of epinephrine in the local anesthetic.
      (2) Because of the inaccessibility of the face to the anesthesia provider and the need for sedation, careful airway evaluation and a history of sleep apnea should be identified.
   b) Patient preparation
      (1) Laboratory tests: As indicated by the history and physical examination
      (2) Diagnostic tests: Electrocardiogram if indicated by the history and physical examination
      (3) Premedication: Standard

3. **Room preparation**
   a) Monitoring equipment is standard, including an end-tidal carbon dioxide nasal cannula or a second nasal cannula attached to the capnograph.
   b) Additional equipment: An extra long anesthesia circuit should be available because of the turning of the table 90 to 180 degrees, and an oral right-angled endotracheal tube is indicated if general anesthesia is to be used.
   c) Drugs: Standard emergency and standard tabletop agents are used.
   d) Intravenous fluids: Because of the use of vasoconstrictors in local anesthesia, blood loss should be minimal.
   e) One 18-gauge intravenous line with normal saline or lactated Ringer's solution at 2 mL/kg/hour is used, or keep vein open, with replacement of the NPO (nothing by mouth) deficit.

4. **Perioperative management and anesthetic technique**
   a) Most facelifts are done with deep sedation. The surgeon will need the patient to remain asleep throughout the procedure.
   b) The choice depends on the patient and surgeon's preference.
   c) If a general anesthetic technique is chosen, an oral right-angled endotracheal tube may be used to facilitate exposure of the surgical field.
   d) If a local anesthetic with intravenous sedation is the technique chosen, a nasal airway may be placed if the patient easily obstructs.
   e) Induction: Routine. If a local anesthetic with sedation is chosen, a short-acting agent (i.e., propofol) should be used because most of these surgical procedures are done on an outpatient basis, with the patient going home the same day.
   f) Before administration of local anesthetic, the patient must be motionless and deeply sedated.
   g) Maintenance: Routine. Deep sedation can be maintained with an infusion. Hypertension should be controlled because this may result in hematoma. Vital signs should be maintained within normal limits. Depending on the patients' anatomy and the skill and experience of the surgeon, this procedure could last up to 6 hours.
   h) Emergence: No special considerations exist.

5. **Postoperative complications**
   a) Hematoma is the most common complication of this procedure, usually occurring at the end of the procedure; but it may also present within the first 10 to 12 hours.
      (1) The cause of this is usually intraoperative hypertension.
      (2) This complication most commonly presents itself with the patient's appearing restless and having unilateral pain to the face or neck.
      (3) The patient should be relatively pain free.
      (4) However, if these symptoms are noticed, the surgeon should be notified, because treatment must be surgical.
      (5) If left untreated, this could compromise the patient's respiratory status.
      (6) A general anesthetic technique or intravenous sedation technique may be done for evacuation of the hematoma. If the hematoma is large, a general technique may be performed if the patient is restless and anxious.
   b) This procedure disrupts branches of the sensory nerves to the face. Numbness may last several months postoperatively, usually 2 to 6 months. This numbness is usually limited to the area of the lower two thirds of the ear, the preauricular area, and the cheeks.

L. Thyroidectomy

1. **Introduction**
   Hyperthyroidism results from excess secretion of triiodothyronine (T_3) and thyroxine (T_4) by the thyroid gland. Subtotal thyroidectomy may be used in the treatment of hyperthyroidism as an alternative to prolonged medical therapy. Extensive but incomplete removal of the thyroid gland induces remission in most patients.
2. **Preoperative assessment and patient preparation**
   a) History and physical examination: Individualized
      (1) Respiratory: Palpate the thyroid gland to determine its size and relationship to the trachea.
      (2) Cardiac: Assess the heart rate, blood pressure, and electrocardiogram.
   b) Diagnostic tests
      (1) Complete blood count, electrolytes, glucose, blood urea nitrogen, creatinine, calcium, electrocardiography, chest radiography are obtained.
      (2) Radiographs may be needed to visualize the trachea and thyroid gland.
      (3) Tests specific to the thyroid gland are obtained: T_3, T_4, and thyroid-stimulating hormone levels.
   c) Preoperative medication and intravenous therapy
      (1) Maintain a euthyroid state and control hyperkinetic circulation. Propylthiouracil, methimazole, potassium iodide, and β-adrenergic antagonists may be used.
      (2) Continue all antithyroid medications.
      (3) Normal thyroid function tests and a resting heart rate of less than 85 beats/min are recommended before surgery. If the systolic blood pressure is higher than 140 mm Hg and the heart rate is higher than 100 beats/min, surgery may be canceled, and more antithyroid medication may be given. With tachycardia associated with cardiac irregularities, surgery may be postponed.

    (4) Give adequate premedication to prevent an increase in sympathetic activity.

    (5) Consider two large-bore (16- to 18-gauge) intravenous lines. The proximity of surgery to vessels of the neck could necessitate aggressive fluid resuscitation if a vessel is accidentally incised.

3. Room preparation

  a) Monitoring equipment: Standard

  b) Pharmacologic agents: β-adrenergic blockers

  c) Position: Supine with the arms tucked at the side, with a small pad possibly placed between the shoulder blades to hyperextend the neck

4. Anesthetic technique

  a) General anesthesia: Endotracheal intubation is required.

  b) The goal of anesthetic management is to achieve a depth of anesthesia that prevents an exaggerated sympathetic response to surgical stimulation and to avoid the administration of medications that stimulate the sympathetic nervous system.

5. Perioperative management

  a) Induction

    (1) Awake fiberoptic intubation may be indicated if the gland impinges on the airway.

    (2) An anode tube may be used to decrease the risk of kinking and airway obstruction.

    (3) Lidocaine and narcotics may be used before laryngoscopy to blunt the sympathetic nervous system response to intubation. An inhalational agent may be used to increase the depth of anesthesia before intubation.

    (4) The induction agent of choice is thiopental because of its antithyroid properties. Avoid ketamine because of its tendency to elicit sympathetic nervous system stimulation.

    (5) Administer muscle relaxants that lack effect on the cardiovascular system.

  b) Maintenance

    (1) Inhalational agents or opioids combined with nitrous oxide are recommended to blunt the sympathetic nervous system response to surgical stimulation.

    (2) If the patient is not euthyroid, maintenance of β-blockade is highly desirable.

    (3) The incidence of myasthenia gravis is increased in hyperthyroid patients.

    (4) Treat hypertension with direct-acting agents.

    (5) Patients with exophthalmos are susceptible to corneal ulceration and drying. Care must be taken to ensure protection of the eyes.

    (6) Monitor temperature, which may indicate thyroid storm or a hypermetabolic state.

  c) Emergence

    (1) Reverse muscle relaxation completely. Use glycopyrrolate (Robinul) rather than atropine (less chronotropic effect) in combination with neostigmine.

    (2) Extubate the patient wide awake with protective reflexes intact. Assess the vocal cords by direct visualization for bilateral or unilateral paralysis from recurrent laryngeal nerve damage.

    (3) Potential complications

      (a) Injury to cricoid or thyroid cartilages, with the potential for laryngeal stenosis

      (b) Injury to the esophagus

      (c) Hemorrhage from the anterior jugular vein

      (d) Injury to the carotid artery or internal jugular vein

      (e) Infection at the cricothyroid incision

6. Postoperative considerations

  a) Complications include recurrent laryngeal nerve damage, tracheal compression, hematoma formation, and hypoparathyroidism.

  b) Thyroid storm may occur intraoperatively but is more likely in the first 6 to 18 hours after surgery.

    (1) The signs and symptoms include tachycardia, hyperthermia, congestive heart failure, dehydration, shock, full bounding pulse, hypertension, atrial fibrillation, sweating, tremors, vomiting, and diarrhea.

    (2) Treatment must be instituted immediately because of the high mortality associated with thyroid storm and should be aimed at both the symptoms and precipitating cause.

    (3) β-Blockers (e.g., propranolol or esmolol) are given to control heart rate and blood pressure.

    (4) Sodium iodide or ipodate helps in reducing the size and activity of the thyroid gland.

    (5) Antithyroid drugs (e.g., propylthiouracil or methimazole) should be given several hours before the iodides to prevent accumulation in the thyroid gland.

    (6) Steroids may also be given.

    (7) Other supportive measures should be aimed at maintaining optimal oxygen levels, cooling the patient, and keeping the patient relaxed.

    (8) Aspirin should be avoided for temperature control because of its tendency to remove T_4 from its carrier protein.

M. Tonsillectomy and Adenoidectomy

1. Introduction

Tonsillectomy and adenoidectomy are among the most common surgical procedures performed in the United States. Such surgical procedures are indicated for the treatment of hypertrophic tonsil and adenoids and recurrent or chronic upper respiratory tract and ear infection.

2. Preoperative patient assessment and patient preparation

  a) History and physical examination

    (1) Upper airway: Externally inspect tonsillar and adenoid hypertrophy. Adenoid hypertrophy can be determined by having the patient breathe with the mouth closed and evaluating the degree of nasal airway obstruction.

    (2) Oral: Because most of these procedures are performed in children, careful inspection for loose or missing teeth is necessary.

  b) Diagnostic tests: Routine laboratory tests

  c) Preoperative medication and intravenous therapy

    (1) Light sedation with a benzodiazepine is used.

    (2) Administration of an antisialogogue may assist in improving the surgical view.

    (3) Minimal blood loss is expected, but massive hemorrhage can occur. One large-bore intravenous catheter is suitable.

3. Room preparation

  a) Monitoring equipment: Standard

b) Pharmacologic agents
  (1) Standard agents are used.
  (2) Short-acting muscle relaxants may or may not be used for maintenance.
c) Position: Supine, arms tucked to the sides; table turned 90 degrees

4. Anesthetic technique
General anesthesia with endotracheal intubation is used. The major goals of anesthesia are to provide an adequate depth of anesthesia such that protective reflexes are blunted, these reflexes return rapidly after the procedure, and postoperative analgesia is adequate.

5. Perioperative management
a) Induction: Nonspecific; intubation with an oral right-angled endotracheal tube is beneficial but not necessary. Confirm the surgeon's preference in type of tube and placement after intubation.
b) Maintenance: Nonspecific; the use of short-acting agents is suggested. Muscle relaxants may or may not be used. If used, they must be completely reversed before extubation. Close monitoring of breath sounds is essential. The tube can easily be dislodged during placement of a mouth gag or during manipulation of the patient's head.
c) Emergence
  (1) Before the end of surgery, the surgeon may release the mouth gag to ensure hemostasis. At this time, an orogastric tube should be inserted gently by the surgeon or anesthesia provider, and the stomach is decompressed. Extubate awake after careful suction of oral pharynx with tonsil suction. Never suction the nasopharynx after adenoidectomy. Gently suction the oropharynx. The airway should be free from blood and secretions before extubation is performed.
  (2) Maintain the patient in a head-down Sims' position (also referred to as the "tonsil position") to facilitate drainage of secretions.

6. Postoperative implications
Postoperative bleeding is the most significant complication. This usually happens 4 to 9 hours or 5 to 10 days postoperatively (the latter time frame is usually the result of infection). These patients should be rehydrated and transfused if necessary. The extent of bleeding is often hidden because of swallowing of blood. Rapid sequence induction should be performed because these patients should always be considered as having full stomachs from the presence of swallowed blood.

N. Tracheotomy

1. Introduction
Tracheotomy is an incision into the trachea to form a temporary or permanent opening, the latter of which is called a tracheostomy. The incision is made through the second, third, or fourth tracheal ring, and a tube is inserted through the opening to allow passage of air and the removal of tracheobronchial secretions. Except in cases of head, neck, and face trauma, tracheotomy is rarely performed as an emergency procedure.

2. Indications for tracheostomy
a) To relieve upper airway obstruction
  (1) Foreign body
  (2) Trauma
  (3) Acute infection: acute epiglottitis, diphtheria

(4) Glottic edema

(5) Bilateral abductor paralysis of the vocal cords

(6) Tumors of the larynx

(7) Congenital web or atresia

b) To improve respiratory function

(1) Fulminating bronchopneumonia

(2) Chronic bronchitis and emphysema

(3) Chest injury with or without flail chest

c) Respiratory paralysis

(1) Unconscious head injury

(2) Bulbar poliomyelitis

(3) Tetanus

3. Tracheostomy technique

a) Patient positioned supine with sandbag between scapulae

b) Transverse cervical skin incision 1 cm above sternal notch

c) Incision extending to the sternomastoid muscles

d) Dissection through fascial planes and retraction of anterior jugular veins

e) Retraction of the strap muscles

f) Division of the thyroid isthmus and oversewing to prevent bleeding

g) Placement of a cricoid hook on the second tracheal ring

h) Stoma fashioned between the third and fourth tracheal rings

i) Removal of the anterior portion of the tracheal ring

j) No advantage in creating a tracheal flap

k) Endotracheal tube withdrawn to the subglottis

l) Tracheostomy tube inserted using an obturator

m) When correct position confirmed, removal of the endotracheal tube

n) Securing of the tube with tapes

4. Preoperative assessment and patient preparation

a) History and physical examination: These patients may or may not be already intubated. If the patient is not intubated, the patient's airway should be carefully assessed. Information regarding any abnormal pathologic features that may make intubation difficult should be sought from the surgeon or reports from specific tests such as triple endoscopy. If intubated, the patient's respiratory status and the following should be assessed: vent settings, peak airway pressures, respiratory rate, amount and color of tracheal secretions, need for and frequency of suctioning, lung sounds, arterial blood gases, chest radiography, and the presence of pulmonary infections.

b) Diagnostic tests

(1) Electrocardiography, chest radiography

(2) Laboratory tests: as indicated by the patient's medical condition

c) Preoperative medication and intravenous therapy

(1) Preoperative medication as tolerated by patient.

(2) One 16- or 18-gauge intravenous line with minimal fluid replacement

5. Room preparation

a) Monitoring

(1) Monitoring is routine, with a central venous pressure or pulmonary arterial catheter, as well as an arterial line as indicated by patient's history.

(2) If peak airway pressures are greater than 60 mm Hg, the patient may need a vent from the intensive care unit.

(3) A sterile 6-inch connector is used to attach the endotracheal tube to the vent or sterile circuit.

(4) Consider a bronchial adapter. Patients frequently have a bronchoscopy after tracheotomy placement.

(5) Warming modalities are used.

b) Pharmacologic agents: No special considerations

6. **Anesthetic technique and perioperative management**

Use general anesthesia and skeletal muscle paralysis or local anesthesia.

a) Induction: If a difficult airway is anticipated, awake fiberoptic intubation should be performed. The surgeon should be on standby for an emergency tracheotomy in the event that intubation attempts are unsuccessful. If the patient is already intubated, titrate anesthetic agents to the patient's need.

b) Maintenance

(1) Adjust the oxygen/air mixture to maintain saturation at greater than 95%.

(2) If the patient is stable, nitrous oxide, an inhalation agent, and a narcotic may be introduced.

(3) Avoid 100% oxygen because this increases the chance of airway fires.

(4) If an airway fire occurs

(a) Pour saline into the pharynx to absorb the heat.

(b) Temporarily discontinue the oxygen source.

(c) Extubate and reintubate with a new endotracheal tube.

(d) Follow-up with chest radiography, bronchoscopy, steroids, and blood gas measurements.

(5) Maintain constant communication with the surgeon. Use a team approach. Use hand ventilation with 100% oxygen during insertion of the tracheotomy tube. The surgeon will ask the anesthesia provider to gently pull back the oral endotracheal tube before insertion of the tracheostomy tube.

c) Emergence

(1) The patient may be transferred to the intensive care unit after the procedure. The nondepolarizing muscle relaxant may not have to be reversed if prolonged ventilation is planned.

(2) The patient has 100% oxygen through an Ambu bag, with monitoring devices functioning, and is returned to the unit.

7. **Postoperative implications**

a) Assess patients for any symptoms suggesting pneumothorax, pneumomediastinum, cardiac tamponade, hemorrhage, and subcutaneous emphysema.

b) Suction the airway as often as necessary to maintain airway and remove secretions.

O. Uvulopalatopharyngoplasty

1. **Introduction**

Uvulopalatopharyngoplasty is performed primarily for the treatment of obstructive sleep apnea. Tonsillectomy is often performed concurrently. Nasopharyngeal airway obstruction is relieved by removing redundant and obstructing tissues of the posterior pharynx.

Inspiratory muscle tone is lost during rapid eye movement sleep, resulting in relaxation of the pharyngeal muscles, thus creating airway obstruction. Adults with obstructive sleep apnea are often obese.

2. **Preoperative assessment**
   a) History and physical examination
      (1) Cardiac: Hypoxia and hypercapnia may lead to pulmonary hypertension, cor pulmonale, cardiac arrhythmias, and failure of the right side of the heart.
      (2) Respiratory: Frequent nocturnal arousals (up to 50 times per hour) are common. Periods of apnea may last up to 2 to 3 minutes. These patients often have a long history of snoring.
      (3) Neurologic: Loss of rapid eye movement sleep results in excess daytime somnolence, fatigue, and impaired judgment.
   b) Patient preparation: Medical management includes weight reduction in obese patients, decreasing alcohol consumption, and nasal continuous positive airway pressure.
      (1) Laboratory tests: These are as indicated by the history and physical examination.
      (2) Diagnostic tests: These are as indicated by the history and physical examination.
      (3) Medications: Use minimal preoperative narcotics or sedatives because these patients have heightened sensitivity to them. Anticholinergics are helpful to decrease secretions.
3. **Room preparation**
   a) Standard monitoring equipment
   b) Additional equipment: airway adjuncts, difficult airway cart
   c) Positioning devices
   d) Operating room table: Ensure appropriate weight limit
   e) Drugs
      (1) Intravenous fluids: 0.9% normal saline or lactated Ringer's solution, 4 mL/kg/hour through an 18-gauge intravenous line
      (2) Blood: Type and screen
      (3) Tabletop: Rapid sequence induction setup
4. **Perioperative management and anesthetic technique**
   a) Induction
      (1) Awake fiberoptic laryngoscopy and intubation may be indicated.
      (2) Inhalation agents are used with maintenance of spontaneous respiration and succinylcholine only after visualization of the larynx.
      (3) Intravenous rapid sequence induction is performed after 3 to 4 minutes of preoxygenation, cricoid pressure, and elevation of the head of the bed.
   b) Maintenance
      (1) Inhalation agent: isoflurane or desflurane
      (2) 50% oxygen (may require high fractional inspired oxygen)
      (3) Rose position: Supine, shoulder roll, head extension
      (4) Operating table turned 90 to 180 degrees
   c) Emergence
      (1) Lidocaine, 1 to 1.5 mg/kg before extubation
      (2) As with tonsillectomy, the surgeon may release the mouth gag to see whether there is any uncontrolled bleeding. At this time, patients should have an orogastric tube placed, and the stomach should be suctioned. The nasal and oropharynx should also be gently suctioned and care taken not to dislodge any clots that may precipitate bleeding and incur laryngospasm.
      (3) Extubation criteria
         (a) The patient is awake, alert, and following verbal commands.

      (b) Muscle relaxant reversal is adequate.

      (c) Respiratory mechanics are acceptable.

5. Postoperative implications

  a) Head of the bed elevated

  b) Humidified oxygen

  c) Hemoglobin and hematocrit if blood loss was excessive

  d) Careful titration of narcotics

6. Postoperative complications

Airway obstruction resulting from swelling is the most common postoperative complication of a uvulopalatopharyngoplasty. Typically, a patient will receive a dose of steroids intraoperatively to aid in reducing this swelling. Patients who undergo this procedure are usually admitted to the hospital, where their respiratory and airway status may be monitored carefully. If the tonsils have been removed, the possibility of recurrent bleeding must also be considered.

INTRATHORACIC AND EXTRATHORACIC

A. Breast Biopsy

1. **Introduction**

   Breast cancer is diagnosed by excisional breast biopsy (by needle aspiration or open excision), followed later by a more definitive surgical procedure designed to decrease tumor bulk and thus enhance effectiveness of systemic therapy (chemotherapy, hormonal therapy, or radiation). Carcinoma of the breast is an uncontrolled growth of anaplastic cells. Types include ductal, lobular, and nipple adenocarcinomas.

2. **Preoperative assessment and patient preparation**

   a) History and physical examination

      (1) The most common initial sign of carcinoma of the breast is a painless mass.

      (2) Bloody discharge is more indicative of cancer than is spontaneous unilateral serous nipple discharge.

      (3) Signs of advanced breast cancer include dimpling of skin, nipple retraction, change in breast contour, edema, and erythema of the breast skin.

   b) Diagnostic tests

      (1) Mammography, thermography, ultrasonography are used.

      (2) Metastases to bone are frequent; therefore, a bone scan and measurement of alkaline phosphatase may be indicated.

      (3) Laboratory tests are as indicated by the patient's medical condition.

   c) Preoperative medications and intravenous therapy

      (1) The patient may be receiving hormone therapy.

      (2) Use light sedation and short-acting narcotics preoperatively because the procedure lasts less than 1 hour.

      (3) Metoclopramide (Reglan): Outpatients have an increased gastric volume, and there may be insufflation of air into the stomach if one is using a mask technique.

      (4) One 18-gauge intravenous tube with minimal fluid replacement is used.

3. **Room preparation**

   a) Monitoring equipment

      (1) Standard

      (2) Noninvasive blood pressure cuff on the side opposite of surgery

   b) Pharmacologic agents: Standard

   c) Position: Supine; may need to tuck the surgical arm to the side

4. **Anesthetic technique**

   a) Local infiltration and general anesthesia are used.

   b) The technique of choice is general anesthesia with mask technique.

5. **Perioperative management**

   a) Induction: Consider rapid sequence induction and endotracheal intubation with a patient who is obese or has a full stomach.

b) Maintenance: No indications are needed.

c) Emergence: If rapid sequence induction is used, perform an awake extubation.

6. **Postoperative implications**
None are reported.

B. Bronchopulmonary Lavage

1. **Introduction**
Bronchopulmonary lavage consists of irrigation of the lung and bronchial tree. It is performed with the patient under general anesthesia with a double-lumen tube. Bronchopulmonary lavage can be used to treat alveolar proteinosis, cystic fibrosis, bronchiectasis, radioactive dust inhalation, and asthma or bronchitis.

2. **Preoperative assessment and patient preparation**
Preoperative assessment is routine, including a ventilation-perfusion scan. The lavage is performed on the most severely affected lung first. If both lungs are affected equally, the left lung is lavaged first because of better exchange in the larger right lung.

3. **Room preparation**
a) A fiberoptic bronchoscope is needed to check for accurate placement of the double-lumen tube.

b) Monitors are routine, with an arterial line.

c) A stethoscope should be placed over the nondependent lung to check for rales, which may indicate leakage of the lavaged fluid into this lung.

d) The patient is positioned in the left or right downward position.

4. **Perioperative management and anesthetic technique**
a) After intravenous induction, anesthesia is maintained with an inhalation agent.

b) Keep the fractional inspired oxygen as high as possible.

c) The cuff seal on the double-lumen tube should be checked and should maintain perfect separation at a pressure of 90% of the lavage fluid cm H_2O to prevent leakage of fluid from around the cuff.

d) With the patient in the head-up position, 700 to 1000 mL of warmed heparinized isotonic saline is instilled from a reservoir 30 cm above the midaxillary line into the catheter to the dependent lung. When the fluid ceases to flow, the patient is placed in the head-down position, and the fluid is allowed to drain out.

e) With each lavage, inflow and outflow volumes are measured to prevent excess absorption and leakage to the ventilated side. At least 90% of the fluid should be recovered with each lavage. Two-lung ventilation is reestablished; as compliance improves, air may be added to maintain alveolar patency. Patients can be extubated in the operating room if they are stable.

C. Bronchoscopy

1. **Introduction**
Bronchoscopy permits direct inspection of the larynx, trachea, and bronchi. Indications include collection of secretions for cytologic or bacteriologic examination, tissue biopsy, location of bleeding and

tumors, removal of a foreign body, and implantation of radioactive gold seeds for tumor treatment. A common indication for bronchoscopy is suspicion of bronchial neoplasm (see the following box).

2. Preoperative assessment
  a) History and physical examination
    (1) Respiratory: Evaluate for chronic lung disease, wheezing, atelectasis, hemoptysis, cough, unresolved pneumonia, diffuse lung disease, and smoking history.
    (2) Cardiac: Question underlying dysrhythmias because they may arise with stimulation from the scope, or they could be a sign of hypoxemia during the procedure.
    (3) Gastrointestinal: Assess the patient's drinking history and nutritional intake.
  b) Diagnostic tests
    (1) Chest radiography
    (2) Computed tomography
    (3) Pulmonary function test with lung disease
    (4) Laboratory tests including complete blood count, electrolytes, glucose, and others as indicated by patient's medical condition
  c) Preoperative medications and intravenous therapy
    (1) The patient may already be taking sympathomimetic bronchodilators and aminophylline.
    (2) Sedatives and narcotics are to be used with caution in patients with poor respiratory reserve.
    (3) Cholinergic blocking agents reduce secretions.
    (4) Intravenous lidocaine, 0.5 to 1.5 mg/kg, decreases airway reflexes.
    (5) Topical anesthesia involves 4% lidocaine using a nebulizer to anesthetize the airway by spraying the palate, pharynx, larynx, vocal cords, and trachea.

Consideration for Rigid versus Fiberoptic Bronchoscopy

Rigid
1. Has been used extensively for removal of foreign bodies
2. In moderate or massive hemoptysis, provides better opportunity to suction
3. When airway patency is compromised by granulation tissue or tumor, instrument able to pass the point of obstruction
4. Preferred for visualization of the carina and for the assessment of its mobility and sharpness
5. Allows the endoscopist to obtain a larger bronchoscopy specimen
6. Preferred in infants and small children

Fiberoptic
1. May require fragmentation of the aspirated object
2. Provides a better yield than rigid bronchoscopy in diagnosing bronchogenic carcinoma
3. Allows detailed visualization of the tracheobronchial tree
4. Facilitates intubation in patients who have difficult anatomic features
5. Improves patient comfort
6. Provides video imaging

(6) One 18-gauge peripheral intravenous line with minimal fluid replacement is used.

3. Room preparation
a) Monitoring equipment is standard: An arterial line is used if thoracotomy is planned or the patient is unstable.
b) Pharmacologic agents: Lidocaine and cardiac drugs are used.
c) Position: Supine; the table may be turned. One must manage an upper airway that is shared with the surgeon.

4. Anesthetic technique
a) Local infiltration or general anesthesia is used.
b) The technique of choice is general anesthesia. One must discuss with the surgeon whether a rigid or flexible fiberoptic bronchoscopy will be performed.
c) Nerve blocks
   (1) Transtracheal: 2 mL of 2% plain lidocaine through the cricothyroid membrane using a 22-gauge needle attached to a small syringe
   (2) Superior laryngeal: 25-gauge needle anterior to the superior cornu of the thyroid cartilage
d) If topical anesthesia is employed, consider total dosage of local anesthetic and be prepared to treat local anesthetic toxicity.

5. Perioperative management
a) Induction
   (1) Flexible bronchoscopy
      (a) The endotracheal tube must be large enough (8 to 8.5 mm) to permit the endoscope to pass easily.
      (b) Do not administer oxygen through the suction channel of the flexible bronchoscope, to avoid gas trapping and inducing barotrauma.
   (2) Rigid bronchoscopy
      (a) Conventional ventilation
         (i) Ventilation through the side port requires high gas flow rates and an intact glass eyepiece.
         (ii) Suction, biopsy, and foreign-body manipulation require removal of the glass and loss of ventilation.
      (b) Jet ventilation
         (i) Give patients high inspired oxygen and hyperventilate them before apneic oxygenation.
         (ii) Perform jet ventilation through the side port of a catheter alongside the bronchoscope.
         (iii) Place the tracheal tube to the left side of the mouth because the surgeon will insert the scope down the right side.
         (iv) The endotracheal tube must be smaller in diameter to allow surgical access.
   (3) After preoxygenation, general anesthesia is induced with the insertion of an oral endotracheal tube.
   (4) Succinylcholine may be contraindicated if the patient has severe muscle spasm, wasting, or complains of myalgia.
b) Maintenance
   (1) General anesthesia must provide good muscle relaxation without patient movement: coughing, laryngospasm, or bronchospasm.
   (2) Cardiac dysrhythmia may be a problem (i.e., supraventricular tachyarrhythmias, premature ventricular contraction, and atrial dysrhythmias). Plan appropriate treatment modalities.

PART II Common Procedures

(3) Volatile anesthetics are useful to provide adequate suppression of upper airway reflexes and permit high inhaled concentrations of oxygen.

(4) Air leaks around the bronchoscope may be minimized by having an assistant externally compress the patient's hypopharynx.

(5) Spontaneous ventilation is preferred in cases of foreign body removal; positive airway pressure could push the foreign body deeper into the bronchial tree.

c) Emergence

(1) The patient should be awakened rapidly with complete return of airway reflexes before extubation.

(2) The patient needs to have a cough to clear secretions and blood from the airway.

6. Postoperative implications

a) If nerve blocks are administered, keep the patient from eating or drinking for several hours postoperatively; the blocks cause depression of airway reflexes.

b) Subglottic edema may be treated with aerosolized racemic epinephrine and intravenous dexamethasone (0.1 mg/kg).

c) Chest radiographs are obtained to detect atelectasis or pneumothorax.

7. Complication

A toxic reaction to local anesthetic is possible.

D. Lung and Heart/Lung Transplantation

1. Introduction

Heart/lung transplants are performed primarily for combined heart and lung disease, such as Eisenmenger's syndrome from congenital heart defect with irreversible pulmonary hypertension, and for certain types of diffuse lung disease, such as primary pulmonary hypertension without significant heart failure and cystic fibrosis. A single-lung transplant is usually performed for end-stage pulmonary disease without significant sepsis, including interstitial fibrosis, lymphangioleiomyomatosis, and emphysema (including α_1-antitrypsin deficiency). Pulmonary vascular diseases, such as primary pulmonary hypertension or pulmonary hypertension associated with an atrial septal defect may also be an indication for single-lung transplantation. Bilateral lung transplantation that is done as a sequential single-lung transplant is performed for septic lung disease, such as chronic bronchiectasis, severe bullous emphysema, pulmonary vascular disease with or without cardiac repair, and cystic fibrosis. One-year survival rates average between 60% and 70%.

End-stage pulmonary disease resulting from destruction of the pulmonary parenchyma or vasculature is a leading cause of mortality and morbidity among adults. Several transplantation operations have been devised to treat end-stage pulmonary disease, each with particular conceptual or practical advantages. These include the heart/ lung, en bloc double-lung, single-lung, and bilateral sequential lung procedures.

2. Incidence and prevalance

Lung transplants of the various types have increased in recent years, with approximately 700 single-lung, 200 double-lung, and 60 heart/lung transplants performed in the United States each year. Recipients range in age from 3 months to 65 years, with male and female patients having equal representation. There are approximately 2200 heart transplants performed annually.

3. **Organ donation**

Donor lungs may be jeopardized by massive fluid resuscitation, aspiration, contusion, and exposure to nonphysiologic oxygen tensions because most organ donors are trauma victims. Ideally, the donor's history should indicate early tracheal intubation with no evidence of aspiration, minimal fluid administration in the course of resuscitation, and absence of chest tubes, pleural disease, or tracheostomy at any time. If bronchoscopy fails to find any pathologic process, intravenous glucocorticoids and antibiotics are administered, and the lungs are harvested. First the heart is removed, followed by the lungs. Some centers may administer a pulmonary vasodilator (prostaglandin E_1) to improve the distribution of the preservative solution. The lungs may also be inflated before immersion in the preservative.

4. **Preoperative assessment and patient preparation**
   a) History and physical examination: Standard preoperative evaluation is supplemented with consideration for the fact that these patients are usually terminally ill, although some are still able to perform limited activity. Thorough documentation of the progression of the disease is indicated.
      (1) Respiratory
         (a) Severe pulmonary hypertension (80/50 mm Hg) results in enlarged pulmonary arteries that may cause vocal cord dysfunction (hoarseness, inability to phonate "e") because of an enlarged pulmonary artery (PA) that stretches the left recurrent laryngeal nerve and results in an increased risk for pulmonary aspiration.
         (b) Assess the patient's ability to undergo one-lung ventilation (OLV). If little perfusion of nonoperative lung is present as indicated by a ventilation-perfusion scan, anticipate the need for cardiopulmonary bypass (CPB). Room air arterial oxygen tension (PaO_2) of less than 45 mm Hg predicts need for CPB.
         (c) Obtain arterial blood gas determinations, pulmonary function tests, and a ventilation-perfusion scan.
      (2) Cardiac
         (a) Assess for recent exacerbation of symptoms. Cardiac catheterization data are reviewed, and responsiveness to specific vasodilators during catheterization is assessed along with the severity of pulmonary hypertension.
         (b) Assess for evidence of right ventricular dysfunction with tricuspid regurgitation.
         (c) Obtain an electrocardiogram, cardiac catheterization, and echocardiogram. The need for partial CPB in lung transplantation is indicated by a mean PA pressure greater than 40 mm Hg and peripheral vascular resistance greater than 5 mm Hg/min/L.
      (3) Neurologic: The patient with pulmonary hypertension may have right-to-left shunting, so a history of embolic episodes must be evaluated. Avoid injection of even small amounts of intravenous air.
      (4) Hematologic
         (a) Assess for the use of anticoagulants.
         (b) Obtain values for hematocrit, partial thromboplastin time, prothrombin time, platelet count, and fibrinogen.
         (c) Polycythemia resulting from chronic hypoxemia is common.

b) Patient preparation
  (1) Laboratory tests
    (a) Assess for renal and hepatic dysfunction.
    (b) Hematocrit, coagulation profile, and others are obtained as indicated.
    (c) Hypokalemia is usually not treated because the heart/lung transplant graft is preserved with potassium, and implantation will reverse hypokalemia.
    (d) Gases often show resting hypoxemia of PaO_2 lower than 50 mm Hg with carbon dioxide retention.
    (e) Pulmonary function tests, heart catheterization, ventilation-perfusion scans, and arterial blood gases are done to predict the difficulties likely to be encountered during and after induction.
    (f) Diminished expiratory flow rates and air trapping may worsen hypoxemia and hypercapnia and may cause hemodynamic instability with induction.
    (g) Elevated PA pressures may indicate CPB to be necessary to prevent right-sided heart failure.
  (2) Premedications
    (a) No premedication is usually required by these patients because most of them are well motivated and psychologically prepared. Because of the respiratory status of these patients, sedation is not usually administered until in the operating room.
    (b) Patients may be hypoxic and receiving continuous oxygen therapy.
    (c) An increased risk of pulmonary aspiration results from the use of oral cyclosporine immediately preoperatively, the unscheduled nature of the surgery, and the incidence of recurrent laryngeal nerve damage.
    (d) Metoclopramide (10 mg) and ranitidine (50 mg) are given intravenously before surgery.
    (e) Cyclosporine, orally 1 to 2 hours before surgery, and azathioprine, intravenously 1 hour before surgery or before induction, are administered. The immunosuppressive regimen varies from center to center.
    (f) Continue with a specific antibiotic regimen. Cefazolin, 1 g intravenously, is given for single-lung transplantation. Coverage for *Pseudomonas* infection is used in patients with cystic fibrosis.
    (g) An epidural catheter may be placed for postoperative pain management unless the patient needs CPB and full heparinization.
c) Preoperative transplant concerns
  (1) Size matching is achieved with x-ray dimensions.
  (2) Organs are also matched based on ABO compatibility because the need for histocompatibility is still unknown and the tolerable ischemic time for lungs is relatively short (4 hours).

5. Intraoperative management of lung transplantation
  a) Monitors and equipment
    (1) Standard monitors are used.
    (2) Arterial line: Blood gases are sampled every 10 minutes.
    (3) A PA catheter is used.

(4) An additional ventilator may be needed to ventilate each lung optimally.

(5) Double-lumen tube (DLT): For double-lung transplant, a left-sided tube is used, and the left-sided bronchial anastomosis is performed distal to the tip.

(6) Use fiberoptic bronchoscopy to verify proper tube placement. Have the equipment to add continuous positive airway pressure and positive end-expiratory pressure (PEEP) intraoperatively.

(7) Agents to treat bronchospasm, right ventricular failure, and pulmonary hypertension should be available.

(8) Two 14- or 16-gauge intravenous tubes are used. Crystalloids should be kept to a minimum because transplanted lung has no lymphatics and cannot drain excess fluid.

(9) Have an axillary roll and beanbag for lateral decubitis position for OLV.

b) Anesthetic technique

(1) General endotracheal anesthesia is used, usually OLV with a DLT for single-lung transplants.

(2) Induction will include a modified rapid sequence induction with a slightly head up position.

(3) Aseptic technique is very important with these immunosuppressed patients.

(4) A slow induction with etomidate, ketamine, or narcotic helps to avoid severe drops in blood pressure. Propofol or thiopental (Pentothal) may also be used.

(5) Succinylcholine or a fast-acting nondepolarizing muscle relaxant is used for laryngoscopy. Preferably, drugs that do not release histamine or depress the myocardium are used (etomidate, vecuronium).

(6) Usually, a left-sided DLT is used for both single- and double-lung transplants, although a single-lumen tube may be used with double-lung procedures (airway separation at the tracheal level).

(7) Nitrous oxide is avoided. Oxygen and air may be used to maintain an oxygen saturation of more than 90% with a minimum inspired oxygen fraction (FiO_2) as tolerated.

(8) A low-dose volatile agent is used for maintenance, to provide some bronchodilation. A narcotic infusion is also used.

(9) Expect ventilation difficulties and progressive carbon dioxide retention, especially after OLV. Adjust ventilation to maintain normal arterial pH to prevent metabolic alkalosis.

(10) Central lines are placed after induction because most patients are unable to lie flat while awake. PA catheter should be withdrawn into its sterile sheath before lung resection (if floated on operative side) and may be refloated back after transplantation.

(11) Single-lung transplants are usually performed with the patient in a lateral position without CPB. With this method, the most critical time is the cross-clamping of the PA. In patients with restrictive disease, pulmonary hypertension, or poor right ventricular function, the sudden increase in pulmonary resistance may precipitate heart failure and hemodynamic collapse. Prostaglandin E_1, milrinone, nitroglycerin, and dobutamine may be used to control pulmonary hypertension and prevent right ventricular failure. If hemodynamic instability ensues, CPB is initiated as a last resort.

(12) Double-lung transplants are performed with the patient supine, and CPB is mandatory. Because systemic arterial supply to

the trachea is permanently interrupted, an omental wrap may be added.

(13) Following anastomosis of the organ, ventilation to both lungs is resumed. Peak inspiratory pressures should be kept to the minimal compatible with good lung expansion and FiO_2 of less than 60%.

(14) Steroids may be given, although studies indicate a decrease in anastomosis healing. Hyperkalemia may result from the preservative solution.

(15) The pulmonary catheter may be reinserted. Transesophageal echocardiography may be helpful in determining right or left ventricular dysfunction and evaluating pulmonary blood flow.

(16) Extensive retrocardiac dissection often leads to cardiac denervation and postoperative bleeding that is difficult to control. Loss of lymphatic drainage increases extravascular lung water and predisposes the transplanted lung to pulmonary edema, so fluids should be kept to a minimum.

(17) Emergence: Lungs are inflated to 35 cm H_2O before closure of the chest to reinflate atelectatic areas and check adequacy of bronchial closure. When surgery is done, both lumina of DLT are aspirated, and the tube is replaced with a single-lumen endotracheal tube.

(18) The patient goes to the intensive care unit intubated and ventilated.

c) Lung isolation: Achieved with a DLT (see the later discussion of thoracotomy)

d) Pulmonary artery clamping

(1) The PA is clamped to improve ventilation-perfusion mismatch and oxygenation, but severe pulmonary hypertension and right ventricular failure may develop.

(2) Treat pulmonary hypertension and reduce right ventricular afterload with vasodilators, but take care to avoid systemic hypotension. The patient may need inotropic support.

(3) One may need to unclamp the PA temporarily to allow further pharmacologic therapy. CPB may be needed if right ventricular failure cannot be controlled pharmacologically.

e) CPB

(1) This is performed if a patient with pulmonary hypertension cannot tolerate unilateral PA clamping.

(2) Indications: Arterial oxygen saturation less than 90% following clamping of PA, cardiac index less than 3 L/min/m^2 despite therapy with dopamine and nitroglycerin, or systolic blood pressure less than 90 mm Hg.

f) Position: Supine to lateral decubitus for single-lung and supine with arms above head for bilateral subcostal incision for double-lung transplantation

6. **Postoperative management of lung transplantation**

a) Infusion of narcotics is through an epidural catheter for postoperative analgesia.

b) If CPB was performed, an epidural catheter should be delayed until normal coagulation is determined.

c) Complications include pulmonary edema resulting from the lack of lymphatic drainage in the transplanted lung, and infection.

d) Keep the patient intubated (24 to 72 hours) until the transplanted lung begins to function properly and there are no symptoms of pulmonary edema and acute rejection.

e) Ventilation with PEEP is essential, but consideration of new anastomoses necessitates using minimal inflation pressures. Some centers may leave the DLT in place for several days and ventilate each lung individually to avoid overinflation of the native lung, gross ventilation-perfusion mismatching, and mediastinal shift.

f) Assess for signs of acute renal failure caused by toxicity from immunosuppressive therapy.

7. Complications of lung transplantation

a) These often include acute rejection, infections, and renal and hepatic dysfunction.

b) Frequent bronchoscopy with biopsies and lavage are used to differentiate between rejection and infection.

c) Other complications include damage to the phrenic, vagus, and recurrent laryngeal nerves and hemorrhage.

8. Intraoperative management of heart/lung transplantation

a) Monitors and equipment
   (1) Standard monitors are used.
   (2) An arterial line is placed.
   (3) Central venous pressure/PA catheter: Invasive monitors are usually placed before induction, but if the patient is very dyspneic in the supine position, monitors may be inserted following induction.
   (4) Transesophageal echocardiography may be used to optimize selection of fluid therapy, vasodilators, chronotropic, and inotropic agents.
   (5) Two 14- or 16-gauge intravenous tubes are used. One needs to anticipate a large blood loss; bleeding can be a major problem following termination of CPB.

b) Anesthetic technique
   (1) General endotracheal anesthesia is used.
   (2) Aseptic technique is very important with these immunosuppressed patients.
   (3) Airway equipment is presterilized, and bacterial filters are used.
   (4) Anesthesia is not induced until harvesting of graft is deemed normal by direct inspection.
   (5) Induction: Avoid further increases in peripheral vascular resistance by protecting against respiratory acidosis, light anesthesia, nitrous oxide, hypoxia, and extremes of lung volume. If the patient is hemodynamically stable, fentanyl is used to blunt pulmonary vascular response to intubation.
   (6) Do not use nitrous oxide because of exacerbation of pulmonary hypertension, reduction in the FiO_2, and expanding intravascular air bubbles.
   (7) Use cricoid pressure because of the risk of aspiration.

c) Termination of CPB
   (1) When tracheal anastamosis is complete, the lungs are ventilated with FiO_2 at 0.21 at 5 breaths/min and tidal volume (TV) of 6 mL/kg. When the bladder temperature reaches 36° C, increase ventilation to 10 breaths/min and TV of 12 mL/kg.
   (2) TV is adjusted to eliminate atelectasis and to obtain peak inflation pressure of 25 to 30 cm H_2O with the chest open.
   (3) Adjust FiO_2 in relation to pulse oximetry and arterial blood gases.
   (4) PEEP may be used to enhance oxygenation.
   (5) Avoid hypoxemia.

(6) A junctional rhythm is common in a denervated heart. Treat with isoproterenol to obtain a heart rate of 100 to 120 beats/min. It is common to see two P waves with sinus rhythm.

(7) Atropine and neostigmine have no affect on the heart rate in denervated heart. Hypertension will not cause reflex bradycardia.

(8) A denervated heart responds normally to norepinephrine, epinephrine, and isoproterenol.

(9) Care should be taken with intravenous fluids and vasodilators because cardiac output of denervated heart is very sensitive to preload.

(10) Use dopamine, isoproterenol, and epinephrine for inotropic support if pulmonary hypertension and right ventricular failure are present.

(11) Methylprednisolone, 500 mg, is given after CPB.

(12) Exacerbation of postbypass bleeding may result from the use of anticoagulants, the trauma of CPB, and depressed liver synthesis function. Coagulation therapy may be needed such as protamine, platelets, blood components, fresh-frozen plasma, ε-aminocaproic acid, desmopressin, and aprotinin. Severe bleeding may require cryoprecipitate or factor IX concentration.

9. **Postoperative management of heart/lung transplantation**
   a) Patient-controlled analgesia for postoperative pain management.
   b) Oliguria may be present; treat with mannitol and furosemide.
   c) Pulmonary edema may be present because of a lack of lymphatic drainage in the transplanted lung.
   d) The patient may have right ventricular failure from pulmonary hypertension and high right ventricular afterload.
   e) Avoid exacerbation of pulmonary hypertension by controlling for hypoxia, acidosis, and extremes of lung volume.

10. **Complications of heart/lung transplantation**
   a) Infection is a potential complication.
   b) There is the potential for nephrotoxicity from cyclosporine therapy.
   c) Complications of corticosteroid use include glucose intolerance, hypertension, hyperlipidemia, aseptic necrosis of the hip, bowel perforation, infection, and obesity.
   d) Complications of azathioprine include thrombocytopenia, leukopenia, hepatotoxicity, and anemia.

E. Mastectomy

1. **Introduction**
   Total mastectomy (simple or complete mastectomy) removes only the breast; no axillary node dissection is involved. It is used for the treatment of ductal carcinoma in situ. Radical mastectomy involves removal of the breast, underlying pectoral muscles, and axillary lymph nodes. There are two major alternatives to radical mastectomy: modified radical mastectomy and wide local excision of the tumor (partial mastectomy or lumpectomy) with axillary dissection. This treatment is followed by postoperative radiation therapy to the remaining breast.

2. **Preoperative assessment**
   Patients often have no other underlying medical problems. The anesthetic implications of metastatic spread to bone, brain, liver, lung, and

other areas should be considered. Preoperative assessment should be routine, with special consideration to the following:

a) Cardiac: Cardiomyopathies may result from chemotherapeutic agents (e.g., doxorubicin at doses greater than 75 mg/m^2). Patients exposed to this type of drug may experience cardiac dysfunction, and a cardiac consultation may be needed to determine ventricular function.

b) Respiratory: If the patient has undergone radiation therapy, there may be some respiratory compromise. Drugs such as bleomycin (greater than 200 mg/m^2) can cause pulmonary toxicity and necessitate administration of a low fractional inspiration of oxygen (0.30).

c) Neurologic: Breast cancer often metastasizes to the central nervous system, and there could be signs of focal neurologic deficits, altered mental status, or increased intracranial pressure. If mental status is altered, a full medical workup should be undertaken without delay. Postpone surgery until the cause is found.

d) Hematologic: The patient may be anemic secondary to chronic disease or chemotherapeutic agents.

3. **Room preparation**
Monitors and equipment are routine. If the procedure is for a superficial biopsy, monitored anesthesia care with sedation can be used. Be sure to place the blood pressure cuff on the arm opposite the operative site. The patient is placed in the supine position during the procedure.

4. **Perioperative management and anesthetic technique**
a) Routine induction and maintenance are used.

b) Pressure dressings are often applied with the patient anesthetized and "sitting up" at the conclusion of the procedure. Communicate with the surgeon if this type of dressing will be used, to time emergence more appropriately. If there are no further considerations, the patient may be extubated in the operating room.

5. **Considerations**
a) Deep surgical exploration may inadvertently cause a pneumothorax. The patient should be monitored for signs and symptoms of pneumothorax, which include increased peak inspiratory pressures, decreased arterial carbon dioxide pressure, asymmetric breath sounds, hemodynamic instability, and hyperresonance to percussion over the affected side.

b) Diagnosis is concluded by a chest radiograph.

c) Treatment includes placing the patient on a fractional inspired oxygen of 100% and insertion of a chest tube.

6. **Postoperative implications**
a) If the patient is unstable hemodynamically (which may suggest a tension pneumothorax), place a 14-gauge angiocatheter in the second intercostal space while the surgeons prepare for chest tube placement.

b) A postoperative chest radiograph may be needed if a pneumothorax is suspected.

F. Mediastinoscopy

1. **Introduction**
Mediastinoscopy is performed to diagnose and stage the spread of carcinoma of the bronchus. It permits biopsy of the subcarinal, peritracheal, and superior tracheobronchial lymph nodes under direct

visualization. It may also be used to place electrodes for atrial pacing of the heart. A small transverse incision is made above the suprasternal notch. The patient's head is turned to the left, and the mediastinoscope is placed in the space between the anterior surface of the trachea and the posterior border of the suprasternal notch.

2. **Contraindications**
    a) Absolute
        (1) Anterior mediastinal tumors
        (2) Inoperable tumor
        (3) Previous recurrent laryngeal nerve injury
        (4) Extreme debilitation
        (5) Ascending aortic aneurysm
        (6) Previous mediastinoscopy
    b) Relative
        (1) Thoracic inlet obstruction
        (2) Superior vena cava syndrome
3. **Preoperative assessment and patient preparation**
    a) History and physical examination
        (1) Respiratory
            (a) Assess for potential airway obstructions and distortions.
            (b) Assess the patient's smoking history.
            (c) There may be significant airway edema in patients with superior vena cava syndrome (edema, venous engorgement of head, neck and upper body, supine dyspnea, headache, and mental status changes).
            (d) A history of oat cell carcinoma may be associated with Eaton-Lambert syndrome, which may prolong the effects of nondepolarizing muscle relaxants.
        (2) Cardiac
            (a) Assess for hypertension, angina, dysrhythmias, and congestive heart failure, among others.
            (b) Reflex bradycardia and arrhythmias may be caused by mechanical compression on the aorta.
        (3) Neurologic
            (a) Assess for evidence of impaired cerebral circulation: stroke, carotid bruits, and transient ischemic attacks.
            (b) The mediastinoscope can exert pressure against the innominate artery and cause diminished blood flow to the right carotid and subclavian arteries.
    b) Diagnostic tests
        (1) Chest radiography is obtained.
        (2) Laboratory tests: Complete blood count, electrolytes, glucose, coagulation profile, type and cross-match, and others are used as indicated by the patient's condition.
        (3) Flow volume loops are helpful in determining whether an obstruction is fixed or intrathoracic or extrathoracic.
    c) Preoperative medications and intravenous therapy
        (1) Sedatives and narcotics: Use with caution in patients with poor respiratory reserve.
        (2) An 18-gauge peripheral intravenous line with minimal fluid replacement is used.
4. **Room preparation**
    a) Monitoring equipment: Standard

(1) Place the pulse oximeter on the right and a noninvasive blood pressure monitor on the left arm.
(2) Continuous assessment of the pulse oximetry waveform is done to identify compression of the innominate artery, with repositioning of the mediastinoscope as necessary.
(3) An arterial line may be placed on the right side.
(4) For patients with superior vena caval obstruction, placing the intravenous line in the lower extremity ensures venous access below the level of obstruction.
(5) Invasive monitors may be required in patients with large mediastinal masses.
  b) Pharmacologic agents
    (1) Atropine: Vagal-mediated reflexes
    (2) Cardioactive drugs
  c) Position: Supine; arms may need to be tucked to the side; supine with the table turned 90 degrees away from the anesthesia provider
5. **Anesthetic technique**
Local anesthetic with intravenous sedation and general anesthetic are used.
  a) Local anesthetic with sedation: The mediastinum has an extensive autonomic nerve supply but few pain fibers. This technique allows continuous monitoring of the level of consciousness in a patient with cerebrovascular disease or an airway obstruction.
  b) General anesthetic: Endotracheal intubation is used.
  c) Technique of choice: General anesthesia is used, with short to intermediate muscle relaxation.
  d) No nitrous oxide is used because of the pneumothorax risk.
6. **Perioperative management**
  a) Induction: Consider the use of reinforced or armored tubes, to avoid tracheal compression from the mediastinoscope.
  b) Maintenance
    (1) After endotracheal intubation, either an inhalation technique or a balanced anesthetic may be used.
    (2) Although the procedure is not very stimulating, the patient must remain motionless.
    (3) A muscle relaxant may be used to prevent the patient from coughing because this may produce venous engorgement in the chest or trauma by the mediastinoscope.
    (4) Patients with Eaton-Lambert syndrome are sensitive to succinylcholine and nondepolarizing muscle relaxants; therefore, the dosage should be reduced.
    (5) Positive-pressure ventilation of the lungs minimizes the risk of venous air embolism.
  c) Emergence
    (1) Extubate after full return of airway reflexes.
    (2) Consider an evaluation of vocal cord movement (extubate under direct vision).
7. **Postoperative implications**
Obtain chest radiographs: Pneumothorax is a complication; it is usually right sided. Signs and symptoms are tracheal shift, decreased blood pressure, cyanosis, decreased oxygen saturation, decreased chest movement, and decreased blood glucose. Treatment is with 100% oxygen, and prepare the patient for chest tube insertion.

8. **Complications**
   a) Sudden or massive hemorrhage from the innominate artery, the azygos vein, or aorta
   b) Recurrent nerve injury, infection, tumor spread, phrenic nerve injury, esophageal injury, chylothorax, air embolism, and hemiparesis

G. One-Lung Ventilation

1. **Introduction**
   One-lung ventilation (OLV) has numerous uses in thoracic surgery.
2. **Indications**
   a) Absolute: Control of ventilation and prevention of contamination of healthy lung
   b) Relative: Surgical exposure and removal of chronic pulmonary emboli
3. **Lung separation methods**
   a) Bronchial blockers: Univent tube. This is a single-lumen endotracheal tube with a built-in movable endobronchial blocker that is then manipulated into the right or left mainstem bronchus with the aid of a fiberoptic bronchoscope.
   b) Double-lumen endobronchial tubes: These are the most commonly used tubes for OLV. Two catheters are bonded together, with one lumen long enough to reach to the mainstem bronchus while the other, shorter portion of the catheter remains in the trachea above the carina. Inflation of both the tracheal and bronchial tube results in lung separation. In a right-sided tube, the bronchial tube is slotted to allow ventilation of the right upper lobe. Use a left-sided tube. A right-sided tube is indicated only when the left-sided double lumen tube is contraindicated (large lesion of left mainstem, tight left mainstem stenosis, and left mainstem bronchus distortion).
   c) Robertshaw: This is a double-lumen tube with no carinal hook. It is available as a left- or right-sided tube.
4. **Insertion of a double-lumen tube (Robertshaw)**
   a) Insert with the distal concave curvature facing anteriorly. Once tip of tube is past the vocal cords, the tube is rotated 90 degrees toward the desired mainstem. Advance the tube until resistance is met (about 29 cm).
   b) The proper position is then checked by inflating the trachea cuff and confirming bilateral, equal breath sounds. The bronchial cuff is then inflated, and bilateral equal breath sounds are confirmed. Then clamp each lumen individually and confirm OLV. A fiberoptic bronchoscope is then used to verify placement.
5. **Management**
   a) Maintain two-lung ventilation as long as possible. After the patient is placed in the lateral decubitus position, the position of the tube should be checked again.
   b) Verify proper placement of the tube using fiberscope if arterial hypoxemia occurs during OLV.
   c) If arterial hypoxemia persists despite proper tube placement, consider use of continuous positive airway pressure or positive end-expiratory pressure.
   d) A sudden increase in airway pressure may indicate tube displacement
   e) Reinstitute two-lung ventilation if needed.

H. Open Lung Biopsy (Wedge Resection of Lung Lesion)

1. **Introduction**

   Open lung biopsy involves the removal of a mass that does not require the removal of an entire pulmonary segment. This procedure is appropriate for a patient with limited pulmonary reserve who cannot tolerate lobectomy.

2. **Preoperative assessment**

   a) Cardiovascular: Electrocardiography; watch for right ventricular hypertrophy, conduction defects, and prior ischemia.

   b) Respiratory: Pulmonary function tests and chest radiographs if computed tomography of the chest is not available. Look for airway obstruction, which could interfere with double-lumen tube placement.

   c) Musculoskeletal: Patients diagnosed with lung cancer may have a myasthenic (Eaton-Lambert) syndrome, causing an increased sensitivity to succinylcholine and nondepolarizing muscle relaxants.

   d) Hematologic: Patients are often anemic because of their primary disease. Preoperative blood transfusions may be a consideration.

   e) Premedication: When epidural opioids are planned, avoid opioid or other sedative medications, which may potentiate the respiratory effects of the spinal opioids.

3. **Room preparation**

   a) Routine monitors and room setup are used.

   b) Consider a double-lumen tube if one-lung ventilation is needed. If so, have a fiberoptic bronchoscope available for checking tube placement.

   c) An arterial line may be required.

   d) Position: The patient is in the lateral decubitus or supine position. If the patient is supine, a wedge is placed under the back of the operative side.

   e) One large-bore intravenous catheter is needed.

   f) Fluid requirements are normal saline or lactated Ringer's solution at 2 mL/kg per hour.

4. **Perioperative management and anesthesia**

   a) Induction and maintenance are routine.

   b) Use a balanced technique of oxygen, isoflurane, and intravenous opioids (if an epidural catheter is not used).

   c) Nitrous oxide may be used with two-lung ventilation, but discontinue it with one-lung ventilation.

   d) Extubate the patient in the operating room, and transfer the patient in the head-up position to the postanesthesia care unit or intensive care unit with oxygen by mask.

5. **Postoperative management**

   Postoperative complications include atelectasis, pneumonia, and fluid overload.

I. Sympathectomy

1. **Introduction**

   Today, sympathectomy has become the method of choice to cure moderate and severe hyperhidrosis of the palms and the face, indicated especially if other therapies have not given an acceptable result. It is also the most efficient way to stop facial blushing, which causes considerable social difficulties and embarrassment in many persons affected by this disturbance. Open sympathectomy requires long periods of hospitalization and recovery. The endoscopic technique is very safe, if performed by a surgeon familiar with this type of procedure, and it leads to definitive cure in nearly 100% of patients.

2. **Preoperative considerations**
   a) Airway assessment
   b) Respiratory assessment: In patient with a history of lung disease, pulmonary function tests
   c) Patent large-gauge intravenous line
   d) Type and cross-match 2 units of blood
3. **Intraoperative considerations**
   a) Avoid nitrous oxide.
   b) Use 100% inspired oxygen fraction in one-lung ventilation.
   c) The procedure is performed with the patient under general anesthesia.
   d) Double-lumen tube: Use a fiberoptic technique to check placement.
   e) Use one-lung ventilation principles.
   f) Consider an arterial line.
4. **Complications**
   a) Horner's syndrome: This is the most feared complication, leading to a slightly smaller pupil and a disfiguring assymmetry of the face resulting from a slightly drooping upper eyelid caused by damage to the uppermost thoracic nerve node, the so called ganglion stellatum. The risk for this event depends mainly on the surgeon's familiarity with the procedure, ranging from less than 0.3% when the operation is performed by a surgeon with great experience. To correct this complication, a plastic surgery procedure (blepharoplasty, which involves shortening of the upper eyelid) is required.
   b) Treatment failure: This is a rare occurrence as long as the patient has not had a severe pleural disease rendering access to the ganglia difficult or impossible.
   c) Pneumothorax: This is a residue of air remaining between the lung and the thoracic wall, either from incomplete removal of the inflated gas or from minor leakage from the lung. Small amounts of air are generally reabsorbed spontaneously and need no further treatment (the patient should, however, avoid taking a flight during the next day or as long as the pneumothorax persists). Greater amounts (very infrequent) may require suction drainage for a day or two. With proper technique, when entering the thoracic cavity and when aspirating the gas at the end of the procedure, the surgeon can almost always avoid this complication. In any case, it can be easily treated.
   d) Compensatory sweating: Up to half of the patients may notice compensatory sweating in other locations (usually on the trunk or on the thighs, especially during physical exercise or high outside temperatures), which may range from barely noticeable to quite disturbing.
5. **Contraindications**
   Severe cardiocirculatory or pulmonary insufficiency, severe pleural diseases (tuberculous-pleuritis, empyema), and untreated hyperthyroidism are contraindications.

J. Thoracotomy

1. **Introduction**
   Thoracotomy is usually performed in an attempt to resect malignant lung tissue, but it may also be performed for trauma, infections, and parenchymal abnormalities, such as recurrent blebs. Because thoracotomy involves incising the pleura, all patients require a chest tube postoperatively. Most patients are older than 40 years and have a history of smoking. Many also have associated cardiovascular disease.

2. **Preoperative assessment**
   a) Cardiac: Exercise tolerance is an excellent assessment for cardiopulmonary reserve. Also question the patient about heart failure or arrhythmias. A 12-lead electrocardiogram is needed. Echocardiography and cardiac catheterization may also be useful in certain patients.
   b) Respiratory: Pulmonary function tests are routine for elective cases involving resections. Arterial blood gases are mandatory but cannot often predict postoperative functioning. Chest radiographs are mandatory. Most patients also have computed tomography of the chest. Question the patient about smoking history, bronchospasm, exercise tolerance, and pneumonia. Auscultate the chest carefully immediately preoperatively. Confer with the surgeon about one-lung anesthesia preferences and whether there are any foreseeable problems with tube placement (e.g., tumor in the mainstem bronchus).
   c) Neurologic: The incidence of Eaton-Lambert syndrome is increased in patients with lung cancer. Assess patients for any generalized weakness or any focal weaknesses that may be the result of stroke.
   d) Gastrointestinal, renal, and endocrine: These assessments are routine.

3. **Patient preparation**
   a) Laboratory tests include complete blood count, electrolytes, blood urea nitrogen, creatinine, glucose, prothrombin time, partial thromboplastin time, arterial blood gases; type and cross-match for at least 2 units (depending on the type of surgery and the patient's hemoglobin).
   b) Keep preoperative medications, especially narcotics, to a minimum in patients who are carbon dioxide retainers.
   c) Digitalization is recommended prior to pneumonectomy to help prevent postoperative heart failure. It will also reduce tachyarrhythmias intraoperatively.
   d) Have inhaled bronchodilators readily available. Many practitioners administer them prophylactically.
   e) Administer an antisialagogue, such as glycopyrrolate, to ease placement and verification of the double-lumen endobronchial tube.

4. **Room preparation**
   a) Monitoring: This is standard, with an arterial line. A central venous pressure or pulmonary arterial catheter is placed in patients with preexisting heart disease. Keep in mind that central venous pressure readings may be inaccurate while the chest is opened, and the pulmonary arterial catheter may interfere with pneumonectomy.
   b) Additional equipment includes double-lumen endobronchial tubes, at least two. (Balloon rupture on insertion is common.) A fiberoptic endoscope is used to check tube placement. Equipment is needed to

add continuous positive airway pressure and positive end-expiratory pressure intraoperatively. Epidural catheter insertion and infusion supplies are indicated, if used. Warming devices are needed for the patient and fluids.

c) Positioning: Lateral or supine with lateral tilt. A beanbag, arm "sled," and axillary rolls may be used. Check for lack of pressure on the downward arm, eye, and ear. Ensure that the patient's arms are not hyperextended.

d) Drugs and fluids: It is preferable to err on the side of underhydrating because these patients are prone to pulmonary edema. Usually, one gives use no more than 4 to 5 mL/kg per hour. Have ephedrine/phenylephrine available to treat hypotension.

5. **Perioperative management and anesthetic technique**
   a) Use standard induction techniques, keeping in mind that the positioning and placement of a double-lumen endobronchial tube require more time than does standard tube placement.
   b) Preoxygenate these patients.
   c) Arterial blood gases are obtained after induction for baseline so they may be compared with later results on one-lung ventilation.
   d) During one-lung ventilation, maintain tidal volume and place the patient on 100% oxygen. If hypoxemia is present (verify tube placement first), add 5 cm of continuous positive airway pressure to the "upward" (surgical) lung. If hypoxemia is still present, add 5 cm of positive end-expiratory pressure to the "downward" (ventilated) lung.
   e) Extubation at the end of the procedure is preferable unless the patient had a preoperative respiratory indication for remaining intubated (e.g., bronchospasm) or there were large fluid shifts. If the patient needs to remain intubated, the double-lumen tube must be replaced with a standard endotracheal tube.

6. **Postoperative considerations**
   Epidural anesthesia, patient-controlled analgesia, or another type of pain control (e.g., nerve block) should be planned preoperatively. The patient must understand and be able to perform deep-breathing exercises. Institute intensive care unit monitoring for at least 24 hours.

K. Thymectomy

1. **Introduction**
   The thymus gland is a bilobate mass of lymphoid tissue located deep to the sternum in the anterior region of the mediastinum. Thymectomy involves two surgical approaches: median sternotomy or transcervical.

   The thymus gland is believed to play a role in myasthenia gravis. This is a neuromuscular disorder in which postsynaptic acetylcholine receptors are attacked, inducing rapid receptor destruction.

2. **Preoperative assessment and patient preparation**
   a) History and physical examination
      (1) Respiratory (based on the patient with myasthenia gravis)
         (a) Weakness of pharyngeal and laryngeal muscles is associated with a high risk of aspiration. Assess the patient's ability to cough and handle secretions.

(b) "Myasthenic crisis": This exacerbation involves the respiratory muscles to the point of inadequate ventilation.
(2) Cardiac: Potential cardiomyopathy
(3) Neurologic
(a) Fatigability and fluctuating motor weakness of voluntary skeletal muscles worsen with repetitive use and improve with rest.
(b) Ptosis and diplopia are initial symptoms.
(4) Endocrine: Potential hypothyroidism
b) Diagnostic tests
(1) Pulmonary function studies are obtained as indicated.
(2) Laboratory tests include electrolytes, complete blood count, type and screen, and others as indicated by the patient's medical condition.
c) Preoperative medications and intravenous therapy
(1) Cholinesterase inhibitors retard the enzymatic hydrolysis of acetylcholine at cholinergic synapses and cause acetylcholine to accumulate at the neuromuscular junction. Continue up to the morning of scheduled surgery.
(2) Immunosuppressive drugs
(a) These drugs interfere with production of antibodies that are responsible for degradation of cholinergic receptors.
(b) Patients who have been receiving these drugs for more than 1 month in the past 6 to 12 months need supplementary steroids.
(3) Antisialogogues and H_2 (histamine$_2$-receptor) blockers: Patients with bulbar involvement should be evaluated to determine the safety of these drugs.
(4) Sedatives and narcotics: Use with caution in patients with poor respiratory reserve.
(5) Antibiotics are used.
(6) An 18-gauge intravenous catheter with moderate fluid replacement is used.

3. Room preparation
a) Monitoring equipment: Standard
(1) An arterial line is placed if blood gas monitoring is necessary.
(2) Some suggest placing the arterial catheter in the left radial artery for continuous monitoring in case the innominate artery is damaged.
b) Pharmacologic agents
(1) Standard agents are used.
(2) Depolarizing muscle relaxants are not to be used in patients with myasthenia gravis.
(3) Nondepolarizing muscle relaxants: Patients with myasthenia gravis have varying responses.
c) Position: Supine

4. Anesthetic technique and perioperative management
General anesthesia is used, and endotracheal intubation is required.
a) Induction
(1) When anesthetizing patients with myasthenia gravis, avoidance of all muscle relaxants is preferred.
(2) An inhaled anesthetic by itself should provide sufficient relaxation of skeletal muscle for intubation of the trachea.
b) Maintenance
(1) The ability to dissipate the effects of inhaled drugs at the conclusion of anesthesia is important for evaluation of muscle strength.

(2) The prolonged effects of narcotics, especially on ventilation, detract from the use of these drugs for maintenance.

c) Emergence

(1) Before extubating the patient, it is important to know that respiratory ability is adequate.

(2) Minimal extubation criteria must be met.

(3) Reversal of neuromuscular blockade is controversial; the additional anticholinesterase may increase weakness and precipitate a cholinergic crisis.

5. **Postoperative considerations**

a) Patients may need to be observed in an intensive care unit.

b) Anesthesia and surgery often decrease the need for anticholinesterase drugs in the postoperative period.

c) Discuss postoperative ventilation possibilities with the patient.

NEUROLOGIC SYSTEM

A. Arteriovenous Malformation Neurosurgery

1. Introduction

Arteriovenous malformations are congenital, intracerebral networks in which arteries flow directly into veins. The patient population with these malformations generally is younger than that with aneurysms. Patients may have bleeding, seizures or, less commonly, cerebral ischemia resulting from "steal" from normal areas or have high-output congestive heart failure. Neurosurgery is performed to correct arteriovenous malformations.

2. Anesthetic management

The anesthetic problems parallel those associated with patients undergoing aneurysm surgery (see the following discussion of cerebral aneurysm). Notably, arteriovenous malformations do not autoregulate their blood flow. The operation is likely to be longer and bloodier than that of aneurysm clipping. Surgery may be preceded by an attempt at embolization by the neuroradiologist, to diminish the risk of surgery. The neurologic examination should be repeated after embolization to document new deficits that otherwise could be attributed to anesthesia and surgery.

B. Cerebral Aneurysm

1. Introduction

An intracranial aneurysm is a localized dilation most frequently located at vessel bifurcations that develops secondary to a weakness of the arterial wall. No single mechanism has been identified in the pathogenesis of an intracranial aneurysm. Possible causes are as follows: congenital structural defects in the media and elastica of the vessel wall; incomplete involution of embryonic vessels; and secondary factors such as arterial hypertension, atherosclerotic changes, hemodynamic disturbances, and polycystic disease.

Approximately 5 million people in North America have cerebral aneurysms, with approximately 30,000 new cases of subarachnoid hemorrhage occurring annually. The peak age for rupture of a cerebral aneurysm is 55 to 60 years. There is also a slight female predilection, with aneurysmal rupture occurring in three women for every two men.

More than one third of patients with subarachnoid hemorrhage die or develop significant and lasting neurologic disabilities before they receive any treatment. A small hemorrhage occurs in approximately 50% of patients and is often tragically ignored or misdiagnosed. Even in patients who receive prompt care, only half remain functional survivors; the remaining patients die or develop serious neurologic deficits.

Aneurysmal rupture is prevented by maintaining a stable or low transmural pressure (TMP) within the aneurysm. TMP is defined as the difference between the mean arterial pressure (MAP) and the intracranial pressure (ICP). The relationship between the TMP and the wall stress or tension of the aneurysm is linear. Either an increase in the MAP or a fall in the ICP increases the TMP, the wall stress, and the risk of rupture. Cerebral perfusion pressure (CPP) is also equal to the difference between MAP and ICP; therefore, when one attempts to maintain a low TMP, one should be careful not to decrease the CPP and compromise cerebral blood flow.

Aneurysms may arise at any point in the circle of Willis. The most common locations for the occurrence of aneurysms are shown in the following table. Traumatic aneurysms develop as a result of direct trauma to an artery with injury to the wall.

Location and Occurrence of Cerebral Aneurysms

Location	Occurrence (%)
Internal carotid system	38
Anterior cerebral system	36
Anterior communicating junction	30
Internal carotid at posterior communicating junction	25
Middle cerebral system	21
Vertebrobasilar system	5

Mirror aneurysms of the internal carotid system are common, and other combinations of locations occur. The site of the bleeding aneurysm is best located by computed tomography studies, evidence of vasospasm in the immediate vicinity, and lobulation of the aneurysm wall on angiographic studies (see the table listing the location and occurrence of cerebral aneurysms).

2. **Preoperative assessment and patient preparation**
   a) History and physical examination: The neurologic findings depend on the hemorrhage location.
      (1) Level of consciousness: Brief loss of consciousness to persistent coma
      (2) Meningeal irritation: Nuchal rigidity, positive Kernig's and Brudzinski's signs, fever, irritability, restlessness
      (3) Visual disturbance: Blurred vision, double vision, or both; visual field defects
      (4) Cranial nerve involvement: Ptosis and dilation of the pupil, inability to move the eye upward or inward, papilledema, photophobia
      (5) Autonomic function: Diaphoresis, chills, heart rate and blood pressure changes, slight temperature elevation, altered respiratory rhythm
      (6) Motor function: Onset and worsening of hemiparesis, aphasia, dysphagia, hemiplegia, unilateral or bilateral transient paralysis of the lower extremities

(7) Increased ICP: Restlessness and lethargy, changes in level of consciousness and vital signs (Cushing's response, increased blood pressure, wide pulse pressure, decreased pulse rate), pupillary changes (mydriasis), impaired pupillary reflex, papilledema, vomiting, fluctuations in temperature, seizures, and respiratory changes

(8) Pain: Sudden onset of a violent headache usually beginning locally at the frontal or temporal region, generalizing to the entire head

b) Diagnostic tests

(1) Computed tomography shows blood in the subarachnoid space.

(2) Magnetic resonance imaging shows blood in the subarachnoid space.

(3) Cerebral arteriography identifies local or general vasospasm, outlining the cerebral vasculature.

(4) Skull radiographs reveal calcified walls of aneurysm and areas of bone erosion.

(5) Electroencephalography reveals shifts in midline structure.

(6) A brain scan shows local diminution of flow.

(7) Lumbar puncture is controversial: Features include increased opening pressures, elevated protein count, elevated white blood cells, cerebrospinal fluid with xanthochromia (hemolyzed red blood cells).

(8) Regional cerebral blood flow: Mean flow values are obtained for both hemispheres and for determination of cerebral vasospasm.

(9) Laboratory tests: Complete blood count, electrolytes, glucose, blood urea nitrogen, creatinine, urinalysis, coagulation profile, and type and cross-match are obtained.

c) Perioperative medications and intravenous therapy

(1) Antihypertensives: As indicated

(2) Antifibrinolytic agents: Aminocaproic acid (Amicar); not given with coagulopathies

(3) Corticosteroids: Dexamethasone

(4) Analgesics/antipyretics

(5) Pituitary hormone: Vasopressin injection

(6) Narcotic analgesic: Acetaminophen with codeine

(7) Agents to control vasospasm: Calcium antagonist

(8) Antibiotics

(9) Premedication: Should not obscure signs of neurologic deterioration; however, some sedation possibly needed to prevent anxiety and hypertension

(10) Two large-bore (16- to 18-gauge) intravenous catheters with variable fluid management

3. Room preparation

a) Monitoring equipment

(1) Standard

(2) Central venous pressure or pulmonary artery catheter to monitor cardiac function, adequacy of fluid, and blood replacement and to allow access to treat venous air embolism

(3) Arterial line: Right or left radial artery, depending on access requirement

(4) Foley catheter, to assess global renal function

(5) Peripheral nerve stimulator, to monitor muscle blockade

(6) Warming modalities: Minimal, with hypothermia's enhancing the brain's ability to tolerate ischemia and reducing the cerebral metabolic requirement

PART II Common Procedures

b) Pharmacologic agents
   (1) Prepare infusions of nitroglycerin, nitroprusside, phenylephrine, and dopamine.
   (2) Drugs: Mannitol, furosemide, lidocaine intravenous push, β-blockers (esmolol) are used.
   (3) Volume: Isotonic salt solution; glucose and water solutions are not recommended because they are rapidly and equally distributed throughout total body water.
       (a) Administer minimal volume before aneurysm clipping (2 to 3 mL/kg). The goal is to maintain hemodynamic stability, accounting for preoperative fluid and electrolyte status.
       (b) When the aneurysm is secured, deficits are replaced with additional volume as needed.
       (c) At the time of aneurysm dissection, blood must be available in case of rupture.

c) Position: The patient is placed in one of several positions, depending on the site of the aneurysm.
   (1) Aneurysms arising from the anterior part of the circle of Willis require that the patient be supine for a frontotemporal approach.
   (2) The lateral position for a temporal approach is required for aneurysms arising from the posterior aspect of the basilic artery.
   (3) Aneurysms arising from the vertebral artery or from the lower basilic artery require a sitting or prone position for a suboccipital approach.
   (4) Aneurysms arising from the anterior communicating artery are usually approached from the right, and those from the middle cerebral and posterior communicating arteries are approached from the side where the aneurysm is located.
   (5) Plan on the use of head-holder pins.
   (6) The airway most likely will be away from immediate reach.

4. **Anesthetic technique and perioperative management**
   a) The anesthetic induction should be slow and deliberate. The anesthetic depth should be sufficient to avoid the hypertensive responses that accompany laryngoscopy and endotracheal intubation.
   b) Anesthesia is induced with titrated doses of either thiopental or propofol. The addition of an opioid (5 to 10 mcg/kg of fentanyl or 1 to 2 mcg/kg of sufentanil) and intravenous lidocaine (1.5 mg/kg) further blunts the patient's response to sympathetic stimulation of laryngoscopy and intubation.
   c) Additional dosage of opioid or thiopental is required for the placement of the three-point pin head holder. Prior injection of local anesthetic minimizes the associated sympathetic stimulation. Epinephrine should not be included with the local anesthetic because delayed absorption (up to 30 minutes after injection) may produce significant increases in blood pressure.
   d) Isoflurane may be introduced following hyperventilation before laryngoscopy to increase the depth of anesthesia.
   e) Ventilation is controlled with administration of 100% oxygen to achieve an arterial carbon dioxide tension of 35 to 40 mm Hg with normal intracranial compliance. Mild hyperventilation (end-tidal carbon dioxide of 25 to 30 mm Hg) is instituted when intracranial compliance is impaired.
   f) Intubation can be accomplished with 1 mg/kg of rocuronium or another nondepolarizing muscle relaxant.

g) Anesthesia is maintained with air and oxygen or nitrous oxide in oxygen, with incremental titrated dosages of an opioid (fentanyl, alfentanil, or sufentanil) or an infusion of remifentanil and a muscle relaxant. Isoflurane may also be added in inspired concentrations not to exceed 1%.

h) Patients who have intracranial aneurysms require precise intraoperative control of blood pressure for prevention of recurrent bleeding and for counteraction of vasospasm.

i) Controlled hypotension is commonly used intraoperatively for making aneurysms softer and more pliable at the time of clipping, as well as for minimizing blood loss should aneurysmal rupture occur at this time. Sodium nitroprusside and an inhalation anesthetic agent are the drugs most widely used for inducing hypotension.

j) The safe limit of controlled hypotension has not been definitively established. Because autoregulation is maintained to an MAP of 50 to 60 mm Hg, some argue that this limit should not be exceeded. In addition, because patients with poor-grade aneurysms may not have intact autoregulation, some argue that a lower limit of 60 mm Hg should be adopted. Limits of autoregulation are shifted to higher pressures in patients with preexisting hypertension, so decreases in MAP should probably be limited to no more than 40% of preoperative values.

k) Many neurosurgeons now routinely use temporary proximal occlusion of the parent vessel, rather than induced hypotension, to facilitate clip-ligation of the neck of the aneurysm.

l) Any spontaneous movement during surgery can be disastrous; therefore, adequate depth of anesthesia and muscle paralysis are crucial.

m) Slack brain: This improves lesion exposure, reduces retractor ischemia, and decreases the chance of rupture.
  (1) Hyperventilate the lungs.
  (2) Administer thiopental.
  (3) Administer osmotic diuretics: Mannitol (0.25 to 2 g/kg).
  (4) Optimize venous drainage.

n) Aneurysm rupture can be catastrophic. The likely times of rupture include the following: dura incised and decreased ICP, excessive brain retraction and increased blood pressure, dissection of aneurysm, clip placed onto neck of aneurysm, and removal of clip holder from clip.
  (1) An abrupt increase in blood pressure during or after induction of anesthesia may indicate that an aneurysm has bled. The use of 100 to 200 mg of thiopental or 0.5 to 1 mcg/kg of sodium nitroprusside decreases the transmural pressure of the aneurysm, although hypotension can be detrimental at this juncture.
  (2) Intraoperative aneurysmal rupture necessitates maintenance of the MAP between 40 and 50 mm Hg or lower to facilitate surgical control of the neck of the aneurysm or the parent vessel. Alternatively, one or both carotid arteries may be compressed for up to 3 minutes to produce a bloodless field. Blood that is lost should be continuously replaced with whole blood, blood products, or colloid solution so intravascular volume is maintained.
  (3) Although barbiturates have been used for protection against focal cerebral ischemia, their efficacy has not been demonstrated in this clinical situation. However, some practitioners advocate the administration of thiopental (3 to 5 mg/kg) before temporary clipping.
  (4) Blood losses must be replaced immediately.

PART II **Common Procedures**

o) Emergence
   (1) Patients with good-grade aneurysms may be extubated in the operating room, although care must be exercised so coughing, straining, hypercarbia, and hypertension are avoided.
   (2) At the conclusion of the anesthetic, propofol, lidocaine, or small doses of alfentanil may be used for short-term anesthesia as the procedure is being finished and for reducing the hemodynamic responses to extubation.
   (3) Unless the patient is to be ventilated postoperatively, deep extubation is the preferred method.
   (4) Endotracheal tubes should be retained in patients with poor-grade aneurysms and in those who have had intraoperative complications; these patients will probably require postoperative ventilation.
   (5) Patients require monitoring in the intensive care unit for assessment of hemodynamics and neurologic status.

5. **Postoperative care**
   a) Postoperative care is directed at the prevention of vasospasm through the maintenance of intravascular volume expansion and moderate hypertension (MAP 80 to 120 mm Hg).
   b) Changes in the level of consciousness and the development of focal neurologic deficits are usually early signs of vasospasm. These clinical signs should be aggressively managed with hypertensive hypervolemic hemodilution and the use of dopamine for blood pressure support.
   c) Computed tomography should be used for ruling out other causes of neurologic deterioration, including rebleeding, infarction, and hydrocephalus.

6. **Postoperative complications**
   a) Delayed ischemia: Vasospasm; in areas of dysfunctional autoregulation, cerebral perfusion passively depends on systemic arterial pressure.
   b) Therapy is directed at improving cerebral perfusion by increasing systemic arterial pressure to approximately 150 mm Hg with either dopamine or phenylephrine.
   c) Increase central venous pressure approximately 10 to 12 mm Hg. Colloid is preferred to crystalloid because of the impermeability of the blood-brain barrier to low-molecular-weight proteins.
   d) Use calcium channel blockers, especially nimodipine, to prevent or treat delayed ischemia.
   e) Potential for recurrent bleeding: This usually occurs in the first 24 hours.

C. Cranioplasty

1. **Introduction**
   Cranioplasty can be performed for a bony tumor resulting from traumatic injury (e.g., depressed skull fracture) or, more rarely, from a condition resulting from a congenital malformation (e.g., fused suture lines). These defects may occur anywhere on the head, so the surgical procedure may take place with the patient in varying positions such as supine, sitting, prone, or supine with the head turned. Patients range widely in age, from the newborn to the elderly.

2. **Preoperative assessment and patient preparation**
   These are individualized according to the patient's need.
3. **Patient preparation**
   Complete blood count, electrolytes, blood urea nitrogen, creatinine, glucose, prothrombin time, and partial thromboplastin time (D-dimer or fibrin split products if disseminated intravascular coagulation needs to be ruled out) are used. Type and cross-match (for at least 2 units). Arterial blood gases are measured if the patient is being ventilated.
4. **Room preparation**
   a) Monitoring equipment: Standard. An arterial line and central line are used if suggested by the patient's history. Use a Foley catheter if surgery is scheduled for more than 2 hours. Some patients may have an intracranial pressure (ICP) monitor in place.
   b) Additional equipment: Determine the patient's position during surgery. If the patient is supine or supine with the head turned, a foam support aids in positioning the head. Longer ventilation tubing is needed because the table will be turned. When the patient is in the sitting position, a Doppler device and a central line (with a 60 mL syringe attached) are needed to assess and treat venous air embolism. With the prone position, use prone foam rest shoulder rolls and multiple pads. In all cases, a nasal endotracheal tube assists in clearing the surgical field and in stabilizing the endotracheal tube.
   c) Drugs and tabletop: Thiopental and etomidate are useful in cranioplasty because of their cerebral protective properties. Propofol is known to decrease ICP. Most surgeons desire to administer antibiotics during surgery, and they should be questioned about steroids and diuretics.
   d) Blood and fluid requirements: Glucose-containing solutions are best avoided in neurologic surgery. It is better to err on the side of under-hydration. Fluid is usually replaced with normal saline or lactated Ringer's solution at 2 to 4 mL/kg per hour. Blood loss may be substantial, and blood should be immediately available to avoid hypotension or crystalloid overload.
5. **Anesthetic technique**
   Induction is intravenous, with one of the agents known to decrease ICP. In severe trauma, one may wish to use only oxygen and to paralyze the patient. Avoid nasal intubation if there is any chance of a basilar skull fracture. For maintenance, keep the patient's mean arterial blood pressure slightly below the baseline and maintain normocarbia to slight hypocarbia. A constant infusion of thiopental, etomidate, or propofol with or without inhalation of isoflurane will help to maintain cerebral perfusion and will minimize the cerebral oxygen consumption. Muscle relaxation is not necessary if the procedure is confined to the skull, and the head is immobilized with tongs or some other type of fixator. Most practitioners leave the endotracheal tube in place until the neurologic status is certain to allow for regular respiration. Lidocaine is useful in minimizing cough.
6. **Postoperative implications**
   Assess postoperative neurologic functions. Pain in patients with altered neurologic status is usually controlled with parenteral agents. One must be watchful to avoid hypercarbia in neurologic patients receiving opiates.

PART II **Common Procedures**

D. Craniotomy

1. Introduction

Most intracranial neurosurgical procedures are performed for supratentorial mass lesions. Intracranial masses may be congenital, neoplastic (benign, malignant, or metastatic), infectious (abscess or cyst), or vascular (hematoma or malformation). Although the underlying pathologic process may be different for different lesions, the anesthetic considerations are the same. A craniotomy, or opening into the cranium, is made for removal of a tumor, relief of intracranial pressure (ICP), or to control bleeding. A flap is created by leaving the bone attached to the muscle so the tissue can be turned down. The dura is then incised in the opposite direction so its base is near the midline. After the surgery is complete, closure is performed in layers: dura, muscles, fascia, galea, and scalp.

2. Perioperative assessment and patient preparation

a) History and physical examination: The clinical signs of a supratentorial mass include seizures, hemiplegia, and aphasia. The clinical signs of infratentorial masses include cerebellar dysfunction (ataxia, nystagmus, dysarthria) and brain stem compression (cranial nerve palsies, altered consciousness, abnormal respiration). When ICP increases, frank signs of intracranial hypertension can also develop.

b) Preanesthetic evaluation should attempt to establish the presence or absence of intracranial hypertension. Computed tomography or magnetic resonance imaging data should be reviewed for evidence of brain edema, midline shift greater than 0.5 cm, and ventricular size. A neurologic assessment should evaluate the current mental status and any existing neurologic deficits.

c) Medications prescribed for the control of ICP (corticosteroids, diuretics) and anticonvulsant therapy should be reviewed to determine whether they have been properly administered.

d) Laboratory evaluation should rule out corticosteroid-induced hyperglycemia and electrolyte disturbances that may develop secondary to diuretic therapy.

e) Diagnostic tests

(1) Computed tomography, magnetic resonance imaging, cerebral arteriogram, electroencephalogram, brain scan, and regional cerebral blood flow

(2) Laboratory tests: Complete blood count, electrolytes, glucose, blood urea nitrogen, creatinine, urinalysis, prothrombin time, partial thromboplastin time, anticonvulsant levels, and type and cross-match

f) Preoperative medications and intravenous therapy

(1) The decision what and when to premedicate should be made only after a thorough patient evaluation.

(2) Benzodiazepines produce respiratory depression and hypercapnia.

(3) Premedication should be omitted in patients with a large mass lesion, a midline shift, and abnormal ventricular size.

(4) Opioids are universally avoided.

(5) If premedication is desired in those patients deemed appropriate, careful titration of intravenous midazolam may begin once the patient has been delivered to the preoperative holding area.

(6) In an attempt to help control ICP in patients with mass lesions, the head of the bed should be elevated 15 to 30 degrees during transport to the preoperative holding area and the operating room.

(7) Steroids and anticonvulsant therapy are continued up to the time of surgery.

(8) Two large-bore intravenous catheters are placed.

3. Room preparation

a) Monitoring equipment

(1) Equipment is routine.

(2) A central venous pressure catheter is used for patients requiring vasoactive drugs; it also allows access for treating venous air embolism.

(3) An arterial line is placed.

(4) Somatosensory-evoked potential testing or electroencephalography evaluates cerebral status and prevents optic nerve damage during resections of large pituitary tumors.

(5) Doppler evaluation monitors venous air embolism.

(6) A Foley catheter guides fluid therapy and frequent use of diuretics.

(7) Peripheral nerve stimulation monitors on the nonaffected side.

(8) ICP is usually assessed by ventriculostomy or subdural bolt.

b) Pharmacologic agents

(1) Prepare infusions of nitroglycerin, phenylephrine, nitroprusside, and dopamine.

(2) Drugs: Mannitol, furosemide, lidocaine, and calcium channel blockers are used.

(3) Volume: Glucose-free isotonic salt solutions are used.

(a) Judicious fluid administration minimizes the occurrence of cerebral edema and ICP, reduced cerebral perfusion pressure, and worsened cerebral ischemia.

(b) In most neurosurgical patients, fluids that contain sodium in a concentration similar to that of serum (e.g., lactated Ringer's solution or 0.9% saline) are administered in a volume that is sufficient for the maintenance of peripheral perfusion but that avoids hypervolemia (0.5 to 1 mL/kg/hour).

(c) Traditionally, less fluid is given than would be administered for nonneurologic surgery, although new recommendations are to keep patient's isovolemic, isotonic, and iso-oncotic.

(d) Avoid dextrose-containing solutions.

(e) Limit the volume of lactated Ringer's solution, and use colloid and normal saline for volume resuscitation.

(f) Limit hetastarch to 1 to 1.5 L to avoid coagulopathy.

(g) Maintain hematocrit at 30% to 35%.

c) Position: Supine

(1) Plan to use head-holder pins.

(2) The patient's head is elevated 15 to 30 degrees to facilitate venous and cerebrospinal fluid drainage.

(3) The head may be turned to the side to facilitate exposure; be careful not to impede jugular venous drainage, which will increase ICP.

(4) The table is usually turned 90 to 180 degrees away from anesthesia personnel. Secure the endotracheal tube and breathing circuit connections.

4. Anesthetic technique and perioperative management

a) Induction

(1) A smooth and gentle induction of general anesthesia is more important than the drug combination used. There is no evidence that one

technique or set of drugs is better than another. A reasonable induction sequence would combine preoxygenation, thiopental (2 to 4 mg/kg) or propofol (1 to 2 mg/kg), and a nondepolarizing muscle relaxant.

(2) There is no evidence that any of the induction agents (midazolam, etomidate, propofol, methohexital) is superior to thiopental.

(3) The hemodynamic response to intubation may be blunted with the administration of fentanyl (10 to 15 mcg/kg total dose) or lidocaine (1.5 mg/kg) administered 3 minutes before laryngoscopy.

(4) The dose of these induction agents may need to be adjusted according to the patient's age and physical status. Whatever agents are selected, the induction should be accomplished without the development of sudden hypertension or hypotension.

(5) Frontal, temporal, and parieto-occipital craniotomies are performed with the patient in the supine position. The head typically is elevated from 15 to 30 degrees to facilitate venous and cerebrospinal fluid drainage. The head may also be turned to the side to facilitate exposure. Excessive neck flexion may impede jugular venous drainage and increase ICP. The endotracheal tube should be stabilized with the anesthetist's hand during positioning.

(6) After positioning is complete, the chest should be auscultated to ascertain proper endotracheal tube position. The endotracheal tube follows the position of the chin: with extension of the neck the chin and endotracheal tube move cephalad; the chin and endotracheal tube move caudad with neck flexion. The anesthesia circuit connections must be firmly secured by simultaneously pushing and twisting to seat the plastic connectors. The risk of unrecognized disconnections may be increased because the operating table is usually turned 90 to 180 degrees away from the anesthetist, and both the patient and the breathing circuit are almost completely covered by surgical drapes.

b) Maintenance

(1) Maintenance of anesthesia may be accomplished with an oxygen/nitrous oxide/opioid technique, with a selected potent inhalation agent, or with oxygen/nitrous oxide and a continuous infusion of propofol.

(2) After endotracheal intubation, mechanical hyperventilation is begun, decreasing end-tidal carbon dioxide to 25 to 30 mm Hg, confirmed with arterial blood gas analysis.

(3) The patient should be covered with blankets or a forced air warming blanket to maintain a core body temperature.

(4) An opioid-based anesthetic technique with nitrous oxide in oxygen with low-dose (less than 1%) isoflurane is a popular choice.

(5) Incremental administration of fentanyl, sufentanil, or alfentanil or an infusion of remifentanil is acceptable. Alternatively, sufentanil, 0.5 to 1 mcg/kg load, followed by either incremental boluses (not to exceed 0.5 mcg/kg per hour) or an intravenous infusion of 0.25 to 0.5 mcg/kg per hour in combination with less than 1% isoflurane in oxygen may be used. Sufentanil administration should be discontinued approximately 45 minutes before the end of surgery to ensure that the patient awakens promptly. The primary advantage of remifentanil is rapid awakening. If the patient experiences hypertension or tachycardia near the end of surgery, the practitioner should consider giving either labetalol or esmolol, not additional opioids.

(6) A volatile agent (preferably isoflurane or sevoflurane) with little or no opioid supplementation can also be used for maintenance of

anesthesia. If isoflurane is used, the concentration should remain less than 1%. Hyperventilation in combination with less than 1% isoflurane generally results in stable intracranial dynamics.

(7) Nitrous oxide may be used in an anesthetic regimen if it is deemed desirable. However, if the patient is suspected to have a pneumocephalus or if there is a potential for air embolism, nitrous oxide use is contraindicated. Nitrous oxide expands both the pneumocephalus and the air embolus.

(8) Hyperventilation is an important adjunct to any neuroanesthetic technique. Hypocapnia decreases ICP before opening of the dura and attenuates the vasodilation produced by the volatile anesthetic agents. Optimal hyperventilation during surgery would yield an arterial carbon dioxide tension of 25 to 30 mm Hg.

(9) Skeletal muscle relaxation prevents patient movement at inappropriate times. It may decrease ICP by relaxing the chest wall, decreasing intrathoracic pressure, and facilitating venous drainage.

(10) In choosing an agent for muscle relaxation, the length of the procedure and the impact of the drug on ICP should be considered.

c) Emergence

(1) Most patients undergoing craniotomy can be extubated at the end of the procedure as long as intracranial hypertension is no longer present.

(2) Patients left intubated should remain sedated, paralyzed, and hyperventilated.

(3) Like induction, emergence must be slow and controlled. Straining or bucking on the endotracheal tube may precipitate intracranial hemorrhage or worsen cerebral edema. A brief period of coughing or gagging is probably not detrimental, provided the blood pressure is optimally controlled.

(4) Uncontrolled hypertension during emergence is associated with an increased incidence of postoperative intracranial hemorrhage.

(5) Judicious titration of short-acting antihypertensives (esmolol, labetalol) has great clinical utility in controlling the blood pressure during emergence.

(6) After the head dressing is applied and full access to the patient is regained, the use of anesthetic gases is discontinued, and the muscle relaxant is reversed.

(7) Intravenous lidocaine (1.5 mg/kg) can be given just before suctioning for cough suppression before extubation.

(8) Rapid awakening facilitates immediate neurologic assessment and can generally be expected after a pure opioid/nitrous oxide technique.

(9) Delayed awakening may result from residual opioid or remaining end-tidal concentrations of potent inhalation agent. Residual opioid may be carefully antagonized when necessary with naloxone in 40-mcg increments to attain a respiratory rate of 12 to 16 breaths/min.

(10) After extubation, the patient is transported to the intensive care unit postoperatively for continued monitoring of neurologic function.

E. Electroconvulsive Therapy

1. Introduction

Electroconvulsive therapy is used in the treatment of endogenous depression in patients in whom an adequate course of antidepressant

PART II **Common Procedures**

drugs has failed and in those who suffer from severe melancholia or are suicidal. It involves placement of electrodes on the scalp and application of a stimulus to elicit a brief grand mal seizure: a 2- to 3-second latent phase, followed by a tonic phase lasting 10 to 12 seconds, and finally by a clonic phase of 30 to 50 seconds. The clinical outcome from electroconvulsive therapy correlates with both duration of individual seizures and cumulative seizure time.

2. **Preoperative assessment and patient preparation**
   a) History and physical examination
      (1) Cardiovascular: Assess baseline status
         (a) Parasympathetic nervous system response to electroconvulsive therapy is immediate and may cause asystole, bradycardia, premature ventricular contractions, hypotension, and ventricular escape.
         (b) Sympathetic nervous system discharge follows within seconds manifested as increased heart rate, premature ventricular contractions, bigeminy, tachycardia, and severe hypertension.
         (c) Myocardial oxygen consumption often increases significantly.
      (2) Individualized based on the patient's history
   b) Relative contraindications: Angina pectoris, congestive heart failure, chronic obstructive pulmonary disease, thrombophlebitis, glaucoma, and retinal detachment
   c) Absolute contraindications: Recent myocardial infarction, recent stroke, intracranial mass, and pheochromocytoma
   d) Laboratory tests: Electrolytes, glucose
   e) Preoperative medications and intravenous therapy
      (1) Antipsychotic agents may compound the sedating properties of anesthesia.
      (2) Monoamine oxidase inhibitors predispose to hemodynamic instability and hypertensive crisis.
      (3) Patients receiving lithium may show delayed awakening, memory loss, and confusion postictally.
      (4) Anticholinergics modify parasympathetic nervous system response; glycopyrrolate causes tachycardia and central nervous system confusion.
      (5) An 18-gauge intravenous line with minimal fluid replacement is used.

3. **Room preparation**
   a) Monitoring equipment: Electrocardiogram, blood pressure cuff, pulse oximeter, and tourniquet
   b) Pharmacologic agents: Standard
   c) Position: Supine, arms safely tucked to the side or secured on armboards

4. **Anesthetic technique and perioperative management**
   Use general anesthesia and skeletal muscle paralysis.
   a) Induction
      (1) Methohexital (0.75 to 1 mg/kg intravenously): Its redistribution is more rapid than that of thiopental, thus decreasing recovery time; etomidate (0.3 to 0.4 mg/kg intravenously) may be an alternative.
      (2) Ventilate lungs with oxygen by mask.
      (3) Inflate a tourniquet on the arm opposite the intravenous catheter; this permits seizure visualization because the arm is isolated from the muscle relaxant.
      (4) Administer a muscle relaxant, usually succinylcholine (1 mg/kg intravenously).

b) Maintenance
  (1) Ventilation continues by mask with 100% oxygen.
  (2) An oral airway may be inserted to prevent tongue and tooth damage.
  (3) An electrical charge is applied to the head; avoid contact with the patient and stretcher.
  (4) Severe hypertension is expected; a short-acting intravenous agent may be needed.
c) Emergence: Mask ventilation is resumed until spontaneous recovery occurs.

5. **Postoperative implications**
  None are reported.

F. Epilepsy Surgery

1. **Introduction**
  Surgery is recommended in the patient with epilepsy when seizure control is intractable to conventional medical treatment. The goal of epilepsy surgery is to remove a focal area of epileptogenesis without causing neurologic deficits. Epilepsy surgery consists of two types. Intracranial electrode placement and testing may be required to localize epileptogenic foci. After localization, surgical resection may be performed. Extensive testing is required to define the focal area and its physiologic activity.

2. **Preoperative assessment and patient preparation**
  a) History and physical examination
    (1) Neurologic: Uncontrollable focal or generalized seizures. Obtain a description of seizure and prodromal symptoms. Obtain list of antiepileptic drugs. A WADA test may be performed (intracarotid injection of a barbiturate) to determine the dominance or speech function in the area of the surgery.
    (2) Gastrointestinal: Antiepileptic drugs may cause liver damage.
  b) Diagnostic tests
    (1) Complete blood count: A low hematocrit can be found in patients taking phenytoin or phenobarbital. A low white blood count can be found in patients taking carbamazepine or primidone. A low platelet count can be found in patients taking carbamazepine, valproate, ethosuximide, or primidone.
    (2) Obtain laboratory levels of antiepileptic drugs as necessary (e.g., phenytoin [Dilantin]).

3. **Room preparation**
  a) Monitoring equipment: A standard arterial line and a central venous pressure catheter are used for general anesthesia. A Foley catheter is used to monitor urine output.
  b) Additional equipment: Determine the position of the patient during surgery (supine, lateral, prone, semisitting, and/or table turned 90 or 180 degrees). A foam support aids in positioning the head. A long circuit, long intravenous tubing, and so on will be needed if the table is turned. Appropriate padding should be used according to the patient's position.
  c) Drugs: Short-acting benzodiazepines, narcotics, and/or a propofol infusion are acceptable for providing conscious sedation. If intraoperative electrocorticography is used, benzodiazepines and anticonvulsants must be avoided. It is best to avoid anesthetics that may trigger

seizure activity (e.g., methohexital, ketamine). Higher drug doses (e.g., muscle relaxants and narcotics) may be needed because of enzyme induction by anticonvulsant therapy. If a semisitting position is used, the anesthetist should be prepared for venous air embolism.

4. **Perioperative management**
   a) Induction: Local anesthesia with sedation and general anesthesia with an oral endotracheal tube are the anesthetic techniques of choice. Local anesthesia with sedation is used when the seizure focus is in the dominant hemisphere or if neurologic injury may be caused by temporal lobectomy. Screening is necessary to determine patients who will be able to tolerate the procedure. Standard induction is used for general anesthesia. If a stereotactic frame is used, fiberoptic awake intubation may be necessary.
   b) Maintenance: If general anesthesia is used, low-dose isoflurane, nitrous oxide, and an opioid infusion are generally used. Isoflurane must be turned off during intraoperative electrocorticography and can be resumed if resection follows. The anesthetist may be asked to elicit a seizure by inducing hyperventilation or administering methohexital. Muscle relaxants generally are not readministered after induction, to facilitate evaluation of motor response.
   c) Emergence: The patient should be emerged smoothly and quickly from anesthesia, to allow assessment for any neurologic deficits.

5. **Postoperative complications**
   Seizure, bleeding, and cerebral edema are postoperative complications. The patient must be monitored carefully for altered mental status. If the patient shows any signs of delayed emergence or altered mental status, a computed tomography scan should be performed.

G. Posterior Fossa Procedures

1. **Introduction**
   Neuropathology within the posterior fossa may impair control of the airway, respiratory function, cardiovascular function, autonomic function, and consciousness. The major motor and sensory pathways, the primary cardiovascular and respiratory centers, the reticular activating system, and the nuclei of the lower cranial nerves are all concentrated in the brain stem. All these vital structures are contained in a tight space with little room for accommodating edema, tumor, or blood. Posterior fossa procedures are discussed here.

2. **Preoperative assessment and patient preparation**
   a) History and physical examination
      (1) Neurologic: The history and physical examination should include a thorough neurologic evaluation with documentation. Pay special attention to signs and symptoms of brain stem involvement, such as focal neurologic deficits, depressed respiration, and cranial nerve palsies. Changes in level of consciousness may be secondary to increased intracranial pressure (ICP) resulting from obstructive hydrocephalus of the fourth ventricle.
      (2) Cardiovascular: Evaluate for cardiovascular disease and hypertension.
      (3) Pulmonary: Assess for a coexisting disease process.
      (4) Renal: Correct fluid and electrolyte abnormalities, if present.

(5) Gastrointestinal: Infratentorial tumors may involve the glossopharyngeal and vagus nerves. This may impair the gag reflex, increasing chances of aspiration.

(6) Endocrine: Steroid therapy may be in use.

b) Laboratory tests: Complete blood count, electrolytes, blood urea nitrogen, creatinine, glucose, prothrombin time, and partial thromboplastin time are obtained.

c) Diagnostic tests: Computed tomography and magnetic resonance imaging are used.

d) Preoperative medications: Anxiolytics may be given to alert and anxious patients. Patients who are lethargic or have an altered level of consciousness do not receive premedication.

e) Intravenous therapy: Central line, two 16- to 18-gauge intravenous catheters; consider a pulmonary arterial catheter. Estimated blood loss is 25 to 500 mL.

3. **Room preparation**

a) Monitoring equipment: Standard monitors, arterial line, central venous pressure, urinary catheter, with possible ICP monitoring, precordial Doppler, electroencephalography, electromyography, and sensory/somatosensory/brain stem auditory–evoked potential monitoring are used.

b) Additional equipment: Depending on the position of the patient, have appropriate padding available (i.e., prone pillow, doughnut, chest and axillary rolls); a fluid warmer is used.

c) Drugs

(1) Miscellaneous pharmacologic agents: Vasoconstrictors, vasodilators, inotropes, adrenergic antagonists, steroids, osmotic and loop diuretics, thiopental, lidocaine, fentanyl, nondepolarizing muscle relaxants, and antibiotics are used.

(2) Intravenous fluids: Use isotonic crystalloid solutions. Avoid glucose- containing solutions. Limit normal saline to less than or equal to 10 mL/kg/hr plus replacement of urinary output. If volume is required, administer 5% albumin or hetastarch and limit to less than or equal to 20 mL/kg. Maintain hematocrit at 30 to 35. Transfuse for a hematocrit of less than 25.

(3) Blood: Type and cross-match for 2 units packed red blood cells.

(4) The tabletop is standard.

4. **Anesthetic technique and perioperative management**

General anesthesia is used.

a) Induction: The goal is to minimize increases in blood pressure and ICP. Once an airway has been established, induce with thiopental (4 to 6 mg/kg), an opioid (fentanyl, 3 to 5 mcg/kg), and a nondepolarizing muscle relaxant (vecuronium, 0.1 to 0.5 mg/kg). To deepen the anesthetic, consider supplementing with fentanyl in 50-mcg increments to a total of 10 to 15 mcg/kg, midazolam, and lidocaine 1.5 mg/kg, 90 seconds before intubation.

b) Maintenance: Most commonly used maintenance anesthetics are opioid, nitrous oxide, and volatile inhalational agents. The most common opioid is fentanyl, and the most common inhalational agent is isoflurane. High-dose narcotic technique may be also considered. Maintain arterial carbon dioxide pressure between 25 and 30 mm Hg. Cardiovascular instability secondary to surgical stimulation of the trigeminal, glossopharyngeal, or vagus nerves is common.

c) Positioning: The patient may be placed in the sitting, lateral, prone, park-bench, or three-quarters prone position. If the sitting position is used, the increased incidence of venous air embolism and cardiovascular instability must be considered.

d) Emergence: Emergence should be as smooth as possible. Avoid bucking or straining on the endotracheal tube. Consider lidocaine, 1.5 mg/kg, 90 seconds before suctioning or extubation. Antihypertensive medications are administered to control systemic hypertension.

5. **Postoperative implications**
   Closely observe for the occurrence of seizures, hemorrhage, edema, increased ICP, neurologic deficits, and tension pneumocephalus. Impairment of cranial nerves or the respiratory center in the brain stem may require postoperative mechanical ventilation.

H. Stereotactic Surgery

1. **Introduction**
   Stereotactic surgery is a neurosurgical technique that makes detailed use of the relationship between the three-dimensional space occupied by intracranial structures or lesions and an extracranial reference system to guide instruments to such targets accurately and precisely. This type of technique is used when the lesion is small or is located deep within brain tissue or as a means of obtaining a biopsy of a lesion for diagnosis.

   Stereotactic procedures can be frame based or image guided (frameless). If the frame-based procedure is used, the frame is anchored to the skull with either four pins or four screws. Application typically takes place outside the operating room using local anesthetic. In the cooperative adult, frame application takes only 5 to 10 minutes. For children, general anesthesia is used. If the image-guided procedure is used, small markers called fiducials are placed on the head with adhesive. An imaging study is then performed to provide a system of reference.

2. **Preoperative assessment**
   a) History and physical examination: Neurologic symptoms vary, depending on the site and size of the lesion; they should be carefully documented. In addition to the routine test, computed tomography is performed preoperatively with the frame in place to determine stereotactic coordinates. Once the coordinates are established, the frame must not be moved on the head until the operation is complete.

   b) Laboratory tests: Complete blood count and other tests are as indicated by the history and physical examination.

   c) Diagnostic tests: Computed tomography of the head and other tests are as indicated by the history and physical examination.

   d) Medication: Usually, medication is not required.

3. **Room preparation**
   a) Monitoring equipment: Standard
   b) Additional equipment
      (1) Stereotactic instruments
      (2) Monitoring, ventilation, and oxygenation equipment during transport
   c) Drugs
      (1) Standard emergency drugs
      (2) Standard tabletop

(3) Intravenous fluids: 18-gauge intravenous line with standard replacement therapy

4. **Anesthetic technique**
   a) General endotracheal anesthesia or monitored anesthesia care is used.
   b) In adults, the stereotactic frame or fiducials are placed the morning of the operation, and the patient is taken to the radiologic suite for computed tomography to determine stereotactic coordinates. The patient is then brought to the operating room with the frame or fiducials still in place. If the operation is to be a biopsy, it is generally done using monitored anesthesia care.
   c) If a complete resection is planned, such as in the removal of an arteriovenous malformation, general endotracheal anesthesia is used. In children, it is usually necessary to induce general anesthesia before placing the frame, thus necessitating the maintenance of general anesthesia during the computed tomography. The child is then moved to the operating room still anesthetized, and the operation is completed.

5. **Perioperative management**
   a) Induction
      (1) If monitored anesthesia care is planned, oxygen is administered by nasal prongs, and the patient is lightly sedated with combinations of droperidol to prevent nausea and vomiting, midazolam to provide amnesia, and meperidine or fentanyl to provide analgesia. The patient must be able to communicate with the surgeon as needed throughout the operation.
      (2) Stereotactic neurosurgery for movement disorders such as Parkinson's disease requires the anesthetist to limit sedation to ensure that the patient will be able to cooperate with the surgeon. If general endotracheal anesthesia is needed with frame-based stereotaxy, fiberoptic laryngoscopy is necessary before inducing anesthesia because the frame precludes intubation by direct laryngoscopy. Once endotracheal intubation is established, anesthesia may be induced with sodium thiopental or propofol, followed by a nondepolarizing blocking drug to facilitate positioning of the patient.
   b) Maintenance
      (1) If general anesthesia is used, the ideal drug is one that decreases intracranial pressure and the cerebral metabolic rate of oxygen, maintains cerebral autoregulation, redistributes flow to the potentially ischemic areas, and provides protection of the brain from focal ischemia.
      (2) If children are to be transported from the site of placement of the stereotactic frame to the radiologic suite and then the operating room, it is best to use inhalational anesthesia with isoflurane and 100% oxygen with spontaneous ventilation to ensure adequate ventilation during transport and study. Opiates and neuromuscular blocking drugs should not be administered until the child is in the operating suite.
      (3) Hyperventilation and diuresis should be avoided in image-guided stereotaxy, because they may cause the brain to shift. If a frame is used, the key to remove it from the patient's head must always be available.
   c) Emergence: No special consideration is reported. The patient is extubated awake and after the return of airway reflexes. If the surgeon

PART II **Common Procedures**

suspects that the patient may have a slow recovery or a neurologic injury, or if the anesthetist believes that recovery from the anesthesia may be delayed, it is advisable to leave the endotracheal tube in place at least overnight.

6. **Postoperative implications**
Focal bleeding may occur postoperatively, causing the onset of a neurologic deficit.

I. Transsphenoidal Tumor Resections

1. **Introduction**
Approximately 10% of intracranial neoplasms are found in the pituitary gland and come to clinical attention because of their mass effects or the hypersecretion of pituitary hormones. These tumors are rarely metastatic and produce local symptoms through bone invasion, hydrocephalus, and compression of a cranial nerve (most often the optic nerve). Frontal-temporal headache and bitemporal hemianopsia are the most common nonendocrine symptoms of enlarging pituitary lesions. Nonsecretory pituitary tumors account for approximately 20% to 50% of lesions in this area and are classified as chromophobe adenomas.

Tumors that secrete excess growth hormone produce acromegaly. Increased growth hormone increases the size of the skeleton, particularly the bones and soft tissues of the hands, feet, and face. The enlarged facial structures may increase the likelihood of difficult intubation. Excess growth hormone may also contribute to the development of coronary artery disease, hypertension, and cardiomyopathy. Hyperglycemia is also a common finding, reflecting a growth hormone–induced glucose intolerance. This discussion focuses on transsphenoidal tumor resection.

2. **Surgical approach**
Medical and surgical therapies exist for both functional and nonfunctional pituitary tumors. Cushing introduced the oronasal midline rhinoseptal transsphenoidal approach to the pituitary in 1910. In 1962, Hardy helped to reintroduce the procedure with the introduction of the surgical microscope and microsurgical dissection techniques. These advances simplified tumor removal by making it easier to distinguish tumor from normal gland.

Transsphenoidal surgery offers several advantages over the intracranial approach. Statistically, morbidity and mortality rates are reduced because of a decrease in blood loss and less manipulation of brain tissue. In addition, the risk of inducing panhypopituitarism is reduced, and the incidence of permanent diabetes insipidus is lower. For patients with large tumors (greater than 10 mm), tumors of uncertain type, and tumors that have substantial extrasellar extension, the transsphenoidal approach is inadequate and a bifrontal intracranial approach is required for successful removal.

3. **Preoperative assessment and patient preparation**
a) History and physical examination: Patients undergo transsphenoidal operations for the treatment of hypersecreting pituitary tumors. Clinical symptoms of pituitary tumors include amenorrhea, galactorrhea, Cushing's disease, and acromegaly.

Each preoperative condition has its own constellation of systemic disorders and accompanying effects on intracranial dynamics that must be considered when an anesthetic technique is selected. Pituitary tumors can damage decussating nasal optic fibers, producing blindness in the temporal half of the visual field of both eyes (bitemporal heteronymous hemianopia). Occasionally, an aneurysm of one of the internal carotid arteries may produce nasal hemianopia on the affected side. Patients who have Cushing's disease may also suffer from hypertension, diabetes, osteoporosis, obesity, and friability of skin and connective tissue. Patients who have acromegaly may have hypertension, cardiomyopathy, diabetes, and osteoporosis, as well as prognathism, cartilaginous and soft tissue hypertrophy of the larynx, and enlargement of the tongue, which may complicate intubation of the trachea. Patients who have panhypopituitarism may exhibit hypothyroidism, requiring preoperative thyroid supplementation.

  (1) Respiratory: Airway changes can occur with acromegaly (the patient may require a smaller oral endotracheal tube). Problems occur with mask fit. Thoroughly evaluate the airway; check for dyspnea, stridor, and hoarseness.

  (2) Cardiac: Common findings are hypertension, coronary artery disease, and congestive heart failure in acromegaly.

  (3) Neurologic: A nonfunctional gland usually is discovered because of increased size, resulting in neurologic changes. A hypersecreting gland is found when small.

  (4) Renal: Electrolyte imbalance is present.

 b) Diagnostic tests: Complete blood count. Patients with panhypopituitarism require hormone replacement before surgery. They should be euthyroid and should be receiving corticosteroids (assess for diabetes mellitus); patients may be taking intranasal vasopressin. Diabetes insipidus may occur after corticosteroid is introduced. Check electrolytes and random blood glucose concentrations as indicated by the history and physical examination.

 c) Preoperative medications and intravenous therapy: Replace deficits and hourly surgical loss; one large-bore intravenous line is needed.

4. **Room preparation**

 a) Monitoring equipment: Standard if the sitting position is used; a central venous pressure catheter and precordial Doppler device are needed; consider an arterial line and a Foley catheter. Visual- or auditory-evoked potentials may be monitored.

 b) Additional medications and continuous infusions: Adjunct medicines to treat hypertension and tachycardia; cocaine, and epinephrine preparation are used.

 c) Position: The transsphenoidal approach usually necessitates that the head and back be elevated 10 to 20 degrees. The patient's head is supported by a three-point pin head holder and centered within a C-arm fluoroscopy unit for radiographic control during surgery. The patient's arms are placed at the sides and padded so injury to the ulnar nerves is avoided.

5. **Anesthetic technique and perioperative management**
Use general anesthesia, oral endotracheal intubation (right-angled endotracheal or anode tube).

 a) Induction and maintenance

  (1) The patient's airway is shared with the surgeon; therefore, great attention must be directed to the proper securing of the

endotracheal tube and anesthesia circuit to prevent unintended extubation and anesthesia circuit disconnection.

(2) Hyperventilation is avoided after anesthetic induction because reductions in intracranial pressure result in retraction of the pituitary into the sella, thus making surgical access difficult.

(3) The anesthetist should also consider the potential for massive hemorrhage because the carotid arteries lie adjacent to the suprasellar area and may be inadvertently injured. Massive bleeding from the carotid artery would probably be fatal.

(4) After anesthetic induction and intubation, the endotracheal tube is typically moved to the left corner of the patient's mouth and is secured to the chin with adhesive and tape. A right-angled endotracheal tube may be effective because these tubes are prebent and curve along the mandible when exiting the mouth.

(5) The esophageal stethoscope and temperature probe are inserted and secured on the lower left as well, leaving the upper lip totally free.

(6) An orogastric tube is placed, aspirated, and then put to gravity drainage during the procedure.

(7) The oropharynx is then packed with moist cotton gauze.

(8) The patient's eyes are first taped closed and then are covered with cotton-padded adhesive patches to prevent corneal abrasion and seepage of cleansing solution and blood into the eyes.

(9) Thiopental, propofol, an opioid (fentanyl, sufentanil, alfentanil, or remifentanil), and a neuromuscular relaxant (either succinylcholine or a nondepolarizing neuromuscular relaxant for intubation, followed by a selected nondepolarizing agent) with a combination of nitrous oxide and oxygen comprise a commonly used anesthetic technique for this procedure.

(10) Isoflurane may be added in low concentrations for blood pressure control; alternatively, it may be used as the primary anesthetic drug (after the establishment of hyperventilation).

(11) The topical use of cocaine and the oral and nasal submucosal injection of local anesthetic solutions containing epinephrine help to constrict gingival and mucosal vessels and dissect the nasal mucosa away from the cartilaginous septum.

(12) Epinephrine use may produce hypertension or dysrhythmias, or both; cocaine interferes with the intraneuronal uptake of catecholamines and can augment both the hypertensive and dysrhythmogenic properties of epinephrine.

(13) A total dose of 200 mg of cocaine should not be exceeded. Persistent dysrhythmias may require treatment with lidocaine or possibly a β-blocker.

(14) Hypertension may be controlled with an increased concentration of the selected inhalation agent or with small intravenous doses of hydralazine, labetalol, or esmolol.

(15) In some cases, it may be necessary to insert a catheter into the lumbar subarachnoid space to facilitate the injection of preservative-free saline to delineate the suprasellar margins. If air is injected, nitrous oxide must be discontinued from the anesthetic mixture because of rapid diffusion into the air now present in the closed cranial vault.

b) Emergence

(1) Deep extubation is the method of choice unless contraindicated by airway management at induction as described for the previously discussed procedures.

(2) Intravenous lidocaine, 1.5 mg/kg given approximately 3 minutes before suctioning and extubation, decreases coughing, straining, and hypertension.

(3) Postoperatively, patients should be responsive to commands in the recovery room. Steroid therapy is continued throughout this period and is tapered over time, if appropriate.

6. Postoperative considerations

a) Postoperative endocrine dysfunction—namely, diabetes insipidus—may occur when the resection involves the suprasellar area.

b) Diabetes insipidus that occurs after most transsphenoidal procedures is usually self-limited and resolves within 1 week to 10 days.

c) Although the onset is usually on the first or second postoperative day, diabetes insipidus may develop during the perioperative period or in the immediate recovery period. Intraoperative diagnosis is made with the sudden onset of diuresis. The diagnosis may be confirmed with concurrent urine and serum osmolalities. If diabetes insipidus persists or if it becomes difficult to match urinary losses, the patient may receive aqueous vasopressin (Pitressin) or desmopressin (DDAVP). Intravenous DDAVP is longer acting and is not associated with the coronary vasoconstriction that follows administration of aqueous vasopressin.

J. Venous Air Embolism

1. Introduction

Although there are numerous physiologic consequences of the seated position, additional clinical considerations involve the choice of anesthetic technique and monitoring devices for the detection of venous air embolism (VAE). The potential for VAE has been traditionally associated with neurosurgical anesthesia. Clinical situations that contribute to the occurrence of VAE are as follows:

Patient positioning (seated, prone, steep Trendelenburg)
Transfusion therapy
Intravenous therapy
Central venous catheterization
Hepatic surgical procedures
Urologic surgical procedures
Posterior spinal procedures
Epidural or caudal catheter insertion
Bone marrow harvesting
Laparoscopy
Radical pelvic surgery

Air may also be entrained from the cranial pin sites of the Mayfield head holder and from improperly connected vascular lines (arterial, central, and intravenous). The occurrence of VAE depends on the development of a negative pressure gradient between the operative site and the right side of the heart. As the gradient between the cerebral veins and the right atrium increases, the potential for air entry increases. The estimated incidence of VAE during neurosurgical procedures ranges from 5% to 50%, with an increased incidence in the seated position.

PART II **Common Procedures**

The physiologic consequences of VAE depend on both the volume and the rate of air entrainment. In the canine model, large cumulative doses of air produce sudden cardiac arrest and death; smaller cumulative doses produce less profound physiologic consequences, including increased pulmonary artery and central venous pressure, decreased cardiac output with accompanying hypotension, progressive hypotension, and dysrhythmias.

2. **Paradoxical air embolism**

Paradoxical air embolism develops with the entry of air into the systemic circulation. Persons with an existing anatomic connection between the right and left sides of the heart (atrial or ventricular septal defect, probe-patent foramen ovale) are particularly at risk. A patent foramen ovale may exist in 30% to 35% of the population. If right-sided heart pressures exceed left-sided pressures, which may occur in the fluid-restricted neurosurgical patient, systemic air may embolize and enter the arterial circulation through a probe-patent foramen ovale.

Patients requiring a seated position for their neurosurgical procedure should be carefully evaluated with echocardiograms if a previous history suggests the presence of an intracardiac defect (presence of heart murmur) or probe-patent foramen ovale. The presence of a probe-patent foramen ovale may be elicited with the injection of contrast material before, during, and after the patient produces a Valsalva maneuver. If a probe-patent foramen ovale is identified, the surgical procedure should be accomplished in an alternative position.

3. **Detection**

a) Air enters the venous circulation as small bubbles that pass through the right side of the heart, entering the pulmonary arterioles. A reflex sympathetic pulmonary vasoconstriction is produced following the release of endothelial mediators, which are ultimately responsible for the clinical manifestations (pulmonary hypertension, hypoxemia, carbon dioxide retention, increased dead-space ventilation, and decreased end-tidal carbon dioxide).

b) Signs and symptoms: These include decreased end-tidal carbon dioxide and nitrogen, hypertension, "mill-wheel" murmur noted by Doppler, dysrhythmias, and increased right atrial and pulmonary arterial pressures.

c) The continued entry of air produces an airlock within the right ventricle and causes right ventricular failure and decreased cardiac output. Altered ventilation-perfusion relationships parallel the hemo-dynamic changes. Obstructed pulmonary blood flow increases dead-space ventilation, resulting in decreased end-tidal carbon dioxide. The entry of a large volume of air in the alveoli may be detected by the sudden appearance of end-tidal nitrogen.

d) The selection of appropriate monitoring for the detection of VAE is based on the various sensitivities of the available monitoring modalities.

e) Precordial Doppler monitoring can detect air entrainment at rates as small as 0.0021 mL/kg/min. The Doppler probe is affixed over the right side of the heart along the right sternal border between the third and sixth intercostal spaces. Proper positioning over the right atrium is confirmed if a change in Doppler signal is elicited when a 10-mL bolus of saline is injected rapidly into a previously placed right central venous catheter.

f) The placement of a right atrial or pulmonary artery catheter affords the means for diagnosis and recovery of intravenous air and also reflects cardiac preload. When a right atrial catheter is placed, it is recommended that either radiographic confirmation or electrocardiographic confirmation of proper placement of the catheter tip be obtained.

g) Advantages and disadvantages of select monitors for detection of venous air embolism are noted in the following table.

h) Capnography complements the capabilities of the Doppler device because small, hemodynamically insignificant air emboli detected with the Doppler device can be differentiated from emboli that may produce arterial hypotension. Capnography is virtually as sensitive as pulmonary artery pressure monitoring but has the added advantage of being noninvasive.

Monitors for Detection of Venous Air Embolism

Monitor	Advantages	Disadvantages
Precordial Doppler	Noninvasive Most sensitive noninvasive monitor Earliest detector (before air enters pulmonary circulation)	Nonquantitative May be difficult to place in obese patients, patients with chest wall deformity, or those in the prone or lateral position False negative if air does not pass beneath ultrasonic beam (about 10% of cases); useless during electrocautery Intravenous mannitol may mimic intravascular air
Pulmonary artery catheter	Quantitative, slightly more sensitive than end-tidal carbon dioxide Widely available Placed with minimum difficulty by experienced clinicians Can detect right atrial pressure greater than pulmonary capillary wedge pressure	Small lumen, less air aspiration than with right atrial catheter Placement for optimal air aspiration may not allow pulmonary capillary wedge pressure measurement Nonspecific for air
Capnography (end-tidal carbon dioxide)	Noninvasive Sensitive Quantitative Widely available	Nonspecific for air Less sensitive than Doppler, pulmonary artery catheter Accuracy affected by tachypnea, low cardiac output, chronic obstructive pulmonary disease

PART II   Common Procedures

Continued

Monitors for Detection of Venous Air Embolism—cont'd

Monitor	Advantages	Disadvantages
End-tidal nitrogen	Specific for air Detects air earlier than does end-tidal carbon dioxide	May not detect subclinical air embolism May indicate air clearance from pulmonary circulation prematurely Accuracy affected by hypotension
Transesophageal echocardiography	Most sensitive detector of air Can detect air in left side of heart and aorta	Invasive, cumbersome Expensive Must be observed continuously Not quantitative May interfere with Doppler

    i) Transesophageal echocardiography is the most sensitive method of air embolism detection, but it is also the most expensive. With transesophageal echocardiography, it is possible to observe both cardiac contractility and air bubbles as they pass through the heart. The detection of a "mill-wheel" murmur through a precordial or esophageal stethoscope is a late sign of air entrainment.

4. Treatment

    a) Detection of venous air embolism should prompt the following steps. First, the surgeon should be notified, and nitrous oxide should be immediately discontinued, 100% oxygen delivered, and the right atrial catheter aspirated.

    b) The surgeon should flood the surgical field with irrigation or pack the area with saline-soaked sponges.

    c) A Valsalva maneuver or bilateral compression of the jugular veins for 5 to 10 seconds increases the cerebral venous pressure and induces bleeding.

    d) The addition of positive end-expiratory pressure also slows air entry. However, 10 to 15 cm H_2O may be required to elevate venous pressure effectively when the patient's head is elevated.

    e) The patient's head should be lowered to decrease air entrainment. This may be accomplished by placing the operating table in Trendelenburg's position. If air entrainment continues, the anesthetist should ask for an assistant. A second pair of hands allows simultaneous jugular vein compression and central catheter aspiration.

    f) Supportive therapy is required for hemodynamic compromise. Administration of ephedrine, 10 to 20 mg intravenously, and an intravenous fluid bolus improves the blood pressure. If this does not restore blood pressure, additional vasopressors (epinephrine) may be required.

    g) Therapy for VAE is listed as follows:

        (1) Notify the surgeon on detection (flood the surgical field with saline, and wax the bone edges).

        (2) Discontinue nitrous oxide administration. Give 100% oxygen

(3) Perform a Valsalva maneuver or compression of the jugular veins.
(4) Aspirate air from the atrial catheter.
(5) Support blood pressure with volume and vasopressors.
(6) Reposition the patient in the left lateral decubitus position with a 15-degree head-down tilt if blood pressure continues to decrease.
(7) Modify the anesthetic as needed to optimize hemodynamics.

K. Ventriculoperitoneal Shunt

1. Introduction
A ventriculoperitoneal shunt is placed to relieve increased cerebrospinal fluid pressure. The hydrocephalus may be caused by a congenital defect, cyst, tumor, trauma, infection, or cerebral blood flow absorption abnormality. Therefore, patients undergoing this procedure range in age from the newborn to the elderly. Besides a conduit to the peritoneum, the ventricle can also be drained into the pleura or right atrium.

2. Preoperative assessment
a) Neurologic; intracranial pressure (ICP) monitoring is routine.
b) Assess for level of consciousness, headaches, nuchal rigidity, seizures, and any presurgical neurologic defects such as stroke, spina bifida, and focal defects.
c) Review results of computed tomography of the head. Review blood pressure and heart rate trends in relation to ICP. Cushing's triad is present: increased ICP, increased blood pressure, and decreased heart rate.

3. Patient preparation
a) Complete blood count, electrolytes (especially if the patient is receiving diuretics), glucose (especially if the patient is on steroids such as dexamethasone), prothrombin time, partial thromboplastin time, and type and screen are obtained.
b) Other diagnostic tests are as indicated. Communicate with the neurologist if steroids and diuretic therapy are anticipated during surgery. Usually, preoperative medication is not given to patients with increased ICP.

4. Room preparation
a) Monitors: Standard. An ICP monitor is also used.
b) Position: Supine with the head turned. A shoulder roll may be used. A foam head rest aids positioning.
c) Additional equipment: The table will probably be turned, thus requiring an adequate length of ventilation tubing. Because much of the patient will be exposed, it is helpful to have a fluid warmer and a higher room temperature.
d) Drugs and tabletop: Standard. Fluids are usually run at approximately 4 mL/hour.

5. Anesthesia and perioperative management
a) Use general anesthesia with endotracheal intubation. Thiopental and etomidate are good choices for induction because of their cerebral protective properties. Muscle relaxation is desirable.
b) Normocarbia aids the surgeon in cannulating the ventricles. It is wise to have the thiopental or etomidate immediately available during the

PART II **Common Procedures**

"tunneling," which is the most stimulating part of this procedure. Extubation is performed at the end of the procedure.

6. Postoperative implications

Assess the patient's neurologic status. Pain can usually be managed with oral preparations.

NEUROSKELETAL SYSTEM

A. Anterior Cervical Diskectomy/Fusion

1. **Introduction**

   Anterior cervical diskectomy or fusion is most commonly performed for symptomatic nerve root or cord compression. Compression may occur from protrusion of an intervertebral disk or osteophytic bone into the spinal canal. An intervertebral disk usually herniates at the fifth or sixth cervical levels. A bone graft may be taken from the iliac crest, or backbone may be used.

2. **Preoperative assessment and patient preparation**

   a) Airway assessment should include thorough assessment of the range of motion of the neck. Neurologic deficits with limited neck movement may require intubation with the head in a neutral position. Intubation can be performed using passive immobilization or in-line traction. Awake intubation with proper positioning is the safest option.

   b) Neurologic deficits should be documented. Patients typically complain of neck pain radiating down one arm, which can progress to weakness and atrophy.

   c) Diagnostic tests include type and screen, complete blood count, and other tests as the patient's condition indicates.

   d) Preoperative medication and intravenous therapy: Patients may have considerable pain preoperatively and require a narcotic with premedication. If a difficult airway is anticipated, premedication should be used sparingly. Use a 16- or 18-gauge intravenous catheter with minimal fluid replacement.

3. **Room preparation**

   a) A standard tabletop setup is used.

   b) The patient is in the supine position, with arms tucked at the side; a small roll may be placed under the shoulders. Pad elbows to avoid ulnar compression, and use slight knee flexion because many patients also have lumbar disease. A doughnut or foam headrest may be used.

   c) Use a single, 18-gauge nonpositional intravenous catheter (arms tucked) with minimal fluid replacement.

4. **Perioperative management and anesthetic technique**

   a) Induction

   (1) General anesthesia with endotracheal intubation is used.

   (2) Tape the endotracheal tube to the side opposite of where the surgeon stands. Keep tape out of the sterile field.

   b) Maintenance

   (1) The trachea and esophagus are retracted laterally while the common carotid is retracted medially. The temporal artery can be palpated to

monitor for carotid artery occlusion. There is the potential risk of damage to the recurrent laryngeal nerve, major arteries, veins, or esophageal perforation.

(2) Blood loss is usually not significant, but epidural venous oozing can occur.

(3) Patients with spinal cord compression have an increased risk for decreased spinal cord perfusion and may not tolerate intraoperative hypotension.

(4) Spinal cord monitoring with somatosensory-evoked potentials may be performed.

(5) The absence of muscle relaxation is required for intraoperative nerve function testing.

(6) If a nerve stimulator is used on the face, limit twitch application to when the surgeon is not operating, because the face may move during stimulation.

c) Emergence

(1) Most patients are extubated in the operating room after the procedure.

(2) Coughing and bucking on the endotracheal tube should be avoided because they can dislodge the bone plug. Intravenous lidocaine can be administered before extubation. The neck must remain in a neutral position. A neck brace may be applied.

(3) Extubate before application of the neck brace; a jaw lift may be required. The patient should be awake before leaving the operating room to allow the surgeon to assess neurologic function.

(4) Consider leaving the patient intubated if there is large blood loss or fluid replacement, difficult intubation, multilevel surgery, or difficult tracheal retraction that can lead to tracheal or airway edema.

(5) Assess the patient's voice for recurrent laryngeal nerve damage, which rarely causes airway obstruction and usually resolves in a few days to 6 weeks.

B. Lumbar Laminectomy/Fusion

1. Introduction

Lumbar laminectomy is most commonly performed for symptomatic nerve root or spinal cord compression. Compression may occur from protrusion of an intervertebral disk or osteophyte bone into the spinal canal. An intervertebral disk usually herniates at the L4 to L5 or L5 to S1 intervertebral space. A laminectomy procedure involves the complete removal of lamina.

Lumbar fusion is performed when there is instability of the spine. Bone graft material can be obtained from the patient's iliac crest or from backbone. Back injuries account for a large percentage of work-related injuries and are a leading cause of work absences. Estimates are that 80% of the population will experience some type of back problem.

2. Preoperative assessment and patient preparation

a) History and physical examination: Assess and document neurologic deficits of the lower extremities.

b) Diagnostic tests: Type and screen blood, and obtain a complete blood count.

c) Preoperative medication and intravenous therapy

(1) Consider a narcotic with premedication if the patient experiences pain.

(2) Consider an antisialagogue because most spinal surgery is performed with the patient in the prone position.

(3) Use a 16- or 18-gauge intravenous catheter with minimal fluid replacement.

3. Room preparation

a) Monitoring equipment: Standard

b) Pharmacologic agents: Vasopressors, steroids, and antibiotics

c) Position

(1) Prone, lateral, and knee-chest positions are used.

(2) Have a foam headrest, doughnut, axillary roll, and indicated padding available.

(3) Specially designed frames may be used to aid in positioning.

4. Anesthetic technique

a) Local infiltration, regional blockade, and general anesthesia are used.

b) Regional blockade: This reduces blood loss and shrinks epidural veins; analgesia to T7 to T8 is required; and regional anesthesia cannot be used if nerve function will be tested.

c) Epidural: This must be in a single dose with the catheter removed.

d) Spinal: Hypotension may be accentuated with position change.

5. Perioperative management

a) Induction

(1) If the prone or knee-chest position is used, anesthesia is induced while the patient is on the stretcher.

(2) Position changes may be done in stages to avoid hemodynamic compromise. It may be necessary to lighten the anesthetic and increase fluids before the position change. A vasopressor may be needed to treat hypotension.

(3) Tape the endotracheal tube to the side of the mouth that will be positioned upward. Confirm endotracheal tube placement after positioning.

b) Maintenance

(1) Question the surgeon regarding the use of muscle relaxants. If nerve function is to be tested, a single dose of an intermediate nondepolarizing muscle relaxant may be used for intubation.

(2) Pad all pressure points and check for pressure on the face every 15 minutes during surgery.

(3) Blood loss is rarely sufficient to necessitate deliberate hypotension. The wound may be infiltrated with an epinephrine solution to decrease intraoperative blood loss.

(4) Sudden profound hypotension may indicate major intra-abdominal vessel (iliac, aorta) damage with bleeding occurring in the retroperitoneal cavity, which may not be visible to the surgeon.

(5) Infiltration of the wound with a local anesthetic will decrease postoperative pain.

c) Emergence

Extubation is performed when the patient is supine. The patient may need to be awake at the end of the procedure to allow the surgeon to assess for neurologic deficits.

6. Postoperative considerations

The patient can usually be transported in any position because stability of the back is rarely compromised.

C. Spinal Cord Injuries

1. Introduction

Spinal cord transection is the description of spinal cord injury that is manifested as paralysis of the lower extremities (paraplegia) or of all extremities (quadriplegia). Spinal cord transection above the level of C2 to C4 is incompatible with survival, because innervation to the diaphragm is likely to be destroyed.

The most common cause of spinal cord transection is the trauma associated with a motor vehicle or diving accident that results in fracture dislocation of cervical vertebrae. Occasionally, rheumatoid arthritis of the spine leads to spontaneous dislocation of the C1 vertebra on the C2 vertebra, producing progressive quadriparesis. These patients can suddenly become quadriplegic. The most frequent nontraumatic cause of spinal cord transection is multiple sclerosis. In addition, infections or vascular and developmental disorders may be responsible for permanent damage to the spinal cord.

2. Preoperative assessment

Spinal cord transection initially produces flaccid paralysis, with total absence of sensation below the level of injury. Temperature regulation and spinal cord reflexes are lost below the level of injury. The phase after the acute transection of the spinal cord is known as spinal shock and typically lasts 1 to 3 weeks. Several weeks after acute transection of the spinal cord, the spinal cord reflexes gradually return, and patients enter a chronic stage, characterized by overactivity of the sympathetic nervous system and involuntary skeletal muscle spasms. Mental depression and pain are pressing problems after spinal cord injury.

a) History and physical examination

   (1) Cardiovascular: Electrocardiograph abnormalities are common during the acute phase of spinal cord transection and include ventricular premature beats and ST–T-wave changes suggestive of myocardial ischemia. Decreased systemic blood pressure and bradycardia are also common secondary to a loss of sympathetic tone. Generally, this condition can be treated effectively with crystalloid and colloid infusion and atropine to increase the heart rate. Around 85% of patients with spinal cord transection above T6 exhibit autonomic hyperreflexia, a disorder that appears after the resolution of spinal shock and in association with the return of the spinal cord reflexes.

   (2) Respiratory: A transection between the levels of C2 and C4 may result in apnea from denervation of the diaphragm. The ability to cough and clear secretions from the airway is often impaired because of decreased expiratory reserve volume. Vital capacity also is significantly decreased if the transection of the spinal cord is at the cervical level. Furthermore, arterial hypoxemia is a consistent early finding during the period after cervical spinal cord injury. Tracheobronchial suctioning has been associated with bradycardia and cardiac arrest in these patients, secondary to vasovagal reflex, a finding emphasizing the importance of establishing optimal arterial oxygenation before undertaking this maneuver. Acute respiratory insufficiency and the inability to handle oropharyngeal

secretions necessitate immediate tracheal intubation. Before intubation is initiated, the neck must be stabilized.

(3) Neurologic: Patients with spinal cord trauma at the T1 level are paraplegic, whereas traumas above C5 may result in quadriplegia and loss of phrenic nerve function. Injuries between these two levels result in varying loss of motor and sensory functions in the upper extremities. Careful assessment and documentation of preoperative sensory and motor deficits are important.

(4) Musculoskeletal: Prolonged immobility leads to osteoporosis, skeletal muscle atrophy, and the development of decubitus ulcers. Pathologic fractures can occur when these patients are moved. Pressure points should be well protected and padded to minimize the likelihood of trauma to the skin and the development of ulcers.

(5) Renal: Renal failure is the leading cause of death in the patient with chronic spinal cord transection. Chronic urinary tract infections and immobilization predispose to the development of renal calculi. Amyloidosis of the kidney can be manifested as proteinuria, leading to a decrease in the concentration of albumin in the plasma.

b) Patient preparation

(1) Laboratory tests: Arterial blood gases substantiate the degree of respiratory impairment; urinalysis, complete blood count, coagulation profile, electrolytes, type and cross-match, and other tests are as indicated by the history and physical examination.

(2) Diagnostic tests: Computed tomography, magnetic resonance imaging, radiography of the injured parts, and other tests are as indicated by the history and physical examination.

(3) Medications: Premedication is useful in this patient population and is individualized based on patient need. Patients with acute spinal cord injury often receive methylprednisolone, 30 mcg/kg loading dose over 15 minutes, then 5.4 mg/hour for 23 hours.

3. **Room preparation**

a) Monitoring equipment

(1) Standard monitoring equipment

(2) Foley catheter

(3) Arterial line

(4) Central venous pressure line as clinically indicated

b) Additional equipment

(1) Patient warming devices

(2) Regular operating table

(3) Cervical traction, tong traction, or pins; shoulder rolls as clinically indicated

c) Drugs

(1) Standard emergency drugs are used.

(2) A standard tabletop is used.

(3) Intravenous fluids are infused through a 16- or 18-gauge intravenous line with normal saline at 4 to 6 mL/kg per hour with a fluid warmer.

(4) Regardless of the technique selected for anesthesia, a drug such as nitroprusside must be readily available to treat precipitous hypertension. Nitroprusside administration, 1 to 2 mcg/kg/min, is an effective method of treating sudden hypertension.

4. **Anesthetic technique**

Use general endotracheal anesthesia. Management of anesthesia in the patient with transection of the spinal cord is largely determined by the duration of the injury. Regardless of the duration of spinal cord transection, preoperative hydration helps to prevent hypotension during the induction and maintenance of anesthesia.

5. **Perioperative management**
   a) Induction

   All trauma patients are considered to have full stomachs, and rapid sequence induction should be performed. Succinylcholine is avoided in patients with spinal cord injury after 24 to 48 hours because of the risk of hyperkalemia from potassium release from extrajunctional receptor sites. Furthermore, succinylcholine-induced fasciculations can exacerbate spinal cord injury. Rocuronium or rapacuronium have a rapid onset and can be used for rapid sequence induction. Ketamine can be used in the hemodynamically unstable patient if head trauma is not suspected. The anesthetist should determine whether the cervical spine x-ray films have been cleared before intubation. Avoid manipulating the head and neck, which can cause further injury. If the patient's neck is unstable, or if difficult intubation is anticipated secondary to a halo device or a body jacket, an awake fiberoptic intubation should be performed. The awake intubation has the advantage of preserving muscle tone, which may protect the unstable spine, and the patient's neurologic status can be assessed after the procedure. Blind nasal, awake fiberoptic nasal, or oral intubations are possible options depending on the patient's condition. A rigid laryngoscopy can be performed with in-line axial stabilization.

   b) Maintenance
      (1) Standard: A single dose of neuromuscular blocking drug (vecuronium 10 mg) may be administered to relax the neck muscles. Additional doses of relaxants are rarely necessary.
      (2) Position: For the anterior approach, the patient is positioned supine with a roll under the shoulders, and the head is moderately hyperextended. Check and pad pressure points. A cervical strap may be placed below the chin to apply continuous cervical traction; avoid pressure on ears and facial nerve. Accidental extubation can result if the chin strap slips off the chin. For the posterior approach, the patient is positioned either prone with horseshoe headrest or three-point stabilization, using a special frame or bolsters that allow the abdomen to hang freely to prevent venous engorgement. Occasionally, the sitting position is used, and this increases the risk of venous air embolism.
      (3) Hypotension: The loss of sympathetic compensation response makes these patients more susceptible to hypotension from positioning, blood loss, and positive-pressure ventilation. One may need to treat with fluids and pressors. The goal is to maintain a systolic blood pressure of 90 mm Hg.
      (4) Autonomic hyperreflexia: Patients with chronic spinal cord injury should be monitored for autonomic hyperreflexia. This condition is associated with injuries above the level of T6. It may be precipitated by cutaneous or visceral stimuli below the spinal cord lesion. Bladder, bowel, or intestinal distention is known to produce autonomic overactivity. An adequate level of general or spinal anesthesia is paramount. Symptoms are hypertension, bradycardia, dysrhythmias, headache, sweating, piloerection below the lesion, vasodilation above the lesion, hyperreflexia, convulsions, cerebral hemorrhage, and

pulmonary edema. Treatment consists of eliminating the stimulus, deepening the anesthetic, raising the head of the bed, and administering vasodilators, α-antagonists, or ganglionic blockers.

(5) Hypothermia: Warming devices are necessary, because the patient's core temperature will approach room temperature because of the interruption in sympathetic pathways to the hypothalamus.

c) Emergence

After a cervical fusion has been performed, the patient may have a halo device or body jacket. The patient should be fully awake and able to manage his or her airway before extubation. Lidocaine can be administered down the endotracheal tube or intravenously to prevent coughing and bucking. The patient should have a tidal volume of greater than 5 mL/kg, a negative inspiratory force of 20 to 25 cm H_2O, and vital capacity of greater than 15 mL/kg. Airway patency can be tested by deflating the cuff to determine whether the patient can breathe around the tube before extubation. The patient should be assessed for airway obstruction secondary to soft tissue occlusion or superior laryngeal nerve damage after extubation.

6. **Postoperative implications**

a) Airway obstruction is usually caused by soft tissue against the posterior pharyngeal wall. The neck fusion or postoperative traction/stabilization device (halo or body jacket) may impair attempts to open the airway. An oral or nasal airway may be required.

b) Pneumonia may result postoperatively.

c) Respiratory insufficiency can result from the development of a tension pneumothorax from entrainment of air through the surgical wound; oropharyngeal laceration during tracheal intubation; or bleeding into the neck at the surgical site, with progressive compression and occlusion of the airway.

d) The patient should be assessed for the presence of neurologic deficits. Reversible causes such as a hematoma should be excluded.

e) Deep vein thrombosis can occur from decreased blood flow and venous stasis. Heparinization and sequential compression stockings should be instituted.

f) Urinary retention may require urinary catheterization.

g) Stress ulcers and gastric ileus can be treated with a nasogastric tube, antacids, and H_2-receptor antagonists.

D. Thoracic and Lumbar Spinal Instrumentation and Fusion

1. **Introduction**

Anterolateral, posterior, or combined anteroposterior approaches can be used to treat pathologic processes of the thoracic and lumbar spine. Spinal instrumentation refers to implanted metal rods affixed to the spine to correct and internally splint the deformed spine. Originally designed for scoliosis, posterior spinal instrumentation is commonly performed simultaneously with spinal fusion for a variety of diagnoses, including fracture, tumor, degenerative changes, and developmental spinal deformity. The original Harrington rod is the simplest and still considered by many to be the standard. Other procedures, such as segmental spinal instrumentation, can distribute correctional forces by sublaminar wiring (Luque) or by hook or screw (Cotrel-Dubousset) procedures that apply multilevel corrective forces on the rods. Bone chips from the posterior iliac crest are placed over the site of fusion. Harrington rodding or similar extensive spinal instrumentation procedures to correct spinal column deformities put the spinal cord at risk for ischemia secondary to mechanical compression of its blood supply. This complication has been mitigated with methods to assess spinal cord function intraoperatively. These include intraoperative testing of neurologic function (wake-up test) and somatosensory-evoked potential (SSEP) monitoring. Wake-up testing requires an informed cooperative patient and a practice trial of patient responses.

The anterior approach may use the Dwyer screw and cable apparatus or Zielke rod. It offers a limited fusion area and less blood loss and can correct significant lordosis. There is a greater risk of damage to the spinal cord when compared with the Harrington rod procedure. The spinal cord can be damaged from the vertebral body screw, especially in the smaller thoracic vertebral bodies and larger number of segmental spinal arteries that require ligation. The patient is positioned laterally, and a transthoracic or retroperitoneal approach is used. The potential for respiratory compromise is significant when using the thoracoabdominal approach. Surgery above the level of T8 requires a double-lumen endotracheal tube to collapse the lung on the operative side. The procedure may require the removal of the tenth and/or sixth rib and diaphragmatic manipulation.

An anteroposterior fusion may be required for patients with unstable spines. Usually, the anterior procedure is performed first, followed by posterior instrumentation after 1 to 2 weeks. Immediate posterior fusion is possible when the area to be fused is small and the primary curvature is below the diaphragm. The anteroposterior approach necessitates an intraoperative position change. Anesthetic considerations are similar to those required for posterior intrumentation. Anesthetic concerns for thoracic and lumbar spine procedures are positioning, replacement of blood and fluid losses, maintaining spinal cord integrity, preventing venous air embolism, and avoiding hypothermia. The wake-up test and SSEPs are frequently used.

2. **Preoperative assessment**

Patients requiring spinal reconstruction usually have either idiopathic or acquired scoliosis. Scoliosis is a deformity of the spine resulting in curvature and rotation of the vertebrae, as well as an associated deformity of the rib cage. Scoliosis can be classified as idiopathic, neuromuscular, myopathic, congenital, trauma or tumor related, and as part of mesenchymal disorders. Most cases are idiopathic, with a male-to-female ratio of 1:4. Surgery is indicated when the curvature is severe: the Cobb angle is greater than 50 degrees or rapidly progressing. Spinal instability requiring surgery may also result from trauma, cancer, or infection. Patients with scoliosis need careful preoperative evaluation of their cardiac, pulmonary, neuromuscular, and renal systems because associated anomalies occur frequently.

a) History and physical examination

   (1) Cardiovascular: Patients have a high incidence of congestive heart disease, right ventricular hypertrophy, pulmonary hypertension, and cor pulmonale. Pulmonary vascular resistance is increased independent of the severity of scoliosis.

(2) Respiratory: Respiratory impairment is proportional to the angle of lateral curvature. Respiratory involvement is more likely when the Cobb angle is greater than 65 degrees. There may be a decreased total lung capacity and vital capacity (restrictive pattern). Ventilation-perfusion mismatch and alveolar hypoventilation may result in hypoxemia. If vital capacity is less than 40% predicted, postoperative ventilation usually is required. Patients with neuromuscular disease may also have impaired protective airway mechanisms and weakness of respiratory musculature.

(3) Neurologic: If an intraoperative wake-up test is planned, the patient should be informed preoperatively and assured that the procedure will involve minimal pain. A practice wake-up test helps to establish a baseline assessment and teaches the patient what to expect. Careful preoperative assessment and documentation of the patient's neurologic status are essential.

(4) Musculoskeletal: Cardiomyopathy is a common finding in patients with muscular dystrophy. These patients are more sensitive to myocardial depression from anesthetic agents, changes in sympathetic tone, and hypercapnia. Patients with muscular dystrophy may require postoperative ventilation secondary to muscle weakness, impaired secretion removal, and atelectasis. The use of succinylcholine is contraindicated in patients with muscular dystrophy, because it may lead to hyperkalemia and cardiac arrest. These patients may be at risk for developing malignant hyperthermia. The use of nontriggering anesthetic agents and careful observation for signs of malignant hyperthermia are essential.

(5) Hematologic: Discontinue platelet inhibitors for 2 to 3 weeks before surgery. Autologous blood donation is recommended. Consider the use of intraoperative hemodilution (hematocrit 30%), controlled hypotension, and cell-saver devices.

b) Patient preparation

(1) Laboratory tests: Complete blood count, prothrombin time, partial thromboplastin time, arterial blood gases, electrolytes, type and cross-match and other tests as indicated by the history and physical examination

(2) Diagnostic tests: Chest radiographs, pulmonary function test, spine studies, eelctrocardiogram, and other tests as indicated by the history and physical examination

(3) Medication: Standard premedication, if appropriate

3. Room preparation

a) Monitoring equipment

(1) Standard monitoring equipment

(2) Arterial line

(3) Foley catheter

(4) Central venous pressure line (if indicated)

b) Additional equipment

(1) Patient warming devices

(2) Cell saver

(3) SSEP monitor (if indicated)

(4) Regular operating table with spinal frame or bolster

c) Drugs

(1) Antibiotics, vasodilators if hypotensive technique

(2) Standard emergency drugs, tabletop

(3) Intravenous fluids through one to two large-bore intravenous catheters with normal saline at 8 to 10 mL/kg per hour with a fluid warmer

(4) Blood loss possibly significant; need for blood to be immediately available

4. **Anesthetic technique**

General endotracheal anesthesia is used. For pediatric cases, preheat the room to 72° to 78° F.

5. **Perioperative management**

a) Induction: Standard; for prone cases, induction is performed while the patient is on the stretcher.

b) Maintenance

(1) Standard: If SSEPs are monitored, a constant state of anesthesia is used; stable hemodynamics and normothermia are essential. Question the SSEP technician regarding the use of nitrous oxide. The concentration of inhalation agents should be kept below 1 MAC. A sufentanil infusion of 0.25 to 1 mcg/kg/hour provides a continuous state of anesthesia and lowers the MAC of volatile agents. Muscle relaxation is acceptable and should be kept constant (1 twitch).

(2) Position: The patient is prone on a spinal frame or bolster. Avoid abdominal compression, which impairs cardiac and pulmonary function as well as increases bleeding through epidural engorgement. Pressure points must be carefully padded and routinely assessed, especially during controlled hypotension. Anterior procedures are often performed with the patient in the lateral position; the dependent limb, ear, and eye should be checked frequently.

(3) Wake-up test: Performed after completion of spinal instrumentation and requires 40 to 60 minutes advance notice from the surgeon. Avoid narcotic or muscle relaxant boluses, decrease inhalation agent; hand ventilate, reverse muscle relaxants and narcotics (naloxone [Narcan], 20-mcg increments) if necessary; monitor train-of-four; request hand squeeze followed by bilateral foot movement. Uncontrolled patient movement during a wake-up test can result in accidental extubation or dislodgment of the spinal instrumentation. Forceful inspiratory efforts may provoke venous air embolism. If the patient moves the hands and not the feet, the surgeon will decrease the spinal distraction. If movement still does not occur, be prepared to increase the blood pressure and transfuse to increase spinal cord perfusion. The possibility of a hematoma should also be considered. After completion of the wake-up test, the anesthetist must be prepared to anesthetize the patient rapidly (have thiopental [Pentothal] or propofol ready).

(4) SSEP indications of spinal cord ischemia should be treated by restoring normal blood pressure and decreasing cord traction. Discontinue volatile agents and ensure adequate oxygenation. Immediate transfusion may be necessary.

(5) Controlled hypotension may be used to decrease blood loss. Inhalation agents, vasodilators, nitroprusside, and/or nitroglycerin are usually used to achieve a mean arterial pressure of 65 mm Hg in normotensive patients or lowering the systolic blood pressure 20 mm Hg from baseline in hypertensive patients. A major concern with hypotensive technique is compromising spinal cord blood supply. Blood pressure should be reduced slowly before the incision and allowed to gradually return to normal after surgery.

(6) Ischemic optic neuropathy can lead to blindness and is associated with deliberate hypotension and anemia. Consider the importance of early blood transfusion in the patient undergoing hypotensive technique.

(7) Hypotensive technique requires an arterial line and Foley catheter to monitor urine output (0.5 to 1 mL/kg/hour).

(8) If a venous air embolism is suspected, the wound is packed, and nitrous oxide is discontinued if in use. Attempt to aspirate air using the central venous pressure catheter; use fluids and pressors; turn the patient supine; and institute cardiopulmonary resuscitation if necessary.

c) Emergence

Emergence usually occurs after the patient is positioned supine. Most patients can be extubated in the operating room if preoperative respiratory status was acceptable. Persistent narcotic or muscle relaxation may delay extubation. Assess neurologic function.

6. Postoperative implications

a) Pulmonary insufficiency: Postoperative ventilation may be required in patients with severe respiratory impairment. A patient with a preoperative vital capacity of less than 40% predicted usually requires postoperative mechanical ventilation. Aggressive postoperative pulmonary care should be emphasized.

b) Neurologic sequelae are the most feared complications, and it is important to assess and document the postoperative neurologic examination.

c) Postoperative pain management allows for early ambulation and compliance with the pulmonary care regimen. Opioids can be administered by the intrathecal, epidural, or parenteral route.

d) Hypothermia may occur.

e) Pneumothorax may occur.

f) Dislodgment of internal fixation is possible.

PART II Common Procedures

OBSTETRICS AND GYNECOLOGY

A. Cesarean Section

1. **Introduction**

   A cesarean section (C-section) is the surgical removal of a fetus through an abdominal/uterine incision. A low transverse incision is the most common; in an emergency, a rapid vertical midline incision may be used. Indications for a C-section are failure of labor to progress, previous C-section, fetal distress, malpresentation of the fetus or umbilical cord, placenta previa, and genital herpes or other local infections.

2. **Perioperative assessment**

   In emergency cases, the time for assessment will be brief. Special attention should be paid to airway assessment because failed intubation is a major cause of maternal morbidity and mortality.

   a) Cardiac

   (1) Full-term pregnancy causes an increase in cardiac output of 30%. Twenty percent of the cardiac output goes to the uterus; with each contraction, blood flow to the uterus increases 15% to 20%.

   (2) Immediately post partum is the largest increase in cardiac output, an up to 80% increase.

   (3) Cardiac output returns to normal 2 weeks post partum.

   (4) By 24 to 34 weeks, blood volume increases 35% to 40% (1000 to 1500 mL). Blood volumes return to normal 1 to 2 weeks after delivery.

   (5) Blood loss for a normal delivery is 500 mL or less; for a twin vaginal delivery or C-section, it is 1000 mL or less.

   (6) There is also, normally, a mild decrease in blood pressure and systemic vascular resistance.

   (7) Evaluate for pregnancy-induced hypertension.

   (8) There is dilutional anemia because of an increase in plasma volume and increased total body water content; hemoglobin is usually greater than 11 g/dL. After delivery there is diuresis, and the hemoglobin returns to normal 2 to 4 weeks post partum.

   (9) Parturients greater than 28 weeks' gestation should not be placed supine without left uterine displacement. Supine hypotension syndrome occurs after the 28th week when patients lie in the supine position, causing diminished venous return that leads to decreases in cardiac output and blood pressure. Symptoms include pallor, nausea and vomiting, sweating, and dizziness. Aortic compression occurs when patients lie in the supine position, causing decreased blood flow to the lower extremities and uteroplacental insufficiency. The arm blood pressure reading does not reflect such changes. Most patients are asymptomatic or feel tingling in the legs with fetal asphyxia. Aortocaval compression occurs as early as 20 weeks; with regional and increased

vasodilation, there is a decrease in venous return. Systemic hypotension, increased uterine venous pressure, and uterine arterial hypoperfusion can compromise uterine and placental blood flow. When these effects are combined with anesthesia, fetal asphyxia may result.

b) Respiratory

(1) Oxygen consumption increases 20% at term, minute ventilation increases 50%, tidal volume increases 40%, respiratory rate increases 20%, and alveolar ventilation is increased, all leading to respiratory alkalosis with arterial carbon dioxide tension decreased to 32 mm Hg.

(2) During labor, the minute ventilation increases 300%, causing hypocarbia and hypoventilation between contractions.

(3) The oxyhemoglobin dissociation curve is shifted to the left, resulting in less oxygen available to the fetus.

(4) Functional residual capacity decreases by 20%, causing a rapid desaturation with apnea; must preoxygenate before induction. Minimum alveolar concentration (MAC) is decreased by 25% to 40%.

(5) There is decreased airway resistance because of progesterone-induced relaxation.

(6) Capillary engorgement of the respiratory mucosa predisposes to upper airway trauma.

(7) Patients have a decreased glottic opening, edematous false cords and arytenoids, and nasal congestion. Never place a nasal airway; use a smaller endotracheal tube (6 to 6.5).

c) Gastrointestinal: All pregnant patients past 16 weeks of gestation are considered to have a full stomach and require pretreatment with 30 mL of a nonparticulate antacid and rapid sequence induction.

d) The enlarged uterus obstructs the inferior vena cava, causing a decrease in the cerebrospinal fluid volume, a decrease in the potential volume of the epidural space, and an increase in the epidural space pressure because of epidural vein engorgement. Decrease the dose of epidural and spinal agents by one third to two thirds. Do not push drugs during contractions, because the pressure in the epidural space increases 6 to 12 times normal.

e) Other: Evaluate for a history of gestational diabetes, HELLP syndrome (hemolysis, elevated liver enzymes, low platelet count), placenta previa, seizures, preterm labor, multiple gestation, drug abuse, pregnancy-induced hypertension, and nonpregnancy-related illnesses and surgical procedures.

3. **Patient preparation**

a) A nonparticulate antacid (such as sodium citrate, 30 mL) is routinely administered at most institutions, regardless of the anesthetic technique chosen. Sedation is best avoided. Benzodiazapines have been implicated as possible teratogens, and it is best to avoid maternal amnesia during childbirth.

b) Laboratory tests should include a type and screen, complete blood count, electrolytes, blood urea nitrogen, creatinine, glucose, prothrombin time, and partial thromboplastin time. In emergency C-sections, there may not be time to complete these tests.

4. **Room preparation**

a) Monitoring

(1) This is standard.

(2) If there is a history of pregnancy-induced hypertension, an arterial line is recommended.

(3) If there is severe preeclampsia, a central line is also recommended, with a pulmonary catheter in cases of hemodynamic instability.
b) Positioning: Supine with left lateral uterine displacement. This is accomplished by placing a wedge under the right hip. Failure to use left lateral uterine displacement can result in aortocaval compression.
c) Drugs and tabletop
(1) The tabletop should be set up for a general anesthetic.
(2) Set out a smaller endotracheal tube (6 to 6.5) as well (because of airway edema).
(3) Have ephedrine and oxytocin drawn up.
(4) Have difficult airway equipment available.
(5) Unless there is maternal hypoglycemia, avoid giving intravenous solutions with glucose because they may lead to neonatal hypoglycemia.

5. **Perioperative management and anesthetic techniques**
a) Always be ready for general anesthesia. Rapid sequence induction should be done after the patient is prepared and draped; notify the surgeon immediately after the endotracheal tube is through the vocal cords. Thiopental (4 mg/kg)/succinylcholine (1.5 mg/kg) is the most common combination for induction. Ketamine (1 mg/kg) is a useful adjunct in cases of instability or bleeding.
b) An oral-gastric tube should be inserted after induction, and the gastric contents should be aspirated.
c) Volatile agents can be used and then substituted with narcotics after the fetus is delivered. Begin at a 0.5 MAC because requirements for obstetrics are typically 30% to 50% reduced. The maximum end-tidal for isoflurane should not exceed 0.5%.
d) Avoid hypotension because uterine flow is pressure dependent.
e) Extubation is always performed with the patient awake because the danger of aspiration will be high.
f) Regional anesthesia is the most common technique used on patients undergoing C-section. For spinal anesthesia, 0.75% bupivicaine, 11 to 12 mg, is usually enough to provide a dense block to T4. Volume loading should be accomplished before performing a spinal block with 1 to 2 L of crystalloid. Ephedrine is also commonly needed in addition to volume loading.
g) An epidural is also an attractive regional anesthetic, especially if the parturient has a catheter in place for laboring. "Topping up" the epidural with 10 to 20 mL of 2% lidocaine or 3% chloroprocaine (Nesacaine) along with narcotic and perhaps ketamine administration just before delivery are two techniques.
h) If the patient is in danger of losing consciousness or reflexes, the airway must be protected and general anesthesia induced.

6. **Postoperative considerations**
a) For pain relief, narcotics may be administered parenterally, with patient-controlled analgesia, orally when tolerated, or intrathecally/epidurally if a catheter is in place.
b) Nausea and vomiting are common in the immediate postpartum period and may be treated with an antiemetic.

7. **Obstetric pharmacology**
a) Placental transfer is dependent on the concentration gradient, molecular weight, lipid solubility, and drug ionization state.
b) Drugs that are nonionized, lipid soluble, and weigh less than 500 d cross the placenta easily.

c) Uterine-stimulating agents are used for the induction and augmentation of labor, the induction of uterine contraction after a C-section or uterine surgery, the induction of a therapeutic abortion, and control of postpartum atony. The uterine vascular bed is not autoregulated. α-Receptors elicit hypertonus when stimulated, and β-receptors elicit a reduction in uterine tone and contractility when stimulated.

   (1) Oxytocin increases intracellular calcium, resulting in a sustained decrease in the uterine resting membrane potential. The frequency and force of contractions increase. The dose for the induction of labor is 1 to 2 milliunits/min and is increased by 1 to 2 milliunits/ min every 15 to 30 minutes until optimum response is achieved. The average dose is 8 to 10 milliunits/min. For control of postpartum bleeding, 10 to 40 milliunits added intravenously may be given after delivery of the placenta.

   (2) Methergine causes an increase in the strength of the contractions, leading to a firm tetanic contraction followed by a series of clonic contractions. α-Agonist effects result in vasoconstriction; coronary artery spasm and myocardial ischemia can occur. Side effects include severe hypertension and bradycardia. The dose is 0.2 mg intramuscularly every 2 to 4 hours.

   (3) Prostaglandins act on specific receptors to stimulate synthesis of cyclic adenosine monophosphate by the activation of adenylate cyclase. This stimulates the smooth muscle of the uterus and results in the induction of strong uterine contractions. Bronchiole smooth muscle contracts in response to prostaglandins and may result in severe bronchoconstriction. The dose is 200 to 500 mcg intramuscularly or intramyometrially.

d) Muscle relaxants are all polar quaternary ammonium compounds that do not cross the placenta in any significant amounts. They are 100% water soluble and have a small volume of distribution. Plasma cholinesterase activity declines with pregnancy because of the patient's expanded blood volume. A modified succinylcholine dose is usually not needed. None of the muscle relaxants relax the uterine muscle.

e) Inhalational agents are lipid soluble, nonionized, and have a low molecular weight. Levels rise quickly in the fetal brain. The degree of neonatal depression is proportional to the depth and duration of the maternal anesthesia. Nitrous oxide has been implicated as a teratogen to the fetus; there is generally little harm at delivery if less than 50% is used.

f) Narcotics cause varying degrees of respiratory depression in the neonate and can prolong the progress of labor. Generally avoid them if delivery is thought to occur within the next 30 to 45 minutes. The peak effect of meperidine occurs 40 to 50 minutes after intramuscular administration, 5 to 10 minutes after intravenous administration. The greatest incidence of respiratory depression occurs 3 to 4 hours after administration. At this time, meperidine is metabolized to the more respiratory-depressing metabolite normeperidine.

g) Benzodiazepines should not be given during the first trimester because of the risk of cleft palate. Avoid in labor and delivery because of the amnesic properties of these drugs.

h) Ephedrine is the drug of choice to treat hypotension because of its mixed α and β effects that maintain maternal cardiac output and uterine perfusion. It can increase the fetal heart rate.

i) Tocolytics are β-adrenergic agonists that are most commonly used to treat preterm labor. All have β_1 and β_2 effects. β_1 stimulation

PART II **Common Procedures**

can result in an increased heart rate and cardiac output; β_2 stimulation can result in hyperglycemia and hypotension. Ritodrine and terbutaline are more specific β_2-agonists that are approved by the United States Food and Drug Administration for the treatment of preterm labor. The intravenous infusion rates are 0.05 to 0.1 mg/min for ritodrine and 0.01 mg/min for terbutaline. These drugs can cause profound tachycardia, and it is recommended that induction be delayed 10 minutes after an infusion is stopped to allow the heart rate to decrease.

j) Magnesium sulfate is a central nervous system depressant that decreases the quantity of acetylcholine released at the motor endplate decreasing neuromuscular transmission, causing smooth muscle relaxation and decreased blood pressure. It is used for preeclampsia, eclampsia, and preterm labor. The dose is 3 to 4 g intravenously over 20 minutes, followed by an infusion of 1 to 1.5 mg/hour; titrate by 0.5 mg/hour until contractions cease. The therapeutic range is 4 to 8 mEq/L. Side effects include sweating, nausea, rag doll syndrome, confusion, and pulmonary edema. As the agent crosses the placenta, there will be a transient decrease in fetal heart rate, low Apgar sores, hypotonia, and respiratory depression. Magnesium increases the sensitivity to depolarizing and nondepolarizing muscle relaxants. Avoid long-lasting muscle relaxants and decrease the dose of all others by one third to two thirds.

B. Dilatation and Curettage

1. **Introduction**

   Dilatation and curettage (D & C) involves dilation of the cervix and scraping of the endometerial lining of the uterus. The procedure is done to diagnose and treat uterine bleeding, cervical lesions, or stenosis. D & Cs are also used to complete an incomplete or missed abortion and are then boarded as suction D & Cs with the gestational week.

2. **Preoperative assessment and patient preparation**

   a) History and physical examination: Assess for any cardiac, respiratory, neurologic, or renal abnormalities. Assess for a history of hiatal hernia or reflux; if a suction D & C, assess the gestational week; if greater than 16 weeks, consider the patient to have a full stomach.

   b) Patient preparation

      (1) Laboratory tests: Human chorionic gonadotropin, urinalysis, complete blood count

      (2) Medications: Evaluation of any medications the patient is taking

      (3) Intravenous therapy: One 18-gauge peripheral intravenous line

3. **Room preparation**

   a) Monitoring equipment: Standard

   b) Additional equipment: Bair Hugger

4. **Perianesthetic management**

   a) Drugs: Anxiolytic agents (midazolam [Versed], 0.01 to 0.02 mg/kg), narcotics (fentanyl, 1 to 2 mcg/kg), oxytocin (Pitocin) for suction D & Cs, induction agents (propofol, 2.5 mg/kg, or thiopental [Pentothal] 4 mg/kg) can be used.

   b) This procedure can be done either with a short-acting spinal or saddle block with lidocaine, 7.5 to 10 mg, as a general anesthetic by mask, laryngeal mask airway, or with an endotracheal tube with inhalation agent/nitrous oxide or with heavy sedation (midazolam [Versed], fentanyl, and propofol).

c) Postoperatively, assess for bleeding, nausea, and cramping. Treat with narcotics, nonsteroidal antiinflammatory drugs, and antiemetics.

C. Gynecologic Laparoscopy

1. **Introduction**
Laparoscopy is a common endoscopic technique in gynecologic procedures. It is frequently used to diagnose or treat pelvic conditions that may include sterilization, adhesions, pain, endometriosis, ectopic pregnancies, ovarian cysts and tumors, infertility, and vaginal hysterectomy. A pneumoperitoneum is achieved by insertion of a trocar and insufflation of carbon dioxide.
2. **Preoperative assessment and patient preparation**
   a) History and physical examination: As indicated by the patient's history and medical condition
   b) Patient preparation
      (1) Laboratory tests: Complete blood count and other tests as indicated
      (2) Diagnostic tests: Pregnancy testing and as indicated
      (3) Preoperative medications: As indicated
      (4) Intravenous therapy: One or two 16- to 18-gauge intravenous catheters
3. **Room preparation**
   a) Monitoring equipment: Standard
   b) Additional equipment: Fluid warmer and Bair Hugger; other equipment as needed
   c) Drugs
      (1) Anesthetic and adjunct agents and antibiotics are used.
      (2) Intravenous fluid: Depends on the procedure performed; calculate as indicated. Estimated blood loss is less than 50 to 100 mL.
      (3) Blood: Type and screen.
      (4) The tabletop is standard.
4. **Perioperative management and anesthetic technique**
   General anesthesia is preferred.
   a) Induction: Standard, as indicated
   b) Maintenance: Inhalational agent/oxygen/opioid and nondepolarizing agent as indicated; antiemetics possible
   c) Position: Lithotomy; Trendelenburg's to improve pelvic exposure
   d) Emergence: Standard
5. **Postoperative implications**
   Complications include nausea, vomiting, and anemia.

D. Hysterectomy: Vaginal or Total Abdominal

1. **Introduction**
Hysterectomy is commonly performed to treat uncontrolled uterine bleeding, dysmenorrhea, uterine myoma, gynecologic cancer, adhesions, endometriosis, and pelvic relaxation syndrome. Frequently, laparoscopy is used; for ovarian cancer prophylaxis, a bilateral salpingo-oophorectomy may be performed as well.

PART II **Common Procedures**

2. **Preoperative assessment**
   a) History and physical examination: As indicated by the patient's history and medical condition
   b) Patient preparation
      (1) Laboratory tests: These are as indicated by the patient's history and medical condition.
      (2) Diagnostic tests: These are as indicated by the patient's history and medical condition.
      (3) Preoperative medications: Anxiolytics are given as indicated; consider prophylaxis for postoperative nausea and vomiting.
      (4) Intravenous therapy: Two 16- to 18-gauge intravenous lines are used; consider a central line and/or an arterial line if the procedure is radical.
      (5) An epidural catheter may be placed for intraoperative or postoperative pain relief.
3. **Room preparation**
   a) Monitoring equipment is standard.
   b) Consider an arterial line and central venous pressure catheter if large blood loss is expected.
   c) Additional equipment includes a fluid warmer and Bair Hugger.
   d) Drugs
      (1) Anesthetic and adjunct agents and antibiotics are used.
      (2) Intravenous fluids: For vaginal hysterectomy, calculate for moderate blood loss; crystalloids at 4 to 6 mL/kg/hour. Estimated blood loss is 750 to 1000 mL. For abdominal hysterectomy, calculate for a moderate to large blood loss; crystalloids at 6 to 10 mL/kg/hour. Estimated blood loss is 1000 to 1500 mL.
      (3) Blood: Type and cross-match for 2 to 4 units of packed red blood cells.
      (4) The tabletop is standard.
4. **Perioperative management and anesthetic technique**
   General or regional anesthesia is used, with a subarachnoid block or epidural with a sensory level of anesthesia of T6 to T8.
   a) Induction: Standard, with the choice as indicated
   b) Maintenance
      (1) General anesthesia: Inhalational agent/oxygen/opioid/anxiolytic and nondepolarizing muscle relaxant
      (2) Regional: Local anesthetic of choice; supplemental anxiolytic and sedation
      (3) Position: Abdominal, supine; vaginal, lithotomy
   c) Emergence: Standard
5. **Postoperative implications**
   a) Complications: Nausea, vomiting, anemia
   b) Pain management: Patient-controlled analgesia; epidural opiates or an epidural local anesthetic such as 0.125% or 0.25% bupivacaine (Marcaine), with fentanyl, 1 mcg/mL at an infusion of 8 to 10 mL/hour.

E. In Vitro Fertilization

1. **Introduction**
   Laparoscopic in vitro fertilization and embryo transfer are frequently performed for the treatment of infertility. This outpatient procedure is indicated for the treatment of tubal disease, endometriosis, and idiopathic infertility.

2. **Preoperative assessment and patient preparation**
   a) History and physical examination: As indicated by the patient's history and medical condition
   b) Patient preparation
      (1) Laboratory tests: Hemoglobin and hematocrit; other tests as indicated
      (2) Intravenous therapy: One 18-gauge intravenous catheter
3. **Room preparation**
   a) Monitoring equipment: Standard
   b) Additional equipment: No special considerations
   c) Drugs
      (1) Miscellaneous pharmacologic agents: Opioid, short-acting non-depolarizing muscle relaxant, anesthetic agent
      (2) Intravenous fluids: Calculated for minimal blood loss; crystalloids at 2 mL/kg/hour; estimated blood loss less than 50 mL
      (3) Blood: No special considerations
      (4) Tabletop: Standard
4. **Perioperative management and anesthetic technique**
   a) General anesthesia is most common and preferred.
   b) Local, regional, subarachnoid block, or epidural techniques can be used.
   c) Induction is standard, as indicated. An outpatient procedure is a consideration.
   d) Maintenance is standard inhalation agent/oxygen/opioid anesthesia.
   e) Consider complications of pneumoperitoneum (i.e., hypercapnia, hypoxia, pneumothorax, ventilation-perfusion mismatch, increased inspiratory pressures, dysrhythmias, altered cardiac output, and hemorrhage).
   f) Position is supine with Trendelenburg's position.
   g) Emergence is standard.
5. **Postoperative implications**
   Complications include abdominal pain and referred shoulder discomfort.

F. Loop Electrosurgical Excision Procedure

1. **Introduction**
   The loop electrosurgical excision procedure is performed for the diagnosis and treatment of cervical intraepithelial neoplasia. This form of electrosurgery uses a loop electrode for excision and fulguration to prevent cervical bleeding. Other types of therapy that may be used to ablate cervical lesions are cryosurgery and carbon dioxide laser surgery.
2. **Preoperative assessment and patient preparation**
   a) History and physical examination: As indicated by the patient's history and medical condition
   b) Patient preparation
      (1) Laboratory tests: Pregnancy test, hemoglobin and hematocrit, urinalysis
      (2) Preoperative medications: Anxiolytics possible if the patient is not pregnant (e.g., midazolam, 0.01 to 0.02 mg/kg)
      (3) Intravenous therapy: One 18-gauge intravenous catheter
3. **Room preparation**
   a) Monitoring equipment: Standard. If a pregnancy is more than 16 weeks' gestation, fetal monitoring may be used.

PART II **Common Procedures**

b) Drugs: Standard tabletop agents are used.

c) Intravenous fluids: Calculate for minimal blood loss, 2 to 4 mL/ kg/hour. Estimated blood loss is 50 to 200 mL.

4. **Perioperative management and anesthetic technique**

   a) Local, monitored anesthesia care, or regional or general anesthesia is used.

   b) Induction: Standard induction is indicated.

   c) In pregnant patients, rapid sequence induction is used.

   d) In nonpregnant patients, mask ventilation may be appropriate.

   e) Maintenance: Standard, inhalational agent/oxygen/opioid. Muscle relaxation is not required.

   f) Position is lithotomy.

   g) Emergence is standard.

5. **Postoperative implications**

   a) Complications include peroneal nerve injury from the lithotomy position, nausea and vomiting, bleeding, postdural headache, and premature labor.

   b) Pain management: Oral analgesics are used if the patient is not pregnant.

G. Pelvic Exenteration

1. **Introduction**

   Pelvic exenteration is performed for the treatment of advanced, recurrent, radioresistant cervical carcinoma. It is considered a radical surgical approach because all pelvic tissues, including the cervix, bladder, lymph nodes, rectum, uterus, and vagina, are resected. Vaginal reconstruction and appropriate colon and urinary diversions are also performed.

2. **Preoperative assessment and patient preparation**

   a) History and physical examination: As indicated by the patient's history and medical condition

   b) Patient preparation

      (1) Laboratory tests: Complete blood count, electrolytes, blood urea nitrogen, creatinine, calcium, magnesium, phosphate, prothrombin time, partial thromboplastin time, urinalysis, and renal function tests

      (2) Diagnostic tests: As indicated by the patient's history and physical examination

      (3) Premedication: Anxiolytics as indicated

      (4) Intravenous therapy: Two 14- to 16-gauge intravenous catheters

      (5) Central and arterial line; pulmonary arterial catheter considered if the patient has a significant cardiac history

      (6) An epidural catheter possible for postoperative pain relief

3. **Room preparation**

   a) Monitoring equipment: Standard; arterial line and central venous pressure and pulmonary arterial catheters considered

   b) Additional equipment: Fluid warmer and Bair Hugger

   c) Drugs: Standard

      (1) Miscellaneous pharmacologic agents include opioid, anxiolytic, nondepolarizing muscle relaxant, local anesthetic, and antibiotics.

      (2) Intravenous fluids: Calculate for major blood loss, 10 to 15 mg/ kg/hour. Estimated blood loss is 1000 to 4000 mL.

4. **Perioperative management and anesthetic technique**

   a) General anesthesia with an epidural block is used.

b) Induction is standard, as indicated.

c) Maintenance is with inhalational agent/oxygen/opioid anesthesia.

d) Consider a local anesthetic through an epidural catheter.

e) Use long-acting nondepolarizing muscle relaxants.

f) Maintain normocarbia, mean arterial pressure of 60 to 88 mm Hg, and urinary output at 0.5 to 1 mL/kg/hour; transfuse as indicated.

g) Position: Both lithotomy and supine positions are used throughout the procedure.

h) Emergence: The patient generally is transported to the intensive care unit for 2 to 3 days; postoperative ventilation may be necessary. If the patient is hemodynamically stable, extubation may be considered.

5. **Postoperative implications**

a) Complications: Bleeding, fluid maintenance from large fluid shifts and mobilizations, and peroneal nerve damage from the lithotomy position

b) Pain management: Epidural, opiates, or both

H. Vaginal Delivery

1. **Preoperative assessment**

See the discussion of cesarean section earlier in this section.

2. **Patient preparation**

a) All patients should have an intravenous catheter placed and should receive a 500- to 1000-mL bolus before an epidural placement.

b) Lumbar epidural anesthesia provides segmental levels of analgesia that block pain impulses from the uterus but maintain sensation in the perineum and avoid motor blockade.

   (1) Generally, this is only administered when labor is well established, and the cervix is dilated 5 to 6 cm in primiparas and 3 to 4 cm in multiparas, with regular contractions.

   (2) Bupivacaine is frequently used because it has little effect on the fetus and a longer duration of action. Solutions commonly used are $\frac{1}{8}$% or $\frac{1}{16}$% with fentanyl, 1 to 2 mcg/mL, with an infusion at 8 to 12 mL/hour and a bolus of 5 to 10 mL.

   (3) Monitor blood pressure frequently for the first half hour, and treat any blood pressure less than 100 mm Hg with ephedrine, fluids, and left uterine displacement.

   (4) Epidural topoffs may be used for forceps delivery or an extensive episiotomy repair with 5 to 10 mL of the infusion or 3% chloroprocaine (Nesacaine).

c) A saddle block may be used for forceps delivery to block the perineum and inner thigh; 7.5 to 10 mg of lidocaine may be given while the patient is in the sitting position.

d) Pudendal nerve block: This blocks the pudendal nerves of S2 to S4 during the second stage of labor and results in low forceps delivery and episiotomy. It is administered transvaginally, with the local anesthetic injected posterior to the ischial spines beneath the sacrospinus ligaments. There is risk of puncture of the fetal scalp.

e) Paracervical block: This is injected into the fornix of the vagina lateral to the cervix. Nerve fibers from the uterus, cervix, and upper vagina are anesthetized; fibers from the perineum are not blocked. There is a high frequency of fetal bradycardia, so it is generally avoided.

ORTHOPEDICS AND PODIATRY

A. Arthroscopy

1. **Introduction**

   Arthroscopic surgery may be performed for diagnostic or therapeutic indications most often involving the ankle, knee, shoulder, or wrist. Advances in arthroscopy permit many procedures to be performed primarily or adjunctively through the arthroscope, and arthroscopic surgery has replaced some procedures that previously were performed through open techniques. Most of these procedures are done in young, healthy patients. The advantages include minimal incisions, decreased postoperative morbidity, and potentially faster rehabilitation.

2. **Preoperative assessment and patient preparation**
   - a) History and physical examination: Individualized
   - b) Diagnostic tests
     - (1) Radiographs of the affected extremity
     - (2) Chest radiograph, electrocardiogram, and laboratory tests as indicated
   - c) Preoperative medicines and intravenous therapy
     - (1) Antiinflammatory medications: Stopped 5 to 7 days before surgery
     - (2) Antibiotics: Cefazolin, 1 g intravenously
     - (3) Sedatives and narcotics
     - (4) One peripheral large-bore intravenous line
     - (5) Epidural catheter placement: Test dose performed on an awake patient.
   - d) Choice of anesthetic method: Local, general, and regional anesthesia have all been used successfully.

3. **Room preparation**
   - a) Standard monitoring equipment
   - b) Standard drugs for general or regional anesthesia
   - c) Special orthopedic tables

4. **Perioperative management**
   - a) Induction: Standard induction with routine medications is used.
   - b) Positioning
     - (1) Most often, arthroscopic procedures for lower extremity joints use the supine position, as do most arthroscopic procedures on the upper extremities.
     - (2) Arthroscopy on the knee requires the supine position with the foot of the operating room bed lowered. The nonoperative leg should either be wrapped with an elastic bandage or have some form of antiembolic stocking in place to reduce pooling of blood and reduce the potential for thrombus formation.
     - (3) Patients undergoing elbow arthroscopy may be placed in the supine, lateral decubitus, or prone position; the position is dictated

by operative necessity and surgeon preference. The prone position is more advantageous primarily because of the better limb stability during the procedure.

(4) Shoulder arthroscopy is usually accomplished by either the modified Fowler's position (beach chair position) or the lateral decubitus position, based on optimal access to the injury and surgeon preference.

(5) Hip arthroscopy is also typically accomplished by the lateral decubitus or the supine positions, with the patient on a fracture table. The fracture table is used to provide greater stability while traction is applied, using either weights and counterweights (lateral decubitus position) or mechanical traction attached to the leg-holding device of the fracture table (supine position).

c) Tourniquet use: See the discussion of knee arthroscopy later in this section.

d) Emergence: The patient is usually extubated in the operating room, unless there was preoperative respiratory compromise.

5. **Postoperative concerns**

a) Pain is usually minimal to moderate, unless reconstruction was performed.

(1) Intraarticular injections of local anesthetics and/or opioids are now widely used in an attempt to provide postoperative analgesia.

(2) Inadequate pain control can lead to decreased mobility and increased incidence of postoperative complications.

b) Swelling/edema: Assess capillary refill in the affected extremity and avoid overhydration intraoperatively.

c) Nerve damage: Assess neurologic function after surgery.

B. Foot and Ankle Surgery

1. **Introduction**

The feet and ankles are the basis of support on which the remainder of the body rests. Surgical correction of maladies and deformities of the feet and ankles falls under the scope of practice of two specialists: the orthopedic surgeon and the doctor of podiatric medicine, or podiatrist. Both these specialists are highly skilled in foot and ankle surgery to correct the multitude of maladies and deformities that occur with the feet and ankles.

The most commonly performed procedures on the ankle involve surgical repair of ankle fractures and fusion of the ankle joint. The Achilles tendon is also a frequent focus of surgery, particularly in more physically active persons. The most widely known surgical procedures on the feet are bunionectomy (with or without fusion), correction of hammertoe deformities (with or without fusion), and plantar fasciotomy (either open or endoscopic).

Open repair of ankle fractures is usually accomplished using plates and screws to hold the bone fragment in proper alignment until the fragments grow back together. Ankle fusion (arthrodesis) is performed for a multitude of medical reasons and may involve two or three bones fused together to provide pain relief and greater joint stability. Incisions are usually made on both the medial and lateral aspects of the ankle joint to allow for optimal surgical access to the involved bones. The fracture is reduced, after which a plate is placed across the fracture site or sites. Holes are drilled with the plate acting as the template, and screws are placed into these holes. For ankle fusions, the incisions are typically made across the medial and lateral aspects of the joint, and Kirschner wires or screws are used to fuse the appropriate bones in place. The incisions are closed, and some type of inflexible stabilizing device is applied (e.g., cast or plaster splints or ambulatory boot) while the patient is under anesthesia. Pneumatic tourniquets are almost always employed to keep blood loss at a minimum and to provide a clear surgical field.

Bunion deformity usually involves the first or great toe. Incision is made along the anterior surface from about midtoe across the metatarsophalangeal joint. The bony deformity is excised. Depending on the variation of the bunionectomy procedure chosen, excision of the bony deformity may be the totality of the procedure, or the angular deformity may be corrected with a screw or Kirschner wire fusion.

Hammertoe deformity correction involves incision of the anterior surface of the malformed toe or toes. The incision crosses the joint containing the bony deformity. The surgeon dissects down to the joint and excises the bony deformity. Depending on the severity of the deformity, the interphalangeal joint may be fused by inserting a Kirschner wire.

Plantar fasciotomy is indicated for severe foot pain during or after ambulating, or on arising after sleep, resulting from chronic plantar fasciitis that has not responded to conservative therapy. Open fasciotomy is accomplished through a small incision along the posterior surface of the calcaneus. The plantar fascia is incised to relieve the tension across the plantar arch. Endoscopic plantar fasciotomy is accomplished via two "miniature" incisions, one medial and one lateral, at the beginning of the plantar arch. A small trocar is inserted through these incisions. The sheath of the trocar is slotted to allow visualization of the plantar fascia with the endoscope. The full thickness of the plantar fascia is incised, and the skin incisions are closed.

2. **Anesthetic management**
   a) Patients scheduled for foot or ankle surgery are excellent candidates for regional anesthesia.
   b) Most surgical procedures on the foot or ankle can be accomplished within a 2-hour time frame, often on an outpatient basis.
   c) Spinal anesthesia provides sufficient surgical anesthesia to allow completion of most procedures. However, the postanesthesia recovery phase may be unacceptably long and may require the patient to spend a night in the hospital or outpatient facility, which may be unacceptable to the patient.
   d) Nerve blocks are especially effective for surgical procedures on the foot or ankle. Posterior tibial nerve block, Mayo blockade, and Bier block are examples of blocks that are effective for foot and ankle procedures.
   e) One may provide intravenous sedation by either continuous infusion or intermittent bolus to provide amnesia and to minimize or eliminate any anxiety the patient may have. The surgeon can inject the surgical site with long-acting local anesthetic (e.g., bupivacaine) to maintain the patient's comfort immediately and for several hours postoperatively.

C. Forearm and Hand Surgery

1. **Introduction**
   Surgical procedures on the hand or forearm may be precipitated by violent trauma resulting in complex or dislocated fractures to the bones of the forearm, hand, or fingers, or they may be performed to alleviate numbness of the hand resulting from compression of the nerves of the forearm or wrist, such as carpal tunnel syndrome. Procedures on the fingers and hand are often relatively quick, requiring 1 hour or less to complete. Surgical correction of complex or dislocated fractures of the forearm may require considerable instrumentation and time to complete. For virtually all the surgical procedures of the hand and forearm, the pneumatic tourniquet is used.

2. **Anesthetic management**
   a) Patients scheduled for surgical procedures on the forearm or hand are excellent candidates for regional anesthesia.
   b) Axillary block and Bier block provide excellent surgical anesthesia for most surgical procedures of the forearm and hand that are anticipated to require 1 hour or less to accomplish.
   c) For procedures precipitated by traumatic injury, such as complex, comminuted fractures or reconstruction of the vascular and nerve structures of the hand or forearm—procedures that may require considerable amounts of time to accomplish—the better anesthetic choice may be general anesthesia.
   d) Tourniquet pain becomes an issue with such longer procedures if regional anesthesia is chosen.
   e) In addition, for the patient requiring surgery as the result of traumatic injury, the issue of the patient's nothing by mouth (NPO) status becomes important. Frequently, trauma patients have eaten or ingested liquids close to the time of the traumatic injury. Alcohol may be a precipitating factor in the traumatic injury as well. For these reasons, rapid-sequence induction of general anesthesia may be a more appropriate anesthetic course.

D. Hip Arthroplasty

1. **Introduction**
   The replacement of joint surfaces is required primarily for inflammatory or degenerative conditions within the joint, such as those accompanying rheumatoid arthritis or osteoarthritis from degeneration of the synovium or cartilage. As normal joint tissues deteriorate or degenerate, the bone ends are exposed, causing pain and limitation of joint movements. Joint stiffness and muscle atrophy follow, further increasing pain, limiting movement, and mobility. Exposed bone surfaces lead to bone growth that may eventually adhere to the opposing bone ends, causing bony ankylosis and loss of joint movement. Therefore, replacement of the deteriorated or degenerated tissues and bones restores movement and relieves pain. Hip arthroplasty is discussed here.

   The hip joint is one of the most frequently replaced joints. Typically, the patient is placed in the lateral decubitus position, which offers greater range of motion and visibility throughout the surgical procedure. This procedure requires a large incision, extending from near the iliac crest across the joint to the midthigh level. Several large muscle groups must be incised and dissected through to gain access to the joint, after which the joint is disarticulated. The femoral head and neck are excised, leaving the femoral canal open. The femur is filled with rich marrow, because it is one of the erythrocyte production areas for the body; therefore, it is also richly vascular. The acetabulum is a part of the pelvic girdle, also one of the erythrocyte production areas, and is richly vascular as well. After the femoral head and neck are removed, the femoral canal is reamed to the appropriate diameter to accommodate the prosthetic head and neck. The acetabulum is then reamed in a similar manner to accommodate its own prosthesis. During the reaming for both prosthetic components, bone is shaved from the canal and acetabulum to produce a smoother bony surface to achieve better adherence of the prosthetic device and cement. Also during the reaming process, venous sinuses within these bony structures are opened, and often destroyed, and this can result in significant blood loss.

After the femoral canal has been satisfactorily prepared, the canal is cleaned out using pulse irrigation, which forces irrigation solution deep within the femoral canal under pressure in a high-frequency, pulsatile manner. The canal is further cleaned with a sponge, after which methylmethacrylate (MMA) cement may be instilled into the femoral canal. For some procedures, usually in younger or very physically active patients, MMA is not used to secure the femoral prosthesis, and the prosthesis is referred to as being "press-fit." After instillation of the MMA cement, the femoral prosthesis is inserted into the canal and is forcibly seated with a mallet. The acetabular component is secured in place with screws and bone grafting. The dislocated joint is reduced, and the soft tissues are returned to normal anatomic position during wound closure.

2. **Preoperative assessment and patient preparation**
   a) History and physical examination
      (1) With this elderly population, assess for coexisting medical diseases.
      (2) Carefully assess blood volume, central venous pressure, and orthostatic hypotension because dehydration may mask hemoglobin changes resulting from hematoma formation.
   b) Diagnostic tests
      (1) Radiographs: Hip and chest film
      (2) Laboratory tests: Complete blood count, electrolytes, glucose, blood urea nitrogen, creatinine, urinalysis, prothrombin time, partial thromboplastin time, bleeding time of the patient on aspirin, and type and cross-match
   c) Preoperative medications and intravenous therapy
      (1) Anticoagulants: Heparin, low-molecular-weight heparin, oral anticoagulants
      (2) Antirheumatic or antiinflammatory medications
      (3) Antibiotics
      (4) Sedatives and narcotics: Used with caution in the elderly population.
      (5) Two peripheral, large-bore (16- to 18-gauge) intravenous lines with moderate fluid replacement
      (6) Epidural catheter placement: Test dose performed on an awake patient

3. **Room preparation**
   a) Monitoring equipment

(1) Standard
(2) Indwelling urinary catheter: Controversial
    (a) Absence of bladder drainage can cause overdistention, affecting bladder function.
    (b) Insertion may cause urinary tract infection.
(3) Central venous pressure: Trend of volume status.
(4) Warming modalities are used.
(5) Electrocardiography leads V_5 and II detect myocardial ischemia and diagnose tachyarrythmias in the elderly population.
(6) Transesophageal echocardiography: Assess fat and bone deposits when the acetabulum is reamed and curetted.
(7) Use x-ray shields for self-protection.
(8) Arterial line monitoring is indicated if hypotensive techniques are used.
  b) Pharmacologic agents: Vasopressors
  c) Position: Lateral; a special orthopedic table may be used.

4. Anesthetic technique
  a) Considerations: Regional blockade, general anesthesia, or a combination of both
  b) Technique of choice
    (1) Regional anesthesia
    (2) Reduced blood loss and postoperative deep venous thrombosis/pulmonary embolism
  c) Regional blockade
    (1) Epidural catheter placement and preoperative test dose OR
    (2) One-time spinal for analgesia to T10
  d) General anesthesia
    (1) Endotracheal tube must be inserted.
    (2) Combination with regional anesthetic allows reduced dosages of agents and control of airway.
  e) Induction
    (1) General anesthesia
      (a) Thorough airway assessment is done in an arthritic population.
      (b) Induction is performed with the patient on the stretcher.
      (c) Succinylcholine may be contraindicated with crush injuries if large amounts of muscle tissue are devitalized.
    (2) Maintenance
      (a) Monitor fluid and blood replacement therapy to minimize blood loss and transfusion that are applicable during hip arthroplasty (e.g., autologous donation and deliberate hypotension).
      (b) Laminar flow is used to minimize infections and can increase evaporative fluid and heat losses from the operative site.
      (c) Controlled hypotensive techniques facilitate surgical exposure and decrease blood loss.
        (i) Blood pressure parameters need to be individualized.
        (ii) Maintain mean blood pressure of 50 to 70 mm Hg.
        (iii) Deepen anesthesia with a volatile anesthetic.
        (iv) Initiate a vasoactive (nitroprusside) drip.
    (3) The nurse anesthetist must be particularly cognizant of the possible occurrence of hypotension, hypoxia, and potential cardiovascular collapse. These complications are observed most often during insertion of the femoral prosthesis during total hip arthroplasty.

(a) Possible causes of these complications include the MMA cement, fat embolism, air embolism, thromboembolism, and bone marrow embolism.

(b) MMA has been demonstrated to produce significant increases in both pulmonary vascular resistance and pulmonary wedge pressure while decreasing systemic vascular resistance, cardiac output, and arterial pressure.

(c) MMA cement is used to distribute the forces of the femoral and acetabular prosthetic components.

  (i) Mixing the cement causes the monomer portion to polymerize—an exothermic reaction.

  (ii) Problems with MMA relate to cementing the femoral prosthesis—unpolymerized monomer can be absorbed into the circulation.

  (iii) It causes direct vasodilation, usually within the first minute; it can last as long as 10 minutes.

  (iv) Venous embolism can occur when the femoral prosthesis is inserted into the femoral canal.

  (v) Hypotension, hypoxia, and cardiovascular collapse following prosthesis insertion have been reported.

  (vi) Prevent complications—communicate with the surgeon regarding application.

  (vii) Use 100% oxygen, decrease the vasodilating agent, maximize fluid status, and have vasopressor support available.

f) Emergence

  (1) If a general anesthetic is implemented, patients are usually repositioned onto the stretcher before emergence.

  (2) Extubation is based on the patient's status.

  (3) Initiate regional blockade through the epidural catheter for postoperative analgesia before the end of the case.

5. **Postoperative implications**

  a) Obtain laboratory results: Hemoglobin and hematocrit; watch for hidden bleeding.

  b) Fat embolism typically appears 12 to 48 hours after a long bone fracture.

    (1) Signs and symptoms

      (a) Arterial hypoxemia

      (b) Adult respiratory distress syndrome

      (c) Central nervous system dysfunction (confusion, coma, seizures)

      (d) Petechiae (neck, shoulders, and chest)

      (e) Coagulopathy

      (f) Fever

    (2) Treatment

      (a) Supportive

      (b) Oxygenation

      (c) Corticosteroids

      (d) Immobilization of long bone fractures

  c) Other potential complications include deep venous thrombosis and pulmonary embolism. Deep venous thrombosis is a precursor to pulmonary embolism development. Deep venous thrombosis has been demonstrated in 40% to 60% of patients undergoing total hip arthroplasty and in approximately 80% of patients having total knee arthroplasty. From within the two patient populations, pulmonary embolism is believed to develop 1% to 5% of the time.

E. Hip Pinning (Open Reduction and Internal Fixation)

⟫·◆·⟪

1. **Introduction**
   Hip pinning involves the open reduction of a hip fracture that is maintained by the application of plates and screws (internal fixation). Bone grafting may be used to repair any defects. Hip fractures may result from high-impact trauma, but most result from minor trauma in elderly persons. If the fracture is related to high-impact trauma, a coexisting trauma should be thoroughly evaluated.

2. **Preoperative assessment and patient preparation**
   a) History and physical examination: Obtain a verbal history from the patient or family member. Note any preexisting disease processes, social history, current medications, past surgical history, and allergies.
   b) Laboratory tests: Hemoglobin, hematocrit, complete blood count, prothrombin time, partial thromboplastin time, and others are obtained as indicated by the history and physical examination.
   c) Diagnostic tests: 12-lead electrocardiography, chest radiography, and others are obtained as indicated by the history and physical examination.
   d) Preoperative medications: These are individualized.

3. **Room preparation**
   a) Monitoring equipment: Standard, arterial line, central venous pressure catheter, pulmonary arterial catheter as indicated
   b) Additional equipment
      (1) Positioning devices and operating table: The patient is usually placed in a lateral position. Aging skin atrophies and is prone to trauma from adhesive tape, electrocautery pads, and electrocardiographic electrodes. Arthritic joints may interfere with positioning; when possible, the elderly patient should be positioned for comfort. Meticulous padding of the axilla and all bony prominences decreases the risk of nerve injury and ischemia. Prevent pressure to the ears and eyes. Maintain the neck in neutral alignment.
      (2) Because of the length of the procedure, the patient's usual age, and surgical exposure, warming modalities should be implemented (fluid warmer, warming blankets).
   c) Drugs
      (1) Continuous infusion: Consider the use of a continuous epidural infusion intraoperatively or for postoperative pain control.
      (2) Intravenous fluids: Estimated blood loss is greater than 1000 mL. Type and cross-match for 2 units of packed red blood cells. Blood loss is replaced 1:1 with blood products or colloid solutions or 3:1 if crystalloid solutions are used. Maintain urine output at 0.5 mL/kg/hour. Keep in mind any preexisting disease processes that may easily place the elderly patient in a state of fluid overload. Consider the use of a cell saver intraoperatively.
      (3) Tabletop: Standard. All equipment needed to implement the anesthetic plan should be available.

4. **Perioperative management and anesthetic technique**
   a) Regional and general anesthesia are both options for the elderly patient.
   b) Hip pinning may be performed using subarachnoid block or continuous epidural infusion extending to the T8 sensory level. Keep in mind the expected length of the procedure, the patient's history

PART II **Common Procedures**

and physical examination findings, and the patient's level of cooperation and ability to lie still. One major advantage of regional anesthesia is a decreased incidence of postoperative thromboembolism. This is thought to be the result of peripheral vasodilation and maintenance of venous blood flow in the lower extremities. Local anesthetics also inhibit platelet aggregation and stabilize endothelial cells. Difficult patient positioning and altered landmarks related to degenerative changes of the spine may increase the technical difficulty of performing a regional block. Postpuncture headaches are not as prevalent in the elderly population.

c) If a general anesthetic is the best choice for the patient, drugs for induction and maintenance should reflect findings from the patient's history and physical examination. One advantage of general anesthesia is that the anesthetic can be induced with the patient on the bed or stretcher before moving to the operating table, thus avoiding painful positioning. A disadvantage of general anesthesia is that the elderly patient cannot be positioned for maximal comfort. Consider the use of nondepolarizing muscle relaxants during induction if there are no airway concerns. Continued muscle relaxation is optional and is left to the discretion of the anesthetist or the request of the surgeon. The effects of nondepolarizing muscle relaxants that are renally excreted may be slightly prolonged in elderly persons because of reduced drug clearance.

d) Emergence: An epidural catheter may be placed for supplemental use with general anesthesia or for postoperative pain control.

e) Fat embolization: See the discussion of pelvic reconstruction later in this section.

5. **Postoperative implications**

a) Consider the use of a continuous epidural infusion for patient-controlled analgesia for postoperative pain control.

b) A marked decrease in blood pressure postoperatively may be related to hematoma formation.

c) Deep venous thrombosis prophylaxis should be instituted postoperatively (support hose and deep venous thrombosis prophylaxis).

F. Knee (Total Knee Replacement) Arthroplasty

1. **Introduction**
Total knee arthroplasty is the other frequently performed joint replacement procedure. A pneumatic tourniquet is typically used to provide a relatively bloodless surgical field. Nevertheless, blood loss as a result of total knee arthroplasty can be up to 2 units. During the procedure, the articulating surfaces of the femur and tibia are excised by precise angular cuts, and the patellar articulating surface is shaved, all to conform the bones to the inner surfaces of the prostheses. Both the femoral and tibial surfaces are covered with methylmethacrylate cement, and the individual prosthesis components are forcibly seated with a mallet. The high-density polyethylene patellar component is cemented and seated with a vise-like clamp. The medial and lateral menisci are replaced with a conforming wedge of high-density polyethylene.

2. **Preoperative assessment**
Assessment is routine, including history and physical examination. These patients have been diagnosed with arthritis of the knee.

a) Respiratory: These patients may have rheumatoid arthritis and associated pulmonary conditions. Pulmonary effusions may be present. Rheumatoid arthritis involving the cricoarytenoid joints may exhibit itself by hoarseness. A narrow glottic opening may lead to a difficult intubation. Arthritic involvement of the cervical spine and temporomandibular joint may also complicate airway management.

b) Cardiovascular: Depending on the severity of the arthritis, the patient may have a lowered exercise tolerance. Rheumatoid arthritis is associated with pericardial effusion. Cardiac valve fibrosis and cardiac conduction abnormalities can occur with possible aortic regurgitation. Test with an electrocardiogram and, if possible, an echocardiogram and dipyridamole thallium imaging.

c) Neurologic: A thorough preoperative neurologic examination may yield evidence of cervical nerve root compression. If indicated, obtain lateral neck films for the determination of stability of the atlanto-occipital joint.

d) Musculoskeletal: Positioning may be difficult because of pain and the decreased mobility of the joints.

e) Hematologic/laboratory: Obtain hemoglobin and hematocrit and other tests related to the history and physical examination.

f) Premedication is individualized based on the patient's need.

3. **Room preparation**
   a) Standard monitoring equipment. A tourniquet may or may not be used.
   b) The patient should have one large-bore intravenous line.
   c) Fluid requirements include normal saline or lactated Ringer's solution at 6 mL/kg/hour.
   d) Standard drugs for general or regional anesthesia are used.

4. **Anesthetic technique**
   a) This procedure can be done using general or regional anesthesia.
   b) Regional anesthesia could be with a subarachnoid block or placement of an epidural catheter.

5. **Perioperative management**
   a) Induction: Standard induction with routine medications. Muscle relaxation is needed for the placement of the prosthesis.
   b) Monitor fluid and blood therapy.
   c) Monitor for physiologic changes that are caused by tourniquets.
   d) Safety measures for preventing tourniquet complications

PART II Common Procedures

Physiologic Changes Caused by Limb Tourniquets

Neurologic Effects
Abolition of somatosensory-evoked potentials and nerve conduction occurs within 30 minutes.
Application for more than 60 minutes causes tourniquet pain and hypertension.
Application for more than 2 hours may result in postoperative neurapraxia.
Evidence of nerve injury may occur at the skin level underlying the edge of the tourniquet.

Muscle Changes
Cellular hypoxia develops within 2 minutes.
Cellular creatinine value declines.
Progressive cellular acidosis occurs.
Endothelial capillary leak develops after 2 hours.

Continued

Physiologic Changes Caused by Limb Tourniquets—cont'd

Systemic Effects of Tourniquet Inflation
Elevation in arterial and pulmonary artery pressures develops. This is usually slight to moderate if only one limb is occluded. The response is more severe in patients undergoing balanced anesthesia that does not include a potent anesthetic vapor.

Systemic Effects of Tourniquet Release
Transient fall in core temperature occurs.
Transient metabolic acidosis occurs.
Transient fall in central venous oxygen tension occurs but systemic hypoxemia is unusual.
Acid metabolites (e.g., thromboxane) are released into the central circulation.
Transient fall in pulmonary and systemic arterial pressures occurs.
Transient increase in end-tidal carbon dioxide occurs.

---

(1) The tourniquet should be applied where the nerves are best protected in the underlying musculature.

(2) Check the proper availability and functioning of the equipment before it is operated.

(3) The tourniquet should be used for no longer than 2 hours.

(4) Only the minimally effective pressure should be used for occluding blood flow to the extremity. For the lower extremity, twice the patient's systolic pressure should be used.

(5) The pressure display must accurately reflect the pressure in the tourniquet bladder.

(6) The cuff must properly fit the extremity.

(7) The limb must be padded, and the cuff must be properly applied to the limb with care and attention.

e) Emergence: These patients are usually extubated in the operating room unless there was preoperative respiratory compromise.

6. **Postoperative implications**
Watch for posterior tibial artery trauma, peroneal nerve palsy (foot drop), hemorrhage from the posterior tibial artery, and tourniquet nerve injury, if indicated.

G. Pelvic Reconstruction

1. **Introduction**
Pelvic reconstruction is a surgical procedure that involves the open reduction of pelvic fractures, which are then maintained by the application of plates and screws. Bone grafting may be used to repair any defects. The surgical time for the procedure is 3 to 6 hours. These fractures may be caused by minor trauma, especially in elderly persons, but most result from high-impact trauma (i.e., motor vehicle trauma). Evaluation of the patient for potential coexisting trauma should include a thorough neurologic, thoracic, and abdominal assessment. The extremities may also be involved.

2. **Preoperative assessment**
a) History and physical examination: Obtain a verbal history from the patient or family member. Note any preexisting disease processes, social history, current medications, past surgical history, and allergies.

(1) Cardiac: Assess for cardiac contusion or aortic tear. Tests include 12-lead electrocardiography, creatine phosphokinase isoenzymes, and chest radiography (wide mediastinal silhouette suggests aortic tear). Transesophageal echocardiography or angiography is indicated if an aortic tear is suspected. Consult with a cardiologist if indicated.

(2) Respiratory: Assess for possible hemothorax, pneumothorax, pulmonary contusion, fat embolism, or aspiration. The patient may require supplemental oxygen or mechanical ventilation to correct hypoxemia. Coexisting trauma to the head or cervical spine may require fiberoptic intubation. Tests include chest radiography and arterial blood gases.

(3) Neurologic: A thorough neurologic evaluation including mental status and peripheral sensory examination. Note any preexisting deficits. Consult with a neurologist if necessary. For tests, computed tomography of the head is indicated before anesthesia for patients who experience a loss of consciousness.

(4) Renal: Renal injury is possible with high-impact trauma. Rule out a urethral tear before the Foley catheter is placed. A suprapubic catheter may be necessary. Intraoperative monitoring of urine output is mandatory to assess adequate renal perfusion. Consult a urologist if necessary. Tests include urinalysis, blood urea nitrogen, serum creatinine, hematuria, and myoglobinuria.

(5) Musculoskeletal: Cervical spine clearance may be required before neck manipulation (i.e., laryngoscopy). Consider evaluating thoracic and lumbar radiographs to rule out any deformity or instability before anesthesia. Tests include cervical spine radiography and others as indicated from the history and physical examination.

(6) Hematologic: Large blood loss associated with traumatic injury may occur. The patient's hematocrit should be restored to greater than 25% before induction of anesthesia. Type and cross-match for 6 units of packed red blood cells. Consider the use of a cell saver intraoperatively.

(7) Gastrointestinal: Patients should be assessed for abdominal injury associated with trauma. The test used is diagnostic peritoneal lavage.

b) Patient preparation

(1) Laboratory tests: Hemoglobin, hematocrit, electrolytes, prothrombin time, partial thromboplastin time, and others are obtained as indicated from the history and physical examination.

(2) Medications: Anxiolytics, narcotics, antibiotics, and others as indicated from the history and physical examination. The patient may also be receiving anticoagulant therapy for the prevention of deep venous thrombosis. A broad-spectrum antibiotic should be administered preoperatively.

3. Room preparation

a) Monitoring equipment: Standard, arterial line, central venous pressure, pulmonary arterial catheter if indicated, two large peripheral intravenous catheters

b) Additional equipment

(1) Positioning devices and operating table: The patient may be placed in the supine, lateral, or prone position. A fracture table may be used. Meticulously pad the chest, axilla, pelvis, and extremities to prevent potential nerve injury and ischemia. Prevent pressure to the downward ear and eye if the patient is in the lateral position. Maintain the patient's neck in neutral alignment.

PART II **Common Procedures**

(2) Because of the length of the procedure and surgical exposure, warming devices should be implemented (i.e., fluid warmer, warming blanket).

(3) A nasogastric tube should be used to decompress the stomach if rapid sequence induction is performed.

c) Drugs

(1) Continuous infusions: Consider the use of an intravenous narcotic infusion. If an epidural catheter is placed for postoperative pain control, consider an intraoperative continuous infusion to decrease anesthetic requirements.

(2) Intravenous fluids and blood: Estimated blood loss is greater than 1000 mL. Type and cross-match the patient for 6 units of packed red blood cells. Blood loss is replaced 1:1 with blood products or colloid solutions or 3:1 if crystalloid solutions are used. Consider the intraoperative use of a cell saver. Maintain urine output at 0.5 mL/kg/hour. Consider the use of deliberate hypotension to control blood loss in those patients without cardiovascular disease or carotid stenosis. Isoflurane, esmolol, sodium nitroprusside, or a combination thereof, titrated to decrease mean arterial pressure by 30% (but not less than 60 mm Hg), is commonly used. Any fluid deficits must be replaced before the institution of deliberate hypotension.

(3) Tabletop is standard.

4. **Perioperative management and anesthetic technique**

a) Induction and maintenance

(1) Rapid sequence induction must be used for trauma patients to decrease the risk of aspiration.

(2) A standard induction may be used if the procedure is performed electively.

(3) Because of the painful nature of the injury, induction is best performed on the patient's bed or stretcher before moving to the operating table.

(4) Drugs for induction and maintenance should reflect the patient's history and physical examination and should account for any significant medical history, current physiologic states, and drug allergies.

(5) Consider the use of a nondepolarizing muscle relaxant during induction if there are no airway concerns.

(6) Anesthetic gases should be warmed and humidified. Continued muscle relaxation is optional and is left to the discretion of the anesthetist or the request of the surgeon.

b) Emergence

(1) An epidural catheter may be placed for supplemental use intraoperatively and for postoperative pain control.

(2) Trauma patients undergoing rapid sequence induction should be fully awake and reflexive before extubation.

(3) Patients who suffer pulmonary complications related to trauma or the surgical procedure (i.e., fat embolism, pulmonary contusion, or aspiration) should not be extubated.

c) Fat embolization

(1) Thirty to 90% of patients with fractures are reported to experience fat embolization. Most patients remain asymptomatic. The incidence of fat embolization is higher in patients with long bone or pelvic fractures.

(2) Signs and symptoms include the following: hypoxemia; tachycardia; tachypnea; respiratory alkalosis; mental status changes;

petechiae on the chest, upper extremities, axillae, and conjunctivae; fat bodies in the urine; and diffuse pulmonary infiltrates.

(3) Treatment is supportive and prophylactic: Oxygen therapy and continuous positive air pressure by mask or endotracheal tube, judicious fluid management to help decrease the severity of pulmonary capillary leaks, heparin, and high-dose corticosteroids may all be considered.

5. **Postoperative implications**

a) Consider the use of continuous epidural infusion or patient-controlled analegesia for postoperative pain control.

b) The L4 to S5 nerve roots may be damaged from the primary traumatic event or the operation. The result is hemiplegia with bladder and bowel dysfunction. Intraoperative pressure on the ilioinguinal ligament may cause neuropathy of the femoral genitofemoral or femoral cutaneous nerve.

c) A marked postoperative decrease in blood pressure may be related to retroperitoneal hematoma formation.

d) Deep venous thrombosis prophylaxis should be instituted postoperatively (i.e., support hose and deep venous thrombosis prophylaxis).

H. Upper Extremity Arthroplasty

1. **Introduction**

Arthroplasty in the upper extremity makes up a low percentage of the number of joint arthroplasties performed each year. Of the two more commonly replaced upper extremity joints, the shoulder and the elbow, shoulder arthroplasty accounts for approximately 5% of the number of total joint replacements performed each year. The primary goal of shoulder arthroplasty is relief of pain, with the secondary goal being improvement in overall joint functioning. Indications for shoulder arthroplasty include glenohumeral joint destruction as a result of osteoarthritis, complex proximal humerus fractures, rheumatoid arthritis, avascular necrosis of the humeral head, and malunion or nonunion of the proximal humerus.

Shoulder arthroplasty is performed with the patient in either the lateral decubitus or modified Fowler's (beach chair) position. Because a pneumatic tourniquet cannot be used, shoulder arthroplasty tends to result in significant intraoperative blood loss.

Elbow arthroplasty is performed with less frequency than shoulder arthroplasty. The goals for elbow arthroplasty are much the same as for shoulder arthroplasty: pain relief and improvement in joint function. The indications for elbow arthroplasty include rheumatoid arthritis, traumatic arthritis, and ankylosis of the joint.

2. **Preoperative assessment**

a) Respiratory

(1) Patients with rheumatoid arthritis may show signs of pleural effusion or pulmonary fibrosis. Hoarseness may result from cricoarytenoid joint involvement. This patient may be difficult to intubate.

(2) Tests: Chest radiography and pulmonary function tests (if indicated; arterial blood gases in compromised patients) are obtained.

b) Cardiovascular: Patients with rheumatoid arthritis may suffer from chronic pericardial tamponade, valvular disease, and cardiac conduction defects.

c) Neurologic
  (1) Arthritic patients may have cervical or lumbar radiculopathies. Preoperative documentation of these conditions is essential. Head flexion may cause cervical cord compression.
  (2) Tests: Cervical spine films to rule out subluxation are indicated in patients with rheumatoid arthritis who have neck or upper extremity radiculopathy.
d) Musculoskeletal: With the possibility of limited neck and jaw mobility, special intubation may be indicated. Special attention must be paid to positioning in patients with bony deformities or contractures.
e) Hematologic: Almost all nontrauma patients will be receiving some type of nonsteroidal antiinflammatory drug, which should be stopped approximately 5 days before the procedure.
f) Endocrine: Patients with rheumatoid arthritis will most likely be receiving some type of corticosteroid and therefore should have a supplemental dose of steroids to treat adrenal suppression (e.g., intravenous hydrocortisone, 100 mg).
g) Laboratory tests: Hemoglobin and hematocrit are obtained from healthy patients; other tests are as indicated from the history and physical examination.
h) Premedication: If a regional block is done, moderate to heavy premedication is indicated.

3. **Room preparation**
   a) Standard monitoring equipment is used.
   b) The patient will be in a semisitting position. A precordial Doppler device may be used to detect venous air embolism.
   c) One large-bore intravenous line will be needed on the nonoperative side.
   d) If the patient is more hemodynamically compromised, hemodynamic monitoring may be indicated.
   e) Fluid replacement involves normal saline or lactated Ringer's solution at 6 mL/kg/hour.

4. **Anesthetic technique: Shoulder**
   a) Patients undergoing total shoulder arthroplasty can be managed by general anesthesia, interscalene block, or supraclavicular block.
   b) If general anesthesia is chosen, caution is advised to observe for the ongoing potential for inadvertent extubation as a result of the surgical manipulations necessary while in close proximity to the patient's head and neck. The patient's neck may be subjected to excessive stretch during the surgical manipulations, and if the patient's head becomes dislodged from the supportive device employed, there is the potential for cervical spine injury.
   c) For the patient undergoing shoulder arthroscopy, pulmonary function will more closely resemble "normal" function as a result of being in the modified Fowler's position. As a result of that position, the potential for venous air embolism is somewhat increased over other positions.
   d) Recognize the risk of fat or bone marrow embolism and thromboembolism incumbent with the required reaming of the shaft of one of the body's long bones. The potential cardiovascular effects of methylmethacrylate cement must also be considered if the humeral component is cemented in place.

e) Blood loss during shoulder arthroplasty can be significant, just as it can with hip arthroplasty. Minimize blood loss and transfusion (e.g., autologous donation and deliberate hypotension).

5. **Anesthetic technique: Elbow**
   a) Elbow arthroplasty can be performed in any of three positions: supine, lateral decubitus, or prone.
   b) The deciding factors on which position will be employed for this procedure are surgeon preference and the health of the patient.
   c) Elbow arthroplasty can be managed by general anesthesia or supraclavicular, infraclavicular, interscalene, or axillary block.
   d) With the patient under general anesthesia, be mindful of the potential complications and physiologic changes associated with each position.
   e) During elbow arthroplasty, the pneumatic tourniquet will probably be used to minimize blood loss and to provide a clear surgical field. Tourniquet: For the upper extremity, the tourniquet is set 70 to 90 mm Hg more than the patient's systolic blood pressure.
   f) Be prepared to treat, insofar as possible, the patient's tourniquet pain whenever regional anesthesia is employed.
   g) Be aware of the increased risk of thromboembolism development when the pneumatic tourniquet is used, particularly in patients with a history of deep venous thrombosis.

6. **Perioperative management**
   a) Induction: Standard. If the patient has limited range of motion, awake fiberoptic intubation may be indicated.
   b) Maintenance: Standard maintenance with muscle relaxation; consider a continuous opioid infusion because of the length of the procedure.
   c) Position: The patient is in the semisitting or lawn chair position or the lateral decubitus position.
   d) Considerations: If using nitrous oxide during placement of the humeral component, discontinue it because of the increased risk of a venous air embolism with moderate muscle relaxation at that time.
   e) Emergence: The patient can be extubated in the operating room. Reverse the muscle relaxant after positioning the patient back to a supine position.

7. **Postoperative implications**
   Consider a patient-controlled analgesia pump or regional block technique for postoperative pain.

PART II Common Procedures

OTHER PROCEDURES

A. Burns

1. Introduction

Burn injuries, regardless of their origin, are classified according to the depth and the extent of the skin and tissue destruction as well as the total body surface area (TBSA) involved. First-degree (superficial) burns are limited to the epidermis, which is the outermost layer of skin. The epidermis is primarily thin and avascular. First-degree burns heal spontaneously and do not usually require any medical intervention. Second-degree burns are also known as deep and superficial partial-thickness burns. They extend into the dermis, which lies below the epidermis. In contrast to the epidermis, the dermis is very vascular and contains numerous blood vessels and nerves. The severity of the type of burn varies, depending on the amount and the depth of the dermal tissues involved. If the epithelial basement membrane of the dermis is intact, the skin will regenerate, and grafting may not be required. Third-degree or full-thickness burns extend into the subcutaneous tissue lying below the dermis. The entire skin thickness is destroyed with third-degree burns. Skin grafting is required for these types of burns because the epithelium and the dermal appendages are destroyed. A fourth-degree burn classification is used by some institutions to describe structures burned below the dermis, such as muscle, fascia, and bone.

A major burn is a second-degree burn involving more than 10% of the TBSA in adults or 20% at extremes of age, a third-degree burn involving more than 10% of the TBSA in adults, and any electrical burn or one complicated by smoke inhalation. A burn formula derived from the National Burn Registry estimating mortality is as follows: if the age of the patient plus the percentage of the TBSA burn exceeds 115, the mortality is greater than 80%. Additionally, from clinical observations, is estimated that the mortality of a burned victim is approximately doubled if there is an inhalation injury sustained in conjunction with a thermal burn.

Patients who sustain full-thickness burns are seen in the operating room, probably repeatedly, for débridement and grafting. The initial assessment of the emergency patient with a burn injury is initiated as for any trauma patient and begins with airway intubation. Keep in mind that airway edema happens rapidly in a burn patient, and intubation after the edema occurs is difficult. Burn patients must have aggressive fluid resuscitation in the first 48 hours. Burns are described according to the rule of nines, which divides the body into areas of 9% or multiples thereof. For example, the head and neck combined, each arm, each leg, the posterior surface of the upper trunk, and the posterior surface of the lower trunk are each considered to be 9% of the surface area of the body. Survival is influenced by the percentage of the surface area involved, and the age of the patient.

2. **Preoperative assessment**
   a) The burn patient requires a thorough and complete preoperative assessment. A complete medical history, including laboratory studies, and a brief physical examination with lung auscultation, assessment of chest compliance, and inspection of the neck and oral cavity to evaluate for difficulties with intubation or reintubation should be implemented.
   b) There are specific data unique to the burn patient that the anesthesia provider should know: knowledge regarding the underlying trauma, the mechanism of burn (electrical, inhalation), the percentage of TBSA burned, the location of the burn sites, the area and the amount that the surgeon intends to débride, and whether the patient will undergo skin grafting during the perioperative course. The assimilation of this information affects the anesthetic plan in terms of anesthetic agents selected, appropriate monitoring, positioning, vascular access, and blood product requirements.
   c) A review of prior anesthetic records can be helpful in determining the anesthetic plan. Quite often, this is possible to do because, more often than not, these patients make several trips to the operating room.
   d) Cardiac: Assess for any preexisting cardiac problems.
      (1) There is also a loss of plasma proteins from within the intravascular compartment resulting from the disrupted endothelium. This persists for up to 36 hours after the initial burn injury. Hypovolemia results with subsequent hypotension and circulatory compromise. Indeed, the size and the extent of the burn determine the magnitude of this development.
      (2) Burn victims can develop "burn shock" within the first 24 to 36 hours following an acute burn injury. A reduction in cardiac output is a hallmark of burn shock, and it appears to occur within minutes after the injury. It is initially preserved by the catecholamine responses of tachycardia and vasoconstriction. However, with the progressive loss of intravascular fluids and proteins, left ventricular filling declines, leading to a reduction in cardiac output.
      (3) Additionally, cardiac output is thought to be depressed from the release of a myocardial depressant factor or proteins by the burned tissues.
      (4) The cardiovascular response to catecholamines is attenuated after a burn injury, owing to a reduction in adrenergic receptor affinity and decreased secondary messenger production. Coronary blood flow can be reduced as a result, further decreasing cardiac function. Systemic vascular resistance increases.
   e) Respiratory
      (1) The pulmonary system is greatly affected in burn patients, with resulting pathophysiologic changes.
      (2) Pulmonary function may decrease markedly, even in the absence of an inhalation injury. Functional residual capacity is reduced, and both lung and chest wall compliance decrease. The latter can be severely compromised if the chest is circumferentially burned.
      (3) With progressive fluid shifts and interstitial edema formation in cases with eschar formation, the inability to expand the lungs adequately impairs ventilation.

PART II Common Procedures

(4) In some cases, escharotomies are necessary to alleviate the pressure in the tissues to improve oxygenation and ventilation.

(5) The oxygen gradient between alveoli and arterial blood increases as well. Ventilation can increase to as much as 40 L/min from a normal rate of 6 L/min.

(6) The lungs are at risk of compromise without an inhalation injury. Many mechanisms are involved. A primary factor is the effect of released mediators on the lung. Plasma oncotic pressure greatly decreases after a burn because of the loss of plasma proteins in both burned and nonburned tissues. Impaired vascular and capillary permeability, combined with the large amount of fluid resuscitation needed, sets the stage for pulmonary edema.

(7) Patients with varying degrees of hypoxemia and respiratory insufficiency require mechanical support and ventilation. High-frequency percussive ventilation may be superior to conventional, volume-controlled mechanical ventilation, presumably because barotrauma is minimized.

(8) In severely burned patients, especially if there is an inhalation injury, prolonged endotracheal intubation and mechanical ventilation are likely. Despite this, early or routine tracheostomy placement in burned patients has not been shown to improve the overall outcome in this patient population.

(9) Assess arterial blood gases with a carboxyhemoglobin level.

f) Neurologic: Assess and document preoperative neurologic function as accurately as possible.

g) Renal

(1) The development of acute renal failure after an acute burn injury is a serious complication, because mortality rates increase. Decreases in renal blood flow can occur immediately after a burn injury, leading to alterations in glomerular filtration.

(2) Causes include the large intravascular depletion, hypovolemia, decreased cardiac output, and increased circulating plasma catecholamine levels. The renin-angiotensin-aldosterone system and the release of antidiuretic hormone are stimulated and act to conserve sodium and water. Subsequently, alterations in electrolyte balance can take place.

(3) Electrical burns with massive muscle necrosis can result in myoglobinemia, which may damage renal tubules and impair renal function. Intravenous administration of sodium bicarbonate to alkalize the urine protects the kidneys by preventing the formation of myoglobin casts. With adequate fluid resuscitation, renal blood flow and glomerular filtration are preserved.

(4) Hourly urine output measurements remain the gold standard for assessing adequate fluid replacement and resuscitation.

(5) Acute renal failure can also occur 2 to 3 weeks after the burn injury. Associated causes include sepsis and delayed wound excision.

h) Gastrointestinal

(1) Caloric requirements for a patient with a 40% thermal injury are estimated to be 132% higher than basal energy expenditure, compared with a 79% increase for sepsis and a 25% increase for major elective surgery.

(2) The increased energy expenditure enhances a period of negative nitrogen balance and causes an erosion of lean body mass,

requiring intensive nutritional support. This nutritional support is essential for the immune system function, wound healing, and the prevention of catabolism.

(3) In patients with large burns and a pronounced hypermetabolic response, carbohydrate is more effective than fat in maintaining body protein.

(4) The burn patient has an injury-induced resistance to the action of insulin in the liver and skeletal muscle. Ongoing assessment of blood glucose with administration of exogenous insulin may be necessary.

(5) The necessity for continued adequate caloric intake cannot be ignored during the preanesthetic evaluation. Because of the importance of nutrition, it is unwise to stop enteral feedings arbitrarily the night before surgery. This can result in an excessive loss of calories, especially if the patient must undergo multiple burn débridements in a short period.

(6) Preoperative nothing by mouth (NPO) status must be kept at a safe minimum, to prevent the patient from reverting to a catabolic state.

(7) Tracheally intubated patients do not need the enteral feedings discontinued before surgery, and unintubated patients can remain on nutritional support as late as 4 hours before the scheduled surgical procedure. This practice improves preoperative nutrition without increasing the risk of aspiration.

(8) On admission to the operating room, the nonintubated patient's nasogastric tube should be suctioned and induction tailored to ensure rapid protection of the airway.

(9) If the patient is not receiving enteral feedings, but rather parenteral feedings through a central venous catheter, the hyperalimentation line should not be used for administration of fluids or drugs during anesthesia. Hyperalimentation and lipid infusions need not be discontinued intraoperatively.

(10) Burn patients demonstrate a decrease in gastrointestinal function. If the percentage of the TBSA involved is greater than 20%, the development of ileus is common.

(11) Another gastrointestinal sequela that burn patients can develop is acute ulceration of the gastric and/or duodenal mucosa. This condition is known as Curling's ulcers. Treatment primarily entails the administration of histamine (H_2)-receptor blockers and antacids. However, there has been an associated increased incidence of pulmonary infection with Pseudomonas in the intensive care unit patient treated with such medication. The clearance of cimetidine, but not ranitidine, is increased, so appropriate dosage adjustments are required.

i) Endocrine

(1) There is an increased level of stress hormones, leading to hyperglycemia and insulin resistance.

(2) There is also a substantial increase in basal metabolic rate resulting from increased catecholamines causing increased oxygen consumption and carbon dioxide production.

j) Hematologic

(1) Coagulopathies have been associated with both the burn process and the relative clotting factor dilution that occurs with volume resuscitation.

(2) Decreased plasma proteins, such as albumin, will increase plasma protein-bound drugs (benzodiazepines).

(3) Blood loss can be extensive, especially with débridements. Estimate blood loss at 4 mL/cm^2 for surface that is excised or harvested. Start infusing blood before beginning the procedure. Because visual estimates are inaccurate, monitor hemoglobin, hematocrit, and urine output.

(4) Patients are susceptible to hypothermia resulting from hypermetabolism, evaporation of fluid, exposure, and multiple blood transfusions.

3. Pharmacologic considerations

a) Burn injury causes considerable changes in plasma protein levels, with significant consequences for the protein binding of drugs. In general, patients with burns exhibit decreased albumin and increased α_1-acid glycoprotein levels.

b) Because the pharmacologic effect is often related to the unbound fraction of a drug, alterations in protein binding can also affect the efficacy and tolerability of drug treatment in patients with burns. This alteration causes the plasma binding of predominantly albumin-bound drugs, such as benzodiazepines, phenytoin, and salicylic acid, to be decreased, resulting in an increase in the free fraction and thus a larger volume of distribution (V_d) for the drug.

c) Drugs primarily bound to α_1-acid glycoprotein (e.g., lidocaine, meperidine, propranolol) have the opposite effect.

d) V_d may be increased or decreased in patients with burns. In general, two factors may cause alteration in V_d: changes in extracellular fluid volume and changes in protein binding.

e) Fluid loss to the burn wound and edema can decrease plasma concentrations of many drugs. After the initial resuscitation state, cardiac output increases as the hypermetabolic phase develops. This increases blood flow to the kidneys and liver with increased drug clearance. Dosage requirements may change if the drug has a small V_d and a narrow therapeutic range. Overall, there is significant patient variability based on fluid status and phase of recovery.

4. Patient preparation

a) A successful anesthetic for the excision and grafting of a burn wound requires planning and preparing needed equipment. Specific anesthetic interventions should be done for these patients before their arrival in the operating room.

b) Preoperative anesthesia planning for the burn patient

(1) Warm up the operating room ahead of time, well before the patient arrives.

(2) Check on the patient's blood status and order more blood if necessary, based on the patient's preoperative hemoglobin and hematocrit values, the size of the burn, and the extent of the planned débridement.

(3) Have the blood in the operating room and checked before surgical débridement is initiated. This is critical in the pediatric patient.

(4) Have at least one blood warmer primed, plugged in, and turned on. If the burn is large, have two.

(5) Make sure that you have adequate intravenous access before the surgeon begins débriding the burn.

(6) Have an adequate supply of narcotics.

(7) Know whether invasive lines will need to be placed and plan ahead of time.

(8) Have a plan, but be willing to modify it if needed.

c) Complete blood count, electrolytes, blood urea nitrogen, creatinine, glucose, urinalysis, prothrombin time, partial thromboplastin time (D-dimer or fibrin split products if disseminated intravascular coagulation is suspected), type and cross-match (number of units depends on the area to be débrided/grafted), chest radiography, and arterial blood gases (with carboxyhemoglobin if indicated) are obtained. Other tests are done as suggested by the history and physical examination.

d) Begin volume replacement with crystalloid or blood, or both, preoperatively. If the patient's condition permits, an anxiolytic (e.g., benzodiazepine) and a narcotic may be useful preoperatively.

5. **Equipment and monitoring**

   a) Burn patients require all the standard monitors intraoperatively. It can be challenging at times to adapt the standard monitors to the burned patient.

   b) Electrocardiogram (ECG) leads are often difficult to place secondary to a lack of intact skin. It may be necessary to staple the leads or use needle electrodes on the patient to obtain an acceptable ECG tracing.

   c) Ideally, blood pressure cuffs should be placed on an unaffected limb or at times, at a nonsurgical site.

   d) The placement of an arterial line for blood pressure monitoring may be warranted even in the healthy patient if the planned amount of surgical débridement is extensive or if manipulation of the patient's limbs intraoperatively limits the accuracy of noninvasive cuff readings. In large burns that are greater than 20% to 30%, invasive blood pressure monitoring should be instituted after induction, if not in place preoperatively. Rapid blood losses, the potential for hemodynamic swings, and the need to check intraoperative laboratory values all validate this requirement.

   e) The standard sites for pulse oximetry placement may not be available. Alternative sites include the nose, the ear, and the cheek.

   f) Any preexisting invasive monitors such as arterial line catheters or central venous or pulmonary artery catheters should be continued in the operating room.

   g) Accurate temperature monitoring is essential, because burn patients can become very hypothermic intraoperatively. Temperature measurements should be obtained through an esophageal stethoscope. Skin temperature devices are highly inaccurate, and there may not be a suitable place to place one.

   h) Patients with burns who are critically ill are usually transported directly to the operating room from the burn intensive care unit and vice versa postoperatively, by the anesthesia provider. These patients are usually intubated, are receiving continuous infusions of pharmacologic agents, and have invasive lines in place. Astute monitoring of the patient's vital signs during transport is mandatory. Care must be taken while transporting the patient to not disrupt or dislodge any invasive or intravenous lines. A portable oxygen delivery system is another component of required transport equipment. Careful handling and vigilant guarding of the airway are vital. The anesthetist must also consider the patient's comfort and privacy during transport. Amnestic and analgesic drugs should be administered as needed.

   i) Monitors: Standard. Needle electrodes may be needed for electrocardiography. Blood pressure can be measured on the lower extremities; an arterial line or a cuff can be placed over the burned area with a sterile lubricated dressing after consultation with the burn specialist. Most patients with burns of more than 40% to 50% require an arterial line, a central line, and a pulmonary arterial catheter if they are hemodynamically unstable. Use caution in placement, and avoid burned areas.

j) Additional equipment: Blood and fluid warmers. A heated circuit and warming blanket are used. Room temperature is increased. Burn patients are poikilothermic.

k) Positioning: Various positions may be required intraoperatively, depending on the area being treated. Assess limb contractures, and stabilize fractures.

6. **Airway management**

a) Any acute airway problems are usually handled on admission to the burn unit. In the patient with a major burn or one who has an inhalation injury, preoperative intubation is likely.

b) In the nonintubated patient without an inhalation injury and whose airway is normal, induction and intubation of the airway can proceed as during any other anesthetic regimen (except no succinylcholine).

c) Preoperative airway evaluation is necessary as with any other patient. The anesthetist should exert good judgment in determining the degree of intubation difficulty. If the airway appears difficult, fiberoptic intubation should be considered or, at least, readily available.

d) In the severely burned patient who is intubated preoperatively, vigilance is required to protect the airway from accidental extubation. Loss of the airway in this patient may be impossible to regain because of edema of the airway structures.

e) Securing of such an airway can be problematic. Tape does not readily stick to burned skin. The use of soft beard straps to secure an endotracheal tube is a good option, especially if the plan is to extubate the patient at the end of the case. Cloth ties encircled around the head are frequently employed in the burn unit to secure endotracheal tubes and should not be disrupted.

7. **Temperature regulation**

a) Depending on the percentage TBSA affected by the burn, temperature regulation can be problematic in the burn patient. These patients are at high risk of hypothermia development resulting from the loss of the skin's insulating mechanisms, radiation and evaporative heat losses, and the large amount of body surface area exposure intraoperatively.

b) The temperature in the operating room should be greater than 28° C.
Intravenous solutions and skin preparations should be warmed. All methods of heat conservation should be employed while the patient is in the operating room.

c) The use of in-line Humidivents or low gas flows reduces evaporative respiratory tract heat loss.

d) Forced-air warming blankets are very effective, but their use can be limited. Over-body heating lamps can be used but need to be at a safe distance above the patient to prevent further skin burns. Plastic bags can also be used to insulate any exposed body parts not being treated surgically.

e) It is suggested that keeping a patient warm is more beneficial than rewarming. With hypothermia, vasoconstriction occurs that may curtail any later warming efforts later. It has been shown that slow rewarming postoperatively in critically ill patients with burn injuries leads to an increase in mortality. If the patient becomes hypothermic even despite the best effort put forth, the surgeon needs to be advised to stop the procedure.

8. **Fluid and blood replacement**

   a) Surgical burn débridements may be extraordinarily bloody operations. Wound management involves removal of the burn eschar layer until brisk bleeding of the dermis is reached.

   b) The surgical team may remove the eschar so rapidly that it becomes difficult to keep up with the massive blood loss, resulting in a suddenly hypovolemic patient. Some institutions stop the surgical procedure after 2 hours, if more than two blood volumes have been lost, or if the body temperature falls to 35° C or by greater than 1.5° C from baseline.

   c) There are many formulas to approximate the amount of potential blood loss for a burn débridement. These vary from 200 to 400 mL of blood loss for each 1% of TBSA excised and grafted to as high as 4% to 15% of the patient's blood volume for every percent of skin débrided.

   d) During and especially after the excision and débridement, gauze pads soaked in a vasoconstrictor (e.g., epinephrine, phenylephrine) are placed on the newly excised wound to control the bleeding. However, this may result in systemic absorption of vasoconstrictors, causing elevation of the patient's blood pressure, even in the presence of hypovolemia. Thrombin-soaked sponges may be preferred for patients in whom systemic absorption of epinephrine may cause myocardial ischemia or arrhythmias.

   e) Adequate venous access is a must before the initiation of surgical débridement. The size and extent of the burn will mandate how much access is needed. It is optimal to have two large-bore peripheral intravenous lines in place to ensure the administration of fluids and blood products quickly.

   f) Critically ill patients often have a central venous catheter in place, especially if the burn is extensive and access is difficult. Although a triple-lumen catheter is adequate in the intensive care unit setting, it may not be ideal in the operating room when fluid and blood replacement is needed quickly.

   g) The readiness of blood products should be ascertained before the patient is brought to the operating room. Ideally, the blood should be in the operating room, checked, and ready to use at the beginning of the surgical procedure. This is particularly necessary in pediatric patients. Some hospitals initiate blood transfusions before the beginning of the surgical débridement and apply compression dressings after excision and grafting.

   h) Careful planning is necessary to manage the hemorrhage and potential complications associated with massive transfusion (citrate toxicity, loss of clotting factors) during the débridement. Visual estimation of the blood loss is subjective at best and is prone to be miscalculated. Suction is not used during débridements. Sponges may be accidentally thrown away or covered up during the procedure. Blood drips onto to the floor, is covered up in the surgical drapes, or leaks under the patient, and it is possible to be lulled into a false sense of security immediately after the eschar incision. Proper monitoring of the patient's urinary output, hematocrit, and hemodynamic status is necessary for keeping the patient's volume within normal limits.

i) One intravenous catheter is adequate for the induction of anesthesia in most burned patients, but at least two large-bore intravenous catheters are necessary before beginning a major excision and grafting procedure. The use of central venous or pulmonary artery catheters is patient dependent. The risk of sepsis in the immunosuppressed patient must be weighed against the benefit of information gained.

9. **Induction and management**
   a) There is no single best anesthetic agent to administer to the burn patient. The anesthetic is individualized and should be based on the patient's preoperative status and medical history.
   b) The patient with an acute burn seldom comes to the operating room immediately after the injury. Patients are usually admitted and stabilized in the burn unit. If the patient requires surgery, the anesthetist must realize that the burn patient is quite "fragile" within the first 24 hours of the injury. Anesthetic agents can exert extreme depressant effects, especially if fluid resuscitation is not adequate or has not been fully completed. The loss of intravascular volume coupled with the potential for a depressed myocardium can result in a hemodynamically unstable patient under general anesthesia.
   c) Careful and slow titration of all anesthetic agents is vital. Premedicating stable patients with a benzodiazepine or a narcotic decreases anxiety and makes transfer to the operating room tolerable. Anxiety, depression, and pain are interrelated in patients with burns.
   d) To minimize patient discomfort, induction can be performed on the patient's intensive care unit bed before moving the patient onto the operating room table.
   e) Regional anesthesia is sometimes considered for burn trauma limited to a small area or an extremity or for surgery during the reconstructive phase.
      (1) One advantage of this technique is prolonged postoperative analgesia. Regional anesthesia is generally limited for a variety of reasons.
      (2) The anesthesia provider must avoid performing any regional technique through burned tissue because of the potential for the spread of infection.
      (3) There is an almost universal presence of hypotension (hypovolemia) and vasodilation with or without sepsis, which is a relative contraindication to the use of spinal or epidural routes for pain control until the burn wound is closed.
      (4) Coagulopathy and cardiorespiratory instability are also reasons to avoid a regional anesthetic technique. The greatest limitation to the use of regional anesthesia is the extent of the surgical field. The anesthetized region must include both the area to be excised and the area to be harvested for donor skin.
      (5) In children, regional anesthesia blocks are sometimes a viable option for postoperative analgesia. A tried and true regional block to institute in children undergoing débridements in the lower extremities or skin harvesting from the buttocks or thighs is a single-shot caudal technique. This can be placed either after the induction of general anesthesia or at end of the case before emergence. Injection of bupivacaine 0.25% and levobupivacaine 0.25% with

epinephrine 1:200,000 added are two options. The volume of local anesthetic injected into the caudal space is determined by the child's weight in kilograms and the analgesia level needed to be covered by the block. If the child is to be admitted postoperatively, the addition of morphine, at 30 to 50 mcg/kg, or clonidine, at 1 to 2 mcg/kg, can be considered.

f) The standard induction drugs are all acceptable to use. Sodium thiopental is well tolerated, but it may require higher than normal dosages. The use of this agent may produce hypotension on induction if the patient has not received adequate intravascular replacement.

g) Etomidate maintains hemodynamic stability during induction with less respiratory depression than barbiturates. However, repeated doses may inhibit adrenocortical function.

h) Propofol has greater negative inotropic effects than does either thiopental or etomidate, which may lead to hypotension after induction. The high lipid content of propofol may limit its use during initial resuscitation and in septic patients.

i) Another intravenous anesthetic is ketamine, a phencyclidine derivative that produces a dissociative anesthetic state of relatively short duration. Ketamine offers the advantage of stable hemodynamics and analgesia. Low doses produce adequate amnesia and analgesia for the débridement of superficial burns; higher doses may be administered for more extensive procedures, such as eschar excisions. Hallucinogenic episodes can be minimized with the administration of benzodiazepines in small doses, and an anticholinergic prevents excessive pharyngeal and tracheobronchial secretions.

j) In the pediatric burn patient, inhalation induction with sevoflurane is certainly acceptable if the child does not have intravenous access before induction and if the airway appears normal.

k) Anesthesia should be maintained with opioid or inhalational agents as the hemodynamic status of the patient permits. Inhaled volatile agents have proved to be safe and effective, allowing rapid adjustment of anesthetic depth and the administration of high oxygen concentrations. The burn patient may be sensitive to the cardiovascular depressant effects of inhaled anesthetics, especially if acute fluid resuscitation is incomplete. Inhaled agents do not provide analgesia during the postsurgical period.

l) Intubated burn patients may require the continuance of specialized critical care ventilators (e.g. percussive ventilators) intraoperatively to maintain adequate oxygenation and ventilation. In this instance, a total intravenous anesthetic is indicated.

m) The main group of anesthetic agents that can exert altered effects in the burn patient are the muscle relaxants. Within the first 24-hour window following the burn injury, the burn is considered stable. Succinylcholine is probably safe to use within this time frame. As stated previously, the postjunctional acetylcholine receptors begin to proliferate soon after a burn injury occurs. This phenomenon is thought to be fully complete by 7 days after the acute injury. Succinylcholine given after the initial first 24-hour window has produced significant hyperkalemia as a result of this up-regulation of receptors.

n) Nondepolarizing muscle relaxants are safe to use in the burn patient. The anesthetist should realize that the patient may demonstrate a

PART II **Common Procedures**

resistance to their effects. Higher dosing or more frequent redosing may be necessary. The origin of the phenomenon again is thought to result from the increase in postjunctional acetylcholine receptors. Because responses to the nondepolarizing muscle relaxants can vary significantly, neuromuscular blockade monitoring should always be used.

10. **Emergence from anesthesia**
    a) The postoperative anesthetic course should be planned in advance and is frequently intuitive. Critically ill and intubated burn patients are kept intubated postoperatively and are directly transported to the burn unit.
    b) The anesthetist should safeguard the airway and be respectful of the patient's need for sedation and analgesia during this terminal phase of the anesthetic.
    c) If the patient is to be extubated, emergence from anesthesia should be planned in advance as well, not unlike any other patient undergoing an anesthetic.
    d) Neuromuscular blockade should be adequately reversed and, if possible, the patient should be allowed to begin spontaneously breathing at an appropriate time.
    e) Narcotics for postoperative analgesia should be titrated according to the patient's respiratory status. Keep in mind that these are painful procedures, and patient's narcotic requirements can be tremendous.

B. Laser Procedures Involving the Airways

1. **Introduction**
   Laser is an acronym for light amplification by stimulated emission of radiation. Laser procedures of the airway usually involve the carbon dioxide (CO_2) laser because such lasers can excise lesions precisely and cause minimal edema. Tumor debulking of lesions found in the lower trachea and bronchi may require the neodymium:yttrium-aluminum-garnet (Nd:YAG) laser, which produces its effects at greater depth. There are many hazards of lasers to both the patient and members of the health care team. Damage can be caused to the lips and skin. Fire and explosion are possible with the use of lasers and volatile anesthetics. Toxins produced by the use of the laser on tissues may be mutagenic. They may also cause infection, acute bronchial inflammation, and altered gas exchange. Because the airway is shared by the surgeon and the anesthesia provider, much communication and cooperation are necessary.

2. **Preoperative assessment**
   a) History and physical examination
      (1) A careful history should be obtained, with great emphasis on airway and respiratory concerns. A thorough airway assessment is necessary. This should include thyromental distance, airway classification, cervical range of motion, dentition, phonation, hoarseness, shortness of breath, pain on swallowing, and edema. The need for awake fiberoptic intubation should be considered. Often, these patients have long smoking histories and may have chronic obstructive pulmonary disease. Such findings should be noted on the history and physical examination. Focus on any history of asthma, emphysema, and respiratory patterns. A complete respiratory assessment should be performed and documented.

(2) Nutritional status should be evaluated because this patient population may have undergone chemotherapy or radiation therapy for the treatment of airway lesions.

(3) Perform a complete systems review.

b) Patient preparation

(1) Laboratory tests: These are based on the history and physical examination.

(2) Diagnostic tests: These are based on the history and physical examination.

(3) Medications: Preoperative sedation is minimal in patients with severe airway obstruction. Additional sedation could cause complete airway obstruction. An antisialagogue should be given to enhance visualization and to decrease secretions. Avoid ketamine because it will increase airway reflexes. Consider dexamethasone (Decadron) to decrease airway inflammation in the postoperative period.

3. Room preparation

a) Monitoring equipment: Standard; arterial line set up and available

b) Additional equipment

(1) Standard emergency drugs are used

(2) The patient's eyes must be protected. They should be taped closed and covered with wet gauze. Do not use oil-based eye lubricants because they are flammable. Others in the room should wear goggles (clear for CO_2, green for argon, and amber for Nd:YAG lasers).

(3) Emergency airway cart and instruments for an emergency cricothyroidotomy and tracheostomy should be available and in the room during induction. A surgeon experienced in tracheostomy should be present during induction for the patient with a compromised airway.

(4) Jet ventilator: A copper tube is attached to the jet ventilator before laryngoscopy; the brass ball tip should be 2 to 3 cm distal to vocal cords. Ventilate at 30 to 35 psi, 10 to 12 breaths/min lasting 1 to 2 seconds. Ensure full expiration to avoid pneumothorax. Contraindications are full stomach, obesity, hiatal hernia, and severe lung or heart disease.

(5) Appropriate endotracheal tubes and a variety of blades and airways should be available to decrease the risk of airway fire, including metal tubes, red rubber, polyvinyl chloride, or silicone tubes. Regardless of the endotracheal tube chosen, one should use the lowest inspired oxygen fraction possible, to decrease the risk of airway fire. Have a 50-mL syringe of normal saline solution on the tabletop.

(6) If an airway fire should occur, ventilation should be stopped, and the oxygen source should be discontinued. Flood the area with water. Remove the burned endotracheal tube. Mask ventilate with 100% oxygen, maintain the anesthetic, and reintubate the patient. Bronchoscopy, laryngoscopy, chest radiography, and arterial blood gas measurements should be performed to determine injury and to provide therapy. The patient should be monitored for at least 24 hours. Short-term steroids may be administered, as should antibiotics and ventilatory support as needed. Also monitor arterial blood gases and chest x-ray films.

(7) Long breathing circuits may be needed if the operating table is to be turned.

(8) Intravenous fluids: An 18-gauge or larger catheter and normal saline or lactated Ringer's solution at 2 to 4 mL/kg/hour are used.

PART II Common Procedures

4. **Perioperative management and anesthetic technique**
   General anesthesia with endotracheal intubation is appropriate. Some surgeons advocate local anesthesia with heavy sedation for certain minor case procedures of the upper airway. However, the patient must not move; remember that sedation may lead to complete airway obstruction.

   a) Induction: Standard intravenous induction is used if the patient does not have airway obstruction. With airway obstruction or an awake patient, fiberoptic bronchoscopy may be performed, and the airway may be secured before induction. Muscle relaxants should be avoided until the airway is secured.

   b) Maintenance: Isoflurane, desflurane, air, and oxygen are standard. Avoid nitrous oxide because it is combustible. Avoid a fraction of inspired oxygen greater than 0.40, to decrease the risk of airway fire.

   c) Emergence: Use awake extubation because there may be some airway edema. Avoid coughing, bucking, and straining on the endotracheal tube to prevent further edema. Consider administering lidocaine intravenously (1 mg/kg).

5. **Postoperative implications**
   Airway complications and postoperative nausea and vomiting may occur.

C. Trauma

1. **Introduction**
   Trauma is the fourth leading cause of death in the developed world. Mortality is related to the age and prior condition of the patient, the type and severity of the trauma, and the rapidity and quality of the emergency treatment received.

2. **Preoperative assessment**
   The time allowed for preoperative assessment is limited and is based on the severity of the trauma. A rapid assessment and review of pertinent patient data available are essential. The availability of blood therapy and the initiation of adequate intravenous lines are to be prioritized.

   a) Cardiac: Assess for symptoms of shock. Assess the chest wall for obvious contusion and assess stability of vital signs.

   b) Respiratory: Assess breath sounds and patterns of respiration.

   c) Neurologic: Assess patient using the Glasgow Coma Scale (GCS). Assume a cervical spine injury until it is definitely ruled out by x-ray examination. There are three categories of the GCS to which a value is assigned: eye opening, motor response, and verbal response. For eye opening: 4 = spontaneous, 3 = to speech, 2 = to pain, 1 = none. For motor response: 6 = to verbal, 5 = localizes to pain, 4 = withdraws to pain, 3 = decorticate flexion to pain, 2 = extends to pain, 1 = none. For verbal response: 5 = oriented, 4 = confused, 4 = inappropriate words, 2 = incomprehensible sounds, 1 = none. A normal GCS score is 15.

   d) Renal: Assess the color and amount of urine.

   e) Gastrointestinal: All trauma patients are considered to have a full stomach. Gastric emptying slows or stops at the time of the trauma. The presence of a nasogastric tube also provides a "wick" that allows gastric fluid to be aspirated.

   f) Endocrine: The release of stress hormones transiently elevates blood glucose levels.

g) Hematologic: Severe physical stress can lead to coagulopathies, as can dilution of clotting factors during massive volume resuscitation.

h) Patient preparation
  (1) Baseline laboratory tests are obtained as available; hemoglobin, hematocrit, and others as indicated by history and physical examination.
  (2) Type and cross-match for at least 4 units.
  (3) Other diagnostic tests are as indicated by history and physical examination.
  (4) Premedication is usually avoided but is individualized in the trauma patient.

3. **Room preparation**
  a) Standard
  b) Arterial line, arterial blood gas measurement, pulmonary artery catheters, blood warmers, rapid infuser, and patient warming equipment
  c) Full range of standard and emergency resuscitative drugs immediately available
  d) Position usually supine unless otherwise indicated.

4. **Anesthetic technique**
  General anesthesia with minimal depressant drugs is used until the patient's status and extent of injury can be determined. Immediate establishment of the airway is the priority. Anesthetics are introduced depending on the stability of the patient.

5. **Perioperative management**
  a) Induction
    (1) This is individualized based on the patient's condition and the severity of trauma.
    (2) Rapid sequence induction and immediate establishment of the airway are necessary.
    (3) Ketamine, propofol, and thiopental (Pentothal) may be administered depending on hemodynamic status.
    (4) If facial or head and neck trauma is evident, then awake intubation, fiberoptic technique, or tracheostomy may be required. Oral intubation is preferable to nasal intubation. If a Philadelphia cervical collar is present, keep the patient's neck in well-maintained axial stabilization of the head.
    (5) If central nervous system trauma is suspected, take precautions to prevent increased intracranial pressure.
  b) Maintenance
    (1) Oxygen and muscle relaxants are required in the critically injured patient.
    (2) After assessment and stabilization, anesthetics are administered as appropriate.
    (3) Aggressive management of fluid (blood 1 mL/1 mL, crystalloid 3 mL/1 mL) electrolyte, blood gas parameters, blood loss, and coagulation status may be required.
  c) Emergence: Continued ventilation and management of all major systems are required in the immediate postanesthesia period.

6. **Postoperative implications**
  Continued ventilation and observation of cardiac, respiratory, renal, and coagulation status are required for at least the first 24 hours in severely injured patients. These patients are transferred to the critical care unit for long-term management of multiple sequelae. Pain control may include narcotics, patient-controlled analgesia, or regional block.

A. Anatomy and Physiology

1. **Cardiovascular physiology**

   a) During fetal development, oxygenation and carbon dioxide (CO_2) elimination are accomplished through the placenta. Oxygenated blood to the fetus travels from the placenta through the umbilical vein through the ductus venosus near the liver, to the inferior vena cava. The foramen ovale, the opening between the right and left atria, allows the oxygenated blood direct access to the left circulation. From the left atrium, the blood is transferred to the left ventricle and then to the body. The blood returns to the placenta through the umbilical arteries. Deoxygenated blood from the superior vena cava is deposited into the right atrium. It is then ejected into the pulmonary artery. Because of high pulmonary vasculature pressure, the blood bypasses the lungs and is instead transferred through the ductus arteriosus to the aorta. The blood travels to the placenta through the umbilical arteries.

   b) Clamping of the umbilical cord increases systemic vascular resistance, increasing aortic and left-sided pressures and allowing the foramen ovale to close and the lungs to assume their role in oxygenation. Pulmonary vascular resistance decreases, and the ductus arteriosus closes as arterial oxygen pressure (PO_2) levels increase.

   c) Hypoxia, hypercarbia, and acidosis lead to persistent pulmonary hypertension and maintenance of fetal circulation. The diagnosis made when right radial (preductal) and umbilical line (postductal) samples reveal a PO_2 difference of 20 mm Hg. Shunting continues across a patent ductus arteriosus, resulting in increased hypoxemia and acidosis.

   d) Treatment of persistent pulmonary circulation includes hyperventilation, maintenance of adequate oxygenation, and alkalosis.

   e) Neonatal cardiac output is heart rate dependent because of a noncompliant left ventricle and fixed stroke volume.

   f) The pediatric basal heart rate is higher than that of adults, although parasympathetic stimulation, hypoxia, or deep anesthesia can cause profound bradycardia and decreased cardiac output.

   g) Sympathetic nervous system and baroreceptor reflexes are immature. Infants have low catecholamine stores and decreased responsiveness to exogenous catecholamines. Infants cannot respond to hypovolemia with vasoconstriction. Therefore, hypovolemia is suspected when there is hypotension in the absence of an increased heart rate.

   h) Normal parameters are given in the following table.

Normal Parameters

Age	Respiratory Rate (breaths/min)	Heart Rate (beats/min)	Systolic Blood Pressure (mm Hg)	Diastolic Blood Pressure (mm Hg)
Neonate	40	140	65	40
1 year	30	120	95	65
3 years	25	100	100	70
12 years	20	80	110	60

i) Physiologic anemia of the newborn: Hematocrit at birth is 50%, 80% of which is fetal hemoglobin. Fetal hemoglobin binds more strongly to O_2 than adult hemoglobin. This facilitates O_2 uptake in utero. After birth, the presence of fetal hemoglobin causes a shift in the oxyhemoglobin curve to the left and a decrease in O_2 delivery to the tissues. At age 1 to 3 months, hemoglobin levels decrease, and levels of 2,3-diphosphoglycerate increase, causing a shift of the oxyhemoglobin curve to the right and increased O_2 delivery to tissues.

2. **Respiratory physiology**
   a) Metabolic rate, CO_2 production, and O_2 consumption are increased.
   b) Functional residual capacity and O_2 reserves are decreased.
   c) Infants have a paradoxical response to hypoxia—initial hyperpnea followed by respiratory depression and depressed response to hypercarbia.
   d) The larynx is at C2 to C4 in children, at C3 to C6 in the adult. This results in increased difficulty in alignment of the pharyngeal and laryngeal axes. A straight blade is useful for laryngoscopy in children.
   e) Children have a stiff, omega-shaped epiglottis. The vocal cords slant up and back.
   f) The narrowest part of the pediatric airway is the cricoid cartilage, as opposed to the adult glottis. The cricoid cartilage can form a seal around the endotracheal tube, eliminating the need for a cuffed tube. The cartilage is funnel shaped. Do not force fit the endotracheal tube. Properly fitted tubes allow a leak at 15 to 25 cm H_2O.
   g) Children have large occiputs that flex the head onto the chest, large tongues, and small chins. Tonsils and adenoids grow rapidly from ages 4 to 7 and may obstruct breathing.
   h) Infants are obligatory nasal breathers. The position of the epiglottis in relation to the soft palate allows simultaneous breathing and sucking/drinking.
   i) The neonatal trachea is 4 cm. Flexion of the head onto the chest forces the endotracheal tube to extend deeper into the right mainstem. Extension of the head may dislodge the tube.
   j) The number of alveoli increases until age 6 years. Mature levels of surfactant are reached at 35 weeks of gestation. Decreased amounts of alveoli and surfactant in the neonatal period increase the risk of infant respiratory distress syndrome.
   k) Increased work of breathing in the infant results from a decreased amount of type I muscle fibers in the diaphragm; this causes predisposition to fatigue. Poor chest wall mechanics, lack of rib cage

rigidity, horizontal orientation of the ribs, weak intercostal muscles, and increased fatigue result in paradoxical chest movements in the newborn.

3. **Nervous system**
   a) Cranial sutures are not fused in the infant; the cranium is pliable. Fluid status is indicated by fullness of the fontanelles.
   b) Myelination of the nervous system continues until age 3. The spinal cord ends at L1 in adults, at L3 in pediatric patients. This is important to consider when using regional anesthesia techniques in the pediatric population.
   c) Preterm and low-birth-weight infants are at risk for intracranial hemorrhage resulting from fragile cerebral vessels. Intracranial bleeding may result from hypoxia, hypercarbia, hyperglycemia or hypoglycemia, hypernatremia, or wide variations in blood pressure.

4. **Renal system**
   a) The total body water in proportion to body weight is higher in neonates than adults. Kidneys function in utero to eliminate urine into the amniotic fluid, whereas the placenta eliminates waste.
   b) Neonates have the complete number of nephrons at birth. Nephrons are immature in function until age 6 to 12 months.
   c) The glomerular filtration rate (GFR) is decreased by renal vasoconstriction, low plasma flow in the renal system, and low blood pressure. GFR increases until age 1 year.
   d) Infants are obligate sodium excretors because of their inability to conserve sodium. Renal tubules are not responsive to the renin-angiotensin-aldosterone system. The infant kidney cannot concentrate urine, leading to an increased risk of dehydration. The ability to reabsorb glucose is also impaired. If excessive glucose is given intravenously, the result is osmotic diuresis.
   e) Pediatric patients have a tendency toward acidosis, because the metabolic rate and CO_2 production are double those of the adult. There is a decreased ability to conserve bicarbonate and to excrete acids.

5. **Hepatic system**
   a) Near birth, the fetal liver increases glycogen stores. Preterm infants are at increased risk for hypoglycemia because of a lack of glycogen stores.
   b) Hepatic metabolism of drugs is decreased in the early weeks of life. The liver functions at the adult level by age 2.

6. **Impaired thermogenesis**
   a) Infants are at risk for hypothermia from the following:
      (1) Increased ratio of surface area to body weight
      (2) Ineffective shivering mechanism
      (3) Decreased amounts of subcutaneous fat present in preterm infants
   b) Heat loss results from the following:
      (1) Radiation: This is the transfer of heat between two objects of different temperatures not in direct contact. Reduce radiant loss by decreasing the temperature gradient (raise the room temperature closer to patient temperature).
      (2) Convection: This is the transfer of heat to moving molecules such as air or liquid. Cover exposed skin.
      (3) Evaporation: This occurs through the skin and respiratory systems, including sweat, insensible water loss through skin, wounds, respiratory tract, and evaporation of liquids applied to the skin.

      (4) Conduction: This is the transfer of heat from the warm infant to a cool object in direct contact.

  c) Patients assume room temperature under anesthesia, a condition termed *poikilothermia.*

  d) Nonshivering thermogenesis: Infants have impaired shivering capabilities. Autonomic nervous system activation during periods of cold results in metabolism of brown fat stores. Brown fat is located around the neck, kidneys, axilla, and adrenals, in addition to spaces between shoulders, under the sternum, and along the spine. Fatty acids in the brown fat stores are oxidated in an exothermic reaction to produce heat. Nonshivering thermogenesis is used until age 1 to 2 years.

  e) Hypothermia in the neonate results in the release of norepinephrine, peripheral and pulmonary vasoconstriction, increasing acidosis, increased pulmonary pressures and right-to-left shunting, and eventually hypoxia, further perpetuating the cycle.

  f) Avoid hypothermia by instituting the following: Increase room temperature, cover the patient's head and exposed extremities, and use overhead warming light. Beware of burns. Use recommended distances for safe use. Heat and humidify delivered gases.

B. Pharmacology

1. Introduction

  a) Neonates have less adipose tissue and muscle in proportion to body weight and have increased total body water. These differences result in higher plasma levels and decreased uptake into inactive tissues.

  b) Infants have decreased renal and hepatic function. Therefore, the half-life of drugs is increased in the neonate.

  c) Neonates have decreased protein binding and a more permeable blood-brain barrier. Therefore, morphine and barbiturates have longer-lasting effects.

  d) Pediatric patients 5 to 13 years of age often have increased metabolism.

2. Inhalation agents

Pediatric patients have an increased cardiac output, low systemic arterial blood pressure, and a greater blood flow per unit to vessel-rich organs. The neonate also has an increased minute ventilation and decreased functional residual capacity. These changes result in a more rapid uptake of inhalation agents and emergence from anesthesia. Minimum alveolar concentration requirements increase the most at ages 1 to 6 months, and they decrease thereafter until puberty. All inhalation agents cause dose-related decreases in myocardial function and ventilation. Halothane or sevoflurane combined with nitrous oxide (N_2O) and oxygen is preferred for mask inductions. Halothane at high concentrations can cause profound bradycardia. Slowly increasing the percentage delivered every couple of breaths helps to prevent bradycardia. Sevoflurane, although less of a cardiac depressant, can cause severe bradycardia in neonates and hypovolemic children. After induction, switching to a less expensive agent such as isoflurane is acceptable. N_2O provides second gas effect for increased agent delivery. N_2O may increase pulmonary vascular resistance and distend open spaces (bowel, middle ear).

PART II **Common Procedures**

3. Intravenous agents

a) Induction agents: See the following table.

Induction Agents

Drug	Induction Dose	Maintenance	Comments
Thiopental (Pentothal)	5–6 mg/kg IV	0.5–2 mg/kg	
Methohexital (Brevital)	1–2 mg/kg IV (1% solution) 5–10 mg/kg IM (3.5% solution) 20–30 mg/kg rectally (10% aqueous solution)		
Propofol (Diprivan)	2.5–3.5 mg/kg IV	125–300 mcg/kg/min	Can cause bradycardia; pretreat with atropine or glycopyrrolate
Ketamine	1–3 mg/kg IV 5–10 mg/kg IM	0.5–1 mg/kg IV	Provides cataleptic, dissociative state with analgesia Pretreat with benzodiazepine to prevent hallucinations

b) Analgesics: See the following table.

Analgesics

Narcotics			
Drug	**Dose: Analgesic**	**Dose: Induction**	**Comments**
Morphine	0.05–0.2 mg/kg		
Meperidine (Demerol)	1–2 mg/kg		Causes less respiratory depression in neonates than morphine
Fentanyl (Sublimaze)	1–3 mcg/kg	10–100 mcg/kg	*Can cause bradycardia and muscle rigidity
Sufentanil (Sufenta)	0.5–2 mcg/kg		*Can cause bradycardia
Remifentanil (Ultiva)	Loading dose: 0.5–1 mcg/kg Continuous infusion: 0.25–0.5 mcg/kg/min		*Bolus can cause bradycardia
Naloxone (Narcan)	0.01 mg/kg		

Nonnarcotic Analgesics	
Drug	**Dose**
Ketorolac (Toradol)	0.4–1 mg/kg IV
Acetaminophen (Tylenol)	10–20 mg/kg orally 30–40 mg/kg rectally

*The use of pancuronium with fentanyl, sufentanil, and remifentanil can help to decrease the incidence of bradycardia.

c) Benzodiazepines: Midazolam (Versed), 0.5 to 0.75 mg/kg orally, 0.08 to 0.5 mg/kg intramuscularly, 0.2 to 0.5 mg/kg nasally, and 0.05 mg/kg intravenously

d) Muscle relaxant reversal: See the following table.

Muscle Relaxant Reversal

Drug	Dose
Neostigmine	0.03–0.07 mg/kg
Pyridostigmine (Regonal)	0.2 mg/kg
Edrophonium	0.7–1.4 mg/kg
Atropine	0.01–0.02 mg/kg
Glycopyrrolate (Robinul)	0.01 mg/kg

e) Miscellaneous agents: See the following table.

Miscellaneous Drugs

Drug	Dose
Epinephrine	0.01 mg/kg
Lidocaine	1–1.5 mg/kg
Sodium bicarbonate	1–2 mEq/kg
Calcium chloride	20 mg/kg

f) Overall, pediatric patients require increased anesthetic doses because of increased metabolic rate, greater cerebral blood flow, greater O_2 consumption, higher extracellular water content, and larger volumes of distribution.

4. **Neuromuscular blockers**
Pediatric patients are resistant to depolarizing muscle relaxants because of increased extracellular water and volume of distribution. Administer succinylcholine, 1 to 2 mg/kg intravenously or 2 to 4 mg/kg intramuscularly. Nondepolarizers are given in mg/kg doses recommended in adults. Theoretically, infants have increased sensitivity to nondepolarizers as a result of limited myelination and immaturity of the neuromuscular junction. This may be offset by the increased extracellular water levels, thus allowing standard doses to be adequate.

C. Fluids

1. **NPO (nothing by mouth) times**
a) 2 to 3 hours after clear liquids
b) 4 hours after breast milk
c) 6 to 8 hours after formula or solid food
d) Less irritability, less hypoglycemia, and less hypotension on induction are benefits of adjusted NPO times.

2. **4-2-1 rule for calculating fluids**
a) Maintenance: See the following table.
b) NPO: Maintenance calculation times number of hours NPO
c) Insensible loss/translocation

Maintenance	
(1) <10 kg	4 mL/kg/hour
(2) 10–20 kg	40 mL/hour + 2 mL/kg >10 kg up to 20 kg
(3) >20 kg	60 mL/hour + 1 mL/kg >20 kg

  (1) Mild (bone marrow transplantation, examination under anesthesia), 0 mL/kg/hour
  (2) Moderate (inguinal hernia repair), 2 mL/kg/hour
  (3) Severe (intraabdominal cases), 4 to 6 mL/kg/hour
  (4) Massive (spinal fusion, craniofacial), 15 to 20 mL/kg/hour
3. **Estimated blood volumes**
   a) Preterm infants, 90 to 100 mL/kg
   b) Newborn, 80 to 90 mL/kg
   c) Age 3 months to 1 year, 75 to 80 mL/kg
   d) Age 3 to 6 years, 70 to 75 mL/kg
   e) Greater than 6 years, 65 to 70 mL/kg
4. **Lowest allowable hematocrit**
   See the following table.

Lowest Allowable Hematocrit

Age	Normal Hematocrit	Lowest Allowable Hematocrit
a) Preterm	40%–45%	36%
b) Newborn	45%–65%	30%–35%
c) 3 months	30%–42%	27%
d) 1 year	34%–42%	24%
e) 6 years	35%–43%	24%

5. **Maximum allowable blood loss**

$$\frac{\text{Patient hematocrit} - \text{Lowest allowable hematocrit (in decimal)}}{\text{Effective blood volume} \times \text{Patient hematocrit (decimal)}}$$

6. **Blood replacement**
   See the following table.

Blood Replacement

Blood Volume Lost	Replacement
10%–20%	Crystalloid 3 mL: 1 mL loss
25%–33%	Colloid 1 mL: 1 mL
50%	Packed red blood cells 1 mL: 1 mL
	Bolus 10 mL/kg intravenous push first, then remainder of calculated replacement
50%–66%	Packed red blood cells along with fresh-frozen plasma (10–15 mL/kg calculated). Fresh-frozen has high citrate content; check for decreased calcium levels posttransfusion
>66%	Packed red blood cells, fresh-frozen, and platelets (0.1–0.3 units/kg or 1 unit/10 kg weight)

D. Equipment

1. **Circuits**
   a) Pediatric circuits are designed to do the following:
      (1) Eliminate valves within the circuit to decrease the resistance to breathing
      (2) Decrease the amount of dead space within the circuit
      (3) Minimize heat loss (Bain circuit)
   b) Commonly used circuits in pediatrics: Mapleson D, Bain, modified T-piece, pediatric circle
   c) Disadvantages
      (1) Require high, fresh gas flows to prevent rebreathing
      (2) Heat and moisture loss in all circuits except Bain
      (3) Pediatric circle lacking valves and CO_2 absorber
2. **Calculation of fresh gas flow**
   a) Fresh gas flow = $2.5 \times$ Minute ventilation
   b) Minute ventilation = Respiratory rate × Tidal volume (6 mL/kg)
3. **Oxygen delivery systems**
   a) Spontaneously breathing patient: Nasal cannula, simple mask, oxygen hood
   b) Patient requiring ventilatory assistance: Positive-pressure delivery system attached to mask or endotracheal tube
4. **Airways**
   See the following table.

Oral Airway Sizes

Age	Size	Centimeters
a) Preterm	000 or 00	3.5 or 4.5
b) Neonate to 3 months	0	5.5
c) 3–12 months	1	6
d) 1–5 years	2	7
e) >5 years	3	8

5. **Laryngoscope blades**
   See the following table.

Laryngoscope Blades

Age	Blade
a) Preterm/newborn	Miller 0
b) Neonate to 2 years	Miller 1
c) 3 years	Miller 2
d) 2–5 years	Wis-Hipple 1.5
e) 3–6 years	Macintosh 2

6. **Endotracheal tubes**
   See table on p. 390.

Endotracheal Tubes

Age	Tube Size
a) Preterm <2 kg	2.5
b) >2 kg	3
c) Neonate	3–3.5
d) 0–6 months	3.5
e) 6–12 months	4
f) 12–18 months	4–4.5
g) 2 years	4.5
h) 2–3 years	4.5–5
i) >4 years	Age (years) + 16/4 or age/4 + 1

E. Congenital Diaphragmatic Hernia

1. **Introduction**

   A congenital diaphragmatic hernia results from abdominal viscera herniating into the chest through a defect in the diaphragm. The left side is affected more frequently. It occurs in 1 of 2000 to 3000 neonates; half are stillborn or die immediately after birth. Stillborn babies have a 95% incidence of other anomalies. Live births have a 20% incidence of other anomalies (patent ductus arteriosus is common). Herniated abdominal contents occupy the thoracic cavity and compromise lung development, leading to hypoplasia and mediastinal shift. The contralateral lung also has decreased amounts of alveoli. Symptoms usually are present after birth (dyspnea, cyanosis, dextrocardia, bowel sounds in the chest, bulging chest, decreased breath sounds). Infants may have to be intubated after delivery and placed in the neonatal intensive care unit.

2. **Preoperative assessment and patient preparation**

   a) History and physical examination

      (1) Cardiac: Check for other anomalies (patent ductus arteriosus). Mediastinal shift may compress the great vessels.

      (2) Respiratory: Check for pulmonary shunting and right-to-left shunting. A pneumothorax of the contralateral lung may occur from high positive inspiratory pressure. Check serial arterial blood gases, end-tidal carbon dioxide, oxygen saturation, chest radiographs, and ventilator setting. Adequate ventilation may correct acidosis.

      (3) Neurologic: Infants may be paralyzed while intubated in the neonatal intensive care unit. Severe hypoxia can lead to neurologic damage.

      (4) Renal: Peripheral perfusion may be increased by dopamine at 1 to 5 mcg/kg/min.

      (5) Gastrointestinal: A nasogastric tube should be placed for intermittent suction to prevent further distention and pulmonary compression.

   b) Patient preparation

      (1) Laboratory tests: Arterial blood gases, complete blood count, and electrolytes

      (2) Diagnostic tests: Chest radiography with bowel gas pattern and mediastinal shift

3. **Room preparation**

   a) Monitoring equipment: Standard. The internal jugular vein can be used for central venous pressure monitoring. The precordial is used on the contralateral side to monitor for pneumothorax. Venous access in the lower extremities is not recommended because of possible vena cava compression.

b) Additional equipment: All warming devices can be used to prevent hypothermia, which increases oxygen consumption and desaturation.

c) Position: Supine. An abdominal incision is usual, but the transthoracic or thoracoabdominal approach may be used.

4. **Perioperative management and anesthetic technique**
   a) General anesthesia is used.
   b) Induction: Rapid sequence or awake intubation is used.
   c) Maintenance: A high oxygen concentration is needed. Avoid nitrous oxide because it can diffuse across the viscera and increase lung compression. High-dose narcotics with low concentrations of volatile anesthetics may be used to maintain cardiovascular stability. High ventilation rates are used for adequate oxygenation. High pressure may increase the incidence of pneumothorax. Perform frequent arterial blood gases, and keep the arterial carbon dioxide pressure at 25 to 30 mm Hg. If sudden hemodynamic compromise, suspect a contralateral pneumothorax. Increase the inspired oxygen concentration to 100%, and obtain a chest x-ray study. A small pneumothorax may spontaneously resolve; larger ones may compromise respiratory and hemodynamic stability, necessitating chest tube placement.
   d) Emergence: Infants usually remain intubated, paralyzed, and ventilated in the neonatal intensive care unit.

5. **Postoperative complications**
   a) These depend on the severity of pulmonary hypertension and hypoplasia. Some infants show a "honeymoon" period followed by deterioration with right-to-left shunting, hypoxia, hypercapnia, acidosis, pulmonary hypertension, and death.
   b) High-frequency oscillation ventilators may be used to reduce pulmonary arterial pressure.
   c) Patent ductus arteriosus may be ligated.
   d) The infant may need extracorporeal membrane oxygenation to decrease the pulmonary workload. The internal jugular vein may be cannulated with one venovenous cannula, or the internal jugular and common carotid may be cannulated with two venoarterial cannulas. The infant is kept paralyzed.
   e) Prostaglandins may be used to decrease pulmonary vascular resistance.
   f) Tolazoline (Priscoline) relaxes vascular smooth muscle with α-adrenergic blockade and is used to treat persistent pulmonary vasoconstriction and hypertension of the newborn. Dilute 100 mg/100 mL for a concentration of 1 mg/mL. Infuse at 1 to 8 mg/kg/hour (usually 1 mg/kg/hour).
   g) Intravenous medication can be used for hemodynamic support.
      (1) Dobutamine: Vasopressor, increases heart rate and contractility 200 mg/250 mL 5% dextrose in water (D5W) (0.8 mg/mL = 800 mcg/mL)
          Infuse at 2.5 to 15 mcg/kg/min (maximum, 40 mcg/kg/min)
      (2) Dopamine: Vasopressor, increases heart rate and contractility 200 mg/250 mL D5W (0.8 mg/mL = 800 mcg/mL)
          Infuse at 1 to 20 mcg/kg/min
      (3) Epinephrine: Inotrope, increases heart rate

1 mg/100 mL D5W (0.01 mg/mL = 10 mcg/mL)
0.1 to 1 mcg/kg/min
(4) Norepinephrine: Inotrope
   Bolus: 0.01 mcg/kg
   Drip: 1 mg/100 mL D5W (10 mcg/mL)
(5) Phenylephrine: a-Agonist
   Drip: 10 mg/250 mL D5W (40 mcg/mL)
   Bolus: 5 to 20 mcg/kg/dose every 15 minutes
(6) Nitroglycerin: Vasodilator, reduces preload
   Drip: 100 mg/250 mL D5W (0.04 mg/mL = 400 mcg/mL)
   1 to 5 mcg/kg/min

F. Genitourinary Procedures

1. **Introduction**
   a) A cystoscopy is usually a brief procedure, allowing for administration of general anesthesia by a mask. A laryngeal mask airway may also be used.
   b) Hypospadias repair, chordee release, and repair of undescended testicles are usually performed with the patient under general anesthesia and with an endotracheal tube. If the testicle cannot be located directly, an intraabdominal approach with muscle relaxation may be required.
2. **Preoperative assessment and patient preparation**
   a) History and physical examination
      (1) Review systems to determine the presence of comorbidities.
      (2) Laboratory tests are as indicated by the history and physical examination.
      (3) Diagnostic tests are as indicated by the history and physical examination.
   b) Patient preparation: Administer midazolam, 0.5 mg/kg orally 30 minutes before the procedure, if desired.
3. **Room preparation**
   a) Monitoring equipment is standard.
   b) Additional equipment includes warming devices for prolonged procedures.
   c) Position: Supine for orchiopexy, chordee release, and hypospadias repair; lithotomy position for cystoscopy. Pad all pressure points, and maintain proper body alignment to prevent nerve and soft tissue injuries.
   d) A standard pediatric tabletop is used.
   e) Intravenous fluids: Depending on the patient's age and size, a 22- or 24-gauge catheter should be sufficient. Infuse normal saline or lactated Ringer's solution at a rate of 2 to 4 mL/kg/hour plus NPO (nothing by mouth) and blood loss replacements.
4. **Perioperative management and anesthetic technique**
   a) Mask induction with oxygen (O_2), nitrous oxide (N_2O), and sevoflurane/halothane. If the patient has a preexisting intravenous line established, administer propofol (2.5 to 3.5 mg/kg) or thiopental (Pentothal; 5 to 6 mg/kg). Muscle relaxation is used if desired for intubation purposes, but muscle relaxation is not required for the procedure.
   b) Obtain a protected airway with appropriately sized endotracheal tube. Ensure proper placement and secure with tape.

    c) Maintenance: O_2, N_2O, and sevoflurane/halothane/isoflurane, with an intravenous fluid rate as calculated. Maintain normothermia. Manipulation of the testicles or peritoneum may produce a profound vagal response. Pretreat with atropine or glycopyrrolate before this occurrence. Caudal anesthesia prevents the response. If bradycardia occurs and is refractory to atropine, treat with a fluid bolus (10 to 20 mL) or epinephrine (10 to 20 mcg) intravenously.

    d) Emergence: Extubate while the patient is awake.

5. Postoperative complications

    a) Pain is a complication.

    b) Opioids may increase the incidence of nausea and vomiting.

    c) Caudal anesthesia is appropriate in children less than 7 years old and may be performed after induction to decrease volatile agent requirements or before emergence.

G. Hernia Repair

1. Introduction

Inguinal hernia repair is the most common procedure performed in children. Premature infants are more likely to have incarcerations, mostly from failure of the processus vaginalis to obliterate. The procedure is performed through an inguinal crease incision. Complications of hernia repairs are rare. Umbilical hernias are more common in African-Americans and may close spontaneously (95% to 98% by age 5 years). Repair is performed through a transverse infraumbilical incision. Intraperitoneal exploration is rarely done.

2. Preoperative assessment

    a) History and physical examination

        (1) Cardiac: These are routine.

        (2) Respiratory: Patients with prolonged ventilation and/or immature lungs are more susceptible to tracheomalacia, subglottic stenosis, and bronchopulmonary dysplasia.

        (3) Neurologic: Premature infants may display transient apneic and bradycardic episodes in response to hypoxemia. Premature infants are more prone to seizure disorders. Complications from general anesthesia may occur from effects on the immature central nervous system.

        (4) Renal: These are routine.

        (5) Gastrointestinal: The patient may have abdominal compression if the umbilical hernia is large. Consider rapid sequence induction for incarcerated hernia and bowel obstructions.

        (6) Endocrine: Premature infants are more prone to hypoglycemia. Check the blood glucose level.

    b) Patient preparation

        (1) Laboratory tests: As indicated from the history and physical examination

        (2) Diagnostic tests: None

        (3) Medications: Midazolam, 0.5 mg/kg orally 30 minutes before surgery for children older than 1 year of age

3. Room preparation

    a) Monitoring equipment is standard.

b) Additional equipment: Use a pediatric circle or Bain circuit. Warm and humidify gases. A warming pad may be used on the table.

c) Position: The patient is supine.

d) Fluids: 0.9% normal saline or lactated Ringer's solution. Dextrose solutions may be used for infants less than 1 month old.

e) Blood loss is negligible.

4. **Perioperative management and anesthetic technique**

a) General anesthesia, mask or endotracheal tube. Caudal block may be performed after induction for postoperative pain and will provide approximately 6 to 12 hours of pain relief postoperatively.

b) Induction: Mask or endotracheal intubation with halothane or sevoflurane/oxygen/nitrous oxide. Obtain an intravenous line after induction. Administer atropine intravenously (0.02 mg/kg) before laryngoscopy, vecuronium (0.1 mg/kg), or cisatracurium (0.1 to 0.2 mg/kg). If applicable, perform a caudal block with bupivacaine (0.25%) 1 mL/kg after induction (onset of 15 minutes).

c) Maintenance: Caudal block will decrease the amount of volatile agent. Increase the MAC before incision to avoid laryngospasm.

d) Emergence: Extubate when the patient is fully awake. Intravenous reversal is with neostigmine (0.07 mg/kg) and glycopyrrolate (0.01 mg/kg).

5. **Postoperative complications**

Postoperative apnea can occur in infants at 50 to 60 weeks of gestational age, especially if they are premature. These patients should be admitted for postoperative observation.

H. Intraabdominal Procedures

1. **Introduction**

Intraabdominal procedures may be indicated for a variety of reasons: pyloric stenosis, necrotizing enterocolitis, omphalocele, gastroschisis, megacolon, biliary atresia, intestinal atresia, incarcerated hernia, malrotation and volvulus, imperforate anus, and exstrophy of the cloaca or bladder.

2. **Preoperative assessment and patient preparation**

a) History and physical examination

(1) Cardiac: Other anomalies (patent ductus arteriosus, ventricular septal defect) may lead to congestive heart failure or murmur. The patient may have a labile blood pressure and hypovolemia from dehydration.

(2) Respiratory: Premature infants may have immature respiratory centers and apneic/bradycardic episodes from hypoxemia. Respiratory compromise is possible with a large abdominal mass.

(3) Neurologic: Premature infants may be prone to seizure disorders, myelomeningocele, and hydrocephalus. Hypoxemia may predispose to intracranial hemorrhage.

(4) Renal: Wilms' tumor may lead to hematuria and other genitourinary anomalies.

(5) Gastrointestinal: The patient may have esophageal/gastric reflux, jaundice, anemia from hepatic disease, diarrhea with malabsorption states, a colostomy, bowel preparation, or intestinal compression.

(6) Endocrine: The patient may have hypochloremia and hypokalemia, or metabolic alkalosis from vomiting. Neuroblastomas are associated with increased catecholamine production.

b) Patient preparation
   (1) Laboratory tests: Vary with pathology, procedure, and the history and physical examination—hemoglobin and hematocrit, type and cross-match, electrolytes, glucose, liver function tests, prothrombin time, and partial thromboplastin time
   (2) Premedication: Midazolam, 0.5 mg/kg orally if at least 1 year old, 30 minutes before the procedure

3. **Room preparation**
   a) Monitoring equipment: Standard. Depending on the procedure and health status, consider an arterial line, central venous pressure catheter, pulmonary arterial catheter, Foley catheter, and peripheral nerve stimulation.
   b) Additional equipment includes a heated humidified circuit, heating pad, hot lamps, and fluid warmers.
   c) Position: The patient is supine.
   d) Fluids: Therapy to address fluid deficit, maintenance, third-space loss, and blood loss. Insensible losses may be elevated because of phototherapy light or radiant heaters.

4. **Perioperative management and anesthetic technique**
   a) General anesthesia is used.
   b) Induction: Decompress the stomach before induction. Preoxygenate for 2 to 3 minutes. Administer atropine (0.02 mg/kg) before laryngoscopy. Use rapid sequence or awake intubation. An upper extremity intravenous catheter is preferred.
   c) Maintenance: Volatile inhalation agents. Nitrous oxide is avoided because of its tendency to distend the bowel. Decreases in central venous pressure of 4 mm H_2O or more are associated with vena cava compression. Use long- or intermediate-acting muscle relaxants: vecuronium (0.05 mg/kg) or pancuronium (0.05 mg/kg). Use narcotic generously (fentanyl, 1 to 2 mcg/kg/dose). Consider intraoperative infusion, especially if postoperative ventilation is planned. Keep the oxygen saturation at 95% to 97%. Avoid hypovolemia. The surgeon may infiltrate the site with local anesthetic before closure. Note the peak inspiratory pressure before abdominal closure.
   d) Emergence: Neostigmine (0.05 to 0.07 mg/kg) and glycopyrrolate (0.01 mg/kg) if postoperative ventilation is not desired. Suction the stomach before extubation. Extubate when the patient is awake.

5. **Postoperative complications**
   a) Postoperative ventilation may be needed.
   b) Residual anesthesia can contribute to postoperative apnea.
   c) Peristalsis is usually delayed; the patient may need total parenteral nutrition.
   d) Sepsis may occur.
   e) Abdominal third-space loss can continue immediately postoperatively; additional fluid resuscitation may be required.

PART II Common Procedures

I. Myringotomy

1. **Introduction**
   Myringotomy is a common outpatient procedure in children. Myringotomy is usually associated with the insertion of ventilation tubes into the tympanic membrane as a treatment for recurrent otitis media.

Typically, a small incision is made with the use of a microscope in the tympanic membrane, and fluid is suctioned through a transcanal approach.

2. **Preoperative assessment**

Other than a history of frequent and recurrent otitis media, this patient population is generally healthy.

a) History and physical examination

   (1) A careful family history should be obtained preoperatively, including any history of family problems with anesthesia.

   (2) Respiratory: Many pediatric patients presenting for myringotomy have a history of frequent upper respiratory tract infections. If currently exhibiting signs and symptoms of upper respiratory tract infections, these children are at greater risk for laryngospasm intraoperatively and postoperatively. Because this procedure is elective, it is commonly recommended to postpone the procedure until the signs and symptoms of upper respiratory tract infection have subsided.

   (3) Dental: Inspection of the airway and questioning of the parents should identify any loose teeth.

b) Patient preparation

   (1) Laboratory tests are as indicated from the history and physical examination.

   (2) Diagnostic tests are as indicated from the history and physical examination.

   (3) Medications: Midazolam, 0.5 mg/kg orally, may be given with 20 to 30 mL of apple juice as a premedication. It is also available as an elixir.

3. **Room preparation**

a) Monitoring equipment is standard.

b) Additional equipment: None is needed.

c) Standard emergency drugs are used (including atropine, lidocaine, epinephrine, and succinylcholine).

d) A pediatric standard tabletop is used.

e) Intravenous fluids: Depending on the age of the patient, expected length of procedure, and history and physical findings, an intravenous catheter may be available for emergency use but is not started routinely. If necessary, use a 20- or 22-gauge peripheral catheter, normal saline or lactated Ringer's solution at 2 to 4 mL/ kg/hour.

4. **Perioperative management and anesthetic technique**

a) Mask general anesthesia is usually adequate for uncomplicated myringotomy of otherwise healthy patients.

b) Induction: Mask inhalation induction with halothane or sevoflurane, nitrous oxide, and oxygen. If an existing intravenous catheter is present, routine intravenous induction is appropriate. Routine intravenous induction is preferred in older children and adults.

c) Maintenance: Standard maintenance with halothane, sevoflurane, or isoflurane, nitrous oxide, and oxygen. Muscle relaxation and opiates are not routinely used. If the patient is an adult, isoflurane or desflurane are preferred to halothane due to increased risk of halothane hepatitis in adults.

d) Emergence: The airway is maintained until the patient is fully awake. In older children and adults, antiemetics should be considered.

5. **Postoperative complications**

a) Nausea and vomiting can be treated with the following:

   (1) Metoclopramide, 0.15 mg/kg/dose intravenously; maximum of 10 mg

(2) Droperidol, 30 to 75 mcg/kg/dose

(3) Ondansetron, 0.05 to 0.1 mg/kg/dose intravenously; maximum of 4 mg

b) These patients are often sensitive to sounds in the immediate post-operative period.

J. Tonsillectomy and Adenoidectomy

1. **Introduction**

   Children may present for tonsillectomy or adenoidectomy with a history of recurrent infections (chronic tonsillitis) or a history of obstruction and sleep apnea.

2. **Preoperative assessment and patient preparation**

   a) History and physical examination

   (1) Cardiac: Echocardiography may be useful to determine the presence of right-sided heart failure from chronic obstruction. These patients are at increased risk for negative pressure pulmonary edema and volume overload.

   (2) Respiratory: Evaluate for potentially difficult airway management. If the child exhibits signs and symptoms of upper respiratory tract infection, there is an increased risk of laryngospasm intraoperatively and postoperatively. It is best to postpone this elective procedure until the upper respiratory tract infection resolves.

   b) Patient preparation

   (1) Judicious use of preoperative medication in children with obstructive apnea

   (2) Midazolam, 0.5 mg/kg orally in children without obstruction

   (3) Laboratory tests: As indicated by the history and physical examination

   (4) Diagnostic tests: As indicated by the history and physical examination

3. **Room preparation**

   a) Monitoring equipment: Standard

   b) Additional equipment: None

   c) Standard emergency drugs: Atropine, lidocaine, epinephrine, and succinylcholine

   d) Standard pediatric tabletop: Endotracheal tubes (RAE or straight), laryngoscope blade and handle, oral airways, lubricant, gauze, and emergency drugs

   e) Intravenous fluids: Depending on age and size of patient, a 22- or 24-gauge catheter probably sufficient; infusion of normal saline or lactated Ringer's solution at 2 to 4 mL/kg/hour

4. **Perioperative management and anesthetic technique**

   a) Mask induction is performed with oxygen (O_2), nitrous oxide (N_2O), and sevoflurane/halothane.

   b) Obtain intravenous access; administer narcotic; give atropine as indicated; and administer muscle relaxant if desired (not necessary).

   c) Intubate with an appropriate-size endotracheal tube. Ensure correct placement by auscultation of breath sounds, movement of chest, and noted end-tidal carbon dioxide wave. Tape in the midline.

   d) An acetaminophen (Tylenol) suppository, 25 to 30 mg/kg, may be given at this point for postoperative pain control.

   e) Maintenance: Standard with sevoflurane, halothane, or isoflurane, O_2, and N_2O. Muscle relaxation is not required. Opiates are given at induction.

PART II **Common Procedures**

f) At the end of the case, reverse the remaining muscle relaxant if used. Carefully suction the stomach and oropharynx. Extubate when the patient is fully awake because of the increased risk of laryngospasm with the presence of blood in the airway. An alternative method is true deep extubation after patient initiates the first breath. Transfer the patient to the recovery unit in lateral-head down position so secretions do not pool in back of airway, thus increasing risk of laryngospasm.

5. **Postoperative complications**
   a) Nausea and vomiting can be treated with the following:
      (1) Metoclopramide, 0.15 mg/kg/dose; maximum of 10 mg
      (2) Droperidol, 30 to 75 mcg/kg/dose
      (3) Ondansetron, 0.05 to 0.1 mg/kg/dose; maximum of 4 mg
   b) Pain
      (1) The severity of pain depends on the history of chronic infections and the surgical technique.
      (2) The site may be infiltrated with local anesthetic.
      (3) Opioids may increase nausea and vomiting.
      (4) Nonsteroidal antiinflammatory agents are not recommended because of the increased risk of bleeding.
      (5) Pain usually resolves in 7 to 10 days with sloughing of tissue.
      (6) Admission to hospital may be required if pain prevents adequate oral intake.
   c) Bleeding
      (1) This occurs in first 8 hours postoperatively or 7 to 10 days postoperatively when the eschar sheds.
      (2) A bleeding tonsil that forces the patient to return to the operating room has several implications:
         (a) The patient is hypovolemic: Establish intravenous access and infuse a balanced salt solution or lactated Ringer's solution.
         (b) The airway may be compromised by the presence of blood and edema. Have an alternative plan for establishing a protected airway. Recommend the use of endotracheal tube 0.5 mm smaller than the original tube because of the presence of edema.
         (c) Plan rapid sequence induction using mivacurium. The patient is considered to have a full stomach because of the presence of blood.

ANESTHESIA FOR THERAPEUTIC AND DIAGNOSTIC PROCEDURES

A. Overall Anesthetic Care Plan

1. Introduction

a) Certain diagnostic and therapeutic procedures performed outside the operating room environment require anesthesia services. These services include providing anesthetic care adhering to the American Association of Nurse Anesthetists/American Society of Anesthesiologists (AANA/ASA) standards and institutional accreditation guidelines, for an overall anesthetic care plan.

b) Examples of areas that use off-site anesthesia services are as follows:

(1) Computed tomography (CT)

(2) Magnetic resonance imaging (MRI)

(3) Nuclear medicine

(4) Interventional radiology

(5) Radiation oncology

(6) Cardiac catheterization laboratory

(7) Endoscopy

2. Monitoring

Follow AANA/ASA/institutional requirements.

3. Check room for essential equipment

a) Oxygen and suction

b) Anesthesia machine and ancillary supplies (i.e., endotracheal tube, laryngoscope/blades, oral and nasal airways, oxygen mask, and nasal cannulas)

c) Adequate monitoring equipment to allow adherence to standards of practice (i.e., electrocardiogram, noninvasive blood pressure equipment, pulse oximeter, capnograph, and thermometer)

d) Intravenous supplies and fluid

e) Sufficient electrical outlets to satisfy anesthesia machine and monitoring equipment requirements

f) Adequate illumination of the patient, anesthesia machine, and monitoring equipment

g) Emergency cart with defibrillator, emergency drugs, and other resuscucitative equipment equivalent to that in the operating room

4. Disadvantages of off-site procedures

a) Physical setup

(1) Unfamiliar and isolated location limits anesthesia department back-up (i.e., emergencies, laboratories, staffing, transportation, and availability of drugs)

(2) Oxygen source: Wall outlet inaccessibility or piped-in gases

(3) Available scavenging system
(4) Availability of wall suction
(5) Availability of electrical outlets
(6) Dim lighting conditions
(7) Recovery staff availability
b) Limited patient access
(1) Crowded spaces
(2) Shields
(3) Fluoroscopy and imaging tables moving and turning
c) Potential contact with hazardous materials
(1) Radiation exposure or exposure to magnetic field
(2) Inhalation agents due to lack of adequate scavenging system
5. **Potential hazards of off-site procedures**
a) Temperature control
(1) Problems include cold rooms and tables and vasodilation under anesthesia.
(2) Temperature monitors are inaccessible.
(3) Turn the internal fans of the MRI unit off during scanning.
(4) Cover the infant's head with a cap.
(5) In MRI, compatible, disposable, crushed warming devices may be used on neonates.
(6) Place patient under warmer after procedure.
b) Monitoring of access and interference from machinery
(1) All monitors must be placed and functioning well before the beginning of procedure.
(2) Monitors should be placed at the point of least distortion.
(3) Equipment should have good artifact suppression characteristics; however, most artifact cannot be eliminated.
(4) Use only MRI-compatible monitors to avoid burns from coiling from an amplified antenna effect.
c) Fluid management
(1) Intravenous access is limited. It is recommended that all pediatric patients less than 1 year old be placed on a Medfusion pump for fluid volume control. Children between ages 1 and 3 years should have intravenous fluids controlled by a Medfusion pump or Buritrol chamber in line to avoid fluid overload. Microinfusion extension tubing has 2 mL volume per 5 ft, and this volume should be considered in fluid calculations.
(2) Intravenous line should be taped securely to avoid loss of access.
(3) Run fluids judiciously according to needs (i.e., bowel preparation or contrast infusion, prolonged fasting, and NPO [nothing by mouth] times).
d) Airway management
(1) There is limited access to the patient, so vigilance and observation are key.
(2) The respiratory pattern may be difficult to observe; monitor end-tidal carbon dioxide and pulse oximetry closely.
6. **Selection of anesthetic agents and techniques**
a) Goals
(1) Ventilation and perfusion of tissues should not be compromised.
(2) The airway should remain patent with spontaneous respirations and protective reflexes intact if using a sedation technique. Protect the airway.

(3) Induction of anesthetic should be rapid, painless, and 100% effective.

(4) The patient should remain motionless for the duration of the procedure.

(5) Recovery should be rapid, and there should be no nausea or dysphoria.

b) Considerations

(1) The patient's condition, age, and underlying medical problems must be evaluated. Many children scheduled for these procedures are chronically ill and may have multiple anomalies and disorders.

(2) The location of the procedure may influence airway and access to the patient and intravenous lines.

(3) Requirements of the procedure, such as duration, position, and the possibility of pain must be considered.

7. Preoperative considerations

a) Patient preparation

(1) All patients should undergo a full preanesthetic assessment to determine their fitness and the type of anesthetic required for the procedure. This should consist of a full history and examination with the appropriate laboratory work.

(2) The parent or guardian must be present for underage children. Adults should have a companion for discharge.

(3) Strict NPO guidelines are adhered to: Children less than 12 months of age should have no solids after midnight on the day of surgery, formula and breast milk are allowed up to 6 hours before surgery, and clear liquids up to 4 hours before surgery. Children 1 to 3 years old should have no solids after midnight; clear liquids may be given up to 6 hours before the time of surgery. Adults should be NPO after midnight.

(4) Appropriate premedication is given for specific procedures; assess patient medical condition and level of maturity and anxiety.

b) Premedication has many purposes: Relief of anxiety, sedation with rapid recovery, analgesia, amnesia, reduction of salivary and gastric secretions, elevation of gastric pH, and decreased cardiac vagal activity.

(1) Midazolam (Versed): Use nasal or oral administration (0.5 to 0.75 mg/ kg); 0.05 mg/kg intravenously.

(2) Methohexital: Use rectally, 20 to 25 mg/kg (diluted to 100 mg/ mL; 7 mg/ kg intramuscularly of 3.5% concentration).

(3) Ketamine: Administer 3 mg/kg intramuscularly or 6 mg/kg orally in conjunction with an antisialagogue (e.g., glycopyrrolate).

(4) Consider atropine (0.01 to 0.02 mg/kg) to provide protection against a cholinergic response.

8. Anesthetic techniques for maintenance

a) Safe choices may include monitored sedation, dissociative, and general anesthesia.

b) Monitored sedation is appropriate for nonpainful, simple diagnostic examinations that require patient cooperation.

c) Total intravenous anesthesia: In children undergoing noninvasive procedures, nonintubated intravenous general anesthesia techniques are commonly used. Light levels of general anesthesia allow for prompt recovery. When a deep level of sedation is obtained, reflex activity is minimized; response to painful stimuli is attenuated; and obstruction, laryngospasm, and apnea are increased.

d) In dissociative anesthesia (ketamine) spontaneous respirations are usually maintained, with anesthesia intramuscularly before intravenous placement. Heart rate and blood pressure are usually increased. Disadvantages include the following: increased airway irritability; painful injection; prolonged, unpredictable, or delirious emergence; nausea; and increased intracranial pressure.

e) General anesthesia is indicated when the airway cannot be assured because of positioning, procedure is lengthy and painful, or airway must be protected (i.e., upper endoscopy). It is also indicated when the patient must remain motionless for long periods or neuromuscular blockade is needed (percutaneous atrial septal defect closure).

9. **Postanesthesia care**
   a) Infants and children generally recover more quickly from anesthesia and are less disturbed by minor complications than adults.
   b) Transport to recovery should include appropriate monitoring, oxygen, and emergency airway equipment and medications.
   c) The ability to deal with adverse reactions in a timely fashion (i.e., contrast dye anaphylaxis, laryngospasm, bronchospasm, cardiovascular collapse) is necessary.

B. Automatic Implantable Cardioverter-Defibrillator

1. **Introduction**
   Indications for use of an automatic implantable cardioverter-defibrillator (AICD) include sustained ventricular tachycardia (VT) and syncope resulting from VT and ventricular fibrillation (VF). Electrical countershock is the only reliable treatment for VF. AICDs resemble large pacemakers and contain a power generator that is implanted over the pectoral muscle under local anesthesia and sedation. AICDs contain a single intracardiac countershocking electrode; this electrode also serves as a ventricular pacing lead. This device senses electrical activity and will emit an electrical countershock if a tachydysrhythmia is sensed.

2. **Preoperative assessment**
   a) Most patients who present for an AICD have severe coronary artery disease, which may include a recent infarct, cardiomyopathy, and coronary artery bypass graft.
   b) History and physical examination
      (1) Document indications for AICD and preexisting medical conditions.
      (2) Evaluate left ventricular function and echocardiogram results.
      (3) Obtain a recent electrocardiogram and cardiac catheterization results if available.
      (4) Assess the chest x-ray film for left ventricular hypertrophy.
   c) Patient preparation
      (1) Obtain electrolytes, prothrombin time, and partial thromboplastin time if the patient is taking anticoagulants.
      (2) Explain to patient that the procedure is performed with local and sedation.

3. **Room preparation**
   a) Fluoroscopy is used during the entire procedure, and lead shields should be worn.
   b) Full monitoring and standard tabletop equipment needs to be available.
   c) Invasive monitoring during the procedure is usually not necessary, unless the patient has preexisting lines.
   d) Know where the crash cart, wall suction, and oxygen source are located.

e) An alternative means of providing emergency pacing should be available.

4. **Perioperative management and anesthetic technique**
   a) Verification of AICD placement involves the induction of VT or VF and tests the device's capability to convert the tachyarrhythmia to a normal sinus rhythm.
   b) While the device is being tested, the patient should be ventilated with 100% oxygen with administration of midazolam (Versed) for amnesia.

5. **Postoperative implications**
   a) Patients with AICDs should not enter a room with a magnetic resonance imaging (MRI) machine, because the MRI magnetic field will deactivate the AICD.
   b) AICDs should be deactivated before lithotripsy.
   c) Be aware of potential pacemaker and AICD interaction with other tachyarrhymthias such as sinus tachycardia or atrial fibrillation.
   d) Patients should be instructed of the need to have the AICD turned off and deactivated before any subsequent surgical procedures, because electrocautery can cause the AICD to discharge inappropriately during surgery.

C. Brachytherapy

1. **Introduction**
   Palladium-103 prostate implants are being used for brachytherapy as an optional treatment for prostate cancer. The sources are permanently implanted directly into the tissue. The seeds are encased in a lead-lined cartridge that attaches to lead-lined placement needles. The seeds are placed by the radiation oncologist through these needles into the prostate through the perineum. Placement is guided by ultrasound.

2. **Preoperative assessment and patient preparation**
   a) The treatment is performed in the radiation oncology department.
   b) Each patient is prescreened and admitted as an outpatient through the short stay unit.
   c) The procedure lasts a maximum of 2 hours.
   d) Patients may undergo a bowel preparation at home before the procedure.
   e) An 18-gauge, 2-inch angiocatheter is placed before the procedure.
   f) Each patient will require intravenous antibiotics before the procedure. One gram of cefazolin (Ancef) is required. If the patient has an allergy to penicillin, then clindamycin (Cleocin), 600 mg, is given.

3. **Room preparation**
   Required monitoring equipment, anesthesia, and airway supplies are provided.

4. **Anesthetic management**
   a) Anesthesia is usually maintained by spinal anesthesia. A minimal T8 level is desired. If the patient is required to have consecutive treatments, an epidural anesthetic may be placed.
   b) Sedation is given as needed.

c) The patient is placed in a lithotomy position for the procedure. A Foley catheter is inserted with Hypaque in the balloon. An ultrasound probe and perineum template are placed before needle placement.

d) The time of treatment is the time of radiation. Everyone must leave the room. Visual contact is always present through monitors. Treatment time is usually 5 to 15 minutes.

5. **Radiation precautions**

   a) Occasionally, seeds can become dislodged from the implanted tissue. Therefore, dressings and linens must not be removed from the room until they have been checked and cleared by the oncology physicist.

   b) If a seed is discovered, *do not* touch it with your hands. Use long forceps to place it in a lead storage container.

   c) Some seeds may pass in the urine for the first few days. Therefore, urine must be strained before being discarded.

   d) Pregnant personnel are not to attend these patients.

   e) All personnel remaining in the room during the procedure should have proper badges. No person or material should leave the room without being surveyed with a Geiger counter.

D. Cardiac Radiofrequency Ablation

1. **Introduction**

   a) Cardiac ablation procedures can be performed either surgically or using radiofrequency techniques through a transvenous catheter.

   b) Transvenous catheter ablation involves the use of radiofrequency energy to deliver direct high-energy current shocks to the heart to ablate atrial and ventricular tachycardia and associated accessory pathways.

   c) Indications for ablation include supraventricular tachycardia and recurrent accessory pathway disorders such as Wolff-Parkinson-White syndrome or Lown-Ganong-Levine syndrome.

2. **Preoperative assessment**

   a) Patients are usually young, with normal ventricular function.

   b) A thorough history and physical examination should be obtained.

   c) Drugs used to treat dysrhythmia are usually discontinued before surgery to make the dysrhythmia more inducible.

   d) External defibrillator-cardioverter pads are placed before the procedure.

   e) Sedation should be given for femoral and internal jugular catheter placement by the cardiologist.

3. **Room preparation**

   Standard monitors and tabletop with fluoroscopy are used.

4. **Perioperative management and anesthetic technique**

   a) Radiofrequency ablation is not considered extremely painful because muscles and nerves are not stimulated. Most patients do experience a burning sensation when ablation is applied, and sedation is necessary at this time.

   b) Mapping of the target foci and accessory pathways requires inducing a reentry tachycardia, using a stimulator to initiate premature atrial and ventricular beats.

   c) The usual procedure time is 4 to 6 hours, with intermittent stimulation used.

5. Postoperative implications
The patient should be monitored overnight for any arrhythmias.

E. Cardioversion

1. Introduction
Synchronized cardioversion is the electrical conversion of a tachyrhythmia, such as atrial fibrillation, atrial flutter, or supraventricular tachycardia, unresponsive to intravenous drugs, to a normal sinus rhythm. A synchronized electrical shock is released through the chest wall; this depolarizes the myocardium and simultaneously makes it refractory, thereby enabling the sinoatrial node to resume its function as a primary pacemaker.

2. Preoperative assessment and patient preparation
a) History and physical examination: Standard
b) Diagnostic tests: 12-lead electrocardiography
c) Preoperative medication and intravenous therapy
    (1) One may desire to hold the daily dose of digoxin.
    (2) One 18-gauge intravenous line with minimal fluid replacement is used.

3. Room preparation
a) Monitoring equipment
    (1) Standard
    (2) Artificial cardiac pacing
b) Pharmacologic agents: Atropine, lidocaine
c) Position: Supine

4. Anesthetic technique
a) Sedation
b) Intravenous sedation: Midazolam, methohexital (Brevital), or propofol in sedative doses until the patient's lid reflex is gone

5. Perioperative management
a) Induction: Preoxygenate the patient with the use of nasal cannula or face mask.
b) Maintenance: As soon as consciousness is lost, the synchronized charge should be delivered with the R wave on the electrocardiogram to avoid causing ventricular fibrillation.
c) Emergence: Support the airway and maintain ventilation until the patient regains consciousness.

6. Postoperative implications
Monitor the electrocardiogram; complex ventricular arrhythmias may appear, especially if the patient was taking digoxin.

F. Computed Tomography Scan and Magnetic Resonance Imaging

1. Introduction
a) To obtain successful computed tomography (CT) and magnetic resonance imaging (MRI) scans, the patient must lie absolutely still throughout the entire procedure.
b) Anesthesia may be needed for cooperative patients with movement disorders and for patients who are confused or uncooperative, such as for patients with closed-head injuries or pediatric patients.

2. Potential problems associated with anesthesia
  a) Patient inaccessibility
  b) Airway management
  c) Effects of the MRI magnetism on the monitoring equipment

3. Considerations on the use of radiopaque dye
  a) Ionic contrast media (sodium meglumin, salts of iodinated acids, or combinations) can be used for imaging studies.
  b) The hyperosmolarity of ionic compounds can cause a typical (nonallergic) reaction characterized by flushing, tachycardia, and nausea, probably caused by endothelial disruption and the subsequent nonimmunologic release of vasoactive substances from mast cells.
  c) Some patients will exhibit a true allergy to iodine. Patients at risk are allergic to shellfish or have iodine, asthma, or drug allergies.
  d) Pretreatment for patients at risk for an allergic reaction includes methylprednisolone (0.5 mg/kg orally) and diphenhydramine (0.5 to 1 mg/kg orally or intravenously).
  e) Treat anaphylaxis with epinephrine (10 mcg/kg).

4. Positioning problems
  a) Examination of the posterior fossa with CT requires extreme flexion of the head, which may obstruct the airway or kink the endotracheal tube.
  b) Patients are secluded in a room away from anesthesia personnel.
  c) Pressure points should be padded to avoid positioning injuries.

5. Recommended anesthesia management
  a) Preprocedure: Midazolam (Versed), 0.5 to 0.75 mg orally 20 minutes before the scan, if the patient is uncooperative.
  b) Start with mask induction with oxygen, nitrous oxide, and halothane or sevoflurane.
  c) Maintenance
    (1) Patients should be spontaneously breathing. Oxygen with nasal cannula or mask can be used. For children younger than 3 months, patients with difficult airways, or patients exhibiting sleep apnea, the airway may be secured with a laryngeal mask airway or an endotracheal tube.
    (2) Propofol: Initial bolus, 1 mg/kg. Atropine may be needed in children to offset cardiac depressive effects.
    (3) Propofol infusion: 5 mg/kg/hour up to a maximum of 10 mg/kg/hour.
    (4) Deepening anesthesia during infusion: Bolus propofol (0.3 to 0.5 mg/kg) and midazolam (Versed, 0.02 mg/kg).

G. Endoscopy

1. Introduction
Endoscopy has become an integral part of modern diagnostic testing.

2. Preoperative assessment and patient preparation
  a) History and physical examination
  b) Preoperative medication and intravenous therapy

3. Room preparation
  a) Positive-pressure oxygen delivery system
  b) Suction and catheters
  c) Standard monitors
  d) Emergency cart with age- and size-appropriate drugs and equipment

4. **Anesthetic technique**
   a) Conscious or deep intravenous sedation is used with the majority of these patients.
   b) Sedation medications can include propofol, midazolam (Versed), and fentanyl.
   c) Lower gastrointestinal procedure intravenous sedation uses midazolam, fentanyl, and propofol at 25 to 75 mcg/kg/hour.
   d) Upper gastrointestinal procedures may require general anesthesia if the patient is at high risk for aspiration because of gastroesophageal reflux disease or esophageal dysfunction.
5. **Postoperative implications**
   a) Respiratory depression
   b) Airway obstruction
   c) Desaturation
   d) Apnea

H. Interventional Cardiology

1. **Introduction**
   Interventional cardiology is indicated for both diagnostic and therapeutic purposes. Angiographic imaging remains an essential component in defining the anatomy of structures that are behind the hilum of the lung and in patients in whom echocardiographic imaging is suboptimal because of poor acoustic windows. Interventional procedures include balloon dilation, coils, stents, atrial septal defect closure, and radiofrequency ablation. Diagnostic procedures include angiography, endomyocardial biopsy, and electrophysiologic study.
2. **Monitoring and room preparation**
   a) Use routine monitors plus an arterial line (check with the cardiologist).
   b) Ensure that emergency medications are drawn up on the tabletop, including vasopressors and antihypertensives.
   c) Have 2 units of blood in the room for interventional procedures.
3. **Preoperative patient preparation**
   a) Preoperative assessment is standard.
   b) Review the cardiac history and any previous diagnostic tests.
   c) The risk of difficult airway is increased in transplant recipients.
      (1) Long-term steroid use may lead to obesity.
      (2) Patients may develop lymphoproliferative disease, resulting in redundant lymphoid tissue in the pharynx and epiglottis leading to airway obstruction.
   d) Type and cross-match for interventional procedures because of the risk of vessel damage and hemorrhage.
4. **Anesthetic considerations**
   a) Use monitored anesthesia care or general anesthesia, depending on the procedure.
   b) Discuss oxygen requirements with the cardiologist. Some procedures require room air for diagnosis of congenital anomalies.
   c) Maintain normothermia.
   d) Watch for signs of allergic reaction to contrast media.
   e) Ask about antibiotics.
   f) Do not allow the patient to emerge from anesthesia until hemostasis achieved.

5. **Complications**
   a) Arrhythmias
   b) Hemorrhage
   c) Hypoxemia
   d) Pulmonary hypertensive crisis
   e) Hypothermia
   f) Contrast reaction/anaphylaxis
   g) Air embolism

I. Nuclear Medicine

1. **Terminology**
   a) Positron-emission tomography (PET) is an advanced imaging system in nuclear medicine that provides a three-dimensional view of human organs to help diagnose disease and other abnormalities. The system is made up of three parts: a cyclotron, a PET scanner, and a computer.
   b) Radionuclides are energy-charged atoms of carbon, nitrogen, oxygen, and fluorine.
   c) Half-life is the period of time it takes for one half of the radioactive material to lose its radioactivity.
2. **Principles**
   a) A PET image is obtained by using a cyclotron-produced radionuclide to make short-lived radiopharmaceutical compounds with half-lives of 2 to 110 minutes. These short half-lives allow lower radiation exposure.
   b) Moments after the radioactive compound is prepared, it is quickly transported to the scanner room through an underground pneumatic tube system. After injection or inhalation by the patient, the compound travels through the patient's bloodstream to the organ being scanned, where it decays and emits positively charged electrons called positrons.
   c) In the body, positrons interact with negatively charged electrons to produce gamma rays that light up at the area being examined. The PET scanner's circular array of detectors is positioned around the patient's body to detect gamma ray activity. The activity is translated by the computer into an image on the computer monitor. The image captures a cross-sectional (tomographic) slice of the organ to show its circulation or metabolism. The glucose base of many compounds used for brain scans will have an uptake quality related to the patient's cerebral metabolic rate. Maintaining the metabolic rate normality is essential to the scanning outcome.
   d) The PET scan image distinguishes parts of the organ to pinpoint where cells are dead or alive, and it helps to determine the best form of treatment for the patient.
3. **Anesthetic considerations**
   a) The PET scan is pain free; however, the patient must be absolutely still during the scanning. The patient lies flat on a table placed in the center of the scanner, and his or her arms may be strapped to the sides to prevent movement. During a brain scan, the patient wears a custom-fitted plastic face mask, and the sides of the mask are hooked onto the PET scanner table to prevent head movements during an examination. This positioning is very difficult for anyone who cannot fully

cooperate (pediatric and claustrophobic patients and those with neuromuscular disease). Anesthesia service will often be requested for head or brain scans.

b) Cerebral metabolism: The outcome of the scan can be affected by depression of cerebral metabolic rates related to anesthesia. The suggested doses of propofol (1 to 2 mg/kg) initial bolus followed by a 5 to 10 mg/kg/hour maintenance infusion have provided excellent scan results, whereas higher doses and other synergistic sedation combinations have resulted in poor cerebral glucose metabolism and the lack of radioactive compound uptake required for scanning.

c) Radiation: The equipment is not the source of radiation. The patient is the source of radiation only after the intravenous injection of the radioactive material. The care provider needs to remain as far from the patient as possible and limit access time of any close or hands-on patient care.

d) Occupational exposure: If an anesthesia provider used complete disregard for radiation safety principles in minimizing exposure, the provider could receive a maximum 4.5 mrem/patient in a 3-hour exposure, which is 0.009% of the legal limit for occupationally exposed individuals and 4.5% of the annual limit to the general public. (Each anesthesia staff member could perform 22 such cases and not exceed the exposure limit to the general public.) In spite of legal concerns, protect staff from any unnecessary radiation exposure.

e) Limited patient access: Assure depth of sedation and ventilatory status; a certified registered nurse anesthetist (CRNA) should be positioned for adequate patient/monitor observation before the patient receiving a radioactive injection.

4. **PET scan room setup**
   a) The CRNA is positioned outside the scanner room and can view the infusion pump, anesthesia monitors, and the patient (assisted by a camera focused on the patient's head) through an observation area. The room may be entered at any time without interfering with the scanning series.
   b) The CRNA can be positioned inside the scanner room, but it is highly recommended that the majority of the observation time be at distances as far from the patient as the room will allow.

5. **Nuclear scan setup**
   a) The CRNA must be positioned inside the scanner room.
   b) Obtain an anesthesia gas machine with a long ventilatory circuit, full monitoring capabilities, anesthesia sedation drugs (i.e., propofol, midazolam [Versed]), portable oxygen, and an oximeter with an Ambu or Jackson-Reese device for transport.
   c) Intravenous maintenance is the preferred method for the scanning period. Avoid oral medications because they will have prolonged cerebral metabolic depression and adversely effect the glucose medium/injectate uptake, resulting in poor scan quality. A brief period of halothane or sevoflurane and nitrous oxide for intravenous start has not affected test outcome, if the expired gas sample is allowed to return to zero before the initial electroencephalogram. Give propofol, initial bolus of 1 to 2 mg/kg and 5 to 10 mg/kg/hour for continuous infusion maintenance.

PART II **Common Procedures**

J. Tracheobronchial Stenting

1. Introduction

Obstruction of the trachea and major bronchi is a complication of bronchogenic carcinoma and extrathoracic malignancies metastatic to the lung and mediastinum. Patients are often symptomatic; they may present with wheezing, dyspnea, or postobstructive pneumonia. Although surgical resection is the preferred treatment of localized lesions, many patients present with extensive and unresectable disease. Other treatment options include chemotherapy, radiation therapy, and laser resection, all of which produce variable and inconsistent relief of the obstruction. For this reason, tracheobronchial stenting using metal stents originally designed for vascular use is being investigated for treatment of this complex clinical problem.

Tracheobronchial stents are indicated for treatment of tracheal and bronchial obstructions, which cause dyspnea, repeated infection, or tracheobronchial fistula. Lesions best suited for stent placement are focal and short segment stenoses or occlusions of the trachea and/or major bronchi that do not extend into the segmental bronchi. Uncovered stents permit air flow through their interstices and therefore can be placed across the orifices of branch airways, although this may impede the clearance of inspissated secretions. Over the course of 1 to 2 months, metal stents become partially or completely incorporated in the tracheal or bronchial wall.

2. Patient preparation

a) A thorough preoperative workup is necessary before anesthesia. The choice of anesthesia is primarily a function of the type of stent used, the comfort of the physician placing the stent, and the comorbid conditions of the patient. In general, silicone stent placement that requires prior airway dilation with rigid bronchoscopy will necessitate general anesthesia. Metallic stents can be placed with topical anesthesia with or without conscious sedation, or general anesthesia may be used.

b) Assess the airway. The patient may have current signs of obstruction including cough, wheezing, and stridor. Check previous respiratory diagnostic examinations, including computed tomography scans and pulmonary function tests. It is very important to understand the patient's current respiratory status and limitations.

c) Assess all other systems for comorbidities.

d) Use standard premedication titrated to effect. Be very cautious to avoid oversedation that could impair ventilation.

e) Glycopyrrolate, 0.2 mg intravenously, is used to decrease secretions and to improve visualization for intubation.

3. Room preparation

Have a difficult-airway cart available.

4. Perioperative management

a) Local sedation

(1) Localize the palate, pharynx, larynx, and trachea with 5 to 7 mL 4% lidocaine using a nebulizer.

(2) Titrate midazolam or propofol with a short-acting opioid to avoid respiratory depression.

b) General anesthesia awake intubation

(1) Localize as previously described.

(2) Preoxygenate for 3 to 5 minutes.

(3) Maintain spontaneous ventilation until the airway is secured with the patient awake or by performing a mask induction.

(4) Intubate with a fiberoptic light.

(5) Position the endotracheal tube 1 cm above the lesion.

(6) If the lesion is near the vocal cords, then a laryngeal mask airway may be used.

c) General anesthesia standard induction

This is used in patients with a small lesion and limited airway obstruction.

d) Maintenance

(1) If muscle relaxation is required, then consider succinylcholine drip.

(2) 100% oxygen is used.

(3) Total intravenous anesthesia or a volatile anesthetic is used.

e) Emergence

(1) The patient is fully awake.

(2) Good suctioning of blood and secretions before emergence will help to prevent coughing at the end of the case.

f) Complications

(1) Hypoxemia

(2) Hypercarbia

(3) Dysrhythmias

(4) Hypertension

(5) Bronchospasm

(6) Stent dislodgement

(7) Bleeding

(8) Tracheobronchial injury

(9) Aspiration

5. **Postoperative considerations**

a) Airway edema

b) Airway obstruction

c) Stent fracture/migration

d) Pneumothorax

e) Secretion retention

K. Transjugular Intrahepatic Portosystemic Shunt

1. **Introduction**

Transjugular intrahepatic portosystemic shunt (TIPS) is simply a shunt between the hepatic and portal veins, created in the liver parenchyma and maintained by placing metallic stents across the tract. The aim is to decrease the portal venous pressure, thereby directing blood flow away from the portosystemic varices, and decreasing the formation of ascitic fluid. Portal hypertension, most commonly from hepatic cirrhosis, leads to development of portosystemic varices and ascites. These varices can develop in a variety of sites, with gastroesophageal the most common. Rupture of gastroesophageal varices leads to massive hemorrhage.

2. **Preoperative assessment**

Refer to Section II of Part 2 for anesthetic implications related to hepatic cirrhosis.

PART II Common Procedures

3. **Patient preparation**
   a) Pretreat with H_2-blockers and nonparticulate antacid.
   b) Type and cross-match 4 units because of the risk of hemorrhage.
   c) Use minimal sedation.
   d) Check laboratory values, including electrolytes, blood urea nitrogen, creatinine, complete blood count, coagulation studies, and liver function tests.
4. **Room preparation**
   a) Standard monitors
   b) Pressure bags or rapid infuser
   c) Vasopressors ready to infuse if needed
5. **Perioperative management and anesthetic technique**
   a) Sedation with local anesthesia
   b) General anesthesia
      (1) Rapid sequence induction
      (2) Standard maintenance
      (3) Awake extubation
   c) Complications
      (1) Portal vein rupture
      (2) Perforation of liver capsule
      (3) Complete heart block
      (4) Congestive heart failure

L. Anesthesia for Therapeutic and Diagnostic Procedures in Pediatric Patients

RADIATION THERAPY

1. **Introduction**
   Radiation therapy uses ionizing photons to destroy lymphomas, pediatric acute leukemias, Wilms' tumor, retinoblastomas, and tumors of the central nervous system. Repeat sessions are typical and require (1) reliable motionlessness and (2) remote monitoring with the child in isolation. As in many off-site locations, the key issue is maintaining an adequate airway because of limited access to the patient.
2. **Preoperative assessment and patient preparation**
   a) The treatment is performed in the radiation oncology department.
   b) Standard preoperative assessment is performed.
   c) Check the previous anesthetic record for any potential problems and anesthetic requirements.
   d) Most children will have some type of medication access port. Flush the catheter with 0.9% normal saline using *sterile* technique. Give a bolus of propofol and start a propofol infusion in the preoperative area. Take the patient to treatment room and maintain the airway.
3. **Room preparation**
   a) Use standard monitoring equipment.
   b) Bring portable oxygen if it is not in the treatment area.
   c) Airway equipment is used.
   d) Emergency medications are available.
   e) Position the patient supine or prone.
   f) Simulations: Use an off-site pediatric anesthesia machine.

4. **Anesthetic management**
   a) Simulations: The case may last up to 60 minutes. General anesthesia with an oral endotracheal tube usually is required. Many procedures are done with the patient in the prone position for brain stem or spinal cord tumors. The purpose of this is to have the child motionless so the clinicians may design a mold to be used to hold the patient in a particular position for the upcoming treatments and for Groshong catheter insertion. Active scavenging through wall suction may be available, but total intravenous anesthesia is frequently used (once an intravenous line and an oral endotracheal tube are established) to expedite emergence and discharge.
   b) Treatments: Pediatric patients come for treatment series after the simulation-established mold and Groshong catheter insertion. Treatment may be as short as 10 minutes or as long as 40 minutes. Use a nasal cannula with end-tidal carbon dioxide tubing or two pediatric nasal cannulas.
5. **Postanesthesia care unit**
   a) Ensure that all standard monitors and equipment are available for recovery of anesthesia.
   b) Have a means of providing 100% oxygen by positive-pressure ventilation.
   c) A resuscitation cart should be available.

DIAGNOSTIC UROLOGY: VOIDING CYSTOURETHROGRAM

1. **Introduction**
   Children requiring a voiding cystourethrogram (VCU) usually have had a failed previous attempt without anesthesia. The test requires placement of a urinary catheter followed by filling of the bladder and voiding. Children usually object to placement of the catheter.
2. **Room preparation**
   a) Pediatric gas machine
   b) Intravenous medication tray
   c) Oxygen tank for transport (optional)
3. **Anesthetic considerations**
   Mask induction is a very quick procedure (less than 10 minutes), and an intravenous line is not usually started. The gas machine should be connected to scavenging through the wall suction pin-index before induction.
4. **Postanesthetic considerations**
   Once the catheter is placed, start waking up the patient, so the patient will be able to go to the bathroom to void. The age of the child is usually about 4 years.

DIMERCAPTOSUCCINIC ACID IMAGING

1. **Introduction**
   Nuclear medicine imaging can be done with dimercaptosuccinic acid (DMSA) to identify renal function, scarring, and pyelonephritis. This requires the patient to remain still. Anesthesia is used for pediatric patients unable to cooperate. The procedure can take 1 to 2 hours.

2. **Room preparation**
   a) Pediatric gas machine
   b) Intravenous medication tray
   c) Oxygen tank for transport optional
3. **Anesthetic considerations**
   a) Standard mask ventilation followed by intravenous insertion
   b) Start propofol infusion at 25 to 50 mcg/kg/min and adjust to maintain spontaneous breathing
   c) Oxygen per nasal cannula

VASCULAR SURGERY

A. Abdominal Aortic Aneurysm

1. Introduction

Surgical treatment of abdominal aortic aneurysm may be required for atherosclerotic occlusive disease or aneurysmal dilation. These processes can involve the aorta and any of its major branches, leading to ischemia or rupture and exsanguination. Elective surgery is indicated when the aneurysm diameter is greater than 5 cm; each centimeter greater than 5 cm increases the chances of rupture.

The primary event in aortic dissection is a tear in the intimal wall through which blood surges and creates a false lumen. The adventitia then separates up and/or down the aorta for various distances. Associated conditions include athlerosclerosis and hypertension (which is present in 80% of these patients), Marfan's syndrome, blunt chest trauma, pregnancy, and iatrogenic surgical injury (e.g., resulting from aortic cannulation during cardiopulmonary bypass).

Aortic dissections involving the ascending aorta are considered type A. Surgical repair is through a median sternotomy using profound hypothermia and total circulatory arrest or cardiopulmonary bypass with moderate hypothermia. Aortic dissections involving the descending aorta (i.e., beyond the origin of the left subclavian artery) are considered type B. Aneurysms can also be classified as saccular, fusiform, or dissecting. Surgical repair involves proximal and distal clamping of the aorta, opening of the aneurysm, evacuation of the thrombus, and placement of a synthetic graft. A midline transabdominal surgical approach or retroperitoneal left thoracoabdominal approach may be used.

The aorta is the main artery from the left ventricle of the heart. It supplies oxygenated blood to all tissues and organs of the body except the alveoli of the lung. The aorta is subdivided into the ascending aorta, the aortic arch, and the descending aorta, which has thoracic and abdominal portions. The abdominal aorta is the second portion of the descending aorta. It descends through the aortic hiatus of the diaphragm, enters the abdomino pelvic cavity, and travels down the ventral surface of the vertebral column. The abdominal aorta terminates at the fourth lumbar vertebra by dividing into the right and left common iliac arteries.

Signs and symptoms include the following: excruciating chest, abdominal, or back pain; a decrease or absence of peripheral pulses; a pulsatile abdominal mass; stroke, paraplegia, and ischemia of extremities; vasoconstriction and hypertension; myocardial infarction; and cardiac tamponade.

Early, short-term treatment includes the use of β-blockers or other cardioactive agents that decrease systolic blood pressure (to approximately

100 mm Hg) and aid in decreasing myocardial contractility and vascular resistance. Ultimately, surgical intervention is often necessary.

2. **Preoperative assessment**

   a) History and physical examination with a special focus on cardiac, renal, and central nervous system function are essential.

   b) Hypertension and diabetes mellitus may also be present. Preoperative analysis of important laboratory work should include hematology, chemistry, type and cross-match, and coagulation profiles. Serum glucose levels should be kept at less than 200 mg/dL.

   c) History and physical examination
      (1) Respiratory: Assess for pulmonary disease—chronic obstructive pulmonary disease, chronic bronchitis, asthma, and emphysema.
      (2) Cardiac: Evaluate for coronary artery disease, angina, hypertension, dysrhythmias, congestive heart failure, and left ventricular dysfunction.
      (3) Renal: Assess the baseline status because the kidneys may be affected with cross-clamping.
      (4) Neurologic
         (a) Spinal cord ischemia may occur with repair of the distal descending thoracic aorta.
         (b) Assess for transient ischemic attacks, strokes, and carotid bruits.
      (5) Endocrine: This patient population is prone to diabetes mellitus.
      (6) Other: Back or flank pain may indicate an expanding or leaking abdominal aortic aneurysm.

   d) Diagnostic tests
      (1) Chest radiography
      (2) Echocardiogram with ejection fraction
      (3) 12-lead electrocardiogram
      (4) Pulmonary function test with abnormal pulmonary histories
      (5) Angiograms: To estimate the difficulty of the procedure and the relationship of cross-clamping to the renal arteries
      (6) Laboratory tests: Complete blood count, electrolytes, glucose, blood urea nitrogen, creatinine, urinalysis, coagulation profile, type and cross-match, and others as indicated

3. **Perioperative medications and intravenous therapy**

   a) Antihypertensives: These are usually needed 24 to 48 hours before surgery.

   b) Antianginals: Nitrates, calcium channel blockers, and β-blockers are used; continue until the day of the procedure.

   c) Digoxin
      (1) Assess the serum level before the procedure.
      (2) Hypokalemia following intraoperative diuresis will increase the likelihood of digoxin toxicity.

   d) Antiarrhythmics: Continue until the day of surgery.

   e) Anticoagulants: Warfarin should be substituted with heparin preoperatively, allowing the patient's prothrombin time to normalize. Plan to hold heparin 4 hours before surgery.

   f) Bronchodilators: Continue until surgery.

   g) Administer antibiotics.

   h) Epidural catheter (for postoperative pain management): Perform a test dose on the awake patient. There is a remote risk of epidural hematoma formation from anticoagulation during surgery.

   i) Preoperative sedatives and narcotics
      (1) Use with caution in patients with poor respiratory reserve.

  (2) The onset of intravenous medications may be delayed because of low cardiac output.
  j) Two peripheral, large-bore (16- to 18-gauge) intravenous lines with variable fluid management are used.
4. **Room preparation**
  a) Monitoring equipment
    (1) Routine monitors should be employed including leads II and V_5 of the electrocardiogram.
    (2) A pulmonary artery catheter (when indicated) monitors cardiac function and the adequacy of fluid and blood replacement.
    (3) Arterial line
      (a) Use the right radial artery, or left radial artery, if the aneurysm involves the innominate artery.
      (b) Maintain mean arterial pressure close to 100 mm Hg in the upper body and greater than 50 mm Hg distal to the aneurysm.
    (4) Somatosensory-evoked potential or electroencephalogram evaluates central nervous system viability during aortic cross-clamping.
    (5) Transesophageal echocardiography monitors left ventricular function during cross-clamping.
    (6) Use a Foley catheter to monitor hourly urine output and assess global renal function.
    (7) Use warming modalities.
    (8) Electrocardiogram leads V_5 and II detect myocardial ischemia.
    (9) Use a Level 1 fluid warmer or similar device for complex cases (i.e., emergency aneurysm procedures).
  b) Pharmacologic agents
    (1) Prepare infusions of nitroglycerin, nitroprusside, phenylephrine, and dopamine.
    (2) Drugs: Use mannitol, fenoldopam, furosemide, sodium bicarbonate, heparin, protamine, and calcium.
    (3) Volume
      (a) Intravascular volume is depleted by hemorrhage, third-spacing into the bowel and peritoneal cavity, and insensible losses associated with a large abdominal incision.
      (b) The greatest blood loss occurs when the aneurysm is opened and the arteries are back-bleeding.
      (c) Crystalloids: Use if electrolytes, glucose, and osmolarity are within normal limits.
      (d) Colloids: Albumin, hetastarch (Hespan), and blood are used.
      (e) Maintain hematocrit in 30% range for oxygen-carrying capacity.
      (f) Autotransfusion: Blood is obtained from the operative field.
  c) Position: Supine
5. **Anesthetic goals**
  a) To minimize morbidity and mortality, the anesthetic goals are to preserve: myocardial (primary), renal, pulmonary, central nervous system, and visceral organ function.
  b) To meet these goals, one must ensure an adequate oxygen supply to the myocardium while reducing myocardial oxygen demand.
6. **Anesthetic technique**
  a) Regional blockade with general anesthesia or general anesthesia
    (1) The technique of choice is general anesthesia with endotracheal intubation because hemodynamic changes are significant.

(2) Regional block: Use epidural catheter placement and a test dose preoperatively, with analgesia to T4 to T5.

(3) With general anesthesia, an endotracheal tube is needed.

b) Induction

(1) Most intravenous induction agents are acceptable, provided they are used judiciously in conjunction with a nondepolarizing muscle relaxant.

(2) The goal is to establish a deep level of anesthesia using a slow, controlled titration of anesthetic agents before induction to minimize hemodynamic fluctuations.

(3) Positioning for surgery is usually supine or lateral, depending on the location of the incision (transabdominal or retroperitoneal approaches).

(4) If the patient is hypotensive with a rupturing abdominal aortic aneurysm, perform an awake intubation or rapid sequence induction with ketamine and succinylcholine.

(5) A slow, "controlled" induction is preferred with an opioid and a nondepolarizing muscle relaxant.

(6) Omit thiopental, propofol (Diprivan), and other cardiac depressors in the patient with poor left ventricular function.

(7) Anticipate exaggerated blood pressure changes; titrate drugs to maintain hemodynamics within 20% of baseline.

(8) Minimize pressor response during intubation of trachea by limiting the duration of laryngoscopy to less than 15 seconds.

c) Maintenance

(1) General anesthesia or a combined technique (i.e., general and epidural) has been used successfully.

(2) Selection of appropriate agents will depend on the patient's physical status.

(3) Use oxygen/air, opioid, and a volatile anesthetic.

(4) Cross-clamping of the thoracic aorta at the suprarenal or supraceliac level is not necessary for surgery.

(5) Maintain normothermia. Heat loss may be considerable.

d) Intravenous fluids

(1) Fluid volume deficits result from hemorrhage, insensible loss, and evaporative loss associated with large abdominal incisions.

(2) Surgically, an abdominal approach will typically require 10 to 15 mL/kg/hour of crystalloid (i.e., balanced salt solutions), and a retroperitoneal approach will require only 10 mL/kg/hour.

(3) Colloids may be necessary in volume-sensitive patients.

e) Aortic cross-clamping and unclamping

(1) Mannitol (25 g) and heparin (5000 to 10,000 units) are administered before cross-clamping.

(2) Activated coagulation times (ACT) are monitored (i.e., baseline before and then 5 minutes after heparin administration). The therapeutic goal is an ACT that is two to three times normal.

(3) Renal perfusion is at risk during cross-clamping and may lead to renal failure. Adequate fluid replacement is the major factor in preventing renal failure. Mannitol, furosemide (Lasix), dopamine, or fenoldopam given before cross-clamping may decrease renal injury. It is important to monitor the hemodynamic parameters and urine output.

(4) Hemodynamics

(a) Blood pressure is maintained slightly below normal before aortic cross-clamping.

(b) If the aorta is clamped below the renal arteries (infrarenal), elevations in afterload and blood pressure are minimal.

(c) If the aorta is clamped above the renal arteries (suprarenal), a greater increase in afterload and blood pressure will be observed.

(d) Should the aorta be clamped above the supraceliac artery, an even greater increase in afterload and blood pressure can be expected.

(e) Systemic blood pressure should be maintained 10 to 15 mm Hg above normal during aortic cross-clamping.

(f) Have vasodilating drugs available (nitroglycerin or nitroprusside) before aortic cross-clamping in anticipation of hypertension.

(5) Blood loss

(a) Surgical blood loss may be replaced with crystalloids, colloids, autologous blood, or packed red blood cells.

(b) Administration of fresh-frozen plasma and platelets depends on coagulation values and the number of packed red blood cells transfused.

(6) Cross-clamp time

(a) Cross-clamp time is usually minimized to 30 to 60 minutes.

(b) Before unclamping, give fluids to increase central venous pressure to more than 5 mm Hg above baseline. This helps to ensure cardiovascular stability, maintenance of blood pressure, and renal preservation.

(7) Unclamping

(a) Anticipate a drop in afterload, preload, and blood pressure following removal of the aortic cross-clamp.

(b) Lighten the depth of anesthesia before unclamping, and allow the blood pressure to climb 30 to 40 mm Hg.

(c) Be prepared to transfuse 1 unit of blood.

(d) Should systemic blood pressure drop precipitously, the surgeon may reclamp until acceptable blood pressure is restored. Release of the clamp one limb at a time may also help with hemodynamic stability.

(e) Use vasopressors as necessary.

(f) As circulation to the lower extremities begins, a negative inotropic effect may be seen because of a washout of anerobic products and systemic acidosis. This response is dependent on the duration of cross-clamp time and the amount of collateral circulation.

f) Emergence

(1) Consider the patient's preoperative physical status, the amount of intraoperative fluid administered, blood loss, the length of procedure, and the presence or absence of any untoward intraoperative events. The patient may require postoperative ventilation for a period of time to limit wide swings in hemodynamic parameters.

(2) Unless the patient's condition is stable, do not reverse muscle relaxants or try to awaken the patient.

(3) Consider initiating regional block through the epidural catheter for postoperative analgesia.

7. Postoperative implications

a) Consider ventilatory support for several hours or overnight.

b) Potential complications include myocardial ischemia/infarction, bleeding, infection, renal failure, peripheral vascular insufficiency, stroke, intestinal ischemia/infarction, paraplegia/monoparesis, fluid shifts, electrolyte imbalance, coagulopathies, and ischemia distal to the site of repair (visceral or spinal cord).

8. **Aortic stent placement**
   a) This is a minimally invasive procedure for repairing abdominal aortic aneurysms. It uses a stent graft (a Dacron tube inside a collapsed metal-mesh cylinder) that is threaded through the arteries, using fluoroscopy, to the site of the aneurysm.
   b) Preoperative assessment: This is the same as for open repair of abdominal aortic aneurysm.
   c) The procedure is performed with the patient under spinal or epidural anesthesia with intravenous sedation.
   d) A central line or pulmonary artery catheter is placed if the patient's history or condition warrants it. Radial arterial and intravenous lines are placed in the right arm, which may be tucked at the patient's side. The left arm and both sides of the groin are used for surgical access.
   e) Intraoperative medications: Heparin will be given, and ACTs should be checked every half hour to maintain level. Mannitol infusion will be used. Infusions of nitroglycerin, phenylephrine, and dopamine should be prepared. Protamine will be used to reverse heparin at the end of the case.
   f) Additional considerations: Keep the patient warm throughout the procedure. Pulmonary artery pressure usually becomes elevated with stent placement.

9. **Emergency aortic abdominal aneurysm surgery**
   a) Signs and symptoms include back pain, syncope, vomiting, and severe hypotension.
   b) Primary goals of emergency surgery are rapid control of blood loss and reversal of hypotension, and the secondary goal is the preservation of myocardial function.
   c) Emergency, stable patients should proceed quickly through the preoperative area. Rapid sequence intubation following preoxygenation should be performed with hypnotic agents, opioids, and muscle relaxants.
   d) Emergency, unstable patients require rapid intravascular volume replacement. Massive blood loss and hypotension can lead to myocardial infarction, acute renal failure, respiratory failure, or mortality in 40% to 50% of patients. Rapid surgical control of the bleeding is the first priority, and placement of invasive monitors should not delay this definitive treatment.

B. Aortobifemoral Bypass Grafting

1. **Introduction**
   Aortobifemoral bypass grafting is commonly performed to correct symptomatic unilateral iliac occlusive disease, which generally occurs in men older than 55 years.

2. **Preoperative assessment and patient preparation**
   a) History and physical examination
      (1) Cardiovascular: 30% to 50% of patients have coexisting coronary artery disease. Other common risk factors are myocardial infarction,

hypertension, angina, valvular disease, congestive heart failure, and arrhythmias.

(2) Respiratory: Most patients have a significant history of smoking and possibly chronic obstructive pulmonary disease.

(3) Neurologic: Check for coexisting cerebrovascular disease.

(4) Renal: Chronic renal insufficiency is common.

(5) Endocrine: Many patients have diabetes and its associated complications.

b) Patient preparation

(1) Laboratory tests: Complete blood count, prothrombin time, partial thromboplastin time, bleeding time, electrolytes, blood urea nitrogen, creatinine, creatinine clearance, and urinalysis are obtained.

(2) Diagnostic tests: 12-lead electrocardiography, pulmonary function tests, arterial blood gases, chest radiography, magnetic resonance imaging, computed tomography, and arteriography are obtained.

(3) Preoperative medications: Knowledge of daily medications is essential. Cardiac medications are continued, and anticoagulant therapy is sometimes held for 4 hours before surgery. Anxiolytics, sedatives, and analgesics are used as indicated.

(4) Intravenous therapy: Have a central line, with two 14- to 16-gauge intravenous lines. The estimated blood loss is 500 mL.

3. Room preparation

a) Monitoring equipment: Standard with arterial line and central venous pressure catheter, pulmonary arterial catheter, or both. ST segment analysis and transesophageal echocardiography are beneficial.

b) Additional equipment: This includes a fluid warmer; consider a cell saver.

c) Drugs

(1) Miscellaneous pharmacologic agents: Osmotic and loop diuretics, local anesthetics, antibiotics, adrenergic antagonists, inotropic agents, vasodilators/constrictors, and heparin are used.

(2) Intravenous fluids: Calculate for major blood loss. Consider rapid infusion of crystalloids, colloids, or both to treat hypovolemic states.

(3) Blood: Type and cross-match for 4 units of packed red blood cells.

(4) Tabletop: This is standard.

4. Anesthetic technique

General anesthesia, epidural anesthesia, or a combination of general and regional anesthesia is used.

5. Perioperative management

a) Induction: Use smooth induction to preserve cerebral perfusion and to maintain hemodynamic stability. For general anesthesia, consider etomidate, fentanyl, lidocaine, and muscle relaxants to decrease episodes of tachycardia and hypotension. For regional anesthesia, consider placing an epidural catheter before beginning anticoagulation.

b) Maintenance: For general anesthesia, consider oxygen/air, volatile agent/narcotic. For regional anesthesia, use local anesthetic/narcotic/anxiolytic. Maintain blood pressure within the high-normal range.

c) Emergence: Maintain hemodynamic stability; prevent hypertension and tachycardia. For general anesthesia, use full reversal of muscle relaxants and smooth extubation.

6. Postoperative implications

Complications include hemodynamic instability, myocardial ischemia, hemorrhage, respiratory failure, renal failure, and neurologic changes.

C. Carotid Endarterectomy

1. Introduction

Surgical excision of fibrous atherosclerotic plaque at or near the bifurcation of the common carotid artery (carotid endarterectomy) is performed for the treatment of transient ischemic attacks. It is reserved for patients with lesions of greater than 80% blockage in the carotid artery. Cerebral angiography is used to determine the location and severity of stenosis. The operative mortality rate is 1% to 2% and results from myocardial infarction; the operative morbidity rate is 4% to 10% and results from stroke.

2. Preoperative assessment and patient preparation

a) History and physical examination
   (1) Cardiac: Assess normal range of blood pressure and heart rate and note asymmetries in blood pressure between arms. Obtain a detailed history of cardiovascular function.
   (2) Neurologic: Assess and document preexisting neurologic deficits to distinguish new deficits.
   (3) Respiratory: Obtain preoperative blood gases if pulmonary disease is suspected. Preoperative arterial carbon dioxide pressure dictates this value during anesthesia.

b) General: Optimal control of hypertension, diabetes, chronic obstructive pulmonary disease, and chronic renal failure is imperative before surgery.

c) Diagnostic tests: Electrocardiogram, complete blood count, blood urea nitrogen, blood sugar, chest radiography, creatinine, electrolytes, type and cross-match, arterial blood gases, other cardiac tests are obtained as needed according to the history.

d) Preoperative medication and intravenous therapy
   (1) Continue all cardiac medications until the time of surgery.
   (2) Two 16- to 18-gauge intravenous lines with moderate fluid replacement are used.
   (3) Premedication is minimal.

3. Room preparation

a) Monitoring equipment
   (1) Equipment is standard, with an arterial line and an electrocardiogram with lead II/V_5 and ST-segment monitoring
   (2) Hemodynamic monitoring is performed.
   (3) Electroencephalogram, somatosensory-evoked potential, and carotid stump pressure monitoring may be used to assess cerebral ischemia.

b) Pharmacologic agents: A standard tabletop setup is used with ephedrine, phenylephrine, esmolol, nitroglycerin, labetalol, heparin, and protamine available.

c) Position: Supine; the patient's arms may be tucked at the sides. A roll may be placed under the shoulder blades to extend the neck. The head may be placed on a doughnut. Determine whether the table will be turned, and attach monitors accordingly.

4. Anesthetic technique

a) Regional block or general anesthesia
b) Regional block: Cervical plexus block at the transverse process of C3 to C4 and along the inferior border of the sternocleidomastoid

muscle offers the advantage of an awake patient, thus allowing for continuous neurologic monitoring.

c) General anesthesia: This allows for control of ventilation, oxygenation, and lack of patient movement. General anesthetics protect the brain by depressing the level of cerebral metabolism and the cerebral metabolic rate of oxygen.

5. **Perioperative management**
   a) Induction
      (1) A slow, controlled induction is preferred with an opioid and non-depolarizing muscle relaxant.
      (2) Anticipate exaggerated blood pressure changes with induction. Adequate hydration is imperative. Use of lidocaine and esmolol will attenuate the response to laryngoscopy.
   b) Maintenance
      (1) Maintain arterial blood pressure in the patient's normal range.
      (2) Before cross-clamping, increase blood pressure by 20 to 30 mm Hg. The patient may need a vasoactive agent (i.e., phenylephrine [Neo-Synephrine]).
      (3) Document the cross-clamping time.
      (4) If a shunt is used, document shunt insertion and removal.
      (5) Maintain arterial carbon dioxide pressure in the patient's normal range.
      (6) If the surgeon stretches the baroreceptor nerve endings, ask the surgeon to inject the area of bifurcation with 1% lidocaine 10 to 15 minutes before carotid artery occlusion.
   c) Emergence
      (1) Smooth emergence is important; use lidocaine to blunt reflexes.
      (2) The patient needs to be awake at the end of the procedure so the surgeon can assess for neurologic deficits.

6. **Postoperative considerations**
   Hypertension is common. Other complications include carotid body damage, hemorrhage with compromise of the airway, myocardial infarction, stroke, and dysfunction of cranial nerves VII, IX, X, and XII.

D. Peripheral Vascular Procedures

1. **Introduction**
   Peripheral vascular procedures include femoral-femoral, femoral-popliteal, femoral-tibial, ileofemoral, axillofemoral, and embolectomies. Obstruction most often is in the superficial femoral artery, followed by common iliac claudication in the gastrocnemius muscle, whereas pain and ischemic ulceration/gangrene occur with severe occlusion.

   Procedures are classified as inflow or outflow vascular reconstruction. The inflow reconstruction procedures bypass the obstruction in the aortoiliac segment (aortoiliac endarterectomy or aortofemoral bypass). These are more stressful procedures requiring cross-clamping of the aorta. Outflow procedures are performed distal to the inguinal ligament to bypass the femoropopliteal or distal obstruction.

Clamping Stage	Goals	Drug to Prepare
Preclamping	Maintain blood pressure 20% baseline (low normal)	Volatile anesthetic Nitroglycerin, nitroprusside (Nipride) If pulmonary capillary wedge pressure is increased and cardiac output is decreased, inotropic support (dopamine, epinephrine) may be needed
	Maximize urinary output	Mannitol, furosemide (Lasix)
	Minimize fluids	Monitor crystalloid administration
	Prevent thrombosis	Heparin—monitor activated clotting times
Cross-clamping	Prevent myocardial infarction	Decrease afterload (nitroglycerin and nitroprusside) Monitor electrocardiogram for ischemia Monitor the cardiac output and expect a decline
	Maintain oxygenation	Oxygen/air or 100% oxygen Monitor oxygen saturation and arterial blood gases
	Maintain urinary output (0.5 mL/kg/hr)	Anuria is rare Dopamine (1 to 5 mcg/kg)
Prerelease	Prevent myocardial infarction from declamping, hypotension	Monitor electrocardiogram Ask surgeon for a 10-min warning before aortic clamp is removed Lighten anesthesia depth Discontinue vasodilating agents (nitroglycerin and nitroprusside) Increase central venous pressure and pulmonary capillary wedge pressure 4 to 6 mm Hg with fluids (and blood if needed) Have vasopressors ready
Postrelease	Maintain blood pressure and vital signs	Use vasopressors (dopamine, epinephrine, phenylephrine).
	Correct acidoses	Mechanical ventilation Bicarbonate administration (pH: <7.25) Calcium chloride administration
	Correct coagulation profile	Protamine
	Maintain urine output	Volume: crystalloids and colloids, dopamine

2. **Preoperative assessment**
   a) History and physical examination
      (1) See the discussion of abdominal aortic aneurysm earlier in this section.
      (2) Musculoskeletal: This includes decreased or absent popliteal and pedal pulses, delayed capillary refill, blanching on elevation of the leg followed by dependent edema after lowering it, and pain with walking relieved by rest.
   b) Diagnostic tests
      (1) See the discussion of abdominal aortic aneurysm earlier in this section.
      (2) Doppler studies
         (a) Determinations of systolic blood pressure at the level of the ankle are compared with brachial determinations.
         (b) Assess the severity of ischemia, urgency of revascularization, and baseline values for evaluation of operative results.
      (3) Angiography: Determine the precise site of the actual lesion.
   c) Preoperative medications and intravenous therapy
      (1) For elderly patients with coexisting medical disease requiring pharmacologic support (i.e., antihypertensives, antianginals, antiarrhythmics, digoxin), these medications may be continued up to the day of the operation.
      (2) Sedatives and narcotics are used.
         (a) Use with caution in patients with poor respiratory reserve.
         (b) The onset of intravenous medications may be delayed because of potentially low cardiac output.
      (3) Two peripheral large-bore (16- to 18-gauge) intravenous lines with moderate fluid management are used.
      (4) Epidural catheter: Test the dose on the awake patient; there is a risk of epidural hematoma from anticoagulation during surgery.
3. **Room preparation**
   a) Monitoring equipment
      (1) Electrocardiogram leads V_5 and II to detect myocardial ischemia and diagnose tachyarrhythmias
      (2) Warming modalities
      (3) Foley catheter
      (4) Arterial line and central venous pressure monitoring possibly necessary
   b) Pharmacologic agents
      (1) Have nitroglycerin, nitroprusside drugs within quick access.
      (2) Drugs include vasopressors, heparin, and β-blockers.
      (3) One may be asked to administer dextran solution.
   c) Position: Supine
4. **Anesthetic technique**
   a) Regional block, general anesthesia, or a combination. The technique of choice is regional anesthesia; it avoids airway problems and sequelae, provides greater hemodynamic stability with coexisting diseases, provides sympathetic block that increases circulation in the lower extremity, reduces the incidence of intravascular clotting, facilitates postoperative pain relief, suppresses the endocrine stress response, and decreases blood loss in selected cases.
   b) Regional block: Analgesia to T10; epidural or spinal
      (1) The elderly population is more sensitive to local anesthetics; reduce the dose by 50%.
      (2) Some practitioners administer ephedrine prophylactically to prevent hypotension.

      (3) The level is slightly above the skin dermatome necessary for the usual incisions (T12), but sympathetic innervation of lower extremities, which contains visceral afferent fibers, is believed to occur at T10 to L2.

5. Perioperative management

  a) Induction

    (1) General anesthesia

      (a) The goals are a smooth transition from awake state to surgical anesthesia and the maintenance of cardiovascular stability.

      (b) A slow "controlled" induction is preferred with an opioid and nondepolarizing muscle relaxant.

      (c) Muscle relaxation may be chosen on the basis of cardiovascular effect.

        i) Pancuronium: If the heart rate is slowed during induction

        ii) Vecuronium: If the heart rate is in the desired range

      (d) The onset of drugs may be delayed with low cardiac output.

      (e) Omit thiopental and other cardiac depressors in patients with poor left ventricular function.

      (f) Anticipate exaggerated blood pressure changes; maintain within 20% of baseline.

      (g) Minimize pressor response during intubation of trachea by limiting duration of laryngoscopy to less than 15 seconds.

    (2) Regional anesthesia

      (a) Review the principles of sympathetic block.

      (b) Consider administering block with the operative side down so that the onset of sympathetic and sensory blockade is faster on the dependent site. Theoretically, the level will be higher on the dependent side. The total volume of anesthetic requirements may be decreased.

  b) Maintenance

    (1) The surgeon will ask that heparin be administered by intravenous push; ensure the patency of the port before injection.

    (2) One may perform intraoperative angiography.

      (a) Allergic reactions may occur with dye.

      (b) The degree of surgical stimulation changes; blood pressure decreases when surgical activity stops in preparation for angiography. Blood pressure and heart rate may increase when dye is injected.

      (c) Repeat injection of contrast dye during multiple attempts at angiography may cause osmotic diuresis.

    (3) Hyperkalemia and acidosis resulting from ischemic extremities are possible, and myoglobin can be released into the circulation.

    (4) Maintain the hematocrit at more than 30 to maximize oxygen-carrying capacity; do not give too many red cells or too few crystalloids because can see an increase in blood viscosity and the possibility of graft thrombosis.

    (5) Unclamping of femoral artery rarely affects hemodynamics significantly. The lower extremity receives arterial blood through collateral vessels even when the femoral artery is occluded.

    (6) Regional anesthesia

      (a) Attention to patient comfort is important.

      (b) Sedation is aimed at reducing patient anxiety without producing respiratory depression or unresponsiveness.

c) Emergence
  (1) Initiate regional block through the epidural catheter for postoperative analgesia before the end of the case.
  (2) Base extubation on the patient's general health, amount of blood loss, and overall status after the procedure.

6. **Postoperative implications**
  a) Obtain hemoglobin and hematocrit values.
  b) Assess the musculoskeletal status of the operative extremity.

E. Portosystemic Shunts

1. **Introduction**
   Portosystemic shunt procedures are performed to prevent or cease variceal hemorrhage resulting from portal hypertension in patients with liver disease, cirrhosis, ascites, and hypersplenism. The redistribution of blood from the portal vein to the inferior vena cava causes variations in flow and resistance of the liver, intestine, and spleen. This hemodynamic alteration aids portal perfusion and oxygenation with net effects of increased venous return and cardiac output. Variations in procedures include portacaval, end-to-end, end-to-side, mesocaval, mesorenal, and splenorenal shunts.

2. **Preoperative assessment and patient preparation**
   a) History and physical examination
   (1) Cardiac: Associated disorders include increased heart rate, circulating blood volume, and intrathoracic pressure. Variations of cardiac output, cardiomyopathy, congestive heart failure, coronary artery disease, and decreased response to catecholamines and systemic vascular resistance may be present.
   (2) Respiratory: Hypoxemia may be related to ventilation-perfusion mismatch, increased closing volume, decreased functional residual capacity, atelectasis, right-to-left pulmonary shunting, increased disphosphoglycerate, pulmonary infections, and impaired hypoxic pulmonary vasoconstriction.
   (3) Neurologic: Manifestations may include hepatic encephalopathy with associated confusion and obtundation.
   (4) Renal: Renal impairment and failure with electrolyte imbalance are frequently observed.
   (5) Gastrointestinal: Gastric or esophageal varices with gastrointestinal bleeding are common.
   (6) Endocrine: Abnormal glucose utilization, increased growth hormone, intolerance to carbohydrates, and irregular sex hormone metabolism may be observed.
   b) Patient preparation
   (1) Laboratory tests: Arterial blood gases, complete blood count, prothrombin time, partial thromboplastin time, bleeding time, electrolytes, blood urea nitrogen, creatinine, creatinine clearance, urinalysis, diffuse intravascular coagulation profile, albumin, bilirubin, serum glutamic-oxaloacetic transaminase, serum glutamic-pyruvic transaminase, ammonia, alkaline phosphatase, and lactate are obtained.
   (2) Diagnostic tests: Electrocardiography, echocardiography, pulmonary function tests, and chest radiography are obtained.

    (3) Preoperative medications: Avoid intramuscular injections. Anxiolytics are administered in small doses as indicated. Consider metoclopramide (10 mg) and ranitidine (50 mg).

    (4) Intravenous therapy: This involves a central line and two 14- to 16-gauge intravenous lines. Consider a pulmonary arterial catheter.

3. Room preparation

a) Monitoring equipment: Standard with arterial line, central venous pressure catheter, and urinary catheter

b) Additional equipment: Fluid warmer, cell saver, Bair Hugger, and rapid infuser

c) Drugs

    (1) Miscellaneous pharmacologic agents: Opioid (fentanyl), midazolam, vasodilators and vasoconstrictors, inotropes, nondepolarizing muscle relaxants, and antibiotics are used.

    (2) Intravenous fluids: Calculate for major blood loss. Estimated blood loss is 1000 to 2000 mL.

    (3) Blood: Type and cross-match for 8 to 10 units of packed red blood cells, platelets, fresh-frozen plasma, and cryoprecipitate.

    (4) Tabletop: This is standard.

4. Anesthetic technique

General anesthesia, epidural anesthesia, or a combination of general and regional anesthesia is used.

5. Perioperative management and anesthetic technique

a) General anesthetic is the technique of choice.

b) Induction: Use rapid sequence induction with thiopental (3 to 5 mg/kg) and succinylcholine (1 to 2 mg/kg). Consider etomidate (0.2 mg/kg) or ketamine (1 mg/kg).

c) Maintenance: Inhalational agent/oxygen/fentanyl/midazolam and nondepolarizing muscle relaxant. Position is supine.

d) Emergence: The patient generally is transported to the intensive care unit.

6. Postoperative implications

a) Complications: Coagulopathy, renal failure, hypothermia, encephalopathy, jaundice, and anemia

b) Postoperative pain management: patient-controlled analgesia.

F. Thoracic Aortic Aneurysm

1. Introduction

Aneurysms that affect the thoracic aorta include ascending and arch defects (60% to 70%) or descending lesions (30%). These dissections are sometimes classified (Crawford) into the segments and arteries that are involved (types 1 to 4). Surgery is performed to prevent rupture, to repair leaking or expansion of the aneurysm, and possibly for acute or chronic dissections. Diseases of the thoracic aorta may be associated with atherosclerosis, connective tissue disorders (Marfan's syndrome), congenital abnormalities, trauma, infection (syphilis), hypertension, and inflammatory processes. Ascending aortic aneurysms typically require a median sternotomy approach with cardiopulmonary bypass. Transverse aortic aneurysms typically require hypothermic circulatory arrest.

2. **Preoperative assessment and patient preparation**
   a) History and physical examination
      (1) Cardiac: Coexisting disorders may include hypertension (70% to 90% of patients), angina, coronary artery disease, congestive heart failure, myocardial ischemia, and peripheral vascular disease.
      (2) Respiratory: Manifestations may include hemoptysis, stridor, dyspnea, pleural effusion, tracheal deviation producing difficulties with intubation and ventilation, and recurrent laryngeal nerve damage resulting in vocal cord paralysis and hoarseness.
      (3) Neurologic: Perform a complete neurologic examination because of the high incidence of spinal cord ischemia.
      (4) Renal: The kidneys may be affected secondary to coexisting diseases.
      (5) Gastrointestinal: Bowel ischemia has been associated with descending aneurysms.
   b) Patient preparation
      (1) Laboratory tests: Complete blood count, electrolytes, blood urea. nitrogen, creatinine, prothrombin time, partial thromboplastin time, urinalysis, arterial blood gases, and type and cross-match
      (2) Diagnostic tests: Electrocardiography, echocardiography, Doppler, magnetic resonance imaging, and chest and abdominal radiography
      (3) Preoperative medications: Anxiolytics and analgesics as indicated
      (4) Intravenous therapy: Central line, two 14- to 16-gauge intravenous lines; possibly a pulmonary arterial catheter

3. **Room preparation**
   a) Monitoring equipment: Standard with right arterial line (or left radial artery if aneurysm involves the innominate artery), pulmonary arterial catheter, and Foley catheter
   b) Additional equipment: Fluid warmers, cardiopulmonary bypass, cell saver, and transesophageal echocardiography; possibly also a difficult-airway cart in patients with tracheal deviation
   c) Drugs
      (1) Miscellaneous pharmacologic agents: Heparin, diuretics (furosemide, mannitol, dopamine, or fenoldopam), vasodilators (nitroglycerin or nitroprusside), vasoconstrictors (phenylephrine), inotropes, adrenergic antagonists, opioids, nondepolarizing muscle relaxant, and antibiotics are used.
      (2) Intravenous fluids: Calculate for major blood loss. Use crystalloids at 6 to 8 mL/kg per hour. The estimated blood loss is 1000 mL or greater.
      (3) Blood: Type and cross-match for 8 to 10 units of packed red blood cells.
   d) Position: Supine, or right lateral decubitus if a thoracotomy approach is used

4. **Perioperative management and anesthetic technique**
   Anesthetic technique is general anesthesia with an oral endotracheal tube or an ET or double-lumen tube for thoracotomy approach.
   a) Induction: Smooth induction to maintain hemodynamic stability can be accomplished with etomidate (0.1 to 0.3 mg/kg) or thiopental (4 to 6 mg/kg), high-dose fentanyl (20 to 100 mcg/kg) or sufentanil (5 to 20 mcg/kg), pretreatment with lidocaine (1.5 mg/kg), and vecuronium (0.1 mg/kg). Consider midazolam (50 to 350 mcg/kg) and esmolol as indicated.

b) Maintenance: Maintain the mean arterial pressure at 60 to 80 mm Hg and urinary output at 0.5 to 1 mL/kg per hour. Inhalational agent/oxygen/narcotic anesthesia is used. The aorta is cross-clamped for 25 to 120 minutes, and cardiopulmonary bypass may be instituted for 30 to 150 minutes. The position is supine or lateral decubitus.

c) Emergence: The patient is transported to an intensive care unit intubated and remains ventilated for 24 to 48 hours. If a double-lumen tube is used, replace with a standard endotracheal tube before transfer.

5. **Postoperative implications**

a) Spinal cord ischemia (paralysis): Cross-clamping of the aorta may compromise flow through the artery of Adamkiewicz (found between T8 and T12). Techniques for prevention of ischemia include the following: hypothermia, lowering of cerebrospinal fluid pressure using a lumbar spinal catheter, intrathecal magnesium, cardiopulmonary bypass, and deep hypothermic circulatory arrest.

b) Renal failure: This occurs in up to 25% of cases and corresponds with increased cross-clamp times. Techniques for prevention include mannitol (25 g) before cross-clamp, maintenance of circulating volume, furosemide, dopamine, and fenoldopam, and meticulous monitoring of urine output.

c) Other complications include cardiac, respiratory, hemorrhage, hypertension, coagulopathy, myocardial ischemia, and arrhythmias.

ADENOSINE (ADENOCARD)

Classification
Antiarrhythmic

Indications
Supraventricular tachycardia

Dose
6-mg bolus given over 1 to 2 seconds followed by normal saline line flush; may increase to 12-mg bolus if arrhythmia persists past 2 minutes. May repeat 12-mg bolus once. How supplied: 3 mg/mL 2- and 5-mL vials.

Onset and duration
Onset: 10 to 20 seconds. Duration: 1 minute.

Adverse effects
Flushing, dyspnea, chest pain, headache, nausea, cough, malaise

Precautions and contraindications
Adenosine should not be used in patients receiving methylxanthine therapy (i.e., aminophylline, theophylline). Dipyridamole (Persantine) inhibits cellular uptake of adenosine. Use it with caution in patients with asthma. It is contraindicated in patients with second- or third-degree heart block.

Anesthetic considerations
This is an agent for use preoperatively and postoperatively. It is not used under anesthesia because it produces sinus arrest. It may be given in lieu of or preceding administration of calcium channel blockers for long-term suppression.

ALBUTEROL SULFATE (PROVENTIL, VENTOLIN)

Classification
β_2-adrenergic agonist, sympathomimetic, bronchodilator

Indications
Treatment of asthma and other forms of bronchospasm

Dose

Inhaler (metered dose): two deep inhalations 1 to 5 minutes apart; may be repeated every 4 to 6 hours (daily dose should not exceed 16 to 20 inhalations. Each metered aerosol actuation delivers approximately 90 mcg/puff); oral: 2 to 4 mg three to four times daily (total dose not to exceed 16 mg); syrup: 2 mg/5 mL is available.

Onset and duration

Onset: inhalation: 5 to 15 minutes; oral: 15 to 30 minutes. Peak effect: inhalation: 0.5 to 2 hours; oral: 2 to 3 hours. Duration: inhalation: 3 to 6 hours; oral: 4 to 8 hours.

Adverse effects

Tachycardia, arrhythmias, hypertension, tremors, anxiety, headache, nausea, vomiting, hypokalemia

Precautions and contraindications

Safe use is not established during pregnancy. Use albuterol cautiously in patients with cardiovascular disease, hypertension, and hyperthyroidism. Monitor glucose and electrolyte levels.

Anesthetic considerations

Tolerance/tachyphylaxis can develop with long-term use. It has additive effects with epinephrine and other sympathomimetics. It is antagonized by β-receptor antagonists.

ALFENTANIL HCL (ALFENTA)

Classification

Opioid agonist; produces analgesia and anesthesia

Indications

Perioperative analgesia

Dose

Induction: intravenous: 50 to 150 mcg/kg; infusion: 0.1 to 3 mcg/kg/min.

Onset and duration

Onset: intravenous: 1 to 2 minutes; intramuscular: less than 5 minutes; epidural: 5 to 15 minutes. Duration: intravenous: 1 to 15 minutes; intramuscular: 10 to 60 minutes; epidural: 30 minutes.

Adverse effects

Bradycardia, hypotension, arrhythmias, respiratory depression; euphoria, dysphoria, convulsions, nausea and vomiting, biliary tract spasm, delayed gastric emptying, muscle rigidity, pruritus

Precautions and contraindications

Reduce the alfentanil dose in elderly, hypovolemic, high-risk surgical patients and with the concomitant use of sedatives and other narcotics. It crosses the placental barrier, and use in labor may produce depression of respiration in the neonate. Resuscitation may be required; have naloxone available.

Anesthetic considerations

Circulatory and ventilatory depressant effects are potentiated by narcotics, sedatives, volatile anesthetics, nitrous oxide. Analgesia is enhanced by α_2-agonists. Muscle rigidity in the higher dose range can be sufficient to interfere with ventilation.

ALPROSTADIL, PGE₁ (PROSTIN VR)

Classification

Prostaglandin E

Indications

Neonates: to maintain temporary patency of the ductus arteriosus until corrective or palliative surgery can be performed

Dose

Children: Continuous infusion into large vein: 0.05 to 0.1 mcg/kg/min initially; when a therapeutic response occurs, decrease to lowest possible dose to maintain response (maximum dose: 0.4 mcg/kg/min).

Dosage forms: 500 mcg/mL 1-mL ampules (refrigerate at 2 to 8° C. Must be diluted in 5% dextrose in water (D_5W) or normal saline for continuous infusion to a final concentration of 5 to 20 mcg/mL.

Onset and duration

Onset: 30 minutes. Elimination half-life: 5 to 10 minutes. Duration: 30 minutes to 2 hours.

Adverse effects

Apnea (10% to 12%), fever (14%), flushing (10%), bradycardia and seizures (4%), thrombocytopenia (less than 1%), disseminated intravascular coagulation (1%), anemia, tachycardia, hypotension (4%), diarrhea (2%), gastric outlet obstruction secondary to antral hyperplasia (related to cumulative dose)

Precautions and contraindications

Apnea is most frequent in infants under 2 kg within the first hour of alprostadil administration; ventilatory assistance may be required. It is contraindicated in neonates with respiratory distress syndrome. Use it with caution in patients with bleeding tendencies because of alprostadil's ability to inhibit platelet aggregation. In all neonates, monitor arterial pressure; should arterial pressure fall significantly, decrease the rate of infusion.

AMINOCAPROIC ACID (AMICAR)

Classification

Hemostatic agent; prevents the conversion of plasminogen to plasmin

Indications

Control of clinical bleeding in which hyperfibrinolysis is a contributing factor (hyperfibrinolysis should be confirmed by laboratory values such as prolonged thrombin time, prolonged prothrombin time, hypofibrinogenemia, or decreased plasminogen levels); also: open heart surgery; postoperative hematuria following transurethral prostatic resection, suprapubic prostatectomy, and nephrectomy; hematologic disorders such as aplastic anemia, abruptio placentae, cirrhosis, neoplastic diseases, and prophylaxis in patients with hemophilia before and after tooth extraction and other bleeding in the mouth and nasopharynx; reduction of blood loss in trauma and shock; possible prevention of ocular hemorrhaging and bleeding in subarachnoid hemorrhage

Dose

Acute bleeding: 5 g infused during the first hour, followed by a continuous infusion of 1 g/hour for 8 hours or until bleeding is controlled.

Chronic bleeding: 5 g preoperatively by intravenous piggyback over 1 hour, then 5 g by intravenous piggyback every 6 hours. Do not exceed 30 g in 24 hours. Decrease dose by 15% to 25% in patients with renal disease.

Children: 100 mg/kg intravenous piggyback over 1 hour, then 30 mg/kg/hour until bleeding is controlled (maximum dose: 18 g/m^2 in 24 hours).

Dosage forms: 250 mg/mL 20 mL parenteral vial (5 g).

Administration: Dilute each dose in a proper volume of D$_5$W normal saline or lactated Ringer's solution.

Onset and duration

Onset: 1 to 72 hours; half-life 1 to 2 hours in patients with normal renal function. No single concentration fits all. It must be diluted. Consult the package insert, an intravenous reference, or the pharmacy. Duration: 8 to 12 hours.

Adverse effects

Convulsions, myopathy, rarely muscle necrosis, nausea, vomiting; rapid infusion associated with hypotension, bradycardia, arrhythmias

Precautions and contraindications

A definitive diagnosis of hyperfibrinolysis must be made before aminocaproic acid administration. Use caution in patients with cardiac, renal, or hepatic disease. Administration in the presence of renal or ureteral bleeding is not recommended because of ureteral clot formation and the possible risk of obstruction. Owing to the substantial risk of serious or fatal thrombus formation, aminocaproic acid is contraindicated in patients with disseminated intravascular coagulation unless heparin is given concurrently.

Anesthetic considerations

Do not administer without a definite diagnosis of laboratory findings indicative of hyperfibrinolysis.

AMINOPHYLLINE (THEODUL, OTHERS)

Classification

Bronchodilator

Indications

Long-term therapy for bronchial asthma; reversal of bronchospasm associated with chronic obstructive pulmonary disease

Dose

Loading dose: For patients not already receiving a theophylline preparation, intravenous: 5 to 6 mg/kg (given over 20 to 30 minutes); or oral/rectal: 6 mg/kg. Maintenance: intravenous: 0.5 mg/kg/hour; oral: 2 to 4 mg/kg every 6 to 12 hours. Therapeutic range: 10 to 20 mcg/mL.

Dosage forms: injection: 25 mg/mL; tablets: 100, 200 mg; tablets (sustained release): 225 mg; oral solution: 105 mg/5 mL; rectal solution: 60 mg/mL (rectal solution not marketed in the United States); rectal suppositories: 250, 500 mg.

Dilution for infusion loading dose: dilute 500 mg in 500 mL D_5W or normal saline (1 mg/mL).

Children 9 to 16 years: 1 mg/kg/hour for 12 hours, then 0.8 mg/kg/hour. Children 6 months to 9 years: 1.2 mg/kg/hour for 12 hours, then 1 mg/kg/hour.

Onset and duration

Onset: intravenous: 2 to 5 minutes; oral: within 30 minutes. Duration: oral: 4 to 8 hours.

Adverse effects

Palpitations, sinus tachycardia, supraventricular and ventricular tachycardia, flushing, tachypnea, seizures, headache, irritability, nausea, vomiting, hyperglycemia

Elevated serum levels are noted in patients receiving cimetidine, quinolone antibiotics, and macrolide antibiotics and in patients with cardiac failure or liver insufficiency. Decreased serum levels are seen with phenobarbital, phenytoin, rifampin, and smokers. Toxicity occurs with plasma levels greater than 20 mcg/mL. Avoid rapid infusions, which may cause hypotension, arrhythmias, and possibly death.

Anesthetic considerations

Aminophylline potentiates the pressor effects of sympathomimetics and may produce seizures, cardiac arrhythmias, cardiorespiratory arrest, and ventricular arrhythmias with excessive plasma levels or in patients receiving volatile anesthetics. Use isoflurane or sevoflurane in patients who must be given aminophylline or other exogenous sympathomimetic drugs before or during surgery. Use of halothane may potentiate cardiac dysrhythmia.

AMIODARONE (CORDARONE)

Classification

Class III antiarrhythmic

Indications

Treatment of life-threatening ventricular arrhythmias that do not respond to other antiarrhythmics (i.e., recurrent ventricular fibrillation and hemodynamically unstable ventricular tachycardia); selective treatment of supraventricular arrhythmias

Dose

Loading: oral: 800 to 1000 mg/day for 1 to 3 weeks. Maintenance: oral: 200 to 600 mg/day. Therapeutic level: 1 to 2.5 mcg/mL. Dosage form: tablets: 200 mg. Intravenous: 100 to 300 mg.

The recommended starting dose of intravenous amiodarone HCl is about 1000 mg over the first 24 hours of therapy, delivered by the following infusion:

- Loading infusions: *first* rapid: 150 mg over the FIRST 10 minutes (15 mg/min). Add 3 mL of amiodarone HCl intravenously (150 mg) to 100 mL D_5W (concentration = 1.5 mg/mL). Infuse 100 mL over 10 minutes.
- *Followed by* slow: 360 mg over the *next* 6 hours (1 mg/min). Add 18 mL of amiodarone HCl intravenously (900 mg) to 500 mL D_5W (concentration = 1.8 mg/mL).
- Maintenance infusion: 540 mg over the *remaining* 18 hours (0.5 mg/min). Decrease the rate of the slow loading infusion to 0.5 mg/min.

Onset and duration

Onset: 2 to 4 days; half-life between 2 weeks and months. Duration: 45 days.

Adverse effects

Arrhythmias, pulmonary fibrosis or inflammation, hepatitis or cirrhosis, corneal deposits, hyperthyroidism, hypothyroidism, peripheral neuropathy, cutaneous photosensitivity

Precautions and contraindications

Amiodarone increases serum levels of digoxin, warfarin, quinidine, procainamide, phenytoin, and diltiazem. The likelihood of bradycardia, sinus arrest, and atrioventricular block increases with concurrent β-adrenergic antagonist and calcium channel–blocker therapy.

Anesthetic considerations

Antiadrenergic effects are enhanced in the presence of general anesthetics and manifest as sinus arrest, atrioventricular block, low cardiac output, or hypotension. Drugs that inhibit the automaticity of the sinus node such as halothane and lidocaine could accentuate effects of amiodarone and increase the likelihood of sinus arrest. The potential need for a temporary artificial cardiac (ventricular) pacemaker and administration of sympathomimetics such as isoproterenol should be considered in patients receiving this drug.

AMRINONE LACTATE (INOCOR)

Classification

Positive inotrope (phosphodiesterase inhibitor)

Indications

Short-term management of congestive heart failure

Dose

Loading dose: 0.75 mg/kg over 2 to 3 minutes. A second bolus may follow after 30 minutes. Maintenance is by continuous infusion of 5 to 10 mcg/kg/min (maximum 24-hour dose: 10 mg/kg).

Dosage forms: injection: 5 mg/mL. Dilution for infusion: 500 mg in 500 mL normal saline solution.

Onset and duration

Onset: within 5 minutes. Duration: 30 minutes to 2 hours.

Adverse effects

Hypotension, arrhythmia, thrombocytopenia, abdominal pain, hepatic dysfunction

Precautions and contraindications

Use amrinone with caution in hypotensive patients. Avoid exposure of the ampule to light. Do not mix in solutions containing dextrose or furosemide. Use it with caution in patients with allergies to bisulfites. Fluid balance, electrolyte concentrations, and renal function should be monitored carefully during treatment. Monitor platelet counts on a long-term basis. Amrinone contains sodium metabisulfite, a sulfite that may cause allergic-type reactions including anaphylactic symptoms and life-threatening or less severe asthmatic episodes in certain susceptible people. Sulfite sensitivity is seen more frequently in asthmatic than in nonasthmatic people.

Anesthetic considerations

This drug is an alternative to conventional inotropes. It is useful when both inotropic and vasodilating properties are desired and/or to lower pulmonary vascular resistance. Milrinone, another phosphodiesterase-3 inhibitor, is more commonly used.

ATRACURIUM (TRACRIUM)

Classification

Nondepolarizing skeletal muscle relaxant

Indications

Relaxation of skeletal muscles during surgery; adjunct to general anesthesia or mechanical ventilation; facilitation of endotracheal intubation

Dose

Initially for paralyzing: intravenous: 0.3 to 0.5 mg/kg. Maintenance: intravenous: 0.08 to 0.1 mg/kg.

Dosage form: injection: 10 mg/mL.

Onset and duration

Onset: less than 3 minutes. Duration: 30 to 45 minutes. Elimination: plasma (Hofmann elimination, ester hydrolysis). The primary metabolite is laudanosine, produced in low doses, a cerebral stimulant, excreted primarily in the urine.

Adverse effects

Primarily resulting from histamine release: vasodilation, hypotension, sinus tachycardia, sinus bradycardia, hypoventilation, apnea, bronchospasm, laryngospasm, dyspnea, inadequate block, prolonged block, rash, and urticaria

Precautions and contraindications

Use atracurium with caution in patients with conditions in which histamine release may prove hazardous, in patients with myasthenia gravis or other muscle disorders, or in electrolyte disturbances.

Anesthetic considerations

Monitor the patient's response with a peripheral nerve stimulator. Reverse the effects with anticholinesterase. Pretreatment doses may induce sufficient neuromuscular blockade to cause hypoventilation in some patients.

ATROPINE SULFATE

Classification

Competitive acetylcholine antagonist at muscarinic receptor

Indications

Symptomatic bradycardia, asystole, cardiopulmonary resuscitation (CPR); antisialagogue; for vagolytic effects to block bradycardia during surgery from stimulation of the carotid sinus, traction on abdominal viscera, or extraocular muscles; blockade of muscarinic effects of anticholinesterases; adjunctive therapy in the treatment of bronchospasm, peptic ulcer disease

Dose

Adults: sinus bradycardia, CPR: intravenous, intramuscular, subcutaneous, via endotracheal tube (diluted in 10 mL sterile water or normal saline): 0.5 to 1 mg every 3 to 5 minutes as indicated (maximum dose: 40 mcg/kg). Preoperative: 0.4 mg intramuscular, subcutaneous, or oral: 30 to 60 minutes preinduction.

Blockade of muscarinic effects of anticholinesterases: 7 to 10 mcg/kg with edrophonium, 15 to 30 mcg/kg with neostigmine, 15 to 20 mcg/kg with pyridostigmine.

Bronchodilation: inhalation: 0.025 mg/kg every 4 to 6 hours. Dilute to 2 to 3 mL in normal saline and deliver by compressed air nebulizer (maximum dose 2.5 mg/dose). Pediatric bronchodilatory dose: 0.05 mg/kg diluted in normal saline three or four times daily.

Children: sinus bradycardia, CPR: intravenous, intramuscular, subcutaneous, or via endotracheal tube: 0.02 mg/kg every 5 minutes up to a maximum of 1 mg in children and 2 mg in adolescents (minimum dose: 0.1 mg).

Preoperative: oral, intramuscular, subcutaneous: 0.02 mg/kg for neonates, 0.1 mg for children weighing 3 kg, 0.2 mg for those weighing 7 to 9 kg, and 0.3 mg for those weighing 12 to 16 kg.

Dosage forms: injection: 0.05, 0.1, 0.3, 0.4, 0.5, 0.8, and 1 mg/mL; inhalation solution: 0.2%, 0.5%; tablets: 0.4, 0.6 mg.

Onset and duration

Inhibition of salivation occurs within 30 minutes to 1 hour and peaks in 1 to 2 hours following oral or intramuscular atropine administration.

Increase in heart rate occurs within 3 to 10 minutes after intravenous or intramuscular administration. Duration: 15 to 45 minutes after intravenous administration and 2 to 4 hours following intramuscular administration.

Adverse effects

Transient bradycardia resulting from a weak peripheral muscarinic cholinergic agonist effect in small doses (less than 0.5 mg in adults), tachycardia (high doses), urinary hesitancy, retention, mydriasis, blurred vision, increased intraocular pressure, decreased sweating, excitement, agitation, drowsiness, confusion, hallucinations, dry nose and mouth, allergic reactions, constipation.

Children and the elderly are more susceptible to these adverse effects.

Precautions and contraindications

Avoid atropine in situations in which tachycardia would be harmful (i.e., thyrotoxicosis, pheochromocytoma, coronary artery disease). Avoid in hyperpyrexial states because it inhibits sweating. It is contraindicated in acute-angle glaucoma, obstructive disease of the gastrointestinal tract, obstructive uropathy, paralytic ileus or intestinal atony, and acute hemorrhage in patients with unstable cardiovascular status. Use it with caution in patients with tachyarrhythmias, hepatic or renal disease, congestive heart failure, chronic pulmonary disease (because a reduction in bronchial secretions may lead to formation of bronchial plugs), autonomic neuropathy, hiatal hernia, gastroesophageal reflux, gastric ulcers, gastrointestinal infections, and ulcerative colitis.

Anesthetic considerations

Additive anticholinergic effects may occur when atropine is given concomitantly with meperidine, some antihistamines, phenothiazines, tricyclic antidepressants, and antiarrhythmic drugs that possess anticholinergic activity (e.g., quinidine, disopyramide, procainamide).

BRETYLIUM (BRETYLOL)

Classification
Class III antiarrhythmic

Indications
Ventricular fibrillation and other ventricular arrhythmias resistant to initial lidocaine, amiodorone, or procainamide treatment

Dose
Ventricular tachycardia: intravenous loading, intramuscular: 5 to 10 mg/kg over 1 minute or may be repeated in 1 to 2 hours. Ventricular fibrillation: intravenous loading: 5 to 10 mg/kg over 1 minute (every 15 to 30 minutes to maximum 30 mg/kg); infusion: 1 to 2 mg/min. Therapeutic level: 0.5 to 1 mcg/mL.
Dosage form: 50 mg/mL.

Onset and duration
Onset antifibrillatory: few minutes; intravenous/intramuscular suppression of ventricular arrhythmia: 20 minutes to 2 hours. Duration: intravenous/intramuscular: 6 to 24 hours.

PART III **Drugs**

Adverse effects

Hypotension, transitory hypertension and arrhythmias, anginal attacks, shortness of breath, dizziness, syncope, nausea, vomiting, diarrhea, rash, hiccups

Precautions and contraindications

Use bretylium with caution in patients with pheochromocytoma, aortic stenosis, and pulmonary hypertension.

Anesthetic considerations

Tricyclic antidepressants may prevent the uptake of bretylium by adrenergic nerve terminals. Treat severe hypotension with appropriate fluid therapy and vasopressor agents such as dopamine or norepinephrine.

BUMETANIDE (BUMEX)

Classification

Loop diuretic

Indications

Treatment of edema of cardiac, hepatic, or renal origin; hypertension, pulmonary edema; usually reserved for patients who do not respond to thiazide diuretics or in whom a rapid onset of diuresis is desired

Dose

Initial dose: 0.5 to 1 mg intravenously over 1 to 2 minutes. If response is not adequate following the initial dose, a second or third dose may be administered at intervals of up to 2 to 3 hours, up to a maximum of 10 mg/day. Children: Dose: IV, IM, PO: 0.015 to 0.1 mg/kg: max = 2 mg qd

Onset and duration

Onset: intravenous: few minutes. Peak effect: 15 to 30 minutes. Duration: 4 hours with normal doses of 1 to 2 mg and up to 6 hours with higher doses. Elimination half-life: 1 to 1.5 hours.

Adverse effects

Transient leukopenia, granulocytopenia, thrombocytopenia, hypotension, chest pain, dizziness; electrolyte abnormalities such as hyperuricemia, hypomagnesemia, hypokalemia, hypochloremia, azotemia, hyponatremia, metabolic alkalosis; hyperglycemia, diarrhea, pancreatitis, nephrotoxicity, muscle cramps, arthritic pain, ototoxicity (less frequent than with furosemide)

Precautions and contraindications

Patients may have anuria, hypersensitivity to bumetanide, severe fluid and electrolyte imbalance, and hepatic coma, if an increase in blood urea nitrogen or creatinine occurs. Patients allergic to sulfonamides may have hypersensitivity to bumetanide.

Anesthetic considerations

Loop diuretics may increase the neuromuscular blocking effect of nondepolarizing relaxants.

BUPIVACAINE HCL (MARCAINE, SENSORCAINE)

Classification
Amide-type local anesthetic

Indications
Regional anesthesia

Dose
Infiltration/peripheral nerve block: less than 150 mg (0.25% to 0.5% solution). Epidural: 50 to 100 mg (0.25% to 0.75% solution), children: 1.5 to 2.5 mg/kg (0.25% to 0.5% solution). Caudal: 37.5 to 150 mg (15 to 30 mL of 0.25% or 0.5% solution), children: 0.4 to 0.7 mL/kg. Spinal bolus/infusion: 7 to 17 mg (0.75% solution), children: 0.5 mg/kg, with minimum of 1 mg. Do not exceed 400 mg in 24 hours (maximum single dose is 175 mg).

Onset and duration
Onset: infiltration: 2 to 10 minutes; epidural: 4 to 7 minutes; spinal: less than 1 minute. Peak effect: infiltration and epidural: 30 to 45 minutes. spinal: 15 minutes. Duration: infiltration/spinal/epidural: 200 to 400 minutes (prolonged with epinephrine).

Adverse effects
Hypotension, arrhythmias, cardiac arrest, respiratory impairment or arrest, seizures, tinnitus, blurred vision, urticaria, anaphylactoid symptoms; high spinal: urinary retention, lower extremity weakness and paralysis, loss of sphincter control, backache, palsies, slowing of labor

Precautions and contraindications
Use bupivacaine with caution in patients with hypovolemia, severe congestive heart failure, shock, and all forms of heart block. It is not recommended for obstetric paracervical block or in concentrations higher than 0.5% because of the incidence of intractable cardiac arrest. It is contraindicated in patients with hypersensitivity to amide-type local anesthetics.

Anesthetic considerations
Intravenous access is essential during major regional block. Toxic plasma levels of bupivacaine may cause cardiopulmonary collapse and seizures.

CHLOROPROCAINE HCL (NESACAINE)

Classification
Ester-type local anesthetic

Indications
Regional anesthesia; local anesthesia including infiltration, epidural (including caudal), peripheral nerve block, sympathetic nerve block

Dose
Infiltration and peripheral nerve block: less than 40 mL (1% to 2% solution). Epidural: bolus 10 to 25 mL (2% to 3% solution), approximately

1.5 to 2 mL for each segment to be anesthetized. Repeat doses at 40- to 60-minute intervals. Infusion: 30 mL/hour (0.5% solution). Caudal: 10 to 25 mL (2% to 3% solution). Children: 0.4 to 0.7 mL/kg (L2 to T10 level of anesthesia). Repeat doses at 40- to 60-minute intervals.

Onset and duration

Rate of onset and potency of local anesthetic action may be enhanced by carbonation. Onset: infiltration/epidural: 6 to 12 minutes. Peak effect: infiltration/epidural: 10 to 20 minutes. Duration: infiltration/epidural: 30 to 60 minutes (prolonged with epinephrine).

Adverse effects

Hypotension, arrhythmias, bradycardia, respiratory depression or arrest, seizures, tinnitus, tremors, urticaria, pruritus, angioneurotic edema; high spinal: backache, loss of perianal sensation and sexual function, permanent motor, sensory, autonomic (sphincter control) deficit in lower segments, slowing of labor

Precautions and contraindications

Use with caution in patients with severe disturbances of cardiac rhythm, shock, heart block, or impaired hepatic function. Inflammation or infection may occur at the injection site. Elderly and pregnant patients are most at risk. It is contraindicated in patients with hypersensitivity to ester-type local anesthetics and to *para*-aminobenzoic acid/parabens. Do not use for spinal anesthesia.

Anesthetic considerations

Reduce doses in obstetric, elderly, hypovolemic, and high-risk patients and in those with increased intraabdominal pressure.

CIMETIDINE (TAGAMET)

Classification

Histamine (H_2) antagonist

Indications

Treatment of duodenal or gastric ulcers, gastroesophageal reflux disease; prophylaxis of aspiration pneumonitis in patients at high risk during surgery

Dose

Prophylaxis of aspiration pneumonitis: adults: 300 to 400 mg orally 1.5 to 2 hours before induction of anesthesia with or without a similar dose the preceding evening. When a more rapid onset of effect is needed, intravenous: dilute 300 to 400 mg in D_5W or normal saline to a volume of at least 20 mL and inject over a period not less than 5 minutes. A slower infusion, over 15 to 30 minutes, may be preferable owing to association of occasional severe bradycardia and hypotension with rapid infusion. Children younger than 12 years of age: use not indicated.

Dosage forms: tablets: 300, 400 mg; parenteral injection: 150 mg/mL.

Onset and duration

Onset: 15 to 45 minutes. Peak plasma levels: 1 to 2 hours orally. Duration: 2 to 4 hours. Elimination half-life: 2 hours. Plasma cimetidine levels that suppress gastric acid secretion by 50% were maintained 4 to 5 hours following intravenous injection.

Adverse effects

Mental status changes such as delirium, confusion, depression, primarily in elderly patients or those with hepatic or renal impairment; leukopenia, thrombocytopenia, and gynecomastia rarely (1%)

Hypotension and severe bradycardia are associated with rapid intravenous infusion. Serum creatinine and liver enzymes may rise during treatment, although hepatotoxicity and renal dysfunction are usually reversible.

Precautions and contraindications

Caution is suggested in renal or hepatic insufficiency. Microsomal metabolism of many drugs may be inhibited. It is contraindicated in patients allergic to cimetidine or other H_2 antagonists.

Anesthetic considerations

Cimetidine inhibits the hepatic mixed-function oxidase system; therefore, it may prolong the half-life of many drugs, including diazepam, midazolam, metoprolol, propranolol, theophylline, lidocaine, and other amide local anesthetics. Ranitidine may be the drug of choice in patients receiving lidocaine local or regional anesthesia.

CLONIDINE (CATAPRES, DIXARIT); EPIDURAL CLONIDINE (CATAPRES, DURACLON)

Classification

Central-acting α_2-adrenergic agonist; reduces sympathetic outflow by directly stimulating α receptors in the medulla vasomotor center

Epidural action produces dose-dependent analgesia by preventing pain signal transmission at presynaptic and postjunctional α_2 adrenoreceptors in the spinal cord.

Indications

Hypertension; epidural and spinal anesthesia; symptomatic control of alcohol, opiate, nicotine, and benzodiazepine withdrawal; diagnosis of pheochromocytoma; growth hormone stimulation test; cancer-related pain; Tourette's syndrome; attention deficit disorder; migraines.

The use of epidural clonidine in combination with epidural opiate agonists results in a decreased opiate requirement that treats neuropathic pain more effectively than visceral pain.

Dose

Maintenance: 0.2 to 0.6 mg/day orally in two divided doses. Hypertensive emergencies: 0.15 mg intravenously over 5 minutes. Transdermal patch: every 7 days (maximum dose: 2.4 mg/day). The same doses are used in renal impairment.

Epidural: must be preservative free. Postoperative pain: epidural clonidine combined with an opiate analgesic: 150 mcg if added to fentanyl, 450 g/day if added to morphine. Neuropathic pain: continuous epidural infusion combined with an opiate analgesic is 30 mcg/hour. Plain clonidine epidural infusion is from 100 to 900 mcg/day; children: start at 0.5 mcg/kg/hour.

All dosages must be titrated to pain relief and incidence of side effects.

The recommended starting dose of epidurnal clonidine HCl for continuous epidural infusion is 30 mcg/h. Although dosage may be titrated up or down depending on pain relief and occurence of adverse events, experience with dosage rates above 40 mcg/h is limited.

Familiarization with the continuous epidural infusion device is essential. Patients receiving epidural clonidine from a continuous infusion device should be closely monitored for the first few days to assess their response.

The 500 mcg/mL (0.5 mg/mL) strength product must be diluted prior to use in 0.9% sodium chloride for injection, to a final concentration of 100 mcg/mL.

Onset and duration

Onset: intravenous or oral: 30 to 60 minutes. Peak effect: 2 to 4 hours. May take too long for a true hypertensive crisis. Duration: antihypertensive: 6 to 10 hours, dose dependent.

Adverse effects

Rebound hypertension, atrioventricular block, bradycardia, congestive heart failure, orthostatic hypotension, sedation, nightmares, constipation, dry mouth, pruritus, urinary retention, contact dermatitis

The most common noncardiovascular adverse reactions to epidural clonidine include anxiety, asthenia, chest pain, confusion, diaphoresis, dizziness, drowsiness, dyspnea, fever, nausea/vomiting, and xerostomia.

Precautions and contraindications

- Avoid in conduction or sinoatrial disorders, hypersensitivity to clonidine, pregnancy, severe renal or hepatic disease. Concomitant administration of tricyclic antidepressants may increase the serum level.
- If the dose is held or when changing to transdermal application, watch for a rapid increase in blood pressure from unopposed α stimulation.
- It crosses the placenta easily and should be discontinued 8 to 12 hours before delivery.
- Epidural clonidine is *not recommended* for intrathecal administration or as an analgesic during labor and delivery or for postpartum or perioperative analgesia because of the risks of hemodynamic instability.

Anesthetic considerations

- Severe rebound hypertension may result from abrupt withdrawal, with neurologic sequelae and myocardial infarction. Labetalol has been successfully used in treatment of hypertensive crisis. Continue on the day of surgery.
- Hepatic elimination is 50%.
- Clonidine reduces perioperative requirements of narcotics and volatile agents.
- Female patients and lower-weight patients have an increased risk of the hypotensive effects of epidural clonidine (use cautiously in patients with severe cardiac disease or hemodynamic instability). More profound decreases in blood pressure may be seen if the drug is administered into the upper thoracic spinal segments.

COCAINE HCL (COCAINE)

Classification
Topical anesthetic and vasoconstrictor, ester-type local anesthetic

Indications
Topical anesthesia and vasoconstriction of mucous membranes (oral, laryngeal, and nasal)

Dose
Topical: 1.5 mg/kg (1% to 4% solution). Nasal: 1 to 2 mL each nostril (1% to 10% solution). Concentrations greater than 4% increase potential for systemic toxic reactions. Maximum safe dose: 1.5 mg/kg.

Onset and duration
Onset: less than 1 minute. Peak effect: 2 to 5 minutes. Duration: 30 to 120 minutes. It is rapidly absorbed from all areas of application.

Adverse effects
Seizures, sloughing of nasal mucosa, arrhythmias, tachycardia, hypertension

Precautions and contraindications
Cocaine is for topical use only, not for intraocular or intravenous use. It potentiates other sympathomimetics; therefore, use reduced doses (if any at all) in patients receiving pressors or ketamine. Use it with caution in patients with nasal trauma.

Anesthetic considerations
Hypertension, bradyarrhythmias, tachyarrhythmias, ventricular fibrillation, tachypnea, respiratory failure, euphoria, excitement, seizures, and sloughing of corneal epithelium may occur. Use it with caution in patients with a history of drug sensitivities or drug abuse (high addiction potential) and pregnancy. Prolonged use can cause ischemic damage to nasal mucosa. Cocaine is contraindicated for intraocular or intravenous use. It sensitizes the heart to catecholamines (epinephrine and monoamine oxidase inhibitors may increase cardiac arrhythmias, ventricular fibrillation, hypertensive episodes). It potentiates arrhythmogenic effects of sympathomimetics, and it has a high addiction potential.

PART III Drugs

CODEINE

Classification
Opioid agonist

Indications
Preoperative and postoperative analgesia

Dose
Oral: 15 to 60 mg every 4 hours; intramuscular/subcutaneous: 15 to 60 mg every 4 hours.

Onset and duration

Onset: oral: 30 to 60 minutes; intramuscular/subcutaneous: 20 to 60 minutes. Duration: oral: 2 to 4 hours; intramuscular/subcutaneous: 2 to 3 hours.

Adverse effects

Sedation, clouded sensorium, euphoria, dizziness, seizures with large doses, hypotension, bradycardia, nausea, vomiting, constipation, dry mouth, ileus, urinary retention, pruritus, flushing

Precautions and contraindications

Use codeine with caution in patients with head injury, owing to respiratory depression and resulting increased intracranial pressure, in hepatic or renal disease, hypothyroidism, Addison's disease, acute alcoholism, seizures, severe central nervous system depression, bronchial asthma, chronic obstructive pulmonary disease, respiratory depression, and shock. Use it with caution in patients with known hypersensitivity to the drug and in elderly patients. It may produce histamine release.

Anesthetic considerations

General anesthetics, other narcotic analgesics, tranquilizers, sedatives, hypnotics, alcohol, tricyclic antidepressants, or monoamine oxidase inhibitors increase central nervous system depression.

CYCLOSPORINE (SANDIMMUNE, OTHERS)

Classification

Immunosuppressant

Indications

Prevention of rejection of organ/tissue (kidney, liver, heart) allograft in combination with steroid therapy

Dose

Initial: oral: 15 mg/kg as a single dose 4 to 24 hours before transplantation; continue for 1 to 2 weeks. Taper to maintenance dose: 5 to 10 mg/kg/day. Intravenous: 0.5 to 6 mg/kg as single dose 4 to 12 hours before transplantation; continue until the patient is able to take oral medication.

Coadministration of a corticosteroid is recommended, as well as possibly azathioprine.

Onset and duration

Onset: 1 to 6 hours (variable). Duration: 1 to 4 days. After oral administration, onset is variable. Elimination half-life: 10 to 27 hours.

Adverse effects

Hypertension, hirsutism, tremor, acne, gum hyperplasia, headache, blurred vision, diarrhea, nausea, paresthesia, mild nephrotoxicity or hepatotoxicity

Precautions and contraindications

History of hypersensitivity to cyclosporine or polyoxyethylated castor oil. Use it with caution in patients with impaired hepatic, renal, cardiac function, malabsorption syndrome, and in those who are pregnant.

Anesthetic considerations

Altered laboratory values may occur. Cyclosporine may elevate blood urea nitrogen, serum creatinine, serum bilirubin, serum glutamic-oxaloacetic transaminase (aspartate aminotransferase), serum glutamic-pyruvic transaminase (alanine aminotransferase), and lactate dehydrogenase. It may prolong the duration of neuromuscular blockade by nondepolarizing muscle relaxants.

DANTROLENE SODIUM (DANTRIUM)

Classification
Skeletal muscle relaxant

Indications
Treatment of malignant hyperthermia (MHT); prophylaxis of MHT in patients with a family history; control of spasticity secondary to multiple sclerosis, spinal cord injury, cerebral palsy, or stroke

Dose
Adults: MHT: 1 mg/kg rapid intravenous bolus; repeat every 5 to 10 minutes until symptoms are controlled; the dose may be repeated to a cumulative dose of 10 mg/kg; oral doses of 4 to 8 mg/kg/day for 1 to 3 days may be administered in three or four divided doses to prevent recurrence of the manifestations. Prophylaxis of MHT: 2.5 mg/kg intravenous bolus 10 to 30 minutes preinduction, then 1.25 mg/kg intravenous bolus 6 hours later.

Dosage forms: capsules: 25, 50, 100 mg; parenteral injection: 20 mg. Administration: reconstitute by adding 60 mL preservative-free sterile water for injection to each 20-mg vial and shake vial until clear. Avoid diluent that contains a bacteriostatic agent. Protect from light and use within 6 hours. For direct intravenous injection. Avoid extravasation.

Onset and duration
Effective blood concentrations: 100 to 600 ng/mL. Intravenous blood concentrations of the drug remain at approximately steady-state levels for 3 or more hours after infusion is completed. Mean half-life: 5 to 9 hours. Onset: oral: 1 to 2 hours; intravenous: less than 5 minutes. Duration: 8 to 12 hours.

Adverse effects
Hepatotoxicity (hepatitis): 0.5%, with mortality reported as high as 10%; muscle weakness, tachycardia, erratic blood pressure, fatigue, central nervous system (CNS) depression, visual and auditory hallucinations, bowel obstruction, hematuria, crystalluria, urinary frequency, phlebitis, pericarditis, pleural effusion, postpartum uterine atony, myalgias

Precautions and contraindications
Monitor liver function at the beginning of dantrolene therapy. Observe for hepatotoxicity, hepatitis. Owing to the increased risk of hepatotoxicity, use it with caution in patients with severely impaired cardiac or pulmonary function and in women or patients older than 35 years. It is contraindicated in active hepatic disease such as hepatitis or cirrhosis, when spasticity is used to maintain motor function, and in lactation.

Anesthetic considerations

Enhanced CNS and respiratory depression occurs with other CNS depressants. Avoid the concomitant use of calcium channel blockers, which can precipitate hyperkalemia and cardiovascular collapse.

DESFLURANE (SUPRANE)

Classification

Inhalation anesthetic

Indications

General anesthesia

Dose

Titrate to effect for induction or maintenance of anesthesia. Minimum alveolar concentration: 6%.

Dosage forms: volatile liquid.

Onset and duration

Onset: loss of eyelid reflex: 1 to 2 minutes. Duration: emergence time: 8 to 9 minutes.

Adverse effects

Hypotension, arrhythmia, respiratory depression, apnea, dizziness, euphoria, increased cerebral blood flow and intracranial pressure, nausea, vomiting, ileus, hepatic dysfunction, malignant hyperthermia

Precautions and contraindications

Desflurane is contraindicated in patients with known or suspected genetic susceptibility to malignant hyperthermia. Changes in mental function may persist beyond the period of anesthetic administration and the immediate postoperative period.

Anesthetic considerations

Abrupt onset of malignant hyperthermia may be triggered by desflurane; early signs include muscle rigidity, especially in the jaw muscles, and tachycardia and tachypnea unresponsive to increased depth of anesthesia. It crosses the placental barrier.

DESMOPRESSIN (DDAVP)

Classification

Synthetic vasopressin analogue

Indications

Treatment of neurogenic diabetes insipidus, nocturnal enuresis, and, in hemophilia A or von Willebrand's disease, to increase factor VIII activity; reduction of perioperative blood loss following cardiac surgery

Dose

Preoperative: 30 minutes before the procedure. Diabetes insipidus: 2 to 4 mcg intravenously or subcutaneously daily in two divided doses; intranasal: 10 to 40 mcg (0.1 to 0.4 mL) in one to three doses.

Pediatrics: 3 months to 12 years: hemophilia A or von Willebrand's disease: 0.3 mcg/kg intravenously, diluted in saline and infused over 15 to 30 minutes. In children who weigh more than 10 kg, use 50 mL diluent, and in children less than 10 kg, use 10 mL diluent. Repeated doses in less than 48 hours may increase the possibility of tachyphylaxis.

Intranasal: 0.05 to 0.3 mL daily in single or divided doses. Doses should start at 0.05 mL or less and be individualized because an extreme decrease in plasma osmolarity in the very young may produce convulsions.

Dosage forms: injection: 4 mcg/mL; desmopressin acetate for injection should be stored at 4° C; nasal: 10 to 40 mcg; may be divided into three doses, and supplied as 10 mcg/0.1 mL or 100 mcg/mL.

Onset and duration

Onset: intranasal: 1 hour; intravenous: 30 minutes. Duration: 8 to 20 hours. Elimination half-life: 3.6 hours.

Adverse effects

Hypotension, hypertension, transient headache (with higher doses), psychosis, seizures, water retention, hyponatremia, abdominal cramps, nasal congestion, rhinitis, facial flushing, hypersensitivity reactions

Precautions and contraindications

This agent is contraindicated in hypersensitivity to desmopressin acetate and in children younger than 3 months of age. Patients with type IIB von Willebrand's disease should not receive desmopressin because platelet aggregation may be reduced. Owing to an increased risk of thrombosis, use it with caution in patients with coronary artery disease. Fluid intake should be decreased in those who do not need the antidiuretic effects of desmopressin. Seizure activity may be related to rapid decreases in serum sodium concentrations secondary to desmopressin. Avoid overhydration; postoperative abdominal cramping may occur.

Anesthetic considerations

None

DEXAMETHASONE (DECADRON)

Classification

Long-acting corticosteroid

Indications

Croup, septic shock, cerebral edema, respiratory distress syndrome including status asthmaticus, acute exacerbations of chronic allergic disorders, corticosteroid-responsive bronchospastic states, allergic or inflammatory nasal conditions, and nasal polyps

Dose

Initial: 0.5 to 9 mg, intramuscularly or intravenously daily, depending on the disease being treated. In less severe diseases, doses lower than 0.5 mg intramuscularly or intravenously may suffice, whereas in others, doses higher than 9 mg may be required.

Cerebral edema: 10 mg intravenously initially followed by 4 mg intramuscularly every 6 hours. Reduce dose after 2 to 4 days, then taper over 5 to 7 days.

Corticosteroid-responsive bronchospastic states: Respihaler: three inhalations three to four times daily (maximum 12 inhalations daily).

Nasal conditions: Turbinaire: two sprays each nostril two to three times daily (maximum 12 sprays/24 hours).

Children: intramuscular or by intravenous push: 6 to 40 mcg/kg or 0.235 to 1.25 mg/m^2 given one or two times daily. Must be given slowly over 3 to 5 minutes by intravenous push.

Dosage forms: Respihaler inhalation: 0.1 mg/spray dexamethasone phosphate; Turbinaire intranasal: 0.1 mg/spray; solution for injection: 4, 10, 24 mg/mL; tablets: 0.25, 0.5, 0.75, 1, 1.5, 2, 4, 6 mg.

Onset and duration

Onset: intravenous/intramuscular: within 10 to 30 minutes; inhalation: within 20 minutes. Elimination half-life: 200 minutes; however, metabolic effects at the tissue level persist for up to 72 hours.

Adverse effects

Cushing's syndrome, adrenal suppression, hyperglycemia, hyperthyroidism, hypercalcemia, peptic ulcer, gastrointestinal hemorrhage, increased intraocular pressure, glaucoma, irritability, psychosis, osteoporosis

Precautions and contraindications

Dexamethasone is contraindicated in patients with peptic ulcer, osteoporosis, psychosis or psychoneurosis, acute bacterial infections, herpes zoster, herpes simplex ulceration of the eye, and other viral infections. Use it with caution in diabetes mellitus, chronic renal failure, infectious disease, and the elderly. Corticosteroids may increase the risk of developing tuberculosis in patients with a positive purified protein derivative test. They may increase the risk of development of serious or fatal infection in persons exposed to viral illnesses such as chickenpox.

Anesthetic considerations

Short-term administration of intravenous or inhalation steroids may be helpful in shock and asthma. Dexamethasone may have some benefit in anaphylaxis. Toxicity following acute dosing is minimal.

DIAZEPAM (VALIUM)

Classification

Central nervous system agent; benzodiazepine; anticonvulsant and anxiolytic

Indications

Anxiety, alcohol withdrawal, status epilepticus, preoperative sedation, sedation for cardioversion; used adjunctively for relief of skeletal muscle spasm associated with cerebral palsy, paraplegia, athetosis, stiff-man syndrome, tetanus

Dose

Status epilepticus: adults: intramuscular/intravenous: 5 to 10 mg; repeat if needed at 10- to 15-minute intervals up to 30 mg, repeat if needed in 2 to 4 hours; children: intramuscular/intravenous: less than 5 years: 0.2 to 0.5 mg slowly 2 to 5 minutes up to 5 mg, total dose. Children older than 5 years: 1 mg slowly 2 to 5 minutes up to 10 mg; repeat if needed in 2 to 4 hours.

Anxiety, muscle spasm convulsions, alcohol withdrawal: adults: oral: 2 to 10 mg two to four times daily; intramuscular/intravenous: 2 to 10 mg; repeat if needed in 3 to 4 hours; children: oral: older than 6 months: 1 to 2.5 mg two or three times daily.

Dosage forms: tablets: 2, 5, 10 mg; capsules: (sustained release) 15 mg; oral solution: 5 mg/5 mL and 5 mg/mL; injection: 5 mg/mL.

Onset and duration
Onset: oral: 30 to 60 minutes; intramuscular: 15 to 30 minutes; intravenous: 1 to 5 minutes. Peak effect: 1 to 2 hours orally. Duration: intravenous: 15 minutes to 1 hours; oral: up to 3 hours. Elimination half-life: 20 to 50 hours; excreted primarily in urine. It is metabolized in liver to active metabolites.

Adverse effects
Drowsiness, fatigue, ataxia, confusion, paradoxical dizziness, vertigo, amnesia, vivid dreams, headache, slurred speech, tremor, muscle weakness, electroencephalogram changes, tardive dyskinesia, hypotension, tachycardia, edema, cardiovascular collapse, blurred vision, diplopia, nystagmus, xerostomia, nausea, constipation, incontinence, urinary retention, changes in libido

Precautions and contraindications
Diazepam is contraindicated in acute narrow-angle glaucoma, untreated open-angle glaucoma, and during or within 14 days of monoamine oxidase inhibitor therapy. Safe use during pregnancy (category D) and lactation has not been established.

Anesthetic considerations
Diazepam reduces requirements for volatile anesthetics. A potential for thrombophlebitis exists with intravenous administration. Elderly patients have decreased clearance and dosage requirements. Its effects are antagonized by flumazenil. It may cause neonatal hypothermia.

DIGOXIN (LANOXIN)

Classification
Inotropic agent

Indications
Treatment of supraventricular arrhythmias, heart failure, atrial fibrillation, flutter

Dose
Adults: loading: intravenous/oral: 0.5 to 1 mg in divided doses (give 50% of loading dose as first dose, then 25% fractions at 4- to 8-hour intervals until adequate therapeutic response is noted, toxic effects occur, or the total digitalizing dose has been administered). Monitor clinical response before each additional dose. Maintenance: intravenous/oral: 0.0625 to 0.25 mg; dosages should be individualized. Elderly adults (older than 65 years): oral: 0.125 mg or less daily as maintenance dose. Small patients may require less.

Children (older than 2 years): loading: oral: 0.02 to 0.06 mg/kg divided every 8 hours for 24 hours; intravenous: 0.015 to 0.035 mg/kg divided every 8 hours for 24 hours; maintenance: oral: 25% to 35% of digitalizing dose daily, divided into two doses.

Children 1 month to 2 years old: loading: oral: 0.035 to 0.060 mg/kg in three divided doses over 24 hours; intravenous: 0.02 to 0.05 mg/kg; maintenance: oral: 25% to 35% of digitalizing dose daily divided every 12 hours.

Neonates less than 1 month old: loading: oral: 0.025 to 0.035 mg/kg divided every 8 hours over 24 hours; intravenous: 0.015 to 0.025 mg/kg; maintenance: oral: 25% to 35% of digitalizing dose daily divided every 12 hours.

Premature infants: loading: intravenous: 0.015 to 0.025 mg/kg in three divided doses over 24 hours. Maintenance: intravenous: 0.01 mg/kg daily divided every 12 hours.

Dosage forms: tablets: 0.125, 0.25, 0.5 mg; capsules (Lanoxicaps): 0.05, 0.1, 0.2 mg; oral solution: 0.05 mg/mL; injection: 0.1 mg/mL, 1-mL ampule (100 mcg); 0.25 mg/mL, 2-mL ampule (500 mcg).

Onset and duration

Onset: intravenous: 5 to 30 minutes; oral: 30 minutes to 2 hours. Duration: intravenous/oral: 3 to 4 days.

Adverse effects

Enhanced toxicity in hypokalemia, hypomagnesemia, hypercalcemia; wide range of arrhythmias, atrioventricular block, headache, psychosis, confusion, nausea, vomiting, ocular changes, diarrhea, gynecomastia.

Overdosage may cause complete heart block, atrioventricular dissociation, tachycardia, and fibrillation.

Precautions and contraindications

Digoxin is contraindicated in ventricular fibrillation.

Anesthetic considerations

Decrease the dosage in patients with impaired renal function and in elderly patients. Monitor serum potassium, calcium, and digoxin levels. The use of synchronized cardioversion in patients with digitalis toxicity should be avoided because it may initiate ventricular fibrillation.

Digoxin interacts with numerous drugs. Increased serum levels are seen with calcium channel blockers (e.g., verapamil, diltiazem, nifedipine), esmolol, flecainide, captopril, quinidine, amiodarone, benzodiazepines, anticholinergics, oral aminoglycosides, and erythromycin. Succinylcholine may cause arrhythmias in digitalized patients. Additive bradycardia may occur with cardiac depressant anesthetics.

DILTIAZEM (CARDIZEM)

Classification
Calcium channel blocker

Indications
Angina pectoris; supraventricular tachycardia

Dose

Bolus intravenous: 0.25 mg/kg over 2 minutes. If needed, follow after 15 minutes with 0.35 mg/kg over 2 minutes. Maintenance infusion: 5 to 15 mg/hour. Adults: oral: 30 mg three or four times daily before meals and at bedtime. Dosage may be gradually increased to a maximum 360 mg/day in divided doses. Sustained-release capsules: 90 mg; oral: twice daily, titrate dosage to effect (maximum recommended dosage: 360 mg/day).

Dosage forms: oral: 30, 60, 90, 120 mg; sustained release: 60, 90, 120, 180, 240, 300 mg; intravenous: 5 mg/mL, 5- and 10-mL vials.

Onset and duration

Onset: oral: 30 minutes; intravenous: 1 to 3 minutes. Elimination half-life: 3 to 5 hours. Duration: 4 to 6 hours.

Adverse effects

Hypotension, flushing, atrioventricular block, constipation, pruritus, bradycardia, edema, nausea, vomiting, diarrhea, depression, headache, fatigue, dizziness

Precautions and contraindications

Hypotension occurs with coadministration with digoxin, β-blockers, and cimetidine. Diltiazem potentiates the cardiovascular depressant effects of volatile, injectable anesthetic agents.

Anesthetic considerations

Intravenous infusions of diltiazem are useful for intraoperative treatment of atrial tachyarrhythmias.

DIPHENHYDRAMINE (BENADRYL)

Classification

Histamine (H_1) antagonist, ethanolamine class

Indications

Adjuvant with epinephrine in the treatment of anaphylactic shock and severe allergic reactions; treatment of drug-induced extrapyramidal effects, motion sickness; antiemetic

Dose

Antihistamine or antiemetic: 10 to 50 mg intramuscularly or intravenously every 2 to 3 hours (maximum dosage: 400 mg/day).

Recommend increasing the dosing interval to every 6 to 12 hours in patients with moderate renal failure (glomerular filtration rate 10 to 50 mL/min).

Children: 1 to 2 mg/kg up to 150 mg/m²/day in up to four divided doses by slow intravenous push (3 to 5 minutes).

Dosage forms: injection: 10 mg/mL, 50 mg/1 mL Steri-dose syringe or ampule; capsules: 25, 50 mg; elixir and syrup: 12.5 mg/15 mL.

Onset and duration

Onset: oral: 1 hour. Duration: 4 to 6 hours. Elimination half-life: 4 to 8 hours.

Adverse effects

Sedation (most frequent); dizziness, tinnitus, tremors, euphoria, blurred vision, nervousness, palpitations, hypotension, psychotic reactions, hypersensitivity.

Other side effects are probably related to the antimuscarinic actions of diphenhydramine and include dry mouth, cough, and urinary retention.

Precautions and contraindications

Diphenhydramine is contraindicated in patients with a hypersensitivity to it and other antihistamines of a similar chemical structure. Antihistamines are contraindicated in patients taking monoamine oxidase inhibitor therapy. Avoid in patients with narrow-angle glaucoma.

Anesthetic considerations

Concurrent central nervous system depressants may produce an additive effect with diphenhydramine.

DOBUTAMINE HCL (DOBUTREX)

Classification

β_1-adrenergic agonist

Indications

Vasopressor; positive inotrope

Dose

Infusion: 0.5 to 30 mcg/kg/min. *Note:* Must be diluted, and an intravenous pump (syringe pump in pediatric patients) must be used.

Onset and duration

Onset: 1 to 2 minutes. Duration: less than 10 minutes.

Adverse effects

Hypertension, tachycardia, arrhythmias, angina, shortness of breath, headache, phlebitis at injection site

Precautions and contraindications

Arrhythmias and hypertension occur at high dobutamine doses. Use it with caution in patients with idiopathic hypertrophic subaortic stenosis. Do not mix dobutamine with sodium bicarbonate, furosemide, or other alkaline solutions; correct hypovolemia before or during treatment.

Anesthetic considerations

Dobutamine is useful for short-term intraoperative therapy for shock and congestive heart failure. Arterial line monitoring is highly recommended.

DOPAMINE HCL (INTROPIN)

Classification

Naturally occurring catecholamine

Indications

Vasopressor; positive inotrope

Dose

Infusion: 1 to 5 mcg/kg low dose for urinary support; pressor dose range: 5 to 20 mcg/kg, greater than 20 mcg/kg for extreme cases. *Note:* Must be diluted, and an intravenous pump must be used.

Onset and duration

Onset: 2 to 4 minutes. Duration: less than 10 minutes after termination of infusion.

Adverse effects

Nausea, vomiting, tachycardia, angina, arrhythmias, dyspnea, headache, anxiety

Precautions and contraindications

Correct hypovolemia as quickly as possible before or during dopamine treatment.

Anesthetic considerations

Avoid dopamine or use it at greatly reduced dose if the patient has received a monamine oxidase inhibitor. Infuse it into a large vein; extravasation may cause sloughing. Treat extravasation by local infiltration of phentolamine (approximately 1 mg in 10 mL normal saline).

DOXACURIUM CHLORIDE (NUROMAX)

Classification

Nondepolarizing skeletal muscle relaxant

Indications

Adjunct to general anesthesia; skeletal muscle relaxation during surgery

Dose

Paralyzing: intravenous: 0.05 to 0.08 mg/kg. Pretreatment/maintenance: 0.005 to 0.01 mg/kg.

Dosage form: 1 mg/mL injection.

Onset and duration

Onset: less than 4 minutes. Duration: 60 to 120 minutes. Elimination: renal.

Adverse effects

Hypoventilation, apnea, respiratory depression, anuria, rash, urticaria, inadequate block, prolonged block

Precautions and contraindications

Airway and oxygenation must be ensured before doxacurium administration.

Anesthetic considerations

Monitor the patient's response with peripheral nerve stimulator. Reverse the effects with anticholinesterase. Pretreatment may cause hypoventilation in some patients.

DOXAPRAM HCL (DOPRAM)

Classification
Central nervous system agent; respiratory and cerebral stimulant (analeptic)

Indications
Postanesthesia and drug-induced respiratory depression and to hasten arousal and return of pharyngeal and laryngeal reflexes; chronic pulmonary disease associated with acute hypercapnia

Dose
Slow intravenous: 0.5 to 1.5 mg/kg, repeat at 5 minutes (maximum dose: 2 mg/kg). Infusion: 5 mg/min until satisfactory respiratory response is obtained, then 1 to 3 mg/min (maximum total dose: 4 mg/kg, including bolus and infusion).

Onset and duration
Onset: 20 to 40 seconds. Peak effect: 1 to 2 minutes. Duration: 5 to 12 minutes.

Adverse effects
Hypertension, chest pain, tachycardia, bradycardia, arrhythmias, cough, laryngospasm, bronchospasm, hiccups, seizures, hyperactivity, headaches, urinary retention, spontaneous voiding, nausea and vomiting

Delay administration for at least 10 minutes after discontinuation of volatile anesthetics because of sensitization to catecholamines when using halothane. The concomitant use of monoamine oxidase inhibitors or other sympathomimetics may potentiate adverse cardiovascular effects.

Precautions and contraindications
Contraindications to doxapram include head trauma, epilepsy or other seizure disorders, mechanical disorders of ventilation, cerebrovascular accident, significant cardiovascular impairment, severe hypertension, or known hypersensitivity to the drug. Use cautiously in patients with a history of severe tachycardia or cardiac arrhythmia, increased cerebrospinal fluid pressure or cerebral edema, pheochromocytoma, or hyperthyroidism or hypermetabolic states.

Anesthetic considerations
Respiratory depression may recur after doxapram's effects are terminated. Because of the low therapeutic index, repeat dosing is discouraged.

EDROPHONIUM CHLORIDE (ENLON, REVERSOL, TENSILON)

Classification
Anticholinesterase agent

Indications
Reversal of neuromuscular blockade; diagnostic assessment of myasthenia gravis, and supraventricular tachycardia

Dose

Reversal: slow intravenous: 0.5 to 1 mg/kg (maximum dose: 40 mg), with atropine (0.007 to 0.015 mg/kg), administered before the edrophonium.

Assessment of myasthenia/cholinergic crisis: slow intravenous: 1 mg every 1 to 2 minutes until change in symptoms (maximum dose: 10 mg); intramuscular: 10 mg.

Onset and duration

Onset: intravenous: 30 to 60 seconds; intramuscular: 2 to 10 minutes. Duration: intravenous: 20 to 40 minutes; intramuscular: 20 to 60 minutes.

Adverse effects

Bradycardia, tachycardia, atrioventricular block, nodal rhythm, hypotension; increased oral, pharyngeal, bronchial secretions; bronchospasm, respiratory depression, seizures, dysarthria, headaches, lacrimation, miosis, visual changes, nausea, emesis, flatulence, increased peristalsis, rash, urticaria, allergic reactions, anaphylaxis

Precautions and contraindications

Use edrophonium with caution in patients with bradycardia, bronchial asthma, cardiac arrhythmias, peptic ulcer, peritonitis, or mechanical obstruction of the intestines or urinary tract.

Overdosage may induce a cholinergic crisis characterized by nausea, vomiting, bradycardia or tachycardia, excessive salivation and sweating, bronchospasm, weakness, and paralysis. Treatment involves discontinuation of edrophonium and administration of atropine, 10 mcg/kg intravenously every 10 minutes until muscarinic symptoms disappear.

Owing to the brief duration of action of edrophonium, neostigmine or pyridostigmine is generally preferred for reversal of the effects of nondepolarizing muscle relaxants.

Anesthetic considerations

Administer with an anticholinergic to avoid cholinergic side effects (e.g., bronchoconstriction, bradycardia). Edrophonium is not recommended when deep block is present.

EMLA (MIXTURE OF LIDOCAINE/PRILOCAINE)

Classification

Local anesthetic

Indications

Topical local anesthesia

Dose

Adults: A thick layer of lidocaine/prilocaine cream is applied to intact skin and covered with an occlusive dressing, or alternatively, a lidocaine/prilocaine anesthetic disc is applied to intact skin:

- *Minor dermal procedures:* For minor procedures such as intravenous cannulation and venipuncture, apply 2.5 g of lidocaine/prilocaine cream ($\frac{1}{2}$ the 5-g tube) over 20 to 25 cm^2 of skin surface, or 1 lidocaine/prilocaine anesthetic disc (1 g over 10 cm^2) for at least 1 hour.

In controlled clinical trials using lidocaine; prilocaine cream, two sites were usually prepared in case there was a technical problem with cannulation or venipuncture at the first site.
- *Major dermal procedures:* For more painful dermatologic procedures involving a larger skin area such as split-thickness skin graft harvesting, apply 2 g of lidocaine/prilocaine cream per 10 cm^2 of skin and allow to remain in contact with the skin for at least 2 hours.

Pediatrics: 0 up to 3 months or less than 5 kg: 1 g over 10 cm^2 of skin for up to 1 hours maximum; 3 up to 12 months and more than 5 kg: 2 g over 20 cm^2 of skin for up to 4 hours maximum; 1 to 6 years and more than 10 kg: 10 g over 100 cm^2 of skin for up to 4 hours maximum; 7 to 12 years and more than 20 kg: 20 g over 200 cm^2 of skin for up to 4 hours maximum.

Onset and duration

The onset, depth, and duration of dermal analgesia on intact skin provided by EMLA depend primarily on the duration of application. To provide sufficient analgesia for clinical procedures such as venipuncture, EMLA should be applied under an occlusive dressing for at least 1 hour. To provide dermal analgesia for clinical procedures such as split-thickness skin graft harvesting, EMLA should be applied under occlusive dressing for at least 2 hours. Satisfactory dermal analgesia is achieved 1 hour after application, reaches maximum at 2 to 3 hours, and persists for 1 to 2 hours after removal. Absorption from the genital mucosa is more rapid and onset time is shorter (5 to 10 minutes) than after application to intact skin. After a 5- to 10-minute application of EMLA to female genital mucosa, the average duration of effective analgesia to an argon laser stimulus (which produced a sharp, pricking pain) was 15 to 20 minutes (individual variations in the range of 5 to 45 minutes).

Adverse effects

During or immediately after treatment with lidocaine or prilocaine on intact skin, possible erythema, edema, or abnormal sensation of skin at treatment site

Systemic adverse reactions following appropriate use of EMLA are unlikely because of the small dose absorbed.

Precautions and contraindications

Application of EMLA to larger areas or for longer times than those recommended could result in sufficient absorption of lidocaine and prilocaine to result in serious adverse effects. EMLA is contraindicated in patients who exhibit allergies to amide local anesthetics. EMLA should be used with care in patients with conditions or therapy associated with methemoglobinemia.

Anesthetic considerations

EMLA is generally safe. When EMLA is used, the patient should be aware that the production of dermal analgesia may be accompanied by the block of all sensations in the treated skin. For this reason, the patient should avoid inadvertent trauma to the treated area caused by scratching, rubbing, or exposure to extreme hot or cold temperatures until complete sensation has returned.

ENALAPRILAT (VASOTEC IV)

Classification
Angiotensin-converting enzyme (ACE) inhibitor

Indications
Hypertension

Dose
Intravenous: 0.625 to 1.25 mg over 5 minutes every 6 hours.
  Dosage forms: 1.25 mg/mL, 1- and 2-mL vials.

Onset and duration
Onset: 10 to 15 minutes. Duration: approximately 6 hours.

Adverse effects
Cough, hypotension, renal impairment, angioedema

Precautions and contraindications
Patients taking diuretics may have to adjust the dose while they are receiving ACE inhibitors. Enalaprilat is contraindicated during pregnancy.

Anesthetic considerations
This is a useful addition to antihypertensive drug choices for perioperative use.

ENOXAPARIN (LOVENOX, LOW-MOLECULAR-WEIGHT HEPARIN)

See Appendix 1, Table 26

Classification
Anticoagulant (antithrombotic), inhibiting factors Xa and IIa and only slightly affecting clotting times

Indications
Prevention of postoperative pulmonary embolism (PE) and/or deep vein thrombosis (DVT); reduction of ischemic complications in patients with cardiovascular disease who have unstable angina and non–Q-wave myocardial infarctions.

Dose
Immediately after surgery: 30 mg or 40 mg subcutaneously every 12 hours to prevent DVT or PE; 1 mg/kg subcutaneously every 12 hours with 100 to 325 mg oral aspirin daily to treat patients with unstable angina/non–Q-wave myocardial infarction.

Onset and duration
Onset: subcutaneous: 20 to 60 minutes. Peak effect: 3 to 5 hours. Duration: 12 hours. Elimination half-life: 3 to 4.5 hours.

Adverse effects

Hemorrhage; epidural/subarachnoid or injection site hematomas; thrombocytopenia; increased aspartate aminotransferase; alanine aminotransferase; liver enzymes; chills, fever, urticaria

Precautions and contraindications

Avoid intramuscular injections of enoxaparin. Use it with caution in pregnant patients and those with a history of coagulopathies or gastrointestinal bleeding. Enoxaparin is absolutely contraindicated in patients with active bleeding, thrombocytopenia, a history of heparin-induced thrombocytopenia, and pork or heparin sensitivities.

Anesthetic considerations

Central axis blocks or removal of indwelling catheters should not occur at least 12 hours before or after the last administration of enoxaparin or, conservatively, not within the last 24 hours. Coagulation tests do not need to be routinely ordered while the patient is taking enoxaparin. However, if coagulation tests are abnormal or bleeding occurs, anti–factor Xa is the most sensitive test to indicate therapeutic anticoagulation levels. Treat an overdose with protamine sulfate. Each milligram of protamine will neutralize 1 mg of enoxaparin.

EPHEDRINE SULFATE

Classification

Noncatecholamine sympathomimetic with mixed direct and indirect actions as well as central nervous system effects

Indications

Hypotension, bradycardia

Dose

Intravenous: 5 to 25 mg (or 100 to 300 mcg/kg); intramuscular: 25 to 50 mg; oral: 25 to 50 mg every 3 hours.

Onset and duration

Onset: intravenous: almost immediate; intramuscular: a few minutes. Duration: intravenous: 10 to 60 minutes.

Adverse effects

Hypertension, tachycardia, arrhythmias, pulmonary edema, anxiety, tremors, hyperglycemia, transient hyperkalemia and then hypokalemia, necrosis at the site of injection; possible tolerance

Precautions and contraindications

Use ephedrine cautiously in patients with hypertension and ischemic heart disease. It has an unpredictable effect in patients in whom endogenous catecholamines are depleted; it may produce central nervous system stimulation.

Anesthetic considerations

Ephedrine is associated with an increased risk of arrhythmias. It is potentiated by tricyclic antidepressants and monoamine oxidase inhibitors.

EPINEPHRINE HCL (ADRENALINE CHLORIDE)

Classification
Endogenous catecholamine

Indications
Inotropic support; treatment of anaphylaxis; increase duration of action of local anesthetic; hemostasis; cardiac arrest; bronchodilation

Dose
Cardiac arrest: 0.5 to 1 mg intravenous bolus every 5 minutes as necessary. Inotropic support: 2 to 20 mcg/min (0.1 to 1 mcg/kg/min). Anaphylaxis: 100 to 300 mcg intravenous push, depending on severity.

Onset and duration
Onset: intravenous: immediate. Duration: intravenous: 5 to 10 minutes.

Adverse effects
Restlessness, fear, throbbing headache, tachycardia, tachydysrhythmias, premature ventricular contractions, ventricular tachycardia, ventricular fibrillation, severe hypertension, angina, extension of myocardial infarction, pulmonary edema

Precautions and contraindications
Use epinephrine with caution in patients with coronary artery disease, hypertension, diabetes mellitus, or hyperthyroidism and in patients taking monoamine oxidase inhibitors.

Anesthetic considerations
Epinephrine may be administered through the endotracheal tube.

ESMOLOL (BREVIBLOC)

Classification
Cardioselective β-blocker

Indications
Supraventricular tachycardia (SVT); perioperative hypertension

Dose
SVT: loading: 50 to 200 mcg/kg/min for 1 minute; follow by infusion of 50 mcg/kg/min for 4 minutes. If the desired effect is not achieved, repeat loading dose and increase infusion to 100 mcg/kg/min. May repeat the process up to maximum of 300 mcg/kg/min.

Dosage forms: 10 mg/mL in 10-mL vial for direct intravenous injection. 250 mg/mL in 10-mL ampule for intravenous infusion.

Onset and duration
Onset: 1 to 2 minutes. Duration: 10 to 20 minutes. Peak effect: 5 to 6 minutes. Not to be infused for more than 48 hours.

Adverse effects

Hypotension, bradycardia, congestive heart failure, bronchospasm, confusion, depression, urinary retention, nausea and vomiting, rash

Precautions and contraindications

Use esmolol with caution in patients with asthma, chronic obstructive pulmonary disease, atrioventricular heart block, or cardiac failure not caused by tachycardia, and diabetes.

Anesthetic considerations

Esmolol may have additive cardiovascular depressant effects when it is coupled with volatile or intravenous anesthetic agents. Use it with caution in bronchospastic patients, owing to minimal cardioselectivity

ETHACRYNIC ACID (EDECRIN)

Classification

Loop diuretic

Indications

Edema of cardiac, hepatic, or renal origin; hypertension, pulmonary edema; usually reserved for patients who do not respond to thiazide diuretics or in whom a rapid onset of diuresis is desired

Dose

0.5 to 1 mg/kg slowly over several minutes up to a maximum of 100 mg in a single dose. The usual average dose is 50 mg. Children: 1 mg/kg over 20 to 30 minutes.

Dosage forms: 50-mg vial, powder for injection; reconstitute by adding 50 mL D_5W or normal saline; tablets: 25, 50 mg.

Onset and duration

Onset: intravenous: 5 to 15 minutes. Duration: intravenous: 2 hours, but may last 6 to 7 hours. Elimination half-life: 1 to 4 hours.

Adverse effects

Fluid and electrolyte imbalance, including hypomagnesemia, hypocalcemia, hypokalemia, hypochloremia, metabolic alkalosis, hyperuricemia; hypoglycemia and hyperglycemia, thrombocytopenia, agranulocytopenia, vertigo, ototoxicity (associated with rapid intravenous injection), pancreatitis, gastrointestinal hemorrhage, hepatotoxicity, hypotension, diarrhea

Precautions and contraindications

Avoid rapid intravenous injection of ethacrynic acid. Use it with extreme caution in patients with impaired renal or hepatic function. It is contraindicated for use in patients once anuric renal failure is established, as well as in patients with hypotension, dehydration with low serum sodium or metabolic alkalosis with hypokalemia, nursing mothers, and infants and severe watery diarrhea.

Anesthetic considerations

Loop diuretics have been reported to increase the neuromuscular blocking effect of nondepolarizing relaxants, possibly because of their potassium-depleting effects.

ETIDOCAINE HCL (DURANEST)

Classification
Amide-type local anesthetic

Indications
Regional anesthesia: infiltration, peripheral nerve block, epidural, caudal

Dose
Infiltration/peripheral nerve block: 50 to 400 mg (1% solution); epidural: 100 to 300 mg (1% or 1.5% solution); caudal: 100 to 300 mg (10 to 30 mL of 1% solution). Children: 0.4 to 0.7 mL/kg (for L2 to T10 level of anesthesia) (maximum dose: 3 mg/kg without epinephrine, 4 mg/kg with epinephrine).

Onset and duration
Onset: infiltration: 3 to 5 minutes; epidural: 5 to 15 minutes. Peak effect: infiltration: 5 to 15 minutes; epidural 15 to 20 minutes. Duration: infiltration: 2 to 3 hours, 3 to 7 hours with epinephrine; epidural: 3 to 5 hours.

Adverse effects
Myocardial depression, arrhythmias, cardiac arrest, hypotension, respiratory depression, anxiety, apprehension, euphoria, tinnitus, seizures, urticaria, edema, nausea and vomiting

Precautions and contraindications
Use etidocaine cautiously in debilitated, elderly, or acutely ill patients, in those with severe shock or heart block, and in pregnancy. It is contraindicated in patients with hypersensitivity to amide-type local anesthetics.

Anesthetic considerations
Do not use etidocaine for spinal anesthesia. Owing to profound motor blockade, it is not recommended for epidural anesthesia for delivery. Benzodiazepines increase the seizure threshold.

ETOMIDATE (AMIDATE)

Classification
Central nervous system agent; nonbarbiturate hypnotic without analgesic activity

Indications
Induction of general anesthesia

Dose
Adult: intravenous: 0.2 to 0.3 mg/kg over 30 to 60 seconds.
Dosage forms: injection: 2 mg/mL, ampules and prefilled syringe.

Onset and duration
Onset: 1 minute. Duration: 3 to 10 minutes. Metabolized in liver, half-life: 75 minutes; excreted primarily in the urine.

Adverse effects

Myoclonus, tonic movements, eye movements, hypertension, hypotension, tachycardia, bradycardia, and other arrhythmias, postoperative nausea and vomiting, hypoventilation, hyperventilation, transient apnea, laryngospasm, hiccups, snoring, adrenocortical suppression

Precautions and contraindications

Use etomidate cautiously in immunosuppressed patients. Its safety during pregnancy, in nursing women, and in children younger than 4 years has not been established.

Anesthetic considerations

Use etomidate with caution in patients with steroid deficiency. Use the large veins. Myoclonus is reduced by premedication with a benzodiazepine or an opioid.

FAMOTIDINE (PEPCID)

Classification

Histamine (H_2) antagonist

Indications

Treatment of duodenal or gastric ulcers and gastroesophageal reflux; prophylaxis of aspiration pneumonitis in patients at high risk during surgery

Dose

Prophylaxis of aspiration pneumonitis: adults: 20 to 40 mg orally the evening before surgery and/or the morning of surgery before induction of anesthesia. If a more rapid onset is desired, 2 mL of intravenous famotidine (10 mg/mL) may be diluted to a concentration of 5 to 10 mL with D_5W, normal saline, or lactated Ringer's solution and given over at least 2 minutes before induction.

Dosage forms: tablets: 20, 40 mg; parenteral injection: 10 mg/mL in 2- or 4-mL vials.

Onset and duration

Onset: 20 to 45 minutes. Peak serum levels occur 1 to 3 hours orally. Duration: Plasma famotidine concentrations that suppress gastric acid secretion by 50% are maintained for 12 hours following an oral dose of 40 mg and 7 to 9 hours after a 20-mg dose.

Adverse effects

Headache (2% to 4.5%), constipation (1.4%), and drowsiness (most frequently reported); mental confusion in elderly patients (occasionally)

Potential bradydysrhythmias and hypotension may be associated with rapid infusion.

Precautions and contraindications

Caution suggested in patients with hepatic or renal dysfunction (possible dose reductions required). This drug is contraindicated in patients with known hypersensitivity to famotidine or other H_2 antagonists.

Anesthetic considerations
Famotidine is a safe alternative to gastric prophylaxis preoperatively.

FENOLDOPAM (CORLOPAM)

Classification
Antihypertensive (dopamine DA-1-receptor agonist)

Indications
A potent vasodilator that stimulates the postsynaptic dopamine DA-receptors, thereby lowering blood pressure, peripheral vascular resistance, renal vascular resistance, and increasing cardiac hemodynamics; short-term use (up to 48 hours) for patients with severe hypertension/malignant hypertension

Dose
Administer fenoldopam as a continuous infusion; no loading dose is needed. The infusion range is 0.04 to 0.8 mcg/kg/min, titrate slowly for blood pressure reduction. Initial doses less than 0.1 mcg/kg/min are marginally antihypertensive but have less reflex tachycardia. Initial doses higher than 0.3 mcg/kg/min or more have been associated with reflex tachycardia.

Onset and duration
Onset: 5 minutes. Peak effect: 15 minutes. Rapidly metabolized; half-life: 5 minutes.

Adverse effects
Reflex tachycardia with a higher initial dosing regimen possibly causing increased intraocular pressure, hypotension, hypokalemia (infusion time greater than 6 hours can cause potassium to fall to less than 3 mEq), headache, flushing, nausea

Precautions and contraindications
Fenoldopam has no absolute contraindications. Use it with caution in patients with severe hepatic disease. It contains a metabisulfite compound, so do not use this drug in patients sensitive to sulfites (especially asthmatic patients) because allergic reaction may result. The concomitant use of other antihypertensive agents (calcium channel blockers, nitrates, β_1-blockers, and α_2-blockers) may result in unexpected hypotension.

Anesthetic considerations
Titrate the drug slowly to prevent reflex tachycardia. Check the patient's potassium level if titrating a long-term infusion (greater than 6 hours). Review for sulfite allergies, especially in patients with asthma. Use with caution in patients with open globe injuries or glaucoma because fenoldopam may increase intraocular pressure. It is generally used as an alternative to nitroprusside.

FENTANYL (SUBLIMAZE, DURAGESIC, ORALET)

Classification
Opioid agonist

Indications

Analgesia and anesthesia

Dose

Analgesia: intravenous: 1 to 2 mcg/kg.

Induction: 30 mcg/kg; infusion: 0.2 mcg/kg/min. Epidural bolus: 1 to 2 mcg/kg; infusion: 2 to 60 mcg/hour. Spinal bolus: 0.1 to 0.4 mcg/kg. Dosage form: injection: 0.05 mg/mL; transdermal patch: 100 mcg/hour. In conjunction with epidural administration: 1 to 2 mcg/kg. For infusion with epidural: 2 to 60 mcg/hour. In conjunction with spinal anesthesia: bolus dose of 0.1 to 0.4 mcg/kg.

Onset and duration

Onset: intravenous: within 30 seconds; intramuscular: less than 8 minutes; epidural/spinal: 4 to 10 minutes. Duration: intravenous: 30 to 60 minutes; intramuscular: 1 to 2 hours; epidural/spinal; 4 to 8 hours.

Adverse effects

Hypotension, bradycardia, respiratory depression, apnea, dizziness, blurred vision, seizures, nausea, emesis, delayed gastric emptying, biliary tract spasm, muscle rigidity

Precautions and contraindications

Reduce fentanyl doses in elderly, hypovolemic, and high-risk patients and with concomitant use of sedatives and other narcotics. It crosses the placental barrier; it may produce depression of respiration in the neonate. Prolonged depression may occur after cessation of transdermal patch use.

Anesthetic considerations

Narcotic effects reversed by naloxone (0.2 to 0.4 mg intravenously). Circulatory and ventilatory depressant effects potentiated by narcotics, sedatives, volatile anesthetics, nitrous oxide, and possibly monoamine oxidase inhibitors, phenothiazines, and tricyclic antidepressants; analgesia enhanced by α_2-agonists. Muscle rigidity in higher dose range sufficient to interfere with ventilation.

FLUMAZENIL (ROMAZICON)

Classification

Benzodiazepine-receptor antagonist

Indications

Reversal of benzodiazepine-receptor agonist

Dose

Intravenous: 0.2 to 1 mg (4 to 20 mcg/kg), titrate to patient response, may repeat at 20-minute intervals (maximum single dose: 1 mg; maximum total dose: 3 mg in any 1 hour).

Dosage form: injection: 0.1 mg/mL.

Onset and duration

Onset: 1 to 2 minutes. Duration: 30 to 90 minutes, depending on the dose of flumazenil and plasma concentration of benzodiazepine to be reversed.

Adverse effects

Arrhythmia, tachycardia, bradycardia, hypertension, angina, flushing, reversal of sedation, seizures, agitation, emotional lability, nausea and vomiting, pain at injection site, thrombophlebitis

Precautions and contraindications

Institute measures to secure airway, ventilation, and intravenous access before administering flumazenil. Resedation may occur and is more common with large doses of long-acting benzodiazepines.

Anesthetic considerations

Do not use flumazenil until the effects of neuromuscular blockade have been fully reversed. Administer it in a large vein to minimize pain at the injection site. Monitor the patient for resedation.

FUROSEMIDE (LASIX)

Classification

Loop diuretic

Indications

Edema of cardiac, hepatic, or renal origin; hypertension, pulmonary and cerebral edema; usually reserved for patients who do not respond to thiazide diuretics or in whom a rapid onset of diuresis is desired

Dose

Diuresis: adult: 20 to 40 mg intramuscularly or intravenously as a single dose. Intravenous doses should be injected slowly over 1 to 2 minutes. Additional doses of 20 mg greater than the previous dose may be given every 2 hours until desired response is obtained. For intravenous bolus injections, do not exceed 1 g/day given over 30 minutes. Acute pulmonary edema: 40 mg intravenously initially; may repeat in 1 hour with 80 mg if necessary. Children: intramuscular or intravenous: 1 mg/kg single dose initially, increasing by 1 mg/kg every 2 hours or more until desired response is obtained or to a maximum of 6 mg/kg/day.

Dosage forms: tablets: 20, 40, 80 mg; injection: 10 mg/mL; oral solutions: 10 mg/mL and 40 mg/5 mL.

Onset and duration

Onset: intravenous: onset of diuresis usually occurs in 5 minutes. Duration: 2 hours. Elimination half-life: widely variable; normal is $\frac{1}{2}$ to 1 hour, but a period of 11 to 20 hours has been reported in patients with hepatic or renal insufficiency.

Adverse effects

Dehydration, hypotension, hypochloremic alkalosis, hypokalemia, hypomagnesemia, hyperglycemia, hyperuricemia

Ototoxicity has been reported with too rapid intravenous injection of large doses. Rarely reported are thrombocytopenia, neutropenia, jaundice, pancreatitis, and a variety of skin reactions.

Precautions and contraindications

Furosemide is contraindicated in anuria (except for a single dose in acute anuria) and pregnancy. Use it with caution in patients with severe or progressive renal disease and hepatic disease. Discontinue it if renal function worsens. Caution should be used in patients allergic to sulfonamides and patients with severe electrolyte imbalance.

Anesthetic considerations

Monitor electrolytes and fluid balance. Administer furosemide carefully in patients taking digitalis. It may be associated with enhancement of nondepolarizing neuromuscular blocking drugs.

GLUCAGON

Classification

Hormone; antidiabetic agent (antihypoglycemic); diagnostic agent

Indications

Treatment of hypoglycemia or β-blocker overdose; inotropic agent used to relax smooth muscle of gastrointestinal tract for radiologic studies; anaphylaxis resistant to epinephrine

Dose

Diagnostic aid for radiologic examination: intravenous/intramuscular: 0.25 to 2 mg before initiation of radiologic procedure. Hypoglycemia: intravenous/intramuscular/subcutaneous: 0.5 to 1 mg.

Onset and duration

Onset: less than 5 minutes. Peak effect: 5 to 20 minutes. Duration: 10 to 30 minutes.

Adverse effects

Hypertension, hypotension, respiratory distress, dizziness, lightheadedness, nausea and vomiting, urticaria, hypoglycemia, hyperglycemia

Precautions and contraindications

Glucagon is contraindicated in patients with a hypersensitivity to the drug (owing to its protein nature). Use it cautiously in patients with history of insulinoma or pheochromocytoma. Safe use during pregnancy and in nursing women has not been established.

Anesthetic considerations

Rapid intravenous administration may cause a decrease in blood pressure. It potentiates the hypoprothrombinemic effects of anticoagulants. Parenteral glucose must be given because release of insulin may subsequently cause hypoglycemia.

GLYCOPYRROLATE (ROBINUL)

Classification

Competitive acetylcholine antagonist at muscarinic receptor

Indications

Vagolytic premedication to block bradycardia from stimulation of the carotid sinus or traction on abdominal viscera or extraocular muscles during surgery; blockade of muscarinic effects of anticholinesterases; adjunctive therapy in the treatment of bronchospasm and peptic ulcer disease

Compared with atropine, glycopyrrolate has twice the potent antisialagogue activity, less tachycardia, and no clinically significant increases in intraocular pressure at doses used preoperatively. It has no sedative effects.

Dose

Adults: Premedication/vagolysis: intravenous, intramuscular, subcutaneous: 0.1 to 2 mg (4 to 6 mcg/kg) administered 30 to 60 minutes preinduction; may repeat in 2- to 3-minute intervals for vagolysis up to 1 mg total. Blockade of muscarinic effects of anticholinesterase: 0.2 mg for each 1 mg of neostigmine or 5 mg of pyridostigmine. Bronchospasm: inhalation 0.4 to 0.8 mg every 8 hours; dilute injectate solution in 2 to 3 mL normal saline and deliver by compressed air nebulizer.

Children: preoperative 2 years or older: 4 mcg/kg. For oral administration, use injectable solution and dilute in 3 to 5 mL juice or carbonated cola beverage. Oral absorption is erratic. Intraoperative vagolysis: 0.01 mg/kg intravenously not to exceed 0.1 mg; may repeat in 2 to 3 minutes.

Dosage forms: injection: 0.2 mg/mL; tablets: 1, 2 mg.

Onset and duration

Onset: oral: 1 hour; intramuscular/subcutaneous: 15 to 30 minutes; inhalation: 3 to 5 minutes; intravenous administration: less than 1 minute. Duration: antisialagogue effect: 7 to 12 hours, depending on the route of administration and dose; vagal blockade: 2 to 3 hours intravenously, 8 to 12 hours orally.

Adverse effects

Tachycardia (high doses), headache, urinary hesitancy, retention, decreased sweating, dry nose and mouth, constipation

Precautions and contraindications

Avoid glycopyrrolate when tachycardia would be harmful (i.e., thyrotoxicosis, pheochromocytoma, coronary artery disease). Avoid it in hyperpyrexial states because it inhibits sweating. Use it with caution in patients with hepatic or renal disease, congestive heart failure, chronic pulmonary disease (because a reduction in bronchial secretions may lead to formation of bronchial plugs), hiatal hernia, gastroesophageal reflux, gastrointestinal infections, and ulcerative colitis. It is contraindicated in acute-angle glaucoma, obstructive disease of the gastrointestinal tract, obstructive uropathy, paralytic ileus, intestinal atony, and acute hemorrhage in patients whose cardiovascular status is unstable.

Anesthetic considerations

Additive anticholinergic effects may occur with meperidine, some antihistamines, phenothiazines, tricyclic antidepressants, and antiarrhythmic drugs that possess anticholinergic activity (e.g., quinidine, disopyramide, procainamide). It is the preferred agent in pregnant patients over atropine and scopolamine because it does not cross the placental barrier.

PART III **Drugs**

GRANISETRON (KYTRIL)

Classification
Selective serotonin receptor antagonist

Indications
Effective single agent used to control nausea and vomiting induced by cisplatin and other cytotoxic agents and for postoperative nausea and vomiting

Dose
The recommended dosage for prevention of postoperative nausea and vomiting is 1 mg.

Onset and duration
Onset: peak plasma concentrations demonstrate wide interindividual variation. After a 40 mcg/kg dose, nausea and vomiting subside within several minutes. Duration: serum levels decline to less than 10 ng/mL at 24 hours following a single 40 mcg/kg infusion. Antiemetic effects last up to 24 hours following intravenous infusion of 40 mcg/kg.

Adverse effects
Headache and constipation (most common); also somnolence, dizziness, diarrhea, flushing, transient elevation of liver enzymes

Precautions and contraindications
Previous hypersensitivity to granisetron or ondansetron, liver disease (owing to the noted elevation of liver enzymes after repeat administration of granisetron), pregnancy, and breast-feeding are contraindications.

Anesthetic considerations
The injection should not be mixed in solution with other drugs. No specific antidote for overdose exists; give symptomatic treatment. Inducers or inhibitors of cytochrome P450 drug-metabolizing enzymes may change the clearance and duration of granisetron.

HALOTHANE (FLUOTHANE)

Classification
Volatile inhalation anesthetic agent

Indications
Induction and maintenance of general anesthesia

Dose
Induction: 1% to 4%. Maintenance: 0.5% to 1.5%. Supplied: glass bottle, volatile liquid.

Onset and duration
Onset: 5 to 10 minutes to achieve surgical anesthesia. Duration: up to 1 hour after discontinuation; dose-dependent; rapid, pleasant induction and smooth emergence.

Adverse effects

Hypotension, shallow and rapid respiration, arrhythmias (when sympathomimetic agents are used), vomiting, hypoxia, respiratory difficulty, postoperative shivering, liver damage, bradycardia, increased intracranial pressure, malignant hyperthermia

Precautions and contraindications

Arrhythmia may be produced by the combination of halothane and catecholamines. It may potentiate effects of nondepolarizing muscle relaxants. Avoid its use in patients who show evidence of liver damage. Halothane has been associated with liver dysfunction (hepatitis, jaundice), especially in persons with prior hepatic disease or previous exposure to halothane. Changes in mental function may persist beyond the period of anesthetic administration and the immediate postoperative period.

Anesthetic considerations

Use halothane cautiously in patients with severe cardiac disease and during pregnancy (the drug is a potent uterine relaxant). Have drugs available to treat bradycardia and hypotension.

HEPARIN

Classification

Anticoagulant; accelerates the rate at which antithrombin III neutralizes thrombin and factors VII, IX, X, and XI

Indications

Prophylaxis and treatment of deep venous thrombosis (DVT) and pulmonary thromboembolism (PE); acute arterial occlusion, intracardiac mural thrombosis, following myocardial infarction after intravenous thrombolytic treatment, disseminated intravascular coagulation with gross thrombosis, anticoagulation during cardiopulmonary bypass (CPB), prophylaxis of thromboembolism in patients with mitral valve disease or atrial fibrillation; maintenance of patency of indwelling venipuncture devices (lock flush).

The value of this drug in transient ischemic attacks secondary to cerebral embolism has not been established.

Dose

Dosage is highly individualized and based on daily activated partial thromboplastin time (aPTT) compared with aPTT 6 hours after each dosage change. Obtain baseline aPTT and adjust dose according to clinical state. For prophylaxis (i.e., hip surgery, atrial fibrillation, valve disease): the ratio of aPTT to baseline aPTT should be 1.2 to 1.5; for prosthetic heart valves, DVT, PE, recurrent embolism: 1.5 to 2. For CPB, monitor activated clotting time (ACT) and maintain ACT of 400 to 480 seconds. Baseline ACT values are 80 to 150 seconds. ACT should be determined 5 minutes after heparin administration. Adequate heparinization must be ensured before initiation of CPB.

CPB: before induction of anesthesia, 300 units/kg should be prepared in case emergency initiation of CPB is necessary. Intravenous bolus: 350 to 400 units/kg. Up to 500 units/kg may be required to maintain ACT greater than 400 seconds in heparin-resistant patients. Additional heparin will be needed for prolonged CPB. A 100 unit/kg hourly reinforcement dose is given starting 2 hours after the initial dose.

Prophylactic or low-dose subcutaneous therapy: 5000 units subcutaneously every 8 to 12 hours. Baseline aPTT is obtained because bleeding complications are occasionally discovered, but routine PTT monitoring is not necessary. For surgical prophylaxis, ideally started 2 hours preoperatively.

Full-dose continuous intravenous infusion for treatment of DVT or PE is based on ideal body weight: intravenous bolus loading dose: 70 units/kg (3000 to 10,000 units); intravenous maintenance dose: continuous infusion 13 to 16 units/kg/hour (750 to 1300 units/hour). For continuous intravenous infusion, 25,000 units heparin may be mixed in 500 mL D_5W or normal saline. The resulting solution is 50 units/mL.

Dosage forms: injection: 1000, 2500, 5000, 7500, 10,000, 20,000, and 40,000 units/mL; lock flush solution: 10 units, 100 units/mL; premixed infusion in dextrose: 50 units/mL; premixed infusion in normal saline: 50 units, 100 units/mL.

Onset and duration

Onset: intravenous: immediate; subcutaneous: 20 to 30 minutes. Elimination half-life: 1 to 2 hours in healthy adults. Duration: half-life and duration increase with increasing doses; prolonged in liver and renal disease.

Adverse effects

Hemorrhage, thrombocytopenia, white-clot syndrome (rare paradoxical thrombosis), necrotizing skin lesions, elevated liver enzymes, osteoporosis, priapism, hypersensitivity

Precautions and contraindications

Avoid intramuscular injections of heparin. It is contraindicated in patients with hemophilia, thrombocytopenia, acute bleeding, peptic ulcer, esophagitis, diverticulitis, esophageal varices, arterial aneurysm, gastrointestinal or urinary tract malignancy, vascular retinopathy, recent liver or renal biopsy, acute pericarditis, threatened abortion, infective endocarditis, recent regional anesthesia, severe hypertension, recent cerebrovascular accident, recent surgery, or trauma to brain, eye, or spinal cord.

Platelet counts, hematocrit, and occult blood in stool and urine should be monitored during the entire course of therapy. An increased risk of bleeding exists with the concomitant use of aspirin, nonsteroidal antiinflammatory drugs, dipyridamole, thrombolytic agents, dextran, dihydroergotamine, and warfarin. Intravenous nitroglycerin may antagonize the effects of heparin and should be administered via a separate line if possible. Digoxin, nicotine, propranolol, antihistamines, and tetracycline may reduce heparin's effects.

Bleeding and heparin overdosage may be treated with protamine sulfate; 1 mg protamine neutralizes 100 units heparin.

Anesthetic considerations

Regional anesthesia is contraindicated. A heparin continuous intravenous infusion should be discontinued 4 to 6 hours preoperatively, and the aPTT should be checked to ensure return to baseline.

HETASTARCH (HESPAN)

Classification
Plasma expander, anticoagulant

Indications
Adjunct for plasma volume expansion in shock resulting from hemorrhage, burns, sepsis, surgery, or other trauma; mild anticoagulant effects following vascular procedures

Dose
Plasma volume expansion from 500 to 1000 mL. Total dosage does not usually exceed 1500 mL/day (20 mL/kg/day). In acute hemorrhagic shock, rates approaching 20 mL/kg/hour have been used.

Dosage forms: 6% solution in 0.9% sodium chloride, 500-mL intravenous infusion bottle.

Onset and duration
Onset: 15 to 30 minutes. Duration: 24 to 48 hours. Average half-life: 17 days.

Adverse effects
Anaphylactic reactions (periorbital edema, urticaria, wheezing); peripheral edema of the lower extremities, chills, mild temperature elevation, muscle pain

Large volumes may alter coagulation times and may result in transient prolongation of prothrombin time, partial thromboplastin time, bleeding, decreased hematocrit, excessive dilution of plasma proteins.

Precautions and contraindications
Hetastarch is contraindicated in patients with severe bleeding disorders, severe cardiac failure, and renal failure with oliguria or anuria. Hetastarch does not have oxygen-carrying capacity, nor does it contain plasma proteins such as coagulation factors. Therefore, it is not a substitute for blood or plasma.

Anesthetic considerations
Infuse it slowly to avoid volume overload. Check the patient's coagulation profile.

HYALURONIDASE (WYDASE, VITRASE)

Classification
Enzyme

Indications
Adjunct to increase absorption and dispersion of other injected drugs such as local anesthetics; hypodermoclysis; subcutaneous urography

Dose
Adjunct: 150 units to injection medium containing other medication. Hypodermoclysis (adults and children older than 3 years of age): 150 units

injected subcutaneously before clysis or injected into clysis tubing near needle for each 1000-mL clysis solution. Subcutaneous urography (patient prone): 75 units subcutaneously over each scapula, followed by injection of contrast medium at the same sites.

Onset and duration
Onset: immediate. Duration: 30 to 60 minutes.

Adverse effects
Rash, urticaria, local irritation

Precautions and contraindications
Use hyaluronidase with caution in patients with blood-clotting abnormalities or severe hepatic or renal disease. Avoid injecting it into diseased areas, to prevent spread of infection.

Anesthetic considerations
It is useful to prevent thrombus formation during vascular procedures as well as for volume expansion. It is also a useful addition for promoting the spread of local anesthetics.

HYDRALAZINE (APRESOLINE)

Classification
Direct-acting arterial vasodilator

Indications
Antihypertensive; vasodilator

Dose
Intravenous and intramuscular: 2.5 to 40 mg (0.1 to 0.2 mg/kg); oral: 10 to 100 mg four times daily.
　　Dosage forms: injection: 20 mg/mL; tablets: 10, 25, 50, and 100 mg.

Onset and duration
Onset: intravenous: 5 to 20 minutes; intramuscular: 10 to 30 minutes; oral: 30 to 120 minutes. Duration: intravenous: 2 to 4 hours; intramuscular/oral: 2 to 8 hours.

Adverse effects
Hypotension, paradoxical pressor response, tachycardia, palpitations, angina, dyspnea, nasal congestion, peripheral neuritis, depression, anxiety, headache, dizziness, nausea and vomiting, diarrhea, lupuslike syndrome, rash, urticaria, eosinophilia, hypersensitivity, leukopenia, splenomegaly, agranulocytosis

Precautions and contraindications
Use hydralazine cautiously in patients with coronary artery disease and mitral valvular rheumatic heart disease, as well as in patients receiving monoamine oxidase inhibitors.

Anesthetic considerations
One may see a reduced response to epinephrine. Enhanced hypotensive effects occur in patients receiving diuretics, monoamine oxidase inhibitors,

diazoxide, and other antihypertensives. It primarily dilates the arterial vasculature.

HYDROCORTISONE SODIUM SUCCINATE (A-HYDROCORT, SOLU-CORTEF)

Classification
Corticosteroid (glucocorticoid and mineralocorticoid properties)

Indications
Treatment of choice for steroid-replacement therapy; also antiinflammatory and immunosuppressive agent, although glucocorticoids (prednisone) preferred for this use; adjunctive therapy in anaphylaxis to prevent prolonged antigen-antibody reactions; adjunctive treatment of ulcerative colitis (enema)

Dose
Adults: shock: 500 mg to 2 g (succinate) intravenously every 2 to 6 hours until the condition stabilized. Not recommended beyond 48 to 72 hours. Adjunctive therapy in anaphylaxis: hydrocortisone phosphate or succinate intravenously 5 mg/kg initially, then 2.5 mg/kg every 6 hours. Adrenal insufficiency: acute, precipitated by trauma or surgical stress: If adrenocorticotropic hormone testing is not being performed, 200 to 300 mg intravenous hydrocortisone succinate over several minutes, then 100 mg intravenously every 6 hours for 24 hours. If the patient is stable, dosage tapering may begin on the second day. Consider steroid replacement in any patient who has received corticosteroid therapy for at least 1 month in the past 6 to 12 months, with 50 to 100 mg intravenously (succinate) before, during, and after surgery. For intraarticular, soft tissue, and intrasynovial injections, use acetate only (acetate is not for intravenous use): 10 to 50 mg combined with local anesthetic such as procaine. Injections may be repeated every 3 to 5 days (for bursae) to once every 1 to 4 weeks (for joints).

Children: 0.16 to 1 mg/kg or 6 to 30 mg/m^2 (phosphate or succinate) intramuscularly or intravenously one or two times daily. The dose depends on the disease being treated.

Onset and duration
Onset: intravenous/intramuscular: 5 minutes. Duration: approximates the duration of hypothalamus-pituitary-adrenal axis suppression (i.e., 30 to 36 hours); after a single oral dose of hydrocortisone, this is 1.25 to 1.5 days.

Adverse effects
Glaucoma and cataracts (long-term therapy); muscle weakness, sodium retention, edema, hypokalemic alkalosis, hyperglycemia, Cushing's syndrome, peptic ulcer, increased appetite, delayed wound healing, psychotic behavior, congestive heart failure, hypertension, growth suppression, pancreatitis.

Acute adrenal insufficiency may occur with abrupt withdrawal after long-term therapy. Withdrawal symptoms include rebound inflammation, fatigue, weakness, arthralgia, fever, dizziness, lethargy, depression, orthostatic hypotension, dyspnea, anorexia, and hypoglycemia.

PART III **Drugs**

Precautions and contraindications

Hydrocortisone is contraindicated in patients with systemic fungal infections. It may mask or exacerbate infections. Use it with caution in patients with ocular herpes simplex or a history of peptic ulcer disease. In patients with myasthenia gravis, hydrocortisone interacts with anticholinesterase agents to produce severe weakness.

Anesthetic considerations

Hypotension from the stress of anesthesia and surgery may occur if regular doses of steroids were taken within 2 months preceding surgery. Supplemental steroids are indicated commencing with preoperative dose and continuing for 3 days for major surgery, for 24 hours for minor surgery, and one dose for a very brief procedure, then taper to normal therapy.

Because of adrenal suppression, etomidate should be avoided in patients with adrenal insufficiency.

IBUTILIDE FUMARATE (CORVERT)

Classification

Class III antiarrhythmic; cardiac action potential prolongation

Indications

Rapid conversion of atrial fibrillation/flutter of acute onset (less than 90 days) to sinus rhythm

Dose

Adults weighing more than 60 kg: 1 vial (1 mg) infused over 10 minutes (may be repeated once in 10 minutes after completion of first dose). Adults weighing less than 60 kg: 0.01 mL/kg infused over 10 minutes (may be repeated once in 10 minutes after completion of first dose). Not recommended for pediatric patients.

Onset and duration

Onset: intravenous: immediate, for antiarrhythmic properties. Peak effect: 10 minutes. Half-life: 6 hours. Atrial arrhythmias usually convert within 30 minutes after ibutilide therapy begins. Duration: 10 to 30 minutes.

Adverse effects

Ventricular arrhythmias (often sustained torsades de pointes), heart block, congestive heart failure, bradycardia, tachycardia, hypotension, nausea, headache

Precautions and contraindications

The drug is contraindicated with patients sensitive to ibutilide, those with second- or third-degree atrioventricular heart blocks or prolonged QT interval, and during pregnancy.

Anesthetic considerations

The risk of pro-arrhythmias/polymorphic ventricular tachycardia is increased when ibutilide is used with other drugs that prolong the QT interval (phenothiazines, procainamide, quinidine, antihistamines). Electrocardiographic monitoring for 4 hours after drug therapy is mandatory because arrhythmias (premature ventricular contractions, ventricular tachycardia, tachycardia, bradycardia, varying degrees of heart blocks) can take place. Have emergency equipment available to perform overdrive pacing, defibrillate, or cardiovert the patient. Monitor serum potassium and magnesium because deficiencies in these electrolytes can precipitate polymorphic ventricular tachycardia.

INSULIN REGULAR (RAPID-ACTING) (HUMULIN R, NOVOLIN R, REGULAR ILETIN II)

See Appendix I, Table 12.

Classification

Antidiabetic agent

Indications

Diabetic ketoacidosis, treatment of diabetes mellitus, hyperkalemia

Dose

• Diabetes mellitus: in general, therapy is initiated with regular insulin, subcutaneously 5 to 10 units in adults and 2 to 4 units in children 15 to 30 minutes before meals and at bedtime. Dose and frequency are carefully individualized, based on blood glucose monitoring every 4 to 6 hours. After satisfactory control is achieved, an intermediate form of insulin may be substituted; this is given before breakfast in a dose approximately two thirds to three fourths that of the previous total daily dose established for regular insulin. Treatment plans are highly variable and patient dependent.

• Perioperative management of insulin-dependent diabetics: half the usual NPH-isophane insulin dose the morning of the day of surgery. It is critical for the patient who is receiving nothing orally and receiving insulin also to receive an intravenous infusion of dextrose 5 to 10 g/hour (equal to 100 to 200 mL of a 5% dextrose solution) to prevent hypoglycemia.

• Postoperative: sliding scale every 4 to 6 hours. Individualize to the patient.

Blood Sugar	Insulin Regular
Less than 200 mg/dL	0 units
200 to 250 mg/dL	5 units subcutaneously
250 to 300 mg/dL	10 units subcutaneously
300 to 350 mg/dL	15 units subcutaneously

• If blood glucose is greater than 350 mg/dL, give insulin regular, 15 units subcutaneously plus intravenously 1 to 2 units/hour. Monitor blood glucose hourly. Correct electrolyte imbalances (hypokalemia, hypophosphatemia) and acidosis.

• Diabetic ketoacidosis: requires insulin by continuous infusion, hourly blood glucose determination, and correction of acidosis, dehydration, and electrolyte imbalances. After renal function is established, potassium replacement therapy may be needed.

• Dosage form: injection: 100 units/mL. U500 Insulin (500 units/mL) is available but should be used only to fill implanted insulin pumps. It should never be stocked outside the pharmacy.

Onset and duration

	Onset (hr)	Peak (hr)	Duration (hr)
Regular (rapid) insulin	0.5 to 1	1 to 5	5 to 8
Intermediate insulins	1 to 4	4 to 12	24 to 28

PART III **Drugs**

Adverse effects

Dose-related hypoglycemia; local allergic reactions, lipoatrophy, and resistance (overcome by switching to more highly purified sources); anaphylaxis

In general, human insulin is least antigenic and pork is less antigenic than beef-pork or pure beef insulin.

Precautions and contraindications

- Diabetic ketoacidosis is a life-threatening condition requiring prompt diagnosis and treatment.
- Changes in purity, strength, brand, type, or species source may result in the need for a change in insulin dosage.
- Treat hypoglycemia with 0.6 mL/kg 50% dextrose intravenously.
- Hypersensitivity may occur.
- Insulin requirements may increase dramatically with stress, sepsis, trauma, or pregnancy.
- Only regular insulins (clear insulins) may be administered intravenously. Intermediate insulins may only be given subcutaneously.
- Hypoglycemic action is increased by the concomitant administration of alcohol, β-blockers, monoamine oxidase inhibitors, salicylates, and sulfonylureas.
- Hypoglycemic action is decreased by thyroid hormones, corticosteroids, dobutamine, epinephrine, furosemide, and phenytoin.

Anesthetic considerations

Blood glucose levels of 120 to 180 mg/dL should be sought, and blood glucose should be monitored frequently intraoperatively. If it is necessary to administer insulin intraoperatively, continuous intravenous infusion may be the best method. If it is given subcutaneously, variability of skin blood flow during anesthesia may cause unpredictable results.

Large intravenous boluses of insulin can put the patient at risk for dysrhythmias caused by intracellular shifts of potassium, phosphorus, and magnesium.

IPRATROPIUM BROMIDE (ATROVENT)

Classification

Anticholinergic, bronchodilator (parasympatholytic)

Indications

Treatment and prevention of bronchospasm resulting from chronic obstructive pulmonary disease (COPD), including emphysema and chronic bronchitis

Dose

Metered-dose inhaler in adults: two to four sprays (initially, 18 mcg/spray), then two sprays every 4 hours (maximum dose: 216 mcg or 12 sprays/day).

Oral nebulizer in adults: 500 mcg w/2.5 mL normal saline mixed via oral nebulization every 6 to 8 hours; may mix with albuterol in nebulizer if used within 1 hour of mixing.

Onset and duration

Onset: within 15 to 30 minutes. Peak effect: 1 to 2 hours. Duration: 4 to 5 hours.

Adverse effects
Local or systemic anticholinergic effects, angina, blurred vision, headache, dizziness

Precautions and contraindications
Use ipratropium cautiously for patients with narrow-angle glaucoma, bladder obstruction, and benign prostatic hypertrophy. It is contraindicated in patients hypersensitive to soya lecithin or related food products such as soybean and peanut, as well as in patients hypersensitive to ipratropium bromide, atropine, and its derivatives.

Anesthetic considerations
Do not use it for relief of bronchospasm in acute COPD exacerbation as a first-line drug. Use drugs with a faster onset.

ISOFLURANE (FORANE)

Classification
Inhalation anesthetic

Indications
General anesthesia

Dose
Titrate to effect for induction or maintenance of anesthesia. Minimum alveolar concentration: 1.14%.
   Dosage form: volatile liquid: 100 mL.

Onset and duration
Onset: a few minutes, dose-dependent. Duration: emergence time: 15 to 20 minutes.

Adverse effects
Hypotension, tachycardia, arrhythmia, respiratory depression, respiratory irritation, apnea, dizziness, euphoria, increased cerebral blood flow and intracranial pressure, nausea and vomiting, malignant hyperthermia, glucose elevation

Precautions and contraindications
Isoflurane is contraindicated in patients with known or suspected genetic susceptibility to malignant hyperthermia. Changes in mental function may persist beyond the period of anesthetic administration and the immediate postoperative period.

Anesthetic considerations
Anesthetic requirements decrease with age. It crosses the placental barrier. Abrupt onset of malignant hyperthermia may be triggered by isoflurane; early signs include muscle rigidity, especially of the jaw muscles, tachycardia, and tachypnea unresponsive to increased depth of anesthesia.

ISOPROTERENOL HCL (ISUPREL)

Classification
Synthetic sympathomimetic, nonspecific β-agonist

Indications

- For mild or transient episodes of heart block that do not require electric shock or pacemaker therapy
- For serious episodes of heart block and Adams-Stokes attacks (except when caused by ventricular tachycardia or fibrillation)
- For use in cardiac arrest until electric shock or pacemaker therapy, the treatments of choice, is available
- For bronchospasm occuring during anesthesia
- As an adjunct to fluid and electrolyte replacement therapy and the use of other drugs and procedures in the treatment of hypovolemic and septic shock, low cardiac output (hypoperfusion) states, congestive heart failure, and cardiogenic shock

Dose
Intramuscular/subcutaneous: 0.2 mg; intravenous: 0.02 to 0.06 mg; infusion: 2 to 20 mcg/min.

Onset and duration
Onset: intravenous: immediately. Duration: intravenous: 1 to 5 minutes.

Adverse effects
Tachyarrhythmias, hypertension, angina, paradoxical precipitation of Adams-Stokes attacks, pulmonary edema, headache, dizziness, tremors, nausea and vomiting, anorexia; possible exacerbation of ischemia and/or hypertension (when used for chronotropic support)

Precautions and contraindications
Isoproterenol is contraindicated in patients with tachyarrhythmias, tachycardia, or hypertension.

Anesthetic considerations
It is useful as an intravenous infusion for the treatment of refractory brady-cardic states. The bronchodilating effect is better achieved with more specific β_2-agonists.

KETAMINE HCL (KETALAR)

Classification
Intravenous general anesthetic

Indications
Sole anesthetic agent for diagnostic and surgical procedures of short duration; induction of anesthesia in critically ill patients; small doses for outpatient analgesia

Dose

Induction: adult: intravenous: 1 to 4.5 mg/kg slowly over 60 seconds; intramuscular: 4 to 6 mg/kg; oral: 6 to 8 mg/kg. Half of the initial dose may be repeated as needed.

Dosage form: injection: 10, 50, 100 mg/mL.

Onset and duration

Onset: intravenous: 2 to 5 minutes; intramuscular: 3 to 8 minutes; oral: 15 to 20 minutes. Duration: intravenous: 5 to 10 minutes; intramuscular: 12 to 25 minutes; oral: 30 to 60 minutes.

Adverse effects

Hypertension, tachycardia, arrhythmias, apnea with rapid administration, laryngospasm, tonic or clonic movements, emergence delirium, hypersalivation, nausea and vomiting, diplopia, nystagmus, slight elevation in intraocular tension; serious emergence reactions

Precautions and contraindications

Ketamine is contraindicated in hypertension, coronary heart disease or increased intracranial pressure, history of cerebrovascular accident, increased intraocular pressure, and psychiatric disorders. It is contraindicated for surgery or diagnostic procedures of pharynx, larynx, and bronchial tree. Use it cautiously in patients with convulsive disorders.

Anesthetic considerations

Do not mix ketamine with barbiturates in same syringe. Emergence reactions are common in adults with high doses and are reduced by medication with a benzodiazepine. Catecholamine-depleted patients may respond to ketamine with unexpected reductions in blood pressure and cardiac output.

KETOROLAC TROMETHAMINE (TORADOL)

PART III **Drugs**

Classification

Nonsteroidal antiinflammatory agent

Indications

Short-term (less than 5 days) management of moderately severe, acute pain that requires analgesia; generally used in a postoperative setting.

Patients should be switched to alternative analgesics as soon as possible. Ketorolac therapy is not to exceed 5 days because of the potential for increased frequency and severity of adverse reactions. The combined duration of use of ketorolac intravenously/intramuscularly and orally is not to exceed 5 days. Oral ketorolac is indicated only for continuation therapy after intravenous/intramuscular ketorolac.

Dose

Intramuscular (give slowly and deeply into the muscle): patients younger than 65 years old: one dose of 60 mg; patients older than 65 years old, renally impaired, and/or less than 50 kg: one dose of 30 mg.

Intravenous (intravenous bolus over no less than 15 seconds): patients younger than 65 years old: one dose of 30 mg; patients older than 65 years old, renally impaired, and/or less than 50 kg: one dose of 15 mg.

Multiple-dose treatment (intravenous or subcutaneous): patients younger than 65 years old: 30 mg every 6 hours, not to exceed 120 mg/day;

Patients older than 65 years old, renally impaired, and/or less than 50 kg: 15 mg every 6 hours, not to exceed 60 mg/day.

Onset and duration

Onset: intravenous/intramuscular: 15 to 30 minutes with maximum effect in 1 to 2 hours. Duration: 4 to 6 hours.

Adverse effects

Gastrointestinal: peptic ulcers, gastrointestinal bleeding, and/or perforation; renal toxicity; risk of bleeding: inhibition of platelet function; hypersensitivity

Because ketorolac and its metabolites are eliminated primarily by the kidneys, clearance of the drug is diminished in patients with reduced creatinine clearance. Renal toxicity with ketorolac has been seen in patients with conditions leading to a reduction in blood volume and/or renal blood flow, in which renal prostaglandins have a supportive role in the maintenance of renal perfusion. In these patients, administration of ketorolac may cause a dose-dependent reduction in renal prostaglandin formation and may precipitate acute renal failure.

Hypersensitivity reactions ranging from bronchospasm to anaphylactic shock have occurred, and appropriate counteractive measures must be available when administering the first dose.

Precautions and contraindications

Fluid retention, edema, retention of sodium, oliguria, and elevations of serum urea nitrogen and creatinine have been reported. Therefore, ketorolac should be used only with caution in patients with cardiac decompensation, hypertension, or similar conditions. Ketorolac is contraindicated in patients with active peptic ulcer disease or recent gastrointestinal bleeding or perforation and in patients with a history of peptic ulcer disease or gastrointestinal bleeding. Ketorolac is also contraindicated in patients with advanced renal impairment and in patients at risk for renal failure owing to volume depletion. It is contraindicated in patients with suspected or confirmed cerebrovascular bleeding, hemorrhagic diathesis, and incomplete hemostasis and those with a high risk of bleeding. It is contraindicated as a prophylactic analgesic before any major surgery and is contraindicated intraoperatively when hemostasis is critical. Ketorolac is also contraindicated in patients with previously demonstrated hypersensitivity to ketorolac tromethamine or allergic manifestations to aspirin (ASA) or other nonsteroidal antiinflammatory drugs (NSAIDs). It is contraindicated for patients currently receiving ASA or NSAIDs because of the cumulative risk of inducing serious NSAID-related side effects. Ketorolac is contraindicated for intrathecal or epidural administration owing to its alcohol content. It is contraindicated in labor and delivery because it may adversely affect fetal circulation and inhibit uterine contractions. Because of the potential adverse effects of prostaglandin-inhibiting drugs on neonates, ketorolac is contraindicated in nursing mothers.

Anesthetic considerations

Do not use ketorolac as prophylactic analgesia before any major surgery or intraoperatively when hemostasis is critical; in patients with suspected or confirmed cerebrovascular bleeding, hemorrhagic diathesis, incomplete hemostasis, and at high risk of bleeding; in patients currently receiving ASA or NSAIDs; for epidural or intrathecal administration; or concomitantly with probenecid.

The use of ketorolac is not recommended in children.

Ketorolac reduced the diuretic response to furosemide in normovolemic healthy subjects by approximately 20%. Hypovolemia should be corrected before treatment with ketorolac is initiated. Ketorolac possesses no sedative or anxiolytic properties. The concomitant use with opiate-agonist analgesics can result in reduced opiate analgesic requirements. Ketorolac is highly bound to human plasma protein (99.2%).

LABETALOL (NORMODYNE, TRANDATE)

Classification
β- and α-adrenergic antagonist

Indications
Hypertension

Dose
Intravenous bolus: 0.15 to 0.25 mg/kg given over 2 minutes; may repeat every 5 minutes up to 300 mg. Continuous infusion: 2 mg/min; titrate to effect. Oral: 100 mg twice daily alone or with diuretic; may increase to 200 mg twice daily after 2 days; further dose increase may be made every 1 to 3 days to maximal response. Maintenance dose: 200 to 400 mg twice daily.

Onset and duration
Onset: intravenous: 1 to 3 minutes; oral: 20 to 40 minutes. Duration: intravenous: 0.25 to 2 hours; oral: 4 to 12 hours.

Adverse effects
Hypotension, bradycardia, ventricular arrhythmias, congestive heart failure, chest pain, bronchospasm, headache, diarrhea

Precautions and contraindications
Use labetalol cautiously in patients with chronic bronchitis, emphysema, preexisting peripheral vascular disease, pheochromocytoma, and diabetes. It is contraindicated in bronchial asthma, overt heart failure, greater than first-degree heart block, and hepatic failure.

Anesthetic considerations
Inhalation anesthetics may enhance the drug's hypotensive effects.

LANSOPRAZOLE (PREVACID)

Classification
Proton pump inhibitor

Indications
Ulcers and acid reflux

Dose

Oral: 15 to 60 mg daily before meals.

Onset and duration

Onset: within 1 hour. Maximum effect: at 2 hours. Duration: greater than 24 hours.

Adverse effects

Abdominal pain, nausea, diarrhea

Precautions and contraindications

Lansoprazole slows the gastric emptying of solids. Reduce the dose in hepatic disease. It is contraindicated for patients hypersensitive to lansoprazole or similar proton pump inhibitors.

Anesthetic considerations

It is highly protein bound and undergoes liver elimination.

LEVOBUPIVACAINE (CHIROCAINE)

Classification

Amide-type local anesthetic

Indications

Regional anesthesia

Dose

For infiltration/peripheral nerve block: 0.25%, 0.5%, 0.75%. Dosing similar to bupivacaine.

Onset and duration

Onset: infiltration: 2 to 10 minutes; epidural: 4 to 7 minutes; spinal: less than 1 minute. Peak effect: infiltration and epidural: 30 to 45 minutes; spinal: 15 minutes. Duration: infiltration/spinal/epidural: 200 to 400 minutes (prolonged with epinephrine).

Adverse effects

Hypotension, arrhythmias, cardiac arrest, respiratory impairment or arrest, seizures, tinnitus, blurred vision, urticaria, anaphylactoid symptoms; high spinal, urinary retention, lower extremity weakness and paralysis, loss of sphincter control, backache, palsies, slowing of labor

Precautions and contraindications

Use levobupivacaine with caution in patients with hypovolemia, severe congestive heart failure, shock, and all forms of heart block. It is contraindicated in patients with hypersensitivity to amide-type local anesthetics.

Anesthetic considerations

Intravenous access is essential during major regional block. Toxic plasma levels of levobupivacaine may cause seizures and cardiopulmonary collapse.

LIDOCAINE HCL (XYLOCAINE, XYLOCAINE JELLY, XYLOCAINE VISCOUS ORAL SOLUTION)

Classification
Amide-type local anesthetic; topical anesthetic; antiarrhythmic agent

Indications
Regional anesthesia, topical anesthesia, treatment of ventricular arrhythmias, attenuation of sympathetic response to laryngoscopy/intubation

Dose
Caudal or epidural: 20 to 30 mL 1% solution (200 to 300 mg); may also use 1.5% and 2% solutions (maximum dose: 200 to 300 mg/hour [4.5 mg/kg]). With epinephrine for anesthesia other than spinal, maximum safe dose is 500 mg (7 mg/kg).

Spinal: 1.5 to 2 mL 5% solution with 7.5% dextrose (75 to 100 mg).

Antiarrhythmic: slow intravenous bolus: 1 mg/kg (1% to 2% solution), followed by 0.5 mg/kg every 2 to 5 minutes (to maximum dose of 3 mg/kg/hour); infusion (0.1% solution): 1 to 4 mg/min (20 to 50 mcg/kg/min). Use only preservative-free forms for intravenous administration.

Local anesthesia: topical: 0.6 to 3 mg/kg (1% to 4% solution); infiltration/peripheral nerve block: 0.5 to 5 mg/kg (0.5% to 2% solution); transtracheal: 80 to 120 mg (2 to 3 mL of 4% solution); superior laryngeal nerve: 40 to 60 mg (2 to 3 mL of 2% solution on each side); stellate ganglion: 50 mg (5 mL of 1% solution); intravenous (regional): upper extremity: 200 to 250 mg (40 to 50 mL of 0.5% solution), lower extremity: 250 to 300 mg (100 to 120 mL of 0.25% solution).

Onset and duration
Onset: intravenous (antiarrhythmic effects): 45 to 90 seconds; infiltration: 0.5 to 3 minutes; epidural: 5 to 25 minutes. Peak effects: intravenous (antiarrhythmic effects): 1 to 2 minutes; infiltration and epidural: less than 30 minutes. Duration: intravenous (antiarrhythmic effects): 10 to 30 minutes; infiltration: 0.5 to 1.5 hours, with epinephrine: 2 to 6 hours; epidural: 1 to 3 hours (prolonged with epinephrine).

Adverse effects
Hypotension, bradycardia, arrhythmias, heart block, respiratory depression or arrest, anxiety, tinnitus, seizures, postspinal headache, palsies, urticaria, pruritus; high spinal, loss of bladder and bowel control, permanent motor, sensory, autonomic (sphincter control) deficit of lower segments

Precautions and contraindications
Use lidocaine with caution in patients with hypovolemia, severe congestive heart failure, shock, all forms of heart block, and pregnancy. It is contraindicated in patients with hypersensitivity to amide-type local anesthetics and those with supraventricular arrhythmias.

Anesthetic considerations
The dosage should be reduced for elderly, debilitated, and acutely ill patients. Anesthetic solutions containing epinephrine should be used with caution in

patients with peripheral or hypertensive vascular disease. Benzodiazepines increase the seizure threshold. Do not use preparations containing preservatives for spinal or epidural anesthesia or for intravenous administration. Do not inject solutions containing epinephrine intravenously. Transient neurologic symptoms have been reported following spinal use.

LORAZEPAM (ATIVAN)

Classification
Benzodiazepine; antianxiety agent; hypnotic; sedative

Indications
Premedication; amnesia; temporary relief of insomnia

Dose
Intravenous/deep intramuscular: 1 to 2 mg (0.05 mg/kg) (maximum dose: 4 mg), dilute with equal volume D_5W or normal saline solution; oral: 1 to 2 mg, two to three times daily. Preoperative medication: 0.05 mg/kg 2 hours before procedure (maximum dosage: 4 mg).

Dosage forms: tablets: 0.5, 1, 2 mg; injection: 2 mg/mL, 4 mg/mL.

Onset and duration
Onset: intravenous: 1 to 5 minutes; intramuscular: 15 to 30 minutes; oral: 1 to 6 hours. Duration: 6 to 24 hours. Elimination half-life: 10 to 15 hours; metabolized to inactive compounds.

Adverse effects
Hypotension, hypertension, bradycardia, tachycardia, respiratory depression, dizziness, weakness, depression, agitation, amnesia, hysteria, urticaria, visual disturbances, blurred vision, diplopia, nausea and vomiting, abdominal discomfort, anorexia

Precautions and contraindications
Intraarterial lorazepam injection may cause arteriospasm; treat with local infiltration of phentolamine (5 to 20 mg in 10 mL normal saline). Use it with caution in elderly and debilitated patients. It is contraindicated for patients with known hypersensitivity to benzodiazepines and narrow-angle glaucoma.

Anesthetic considerations
Unexpected hypotension and respiratory depression may occur when lorazepam is combined with opioids. Use it with caution in elderly patients and in patients with limited pulmonary reserve. It is not for use in children younger than 12 years old. Treat overdoses with flumazenil. Decreased requirements for volatile anesthetics are noted.

MAGNESIUM SULFATE

Classification
Replacement agent; anticonvulsant

Indications

Prevention and control of seizures in toxemia/eclampsia of pregnancy, epilepsy, nephritis, and hypomagnesemia; treatment of acute magnesium deficiency; tocolytic therapy; adjunctive therapy of acute myocardial infarction, torsades de pointes ventricular tachycardia, and hypokalemia-related arrhythmias; laxative

Dose

Preeclampsia/eclampsia: intravenous: 4 g in 250 mL D_5W or normal saline infused slowly, followed by 2 to 3 g/hour by continuous infusion; blood level should not exceed 7 mEq/L. Hypomagnesemic seizures: mild: 1 g intravenously/intramuscularly every 6 hours for four doses. Total parenteral nutrition: intravenous: 8 to 24 mEq/day.

Onset and duration

Onset: intravenous: immediate; intramuscular: less than 1 hour; oral: 1 to 2 hours. Peak effects: intravenous: few minutes; intramuscular: 1 to 3 hours. Duration: intravenous: 30 minutes; intramuscular: 3 to 4 hours.

Adverse effects

Hypotension, circulatory collapse, heart block, respiratory paralysis, flaccid paralysis, depressed reflexes, hypocalcemia, flushing, sweating, hypothermia

Precautions and contraindications

Magnesium sulfate is not for use in patients with heart block or extensive myocardial damage. Use it with caution in patients with impaired renal function, in digitalized patients, and with concomitant use of other central nervous system depressants or neuromuscular blocking agents. Intravenous administration is contraindicated during the 2 hours preceding delivery. Oral administration is contraindicated in patients with abdominal pain, nausea, vomiting, fecal impaction, or intestinal irritation, obstruction, or perforation.

Anesthetic considerations

Magnesium sulfate potentiates both depolarizing and nondepolarizing muscle relaxants. Periodic monitoring of serum magnesium concentrations is essential during magnesium therapy. Maintain urine output at a minimum of 100 mL every 4 hours. Monitor deep tendon reflexes during magnesium therapy. Stop therapy as soon as the desired effect is reached. Monitor the patient's respiratory function.

PART III Drugs

MANNITOL (OSMITROL)

Classification

Osmotic diuretic

Indications

Reduction of intracranial pressure and intraocular pressure; protection of renal function during periods of hypoperfusion (shock, burn, open heart surgery, kidney transplants, abdominal aortic aneurysm repair); transurethral prostate resection (TURP) irrigation (minimizes hemolytic effects of water and promotes rapid excretion of absorbed irrigants)

Dose

Adults: Reduction of intracranial/intraocular pressure: 1.5 to 2 g/kg of 15% to 25% solution over 30 to 60 minutes. When used preoperatively, give 1 to 1.5 hours preoperatively for maximum pressure reduction. Test dose: Marked oliguria or suspected inadequate renal function: 0.2 g/kg or 12.5 g over 3 to 5 minutes. If satisfactory response not obtained, may repeat. If response still not obtained, *do not use mannitol.* Prevention of oliguric renal failure: 50 to 100 g intravenously over 2 hours. TURP: 2.5% to 5% irrigation instilled into bladder.

Children: 2 g/kg or 60 g/m^2 as 15% to 20% solution over 2 to 6 hours to treat edema and ascites; over 30 to 60 minutes to treat cerebral or ocular edema.

Dosage forms: parenteral injection: 5%, 10%, 15%, 20%, 25%; urogenital irrigation solution: 2.5% to 5%.

Onset and duration

Onset: diuresis in 30 minutes to 1 hour; reduction of intracranial and intraocular pressure in 15 to 30 minutes. Duration: 3 to 8 hours.

Adverse effects

Most serious: fluid imbalance and electrolyte loss; less serious: pulmonary edema, hypertension, water intoxication, congestive heart failure, skin necrosis with extravasation

Precautions and contraindications

Monitor serum osmolarity and electrolytes closely. Discontinue mannitol if there is low urine output. Mannitol may crystallize at low temperatures. Do not use a solution containing crystals—resolubilize in hot water with periodic shaking. The use of mannitol is contraindicated in patients with pulmonary edema, congestive heart failure, severe dehydration, impaired renal function not responsive to test dose, edema associated with capillary fragility, or acute intracranial bleeding (except during craniotomy).

Anesthetic considerations

Mannitol disrupts the blood-brain barrier, enhancing penetration of other drugs into the central nervous system.

MEPERIDINE HCL (DEMEROL)

Classification

Synthetic opioid agonist

Indications

Analgesia

Dose

Intravenous/intramuscular: 25 to 100 mg; intravenous: infusion 1 to 20 mg/hour for short duration, then titrate to patient's need.

Onset and duration

Onset: oral or intramuscular: 20 to 45 minutes; intravenous: 1 to 5 minutes. Duration: oral/intravenous/intramuscular: 2 to 4 hours.

Adverse effects

Hypotension, cardiac arrest, respiratory depression or arrest, laryngospasm, euphoria, dysphoria, sedation, seizures, dependence, constipation, biliary tract spasm, chest wall rigidity, urticaria, pruritus

Precautions and contraindications

Reduce the meperidine dose in elderly, hypovolemic, high-risk surgical patients and with the concomitant use of sedatives and other narcotics. Severe and occasionally fatal reactions can occur in patients who are receiving or have just received monoamine oxidase inhibitors; treat these patients with hydrocortisone. It is not for long-term use. The toxic metabolite of meperidine HCl (normeperidine) is hazardous, especially in elderly patients and those with renal compromise.

Use it with caution with and the elderly in patients with asthma, chronic obstructive pulmonary disease, increased intracranial pressure, or supraventricular tachycardia, or renal failure.

Meperidine crosses the placental barrier. Use during labor may produce depression of respiration in the neonate. If it is used, resuscitation of the neonate may be required; therefore, have naloxone available.

Cerebral irritation and seizures can occur when meperidine is used in large doses. Meperidine potentiates the central nervous system and cardiovascular depression of narcotics, sedative-hypnotics, volatile anesthetics, and tricyclic antidepressants. There is a severe and sometimes fatal reaction with monoamine oxidase inhibitors. Analgesia is enhanced by α_2-agonists. Meperidine aggravates adverse effects of isoniazid. It is chemically incompatible with barbiturates.

Anesthetic considerations

Meperidine is used occasionally for preoperative or postoperative analgesia.

MEPHENTERMINE SULFATE (WYAMINE SULFATE)

Classification

Synthetic noncatecholamine that stimulates α- and β- receptors, both directly and indirectly

Indications

Hypotension

Dose

Intravenous/intramuscular: 10 to 45 mg (0.4 mg/kg); infusion: 0.25 to 5 mg/min.

Onset and duration

Onset: intravenous: 1 to 5 minutes; intramuscular: 5 to 15 minutes. Duration: intravenous: 15 to 30 minutes; intramuscular: 1 to 2 hours.

Adverse effects

Hypertension, arrhythmias, anxiety, seizures, euphoria, paranoid psychosis

Precautions and contraindications

Use mephentermine with caution in patients with hypertension or hyperthyroidism. There is also an increased risk of arrhythmias with use of volatile agents. Mephentermine sulfate may increase uterine contractions, especially during the third trimester of pregnancy. It is not recommended for use in pregnant women.

Anesthetic considerations
Use it with caution in patients receiving monoamine oxidase inhibitors or tricyclic antidepressants.

MEPIVACAINE HCL (CARBOCAINE, ISOCAINE, POLOCAINE)

Classification
Amide-type local anesthetic

Indications
Regional anesthesia: infiltration, brachial plexus block, epidural, caudal

Dose
Infiltration: 50 to 400 mg (0.5% to 1.5% solution). Brachial plexus block: 300 to 400 mg (30 to 40 mL of 1% solution). Epidural: 150 to 400 mg (15 to 20 mL of 1% to 2% solution). Caudal: 150 to 400 mg (15 to 20 mL of 1% to 2% solution).
     Children: 0.4 to 0.7 mL/kg (maximum safe dosage: 7 mg/kg with epinephrine).

Onset and duration
Onset: infiltration: 3 to 5 minutes; epidural: 5 to 15 minutes. Peak effects: infiltration/epidural: 15 to 45 minutes. Duration: infiltration: 0.75 to 1.5 hours, 2 to 6 hours with epinephrine; epidural: 3 to 5 hours (prolonged with epinephrine).

Adverse effects
Myocardial depression, arrhythmias, cardiac arrest, respiratory depression or arrest, anxiety, apprehension, tinnitus, seizures, loss of hearing, urticaria, pruritus

Precautions and contraindications
Use mepivacaine with caution in debilitated, elderly, or acutely ill patients, especially if there is severe disturbance in cardiac rhythm or heart block. Use it with caution in pregnant patients. Mepivacaine is contraindicated in patients with hypersensitivity to amide-type local anesthetics.

Anesthetic considerations
Do not use solutions with preservatives for caudal or epidural block. Mepivacaine is not for use as spinal or obstetric anesthesia.

METARAMINOL BITARTRATE (ARAMINE)

Classification
Synthetic noncatecholamine

Indications

Hypertension; stimulates α- and β-receptors, both directly and indirectly

Dose

Intramuscular/subcutaneous: 2 to 10 mg; intravenous: 0.5 to 5 mg.

Onset and duration

Onset: intravenous: 1 to 5 minutes; intramuscular/subcutaneous: 5 to 15 minutes. Duration: intravenous: 10 to 15 minutes; intramuscular/ subcutaneous: 1 to 2 hours.

Adverse effects

Apprehension, restlessness, dizziness, headache, tremor, weakness, seizures, hypertension, hypotension, precordial pain, palpitations, arrhythmias, bradycardia, premature ventricular contractions, atrioventricular dissociation, nausea and vomiting, decreased urine output, hyperglycemia, flushing, pallor, sweating

Precautions and contraindications

Use metaraminol with caution in patients with hypertension, thyroid disease, diabetes, or cirrhosis, or in those receiving digoxin. It is contraindicated in patients with peripheral or mesenteric thrombosis, pulmonary edema, hypercarbia, or acidosis.

Anesthetic considerations

The risk of adverse cardiac effects with the use of general anesthetics is increased.

METHADONE HCL (DOLOPHINE HCL)

Classification

Synthetic narcotic

Indications

Analgesia; opiate recovery programs

Dose

Analgesia: subcutaneous/intramuscular/oral: 2.5 to 10 mg (0.1 mg/kg) every 4 hours; epidural bolus: 1 to 5 mg. Narcotic abstinence syndrome: oral: 20 to 120 mg/day.

Onset and duration

Onset: intravenous: 5 to 10 minutes; intramuscular: 20 to 60 minutes; oral: 30 to 60 minutes; epidural: 5 to 10 minutes. Duration: intravenous/ intramuscular/oral: about 6 hours; epidural: 6 to 10 hours.

Adverse effects

Hypotension, circulatory depression, bradycardia, syncope, respiratory depression, euphoria, dysphoria, disorientation, urinary retention, biliary tract spasm, constipation, anorexia, rash, pruritus, urticaria

Precautions and contraindications

Reduce the methadone dose in the elderly, hypovolemic, or high-risk surgical patient or with use of narcotics and sedative-hypnotics.

Anesthetic considerations

Do not give pentazocine to heroin addicts receiving methadone. Methadone is ineffective for relief of general anxiety. Use it with caution in patients with asthma, chronic obstructive pulmonary disease, or increased intracranial pressure. Methadone can produce the drug effects of morphine.

METHOHEXITAL SODIUM (BREVITAL SODIUM)

Classification

Ultrashort-acting barbiturate

Indications

General anesthetic for short surgical procedures; induction of hypnosis; supplementation of other anesthetics

Dose

Intravenous: induction: 50 to 120 mg (average 70 mg), 1 to 1.5 mg/kg usual dose in adults.

Dosage forms: powder for injection: mixed as a 1% solution.

Onset and duration

Onset: 30 to 60 seconds. Duration: 5 to 15 minutes.

Adverse effects

Circulatory depression, thrombophlebitis, myocardial depression, cardiac arrhythmia, respiratory depression, central nervous system disturbances, seizures, nausea and vomiting, abdominal pain, rectal irritation (rectal administration), pain at injection site, myoclonus

Precautions and contraindications

Use methohexital with caution in patients with severe cardiovascular disease, hypotension, shock, Addison's disease, hepatic or renal dysfunction, myxedema, increased intracranial pressure, asthma, or myasthenia gravis. Methohexital sodium is contraindicated in patients with variegate porphyria or acute intermittent porphyria or in those with hypersensitivity to barbiturates.

Anesthetic considerations

Consider reducing the dose when it is used in conjunction with narcotics. Overdosage may occur from too rapid or repeated injections. Do not mix methohexital with atropine sulfate or succinylcholine. Use only if it is clear and colorless. Methohexital sodium is not compatible with lactated Ringer's solution.

METHOXAMINE HCL (VASOXYL)

Classification

α-Receptor agonist

Indications

Hypotension

Dose

Intravenous: 1 to 5 mg, given slowly; intramuscular: 5 to 15 mg (0.25 mg/kg).

Onset and duration

Onset: intravenous: almost immediately; intramuscular: 15 to 20 minutes. Duration: intravenous: 15 to 60 minutes; intramuscular: 60 to 90 minutes.

Adverse effects

Reflex bradycardia, hypertension, hypotension, respiratory difficulty, tremors, dizziness, seizures, cerebral hemorrhage, headache

Precautions and contraindications

Use methoxamine with extreme caution in elderly patients and in patients with bradycardia, partial heart block, myocardial disease, or severe arteriosclerosis. Methoxamine contains sulfites and thus may cause allergic-type reactions.

Anesthetic considerations

Infuse it into large veins to prevent extravasation. Treat extravasation with local infiltration of phentolamine (5 to 10 mg in 10 mL normal saline solution) or with sympathetic block.

METHYLENE BLUE (UROLENE BLUE)

Classification

Antidote; diagnostic agent

Indications

Treatment of idiopathic and drug-induced methemoglobinemia; dye effect for tissue staining; urinary antiseptic (oral route); antidote to cyanide poisoning

Dose

Intravenous: 1 to 2 mg/kg (inject over several minutes); oral: 65 to 130 mg three times daily with water.

Onset and duration

Onset: intravenous: almost immediate. Peak effects: intravenous: less than 1 hour. Duration: intravenous/oral: several hours

Adverse effects

Tachycardia, hypertension, precordial pain, cyanosis, confusion, headache, nausea and vomiting, diarrhea, abdominal pain, bladder irritation, hemolytic anemia, methemoglobinemia, hyperbilirubinemia, blue staining of skin

Precautions and contraindications

Safe use during pregnancy is not established. Methylene blue is contraindicated in patients with renal insufficiency, hypersensitivity to methylene blue, glucose-6-phosphate dehydrogenase deficiency (hemolysis), or for intraspinal injection.

Anesthetic considerations

Methylene blue causes discoloration of urine and feces. It may cause artificial readings with pulse oximetry; inject it slowly to prevent a local high concentration from producing additional methemoglobinemia. Monitor intake, output, and hemoglobin.

METHYLERGONOVINE (METHERGINE)

Classification

Oxytocic (ergot alkaloid); adrenergic antagonist; sympatholytic

Indications

Prevention and treatment of postpartum hemorrhage caused by uterine atony or subinvolution

Dose

Intramuscular: 0.2 mg every 2 to 5 hours (maximum 5 doses); intravenous: 0.2 mg/mL (over 1 minute while monitoring blood pressure and uterine contractions); oral: 0.2 to 0.4 mg every 6 to 12 hours for 2 to 7 days.

Onset and duration

Onset: intravenous: immediate; intramuscular: 2 to 5 minutes; oral: 5 to 15 minutes. Peak effects: 3 hours. Duration: intravenous: 45 minutes; intramuscular: 3 hours; oral: 3 or more hours.

Adverse effects

Hypertension, chest pain, palpitations, dyspnea, headache, nausea, vomiting, tinnitus; high doses: possible signs of ergotism

Precautions and contraindications

Use it with caution in patients with hypertension, sepsis, obliterative vascular disease, and hepatic, renal, or cardiac disease. Methylergonovine is contraindicated in patients with hypersensitivity to ergot preparations and in those with toxemia or untreated hypocalcemia.

Anesthetic considerations

Monitor patients for hypertension or other adverse effects. Parenteral sympathomimetics or other ergot alkaloids add to pressor effect and may lead to hypertension. Intravenous administration is not routine, because it can produce sudden hypertension and cerebrovascular accidents.

METOCLOPRAMIDE (REGLAN)

Classification

Dopamine-receptor antagonist; antiemetic; stimulant of upper gastrointestinal motility

Indications

Diabetic and postsurgical gastric stasis; prevention of chemotherapy-induced emesis; facilitation of small bowel intubation; treatment of gastroesophageal reflux; prevention of postoperative nausea and vomiting

Dose

Adults: 10 mg intravenously slowly over 1 to 2 minutes as a single dose; may repeat once. Children: 6 to 14 years old: intravenous: 2.5 to 5 mg; children under 6 years: 0.1 mg/kg.

Dosage forms: intravenous: 5 mg/mL in 2- and 10-mL vials; oral: tablets: 5 mg and 10 mg; syrup: 5 mg/5 mL.

Onset and duration

Onset: 1 to 3 minutes. Duration: 2 to 3 hours. Elimination half-life: 2.5 to 5 hours in patients with normal renal function.

Adverse effects

Anxiety, restlessness, mental depression, gastrointestinal upset, urticaria, allergic reactions, diarrhea; frequent drowsiness

Extrapyramidal side effects such as opisthotonos, clonic convulsions, oculogyric crisis, facial grimacing, involuntary movement of limbs, and rarely stridor and dyspnea (possibly from laryngospasm) occur with 0.2% or less frequency in the foregoing doses but are more common in children. Diphenhydramine may reverse the extrapyramidal effects. Butyrophenones and phenothiazines may potentiate the extrapyramidal side effects.

Precautions and contraindications

Use it with caution in pregnant patients. Metoclopramide may exacerbate Parkinson's disease and hypertension and may increase pressure on suture lines following gut anastomosis or closure. Patients should be cautioned that metoclopramide may impair their ability to perform activities requiring mental alertness, including driving or operating machinery. Alcohol and other central nervous system depressants may enhance these effects.

Do not use metoclopramide with monoamine oxidase inhibitors, tricyclic antidepressants, or sympathomimetics. Metoclopramide should not be used in patients with pheochromocytoma, a history of seizure disorder, or gastrointestinal hemorrhage, obstruction or perforation.

Anesthetic considerations

Metoclopramide may increase the neuromuscular blocking effects of succinylcholine or mivacurium by inhibiting plasma cholinesterase.

MIDAZOLAM (VERSED)

Classification

Benzodiazepine; hypnotic; sedative

Indications

Preoperative sedation; induction of anesthesia; long-term sedation in intensive care unit; sedation before short diagnostic and endoscopic procedures

Dose

Should be individualized based on the patient's age, underlying pathologic features, and concurrent indications. Adolescents (less than 12 years): intravenous: 0.5 mg; can be repeated every 5 minutes until desired effect is achieved. Adults: preoperative sedation: intramuscular: 0.07 to 0.08 mg/kg

PART III **Drugs**

30 to 60 minutes before surgery; usual dose: approximately 5 mg; intravenous: initial: 0.5 to 2 mg slowly over 2 minutes; usual total dose: 2 to 5 mg; decrease dose in elderly patients; reduce dose by 30% if other central nervous system depressants are administered concomitantly.

Dosage form: injection: 1, 5 mg/mL.

Onset and duration

Onset: intravenous: 1 to 5 minutes; intramuscular: 15 minutes; oral/rectal: less than 10 minutes. Duration: 2 to 6 hours. Elimination half-life: 14 hours; excreted in urine.

Adverse effects

Tachycardia, hypotension, bronchospasm, laryngospasm, apnea, hypoventilation, vasovagal episodes, euphoria, prolonged emergence, agitation, hyperactivity, pruritus, rash

Precautions and contraindications

Midazolam is not for intraarterial injection. Its safe use in pregnancy, labor and delivery, by nursing mothers, or by children is not established. Midazolam is contraindicated in patients with intolerance to benzodiazepines and in those with acute narrow-angle glaucoma, shock, coma, or acute alcohol intoxication.

Anesthetic considerations

Use midazolam with caution in elderly patients and in patients with chronic obstructive pulmonary disease, chronic renal failure, or congestive heart failure. Reduce the doses in hypovolemia and with the concomitant use of other sedatives or narcotics. Hypotension and respiratory depression may occur when it is given with opioids; consider smaller doses. Treat overdoses with flumazenil.

MILRINONE (PRIMACOR)

Classification

Inotropic agent; phosphodiesterase-3 inhibitor

Indications

Therapy for congestive heart failure; cardiac bypass procedures and heart transplants

Dose

Intravenous: loading dose: 50 mcg/kg over 10 minutes; maintenance dose: 0.375 mcg/kg/min, 0.5 mcg/kg/min, or 0.75 mcg/kg/min.

Dosage form: intravenous: 1 mg/mL.

Onset and duration

Onset: intravenous: 2 minutes; oral: 1 to 1.5 hours. Duration: 2 hours.

Adverse effects

Thrombocytopenia, arrhythmia, angina, hypotension, headache, hyperthermia

Precautions and contraindications

Use it with caution in patients with renal insufficiency and in those with aortic or pulmonic valvular disease. Milrinone is contraindicated in patients with hypersensitivity to milrinone or amrinone.

Anesthetic considerations

Milrinone is an attractive alternative to conventional inotropics. It may be useful if both an inotropic effect and vasodilation are desirable.

MIVACURIUM (MIVACRON)

Classification

Nondepolarizing skeletal muscle relaxant

Indications

Adjunct to general anesthesia; skeletal muscle relaxation during surgery

Dose

Intravenous: paralyzing: 0.07 to 0.25 mg/kg. Children: 0.1 to 0.2 mg/kg over 5 to 15 seconds.

Dosage forms: 0.5 mg/mL in 5% dextrose; 0.5 mg/mL.

Onset and duration

Onset: 2 minutes. Duration: 15 to 30 minutes.

Adverse effects

Hypotension, vasodilation, tachycardia, bradycardia, hypoventilation, apnea, bronchospasm, laryngospasm, dyspnea, rash, inadequate block, prolonged block

Precautions and contraindications

Mivacurium is contraindicated in patients with hypersensitivity to the drug.

Anesthetic considerations

Use it with caution in patients with sensitivity to the release of histamine. Prolonged neuromuscular blockade may occur in patients with low plasma pseudocholinesterase; one may reverse the effects with an anticholinesterase agent if enough time has lapsed since administration; monitor the patient's response with a peripheral nerve stimulator.

PART III **Drugs**

MORPHINE SULFATE (ASTRAMORPH, DURAMORPH, MORPHINE, MS CONTIN)

Classification

Opioid agonist

Indications

Premedication; analgesia; anesthesia; treatment of pain associated with myocardial ischemia and dyspnea associated with left ventricular failure and pulmonary edema

Dose

Analgesia: intravenous: 2.5 to 15 mg; intramuscular/subcutaneous: 2.5 to 20 mg; oral: 15 to 30 mg every 4 hours as needed; oral extended release: 30 mg every 12 hours; rectal: 5 to 20 mg every 4 hours. Anesthesia induction: intravenous: 1 mg/kg; epidural bolus: 2 to 5 mg; epidural infusion: 0.1 to 1 mg/hour; spinal (preservative-free solution only): 0.2 to 1 mg.

Children: intravenous: 0.05 to 0.2 mg/kg; intramuscular/subcutaneous: 0.1 to 0.2 mg/kg.

Onset and duration

Onset: intravenous: almost immediate; intramuscular: 1 to 5 minutes; oral: less than 60 minutes; epidural and spinal: 1 to 60 minutes. Duration: intravenous/intramuscular/subcutaneous: 2 to 7 hours; epidural and spinal: 24 hours.

Adverse effects

Hypotension, hypertension, bradycardia, arrhythmias, chest wall rigidity, bronchospasm, laryngospasm, blurred vision, syncope, euphoria, dysphoria, urinary retention, antidiuretic effect, ureteral spasm, biliary tract spasm, constipation, anorexia, nausea, vomiting, pruritus, urticaria

Precautions and contraindications

Reduce the morphine dose in elderly, hypovolemic, or high-risk surgical patients and with the concomitant use of sedatives and other narcotics. Morphine sulfate crosses the placental barrier, so use in labor may produce depression of respiration in the neonate. Resuscitation of the neonate may be required; therefore, have naloxone available.

Anesthetic considerations

Central nervous system and cardiovascular depressant effects are potentiated by alcohol, sedatives, antihistamines, phenothiazines, butyrophenones, monoamine oxidase inhibitors, and tricyclic antidepressants. Morphine sulfate may decrease the effects of diuretics in patients with congestive heart failure. Analgesia is enhanced by α_2-agonists.

NALMEFENE HCL (REVEX)

Classification

Opiate antagonist

Indications

Complete or partial reversal of drug effects, respiratory depression, and overdose associated with natural and/or synthetic opioids

Dose

Reversal of opiate depression: titrate to the desired response at increments of 0.25 mcg/kg every 2 to 5 minutes; doses greater than 1 mg/kg give no additional therapeutic effects; titrate at a dose of 0.1 mcg/kg every 2 to 5 minutes in patients with increased cardiovascular risk.

Suspected opiate overdose: first dose 0.5 mg/70 kg; second dose 1 mg/70 kg if required 2 to 5 minutes later; doses greater than 1.5 mg/70 kg do not provide increased therapeutic effects.

Suspicion of opiate dependency: challenge dose of 0.1 mg/70 kg; if signs of withdrawal do not appear within 2 minutes, the recommended dosage guidelines should be followed.

Onset and duration

Onset: intravenous: within 2 minutes; intramuscular, subcutaneous: 5 to 15 minutes; intravenous: administration of a 1-mg dose of nalmefene will block 80% of brain opiate receptors within 5 minutes. The duration of action and opiate receptor occupancy of nalmefene were shown to be significantly greater than those of naloxone, which has half-life of 1.1 hour. Duration: equals that of most opioids. This provides the patient with added protection against possible renarcotization. Elimination half-life: 10.8 hours. It is metabolized in liver via glucuronide conjugation and excreted in the urine. Plasma clearance is reported to be 0.8 L/kg/hour.

Adverse effects

Pulmonary edema, hypotension, hypertension, ventricular arrhythmias, bradycardia, dizziness, depression, agitation, nervousness, tremor, confusion, myoclonus, withdrawal syndrome, nausea and vomiting, diarrhea, dry mouth, headache, chills, pruritus, pharyngitis.

A higher occurrence of adverse effects is reported with amounts exceeding recommended dosages.

Precautions and contraindications

Nalmefene has decreased plasma clearance in patients with liver or renal disease. The dose of nalmefene should be delivered over 60 seconds in patients with renal failure to minimize associated hypertension and dizziness. Dosage need not be adjusted for one-time administration. Recurrence of respiratory depression is possible even after a positive response to initial administration. Use it with caution in patients at increased cardiovascular risk. Acute withdrawal symptoms are associated with administration to opiate-dependent patients. There is incomplete reversal of buprenorphine-induced depression. Animal studies have shown a potential for seizure induction. The potential risk of seizure increases with the coadministration of nalmefene and flumazenil. Nalmefene is contraindicated in persons who display an allergic response related to the drug's administration. Safety and effectiveness of nalmefene for neonates and children have not been established.

Anesthetic considerations

No adverse reactions were noted in studies in which nalmefene was coadministered after benzodiazepines, volatile anesthetics, muscle relaxants, or their reversals.

NALOXONE HCL (NARCAN)

Classification
Opioid antagonist

Indications
Opiate reversal

Dose

Intravenous/intramuscular/subcutaneous: 0.1 to 2 mg titrated to patient response; may repeat at 2- to 3-minute intervals; response should occur with a maximum dose of 10 mg. Children: 5 to 10 mcg/kg every 2 to 3 minutes as needed.

Onset and duration

Onset: intravenous: 1 to 2 minutes; intramuscular/subcutaneous: 2 to 5 minutes. Duration: intravenous/intramuscular/subcutaneous: 1 to 4 hours.

Adverse effects

Tachycardia, hypertension, hypotension, arrhythmias, pulmonary edema, nausea and vomiting related to dose and speed of injection

Precautions and contraindications

Use naloxone with caution in patients with preexisting cardiac disease.

Anesthetic considerations

Titrate naloxone slowly to effect the desired results. Patients who have received naloxone should be carefully monitored because the duration of action of some opiates may exceed that of this drug.

NALTREXONE HCL (REVIA, TREXAN)

Classification

Opiate receptor antagonist

Indications

Reversal of toxic effects of opioid drugs; treatment of opiate and alcohol addiction, Tourette's syndrome, tardive dyskinesia, Lesch-Nyhan disease, and dyskinesia associated with Huntington's disease

Dose

Oral: 25 mg tablet followed by 25 mg in 1 hour if no signs of withdrawal present (withdrawal will begin 5 minutes after oral dose and may last up to 48 hours).

Dosage form: tablet: 25, 50 mg.

Onset and duration

Onset: within 5 minutes. Peak effects: within 1 hour. Duration: 24 to 72 hours.

Adverse effects

Headache, nervousness, confusion, restlessness, hallucinations, paranoia, nightmares, nausea and vomiting, diarrhea, abdominal pain and cramping, phlebitis, epistaxis, tachycardia, hypertension, edema, hepatotoxicity, joint or muscle pain, severe narcotic withdrawal

Precautions and contraindications

Patients addicted to heroin or other opiates should be drug free for 10 days before initiation of naltrexone therapy to avoid precipitation of withdrawal syndrome. Naltrexone contraindication is absolute in patients dependent on narcotics, in patients in acute withdrawal, and in those with liver disease or acute hepatitis. Serious overdose may occur after attempts to overcome the blocking effects of naltrexone.

Anesthetic considerations
Baseline liver function studies should be performed. The primary active metabolite is subject to glucuronide conjugation. Aspartate transaminase levels may be temporarily elevated after initiation of therapy. Patients taking naltrexone may not respond to opiates administered during anesthesia. Blockade of naltrexone may be overcome by large doses of opiates.

NEOSTIGMINE METHYLSULFATE (PROSTIGMIN)

Classification
Anticholinesterase agent

Indications
Reversal of nondepolarizing muscle relaxants; myasthenia gravis

Dose
Reversal: slow intravenous: 0.06 mg/kg (maximum dose: 6 mg), with atropine (0.015 mg/kg) or glycopyrrolate (0.01 mg/kg). Myasthenia gravis: oral: 15 to 375 mg daily (three divided doses); intramuscular/slow intravenous: 0.5 to 2 mg (dose must be individualized).

Onset and duration
Onset: reversal: intravenous: 3 to 15 minutes. Myasthenia gravis: intramuscular: less than 20 minutes; oral: 45 to 75 minutes. Duration: 45 to 60 minutes.

Adverse effects
Bradycardia, tachycardia, atrioventricular block, nodal rhythm, hypotension, bronchospasm; respiratory depression; seizures; dysarthria; headaches; nausea, emesis, flatulence, increased peristalsis; urinary frequency; rash, urticaria, allergic reactions, anaphylaxis; increased oral, pharyngeal, and bronchial secretions

Precautions and contraindications
Use neostigmine with caution in patients with bradycardia, bronchial asthma, epilepsy, cardiac arrhythmias, peptic ulcer, peritonitis, or mechanical obstruction of the intestines or urinary tract. Overdosage may induce a cholinergic crisis characterized by nausea, vomiting, bradycardia or tachycardia, excessive salivation and sweating, bronchospasm, weakness, and paralysis; treatment includes discontinuation of neostigmine use and administration of atropine (10 mg/kg intravenously every 3 to 10 minutes until muscarinic symptoms disappear).

Anesthetic considerations
Neostigmine may increase postoperative nausea and vomiting.

NESIRITIDE (NATRECOR)

Classification
Purified preparation of a new drug class, human B-type natriuretic peptide (hBNP), manufactured from *Escherichia coli* using recombinant DNA technology

Indications
Intravenous treatment of acutely decompensated congestive heart failure in patients who have dyspnea at rest or with minimal activity; reduction of pulmonary capillary wedge pressure and improvement of dyspnea

Dose
Intravenous: 2 mcg/kg bolus, followed by a continuous infusion at a dose of 0.01 mcg/kg/min.

Withdraw the bolus volume from the nesiritide infusion bag, and administer it over approximately 60 seconds through an intravenous port in the tubing. Immediately following the administration of the bolus, infuse nesiritide at a flow rate of 0.1 mL/kg/hour. This will deliver a nesiritide infusion dose of 0.01 mcg/kg/min.

To calculate the appropriate bolus volume and infusion flow rate to deliver a 0.01 mcg/kg/min dose, use the following formulas:

Bolus volume (mL): 0.33 × Patient weight (kg)
Infusion flow rate (mL/hour): 0.1 × Patient weight (kg)

Onset and duration
Onset: 15 to 60 minutes. Duration: 1 to 2 hours after discontinuation of infusion.

Adverse effects
Hypotension

The rate of symptomatic hypotension may be increased in patients with a blood pressure lower than 100 mm Hg at baseline, and nesiritide should be used cautiously in these patients. Combining nesiritide with other drugs that may cause hypotension such as nitroglycerin or an angiotensin converting enzyme inhibitor may increase the potential for hypotension.

Precautions and contraindications
Nesiritide should be administered only in settings where blood pressure can be monitored closely, and the dose of nesiritide should be reduced or the drug discontinued in patients who develop hypotension.

Anesthetic considerations
Nesiritide is not recommended for patients for whom vasodilating agents are not appropriate, such as patients with significant valvular stenosis, restrictive or obstructive cardiomyopathy, constrictive pericarditis, pericardial tamponade, or other conditions in which cardiac output depends on venous return, or for patients suspected to have low cardiac filling pressures.

NICARDIPINE (CARDENE)

Classification
Calcium channel blocker

Indications
Hypertension; chronic stable angina; vasospastic angina

Dose
Angina: initially 20 mg orally three times daily, titrate dosage according to patient response; usual dosage 20 to 40 mg orally three times daily.

Hypertension: initially 20 to 40 mg orally three times daily, increase dosage according to patient response; intravenous: 5 mg/hour, increased by 2.5 mg/hour increments every 15 minutes, up to 15 mg/hour.

Onset and duration
Onset: intravenous: 1 minute; oral: 30 minutes to 2 hours; sustained release: 1 to 4 hours. Duration: intravenous/oral: 3 hours.

Adverse effects
Edema, dizziness, headache, flushing, hypotension

Precautions and contraindications
Use it with caution in patients with hypersensitivity to nicardipine, other dihydropyridines, or other calcium channel antagonists and those with symptomatic hypotension or advanced aortic stenosis.

Anesthetic considerations
Nicardipine is an intravenous calcium channel blocker. It may be useful in controlling perioperative hypertension.

NIFEDIPINE (ADALAT, PROCARDIA)

Classification
Calcium channel blocker

Indications
Hypertension; chronic stable angina; vasospastic angina

Dose
10 to 30 mg three times daily up to 180 mg/day; off-label route: sublingual.

Onset and duration
Onset: oral: 20 minutes; sublingual: 5 to 20 minutes. Duration: oral/sublingual: 12 hours.

Adverse effects
Hypotension, palpitations, peripheral edema, bronchospasm, shortness of breath, nasal and chest congestion, headache, dizziness, nervousness, nausea, diarrhea, constipation, inflammation, joint stiffness, peripheral edema, pruritus, urticaria, fevers, chills, sweating

Precautions and contraindications

Monitor patient's blood pressure carefully during initial administration and titration. Use nifedipine with caution in hypovolemic patients, the elderly, and those with acute myocardial infarction and unstable angina.

Anesthetic considerations

Nifedipine potentiates the effects of depolarizing and nondepolarizing muscle relaxants and provides additive cardiovascular depressant effects with the use of volatile anesthetics or other antihypertensives. Nifedipine increases the toxicity of digoxin, carbamazepine, and oral hypoglycemics. It may bring about cardiac failure, atrioventricular conduction disturbances, and sinus bradycardia with concurrent use of β-blockers; severe hypotension and bradycardia may occur with bupivacaine. The concomitant use of intravenous verapamil and dantrolene may result in cardiovascular collapse.

NITROGLYCERIN (NITRO-BID, NITRO-DUR, NITROGARD, NITROSTAT, NITROL, TRIDIL, NITROCINE, TRANSDERM-NITRO, NITROGLYN, NITRODISC)

Classification

Peripheral vasodilator

Indications

Angina; controlled hypotension, treatment of pulmonary edema and congestive heart failure associated with acute myocardial infarction

Dose

Initially, titrate 5 to 20 mcg/min; thereafter, titrate by 10 mcg/min steps. Tablets: 0.15 to 0.6 mg every 5 minutes as needed to maximum of three doses in 15 minutes (sustained-release buccal, 1 to 2 mg every 3 to 5 hours); place tablet between the lip and gum above the incisors.

Dosage forms: injection: 0.5 and 5 mg/mL: tablets: sublingual: 0.15, 0.3, 0.4, 0.6 mg; sustained-release buccal: 1, 2, 3 mg; oral: 2.5, 6.5, 9 mg; capsules: 2.5, 6.5, 9 mg; aerosol translingual: 0.4 mg/metered dose; transdermal systems: 2.5, 5, 7.5, 10, 15 mg/24 hours; ointment: 2% (1 inch contains 15 mg nitroglycerin). Dilution for infusion: 8 mg diluted in 250 mL D_5W or normal saline (32 mcg/mL), 50 mg in 250 mL, 100 mg in 250 mL (400 mcg/mL).

Onset and duration

Onset: intravenous: 1 to 2 minutes; sublingual: 1 to 3 minutes; oral sustained release: 20 to 45 minutes; transdermal: 40 to 60 minutes. Duration: 30 minutes to 2 hours, depending on route.

Adverse effects

Orthostatic hypotension, tachycardia, flushing, palpitations, fainting, headache, dizziness, weakness, nausea and vomiting

Precautions and contraindications

Use it with caution in patients with hypotension, uncorrected hypovolemia, inadequate cerebral circulation, increased intracranial pressure, head

trauma, cerebral hemorrhage, or severe anemia. Nitroglycerin is contraindicated in patients with compensatory hypertension such as with arteriovenous shunts, coarctation of the aorta, and inadequate cerebral circulation.

Anesthetic considerations

The hypotensive effects of nitroglycerin are potentiated by alcohol,
phenothiazines, calcium channel blockers, β-blockers, other nitrates, and
antihypertensives. Nitroglycerin may antagonize the anticoagulant effect of
heparin. Methemoglobinemia may occur at high doses.

Attenuation of hypoxic pulmonary vasoconstriction may occur with
nitroglycerin. Infusion rates of greater than 3 mcg/kg/min may result in
decreased platelet aggregation. The hypotensive effects of nitroglycerin are
potentiated by volatile anesthetics, ganglionic blocking agents, other
antihypertensives, and circulatory depressants.

NITROPRUSSIDE SODIUM (NIPRIDE, NITROPRESS)

Classification
Peripheral vasodilator

Indications
Hypertension; controlled hypotension; treatment of cardiogenic pulmonary
edema; treatment of cardiogenic shock

Dose
Infusion: 10 to 300 mcg/min (0.25 to 10 mcg/kg/min) (maximum dose:
10 mcg/kg/min for 10 minutes or long-term infusion of 0.5 mcg/kg/min).
Because of light sensitivity, wrap the intravenous solution container in foil.
Monitor plasma thiocyanate concentrations in patients receiving infusions
for more than 48 hours.

Onset and duration
Onset: 30 to 60 seconds. Duration: 1 to 10 minutes.

Adverse effects
Reflex tachycardia; cyanide toxicity possible even with low doses
Treatment of cyanide toxicity: immediately discontinue nitroprusside
use, administer oxygen, treat acidosis with bicarbonate, start sodium nitrate
3% solution 4 to 6 mg/kg over 3 minutes, to produce 10% methemoglobin,
which will reversibly bind free cyanide ion. Follow with an infusion of
sodium thiosulfate (vitamin B_{12}), 150 to 200 mg/kg.

Precautions and contraindications
Use nitroprusside with caution in patients with renal or hepatic failure,
which may lead to increased risk of cyanide toxicity. There is a potential for
fetal cyanide toxicity in pregnant patients.

Anesthetic considerations
Titrate it carefully for short periods of deliberate hypotension. Monitor the
patient for cyanide toxicity. Elevated mixed venous oxygen tension may also
occur.

PART III Drugs

NITROUS OXIDE (N₂O)

Classification
Inhalation anesthetic

Indications
Component of balanced anesthesia or dental analgesia

Dose
Induction: 70% in an oxygen mixture. Maintenance: 50% to 70% in oxygen. Analgesia: 20% to 30%. Supplied in steel cylinders (blue) as a colorless liquid under pressure.

Onset and duration
Onset: 1 to 5 minutes. Duration: 5 to 10 minutes after cessation of continuous inhalation.

Adverse effects
Primarily caused by lack of oxygen from improper administration technique: confusion, cyanosis, convulsions, possible bone marrow depression

Precautions and contraindications
Caution the patient not to drive or operate other machinery until the effects of nitrous oxide have completely disappeared. Inform the patient that confusion, vivid dreams, dizziness, and hallucinations may occur on termination of the drug. Inspired oxygen concentrations of at least 30% should be given.

Anesthetic considerations
Nitrous oxide is nonflammable but will support combustion. There is a noticeable second-gas effect that initially hastens the uptake of other agents when high concentrations are used. Nitrous oxide diffuses into air-containing cavities 34 times faster than nitrogen can leave. This can cause a potentially dangerous pressure accumulation (i.e., middle ear perforation, bowel obstruction, pneumothorax, air embolism, endotracheal tube cuff).

NIZATIDINE (AXID)

Classification
Histamine (H₂)-receptor antagonist

Indications
Treatment of duodenal or gastric ulcers and gastroesophageal reflux disease; prophylaxis of aspiration pneumonitis in patients at high risk during surgery

Dose
For prophylaxis of aspiration pneumonitis in adults: 150 mg orally 2 hours before the induction of anesthesia; may be given with or without a similar dose the preceding evening. For patients with impaired renal function as evidenced by serum creatinine level greater than 2.5 mg/dL, a single dose only is needed.
    Dosage form: 150-mg capsule.

Onset and duration

Onset: 0.5 hour peak plasma levels: 1 to 3 hours after oral administration and less than detectable limits in healthy patients 12 hours later. Elimination half-life: 1 to 2.8 hours.

Adverse effects

Headache (most common), gastrointestinal effects and dizziness (4.5%); rarely, thrombocytopenia, leukopenia, anemia; somnolence (2%) and mental confusion possible in elderly patients

Precautions and contraindications

Caution is suggested in patients with hepatic or renal dysfunction. Nizatidine is contraindicated in patients with known hypersensitivity to nizatidine or other H_2 antagonists.

Anesthetic considerations

Nizatidine is safe for use during anesthesia.

NOREPINEPHRINE BITARTRATE (LEVOPHED)

Classification

Catecholamine

Indications

Vasoconstrictor; inotrope; potent peripheral vasoconstrictor of arterial and venous beds; potent inotropic stimulator of the heart (β_1-adrenergic action) but to a lesser degree than epinephrine or isoproterenol.

It does not stimulate β_2-adrenergic receptors of the bronchi or peripheral blood vessels except at high doses. It increases systolic and diastolic blood pressures and coronary artery blood flow. Cardiac output varies reflexly with systemic hypertension but is usually increased in hypotensive patients when blood pressure is raised to an optimal level. At low doses, increased baroreceptor activity reflexly decreases the heart rate. Norepinephrine reduces renal, hepatic, cerebral, and muscle blood flow.

Dose

Infusion: 8 to 12 mcg/min; use the lowest effective dose.

Onset and duration

Onset: 1 minute. Duration: 2 to 10 minutes.

Adverse effects

Bradycardia, tachyarrhythmias, hypertension, decreased cardiac output, headache, plasma volume depletion

Administer into a large vein to minimize extravasation. Treat extravasation with local infiltration of phentolamine (10 mg in 10 mL normal saline) or sympathetic block.

Precautions and contraindications

Norepinephrine bitartrate is contraindicated in patients with mesenteric or peripheral vascular thrombosis.

Anesthetic considerations

Norepinephrine causes an increased risk of arrhythmias with use of volatile anesthetics or bretylium or in patients with hypoxia or hypercarbia. The pressor effect is potentiated in patients receiving monoamine oxidase inhibitors, tricyclic antidepressants, guanethidine, or oxytocics. Norepinephrine may cause necrosis or gangrene with extravasation.

OMEPRAZOLE (PRILOSEC, LOSEC, OMID)

Classification

Proton pump inhibitor

Indications

Gastroesophageal reflux disease

Dose

Oral: 10 to 40 mg daily before meals.

Onset and duration

Onset: within 1 hour (maximum effect: 2 hours). Duration: up to 72 hours.

Adverse effects

Headache, diarrhea, abdominal pain, nausea and vomiting, rash, constipation, dizziness

Precautions and contraindications

Omeprazole is contraindicated in patients with hypersensitivity to omeprazole or other similar proton pump inhibitors.

Anesthetic considerations

Omeprazole is highly protein bound. It undergoes liver and renal elimination. Omeprazole may prolong the elimination of drugs metabolized by oxidation in the liver (i.e., diazepam, warfarin, phenytoin).

ONDANSETRON HCL (ZOFRAN)

Classification

Gastrointestinal agent; serotonin ($5HT_3$) receptor antagonist; antiemetic

Indications

Prevention of nausea and vomiting associated with cancer chemotherapy; postoperative nausea and vomiting

Dose

With chemotherapy: intravenous: three doses—0.15 mg/kg first dose 30 minutes before chemotherapy, then 4 to 8 hours after first dose (may give as 8 mg bolus, then 1 mg/hour continuous infusion with maximum dose of 32 mg/day). Perioperative nausea and vomiting: 2 to 4 mg.

Onset and duration

Onset: variable; most effective if therapy begins before emetogenic chemotherapy. Peak effects: 1 to 1.5 hours. Duration: 12 to 24 hours.

Adverse effects

Tachycardia, angina, dizziness, lightheadedness, headache, sedation, diarrhea, constipation, dry mouth, rash, bronchospasm, hypersensitivity reactions

Precautions and contraindications

Use ondansetron with caution in pregnant or nursing women and in children younger than 3 years old. Ondansetron is contraindicated in patients with hypersensitivity to the drug.

Anesthetic considerations

Monitor cardiovascular status, especially in patients with a history of coronary artery disease.

OXYTOCIN (PITOCIN, SYNTOCINON)

Classification

Oxytocic; lactation stimulant

Indications

Initiation or improvement of uterine contraction at term or after dilation of cervix and delivery of fetus; stimulation of letdown reflex in nursing mothers to relieve pain from breast engorgement

Dose

Administration of oxytocin is always via continuous intravenous infusion. Augmentation of labor: 10 units (1 mL) diluted in 1000 mL of infusate; infusion rates vary from 1 to 10 milliunits/min.

Minimizing of postpartum bleeding: 20 to 100 milliunits/min; effects appear within 3 minutes, are maximal at about 20 minutes, and disappear within 15 to 20 minutes after discontinuing the infusion. In practical terms, 20 to 40 units is usually added to 1000 mL of fluid and is administered to effect.

Promotion of milk ejection: nasal: 1 spray or drop in one or both nostrils 2 to 3 minutes before nursing or pumping the breasts.

Onset and duration

Onset: intravenous: immediate; nasal: few minutes; intramuscular: 3 to 5 minutes. Peak effects: intravenous: less than 20 minutes; intramuscular: 40 minutes. Duration: intravenous: 20 minutes to 1 hour; nasal: 20 minutes; intramuscular: 2 to 3 hours.

Adverse effects

Hypersensitivity leading to uterine hypertonicity, tetanic contractions, uterine rupture, cardiac arrhythmias, nausea and vomiting, hypertension, subarachnoid hemorrhage, seizures from water intoxication, hyponatremia

510   Part III   Drugs

Precautions and contraindications

Use it with caution with other vasoactive drugs. Oxytocin is contraindicated in patients with hypersensitivity to the drug. Oxytocin is also contraindicated in complications of pregnancy: significant cephalopelvic disproportion, fetal distress in which delivery is not imminent, prematurity, placenta previa, or past history of uterine sepsis or of traumatic delivery. The nasal preparation is contraindicated during pregnancy.

Anesthetic considerations

Administration should follow delivery of the fetus. Oxytocin may increase the pressor effects of sympathomimetics. Prolonged intravenous infusion of oxytocin with excessive fluid volume may cause severe water intoxication with seizures, coma, and death. Infuse oxytocin intravenously only after dilution in large volume, preferably with an infusion pump.

PANCURONIUM (PAVULON)

Classification

Nondepolarizing skeletal muscle relaxant

Indications

Adjunct to general anesthesia; skeletal muscle relaxation during surgery

Dose

Intravenous paralyzing: 0.04 to 0.1 mg/kg; pretreatment/maintenance: 0.01 to 0.02 mg/kg.

Dosage forms: injection: 1 mg/mL in 10-mL vial; ampule: 2 mg/mL.

Onset and duration

Onset: 1 to 3 minutes. Duration: 40 to 65 minutes.

Adverse effects

Tachycardia, hypertension, hypoventilation, apnea, bronchospasm, salivation, flushing, anaphylactoid reactions, inadequate block, prolonged block

Precautions and contraindications

Pancuronium is contraindicated in patients with myasthenia gravis, bromide hypersensitivity or in those with conditions in which tachycardia is undesirable.

Anesthetic considerations

Pretreatment doses of pancuronium may cause hypoventilation in some patients. Monitor the patient's response with a peripheral nerve stimulator. Reverse the effects with anticholinesterase.

PHENTOLAMINE (REGITINE)

Classification

α-Adrenergic blocker

Indications

Controlled hypotension; treatment of perioperative hypertensive crisis that may accompany pheochromocytoma removal; prevention or treatment of dermal necrosis or sloughing after intravenous administration or extravasation of barbiturate or sympathomimetic

Dose

Antihypertensive: intravenous/intramuscular: 2.5 to 5 mg. Antisloughing infiltration: 5 to 10 mg (maximum dose: 10 mg); dilute in 10 mL normal saline.

Dosage forms: injection: 5 mg/mL; dilution for infusion 200 mg in 100 mL D_5W or normal saline.

Onset and duration

Onset: intravenous: 1 to 2 minutes; intramuscular: 5 to 20 minutes. Duration: intravenous: 10 to 15 minutes; intramuscular: 30 to 45 minutes.

Adverse effects

Hypotension, tachycardia, arrhythmias, myocardial infarction, dizziness, cerebrovascular spasm and occlusion, flushing, diarrhea, nausea and vomiting

Precautions and contraindications

Use it with caution in patients with ischemic heart disease. Phentolamine-induced α-receptor blockade will potentiate β_2-adrenergic vasodilation of epinephrine, ephedrine, dobutamine, or isoproterenol.

Anesthetic considerations

Use it with epinephrine, ephedrine, dobutamine, or isoproterenol. Phentolamine may cause a fall in blood pressure.

PHENYLEPHRINE (NEO-SYNEPHRINE)

Classification

Synthetic noncatecholamine; α-adrenergic agonist

Indications

Vasoconstriction; treatment of hypotension, shock, supraventricular tachyarrhythmias; prolongation of duration of local anesthetics

Dose

Intravenous: 10 to 100 mcg; do not exceed 0.5 mg initial dose or repeat sooner than 15 minutes. Intravenous infusion: 20 to 50 mcg/min; titrate to effect.

Onset and duration

Onset: immediate. Duration: 15 to 20 minutes.

Adverse effects

Reflex bradycardia, arrhythmias, hypertension, headache, restlessness, reflex vagal action

Precautions and contraindications

Use phenylephrine with extreme caution in elderly patients and patients with hyperthyroidism, bradycardia, partial heart block, or severe arteriosclerosis.

Anesthetic considerations

Infuse phenylephrine into a large vein; treat extravasation with phentolamine (5 to 10 mg in 10 mL normal saline and/or sympathetic block).

PHENYTOIN (DILANTIN)

Classification

Anticonvulsant

Indications

Convulsions; treatment of cardiac arrhythmias from digitalis intoxication, ventricular tachycardia, and paroxysmal atrial tachycardia resistant to conventional methods; treatment of migraine or trigeminal neuralgia

Dose

- Anticonvulsant: intravenous: 10 to 15 mg/kg in 50 to 100 mL normal saline at a rate not exceeding 50 mg/min or 1.5 g/24 hours.
- Maintenance: intravenous/oral: 100 mg every 6 to 8 hours or 300 to 400 mg once a day.
- Antiarrhythmic: intravenous: 1.5 mg/kg slow push every 5 minutes until arrhythmia is suppressed or undesirable effects appear (maximum dosage: 10 to 15 mg/kg/day).
- Children: anticonvulsant: loading dose 10 to 15 mg/kg, 1 g intravenous piggyback in normal saline up to 20 mg/kg in 24 hours.
- Oral maintenance: 4 to 8 mg/kg daily in two to three equally divided doses.
- Dosage forms: injection: 50 mg/mL; capsules and extended-release capsules: 30, 100 mg; chewable tablets: 50 mg; oral suspension: 30 mg/5 mL, 125 mg/5 mL.

Onset and duration

Onset: intravenous: 3 to 5 minutes Therapeutic levels: 10 to 20 mcg/mL; can be attained in 1 to 2 hours after appropriate loading. Elimination half-life: highly variable; increases as plasma levels increase; ranges from 8 to 60 hours (average 22 hours). Patients with liver disease may have highly variable clearance because of saturation kinetics. Duration: 8 to 24 hours, depending on dose.

Adverse effects

Often dose related: nausea and vomiting, gum hyperplasia, megaloblastic anemia (from folate deficiency), osteomalacia (with long-term therapy), thrombocytopenia, granulocytopenia, toxic hepatitis; rarely, exfoliative dermatitis, Stevens-Johnson syndrome, systemic lupus erythematosus; nystagmus (blood level greater than 20 mcg/mL), ataxia (blood level greater than 30 mcg/mL), and somnolence (blood level greater than 40 mcg/mL)

At rates exceeding 50 mg/min, hypotension, cardiovascular collapse, and central nervous system depression may occur.

Precautions and contraindications

- If a rash occurs during therapy, phenytoin should be discontinued; if the rash is exfoliative, purpuric, or bullous or if systemic lupus erythematosus or Stevens-Johnson syndrome is suspected, phenytoin should not be restarted.

- Phenytoin will precipitate in all solutions other than normal saline. Flush the line before and after administration. Do not mix phenytoin with other drugs. Phenytoin must be administered within 1 hour of mixing, owing to short stability.
- Plasma levels should be monitored during therapy after a steady state is achieved and whenever toxicity is suspected.
- Phenytoin should be administered intravenously only with extreme caution in patients with respiratory depression or myocardial depression. Intravenous use is contraindicated in patients with sinus bradycardia, sinoatrial block, second- or third-degree atrioventricular block, or Adams-Stokes syndrome. Phenytoin is not useful in infantile febrile seizures.
- Abrupt withdrawal in patients with epilepsy may precipitate status epilepticus.
- Phenytoin is highly protein bound and has multiple drug interactions. Serum levels may be increased by diazepam, theophylline, warfarin, cimetidine, acute alcohol intake, and halothane. Serum levels are decreased by chronic alcoholism.

Anesthetic considerations

Phenytoin treatment may increase the dose requirements for all nondepolarizing muscle relaxants except atracurium. Dose-response curves are shifted to the right, and the duration is markedly reduced.

Phenytoin follows Michaelis-Menten kinetics. A small incremental dose can radically increase free drug levels at equilibrium.

PHYSOSTIGMINE SALICYLATE (ANTILIRIUM)

Classification
Anticholinesterase agent

Indications
Reversal of prolonged somnolence and anticholinergic poisoning

Dose
Intravenous/intramuscular: 0.5 to 2 mg (10 to 20 mcg/kg) at rate of 1 g/min, repeat dosing at intervals of 10 to 30 minutes.

Onset and duration
Onset: intravenous/intramuscular: 3 to 8 minutes. Duration: intravenous/intramuscular: 30 minutes to 5 hours.

Adverse effects
Bradycardia, bronchospasm, dyspnea, respiratory paralysis, seizures, salivation, nausea and vomiting, miosis

Precautions and contraindications
High doses of physostigmine may cause tremors, ataxia, muscle fasciculations, and ultimately a depolarization block. Use it with caution in patients with epilepsy, parkinsonian syndrome, or bradycardia. Do not use it in the presence of asthma, diabetes, or mechanical obstruction of the intestine or urogenital tract or in patients receiving choline esters or depolarizing muscle relaxants.

PART III **Drugs**

Anesthetic considerations

Rapid intravenous administration may cause bradycardia and hypersalivation, leading to respiratory problems or possibly seizures. Treatment of
cholinergic crisis includes mechanical ventilation with repeated bronchial
aspiration and intravenous administration of atropine, 2 to 4 mg every 3 to
10 minutes until control of muscarinic symptoms is achieved or until signs
of atropine overdose appear.

PIPECURONIUM BROMIDE (ARDUAN)

Classification

Nondepolarizing skeletal muscle relaxant

Indications

Adjunct to general anesthesia; skeletal muscle relaxation during surgery

Dose

Intravenous paralyzing: 0.07 to 0.10 mg/kg; pretreatment and maintenance:
0.01 to 0.015 mg/kg; children: (3 months to 1 year) adult dosage on an
mg/kg basis.

Dosage forms: powder for injection: 10 mg (10 mL).

Onset and duration

Onset: less than 3 minutes. Duration: 45 to 120 minutes. Elimination: renal.

Adverse effects

Hypotension, hypertension, bradycardia, myocardial infarction, hypoventilation, apnea, depression, anuria, urticaria, rash, inadequate block,
prolonged block, hypoglycemia, hyperkalemia, increased creatinine.

Pipecuronium exhibits enhanced neuromuscular blockade in patients
with myasthenia gravis.

Precautions and contradictions

Patients may exhibit allergy to pipecuronium. Because of the drug's long
duration of action, postoperative ventilation is likely to be required.

Anesthetic considerations

Reverse any effects with anticholinesterase. Monitor the patient's response
with a peripheral nerve stimulator. Pretreatment doses may cause hypoventilation in some patients. Pipecuronium is recommended only for procedures
anticipated to last 90 minutes or longer.

PRILOCAINE HCL (CITANEST)

Classification

Amide-type local anesthetic

Indications

Regional anesthesia: infiltration/peripheral nerve block, topical, epidural,
intravenous regional

Dose

Infiltration/peripheral nerve block: 0.5 to 6 mg/kg (0.5% to 2% solution); topical: 0.6 to 3 mg/kg (2% to 4% solution); epidural: 200 to 300 mg (1% to 2% solution); (maximum safe dosage: 6 mg/kg without epinephrine; 9 mg/kg with epinephrine 1:200,000).

Onset and duration

Onset: infiltration: 1 to 2 minutes; epidural: 5 to 15 minutes. Peak effects: infiltration/epidural: less than 30 minutes. Duration: infiltration: 0.5 to 1.5 hours without epinephrine, 2 to 6 hours with epinephrine; epidural: 1 to 3 hours (prolonged with epinephrine).

Adverse effects

Hypotension, arrhythmia, collapse, respiratory depression, paralysis, seizures, tinnitus, blurred vision, urticaria, anaphylactoid reactions, methemoglobinemia; high spinal, urinary retention, lower extremity weakness and paralysis, loss of sphincter control, headache, backache, slowing of labor

Precautions and contraindications

Use it with caution in patients with hypovolemia, severe congestive heart failure, shock, all forms of heart block, or pregnancy. Prilocaine is contraindicated in patients with hypersensitivity to amide-type local anesthetics and in infants younger than 6 months old (low dose may cause methemoglobinemia).

Anesthetic considerations

Treat methemoglobinemia with methylene blue (1 to 2 mg/kg injected over 5 minutes). In intravenous regional blocks, deflate the cuff after 40 minutes and not before 20 minutes.

PROCAINAMIDE (PROCAN SR, PRONESTYL)

Classification

Class Ia antiarrhythmic

Indications

Treatment of lidocaine-resistant ventricular arrhythmias; arrhythmia control in malignant hyperthermia; treatment of atrial fibrillation or paroxysmal atrial tachycardia

Dose

Loading: slow intravenous push: 100 mg every 5 minutes (maximum: 500 mg); do not exceed 50 mg/min (children: 3 to 6 mg/kg given over 5 minutes). Dilute 1000 mg in 50 mL D_5W. Intramuscular: 100 to 500 mg in doses divided every 3 or 6 hours. Maintenance: infusion: 2 to 6 mg/min (children: 0.02 to 0.08 mg/kg/min). Therapeutic level: 3 to 10 mcg/mL.

Dosage form: injection: 100 mg/mL, 500 mg/mL. Dilution for infusion: 2 g in 500 mL D_5W (4 mg/mL).

Onset and duration

Onset: intravenous: immediate; intramuscular: 10 to 30 minutes. Duration: 2.5 to 5 hours.

Adverse effects

Hypotension, heart block, arrhythmias, seizures, confusion, depression, psychosis, anorexia, nausea and vomiting, diarrhea, systemic lupus erythematosus, pruritus, fever, chills

Precautions and contraindications

Use it with caution in patients with first-degree heart block or arrhythmias associated with digitalis toxicity. Reduce doses in patients with congestive heart failure or renal failure. Procainamide is contraindicated in patients with complete heart block, torsades de pointes, or systemic lupus erythematosus.

Anesthetic considerations

Procainamide requires periodic monitoring of patient plasma levels, vital signs, and electrocardiogram (QRS widening greater than 25% may signify overdosage). Procainamide potentiates the effect of both nondepolarizing and depolarizing muscle relaxants.

PROCAINE HCL (NOVOCAIN)

Classification

Ester-type local anesthetic

Indications

Local anesthetic: infiltration, peripheral nerve block, sympathetic nerve block, regional anesthesia

Dose

Infiltration: less than 500 mg (0.5 to 2% solution); epidural: less than 500 mg (1 to 2% solution); spinal: 50 to 200 mg (10% solution with glucose 5%). Solutions with preservatives may not be used for epidural or spinal block.

Onset and duration

Onset: infiltration/spinal: 2 to 5 minutes; epidural: 5 to 25 minutes. Peak effects: infiltration/epidural/spinal: less than 30 minutes. Duration: infiltration: 0.25 to 0.5 hours (without epinephrine), 0.5 to 1.5 hours (with epinephrine), epidural/spinal: 0.5 to 1.5 hours (prolonged with epinephrine).

Adverse effects

Hypotension, bradycardia, arrhythmias, heart block, respiratory depression or arrest, tinnitus, seizures, dizziness, restlessness, loss of hearing, euphoria, postspinal headache, palsies, urticaria, pruritus, angioneurotic edema; high spinal, loss of bladder and bowel control and permanent motor, sensory, and autonomic (sphincter control) deficits of lower segments

Precautions and contraindications

Use it with caution in patients with severe cardiac disturbances (heart block, arrhythmias) or inflammation/sepsis at injection site. Procaine is contraindicated in patients with hypersensitivity to *para*-aminobenzoic acid/parabens, or ester-type anesthetics.

Anesthetic considerations

Central nervous system effects are generally dose dependent and of short duration. Vasopressors and oxytocics may cause hypertension. Preparations containing preservatives should not be used for epidural and spinal anesthesia.

PROCHLORPERAZINE MALEATE (COMPAZINE)

Classification

Antiemetic; psychotherapeutic; phenothiazine antipsychotic

Indications

Control of nausea and vomiting; management of manifestations of psychotic disorders of excessive anxiety, tension, and agitation

Dose

Antiemetic: oral: 5 to 10 mg three or four times daily; rectal: 25 mg twice daily; intravenous/intramuscular: 5 to 10 mg (5 mg/mL/min) (maximum dose: 40 mg/day). Do not administer subcutaneously because of local irritation.

Onset and duration

Onset: intravenous: a few minutes; intramuscular: 10 to 20 minutes; oral: 30 to 40 minutes; rectal: 60 minutes. Peak effects: intravenous/intramuscular/oral: 15 to 30 minutes. Duration: intravenous/intramuscular/oral/rectal: 3 to 4 hours.

Adverse effects

Extrapyramidal reactions, dystonia, central nervous system depression, hypotension

Precautions and contraindications

Prochlorperazine maleate is contraindicated in pediatric patients and in patients with parkinsonian disease.

Anesthetic considerations

Prochlorperazine maleate may produce an additive central nervous system depression when it is used with anesthetics. Avoid using prochlorperazine maleate with droperidol or metoclopramide because of extrapyramidal effects.

PROMETHAZINE HCL (PHENERGAN, PENTAZINE, PHENAZINE, PROTHAZINE)

Classification

Phenothiazine: antiemetic, antivertigo agent, antihistamine (H_1-receptor antagonist), sedative or adjunct to analgesics

Indications

Motion sickness or nausea; rhinitis; allergy symptoms; sedation; routine preoperative or postoperative sedation; adjunct to analgesics

PART III Drugs

Dose

Intravenous: administer cautiously because of hazard of phlebitis, necrosis, and gangrene of extremities; must dilute with equal volume of compatible diluent and administer slowly. Children: administer no larger dose than 0.5 mg/kg; intramuscular, oral, rectal: 12.5 to 50 mg. *Do not* administer subcutaneously or intraarterially because of the risk of necrosis and gangrene of extremities.

Dosage forms: tablet: 12.5, 25, and 50 mg; syrup: 6.25 and 25 mg/5 mL; suppositories: 12.5, 25, 50 mg; injection: 25 and 50 mg/mL.

Onset and duration

Onset: intravenous: 150 seconds; intramuscular, oral, rectal: 15 to 30 minutes. Duration: intravenous, intramuscular, oral, rectal: 2 to 5 hours.

Adverse effects

Hypotension, bradycardia, bronchospasm, drowsiness, sedation, dizziness, confusion, extrapyramidal reactions, agranulocytosis, thrombocytopenia

Precautions and contraindications

Use it with caution, because the central nervous system and circulatory depressant actions of alcohol, sedative-hypnotics, and anesthetics are potentiated. Promethazine is contraindicated in patients with Parkinson's disease and in those receiving monoamine oxidase inhibitors.

Anesthetic considerations

Anesthetic recovery may be prolonged. Do not use in children younger than 2 years of age.

PROPOFOL (DIPRIVAN; GENERIC FORMULATION ALSO AVAILABLE)

Classification

Anesthesia induction agent

Indications

Anesthesia induction and maintenance; intravenous sedation; prolonged sedation in critical care

Dose

Intravenous bolus: 1 to 2.5 mg/kg. Dilute in suitable intravenous fluid, preferably D_5W. *Do not* dilute the final solution to less than 2 mg/mL in order to protect suspension. *Do not* use any filter with a pore size smaller than 5 mm. Infusion: 25 to 200 µg/kg/min.

Dosage form: 10 mg/mL in 20-mL ampules and 50- and 100-mL vials.

Onset and duration

Onset: immediate. Duration: 5 to 20 minutes, depending on dose.

Adverse effects

Hypotension, bradycardia, respiratory depression, prolonged somnolence, vivid dreams, burning on injection, hiccups, disinhibition, arrhythmias

Precautions and contraindications

Reduce the propofol dose or avoid the drug in patients with cardiac compromise, in elderly patients, and in those with respiratory disease, hypotension, or increased intracranial pressure. Watch for respiratory and cardiac depression when coadministering other central nervous system or cardiac depressant drugs. Strict aseptic technique must be used when handling the drug to avoid bacterial growth in the emulsion vehicle. The generic formulation contains metabisulfate and should be avoided in patients sensitive to these compounds. Infusion of doses larger than 5 mg/kg/hour for longer than 48 hours may result in propofol emulsion syndrome.

Anesthetic considerations

Minimize pain on injection by giving a small dose of plain lidocaine (1%) before propofol injection. Both convulsant and anticonvulsant effects have been reported, so do not use propofol in patients with a history of seizures. The antiemetic properties of propofol may be an advantage in patients at risk for postoperative nausea and vomiting.

PROPRANOLOL (INDERAL, OTHERS)

Classification

Nonselective β-adrenergic receptor antagonist

Indications

Hypertension; angina; ventricular and supraventricular arrhythmias; hyperthyroidism; migraines

Dose

Intravenous: 0.25-mg increments, up to 3 mg; oral: 10 to 80 mg every 6 to 8 hours or 80 to 240 mg/day sustained release.

Dosage forms: injection: 1 mg/mL (1 mL); tablet: 10, 20, 40, 60, 80, 90 mg.

Onset and duration

Onset: intravenous: less than 2 minutes; oral: 30 to 60 minutes. Duration: intravenous: 1 to 4 hours; oral: up to 24 hours sustained release.

Adverse effects

Bradycardia, hypotension, atrioventricular block, bronchospasm, hypoglycemia, claudication, diarrhea, nausea, vomiting, constipation, nightmares, mental depression, insomnia, increased plasma triglycerides and decreased high-density lipoproteins

Precautions and contraindications

Propranolol is contraindicated in asthmatic patients and in patients with reduced myocardial reserve, peripheral vascular disease, diabetes, congestive heart failure, or shock. If the drug is discontinued abruptly, withdrawal may be manifested as increased nervousness, increased heart rate, increased intensity of angina, or increased blood pressure (related to up-regulation). The effects of propranolol may be potentiated by inhalational anesthetics and other cardiodepressant drugs.

Anesthetic considerations

Esmolol is preferred over propranolol for intraoperative use, because of its more controllable duration of action. Propranolol may be useful as an antiarrhythmic because of its membrane-stabilizing properties.

PROTAMINE SULFATE

Classification

Heparin antagonist

Indications

Treatment of heparin overdosage; heparin neutralization after extracorporeal circulation in arterial and cardiovascular surgery

Dose

Dosage is based on blood coagulation studies, usually 1 mg protamine for every 100 units of heparin remaining in the patient, given slowly by intravenous over 10 minutes in doses not to exceed 50 mg.

Because heparin blood concentrations decrease rapidly, the required dose of protamine sulfate decreases based on the elapsed time. One half of the usual dose of protamine should be given if 30 minutes have elapsed since heparin administration, and one fourth of the usual dose should be given if 2 hours or more have elapsed.

Dosage forms: parenteral injection for intravenous use only: 10 mg/mL, 5-mL ampule or vial. Reconstitute a 50-mg vial by adding 5 mL sterile water or bacteriostatic water containing 0.9% benzyl alcohol. The resultant solution contains 10 mg/mL. A protamine solution is intended for intravenous bolus use and not for further dilution. If further dilution is desired, however, 5% dextrose or 0.9% sodium chloride intravenous piggyback may be used and given over 30 minutes.

Children: injections preserved with benzyl alcohol may cause toxicity in the neonate.

Onset and duration

Onset: neutralization of heparin occurs within 5 minutes. Duration: neutralization of heparin persists for approximately 2 hours.

Adverse effects

Rapid intravenous injection: hypotension, bradycardia, flushing; other possible effects: hypersensitivity, anaphylaxis, dyspnea, noncardiac pulmonary edema, circulatory collapse, pulmonary hypertension, "heparin rebound" (in cardiopulmonary bypass).

A paradoxical anticoagulant effect may occur with total doses greater than 100 mg.

Precautions and contraindications

Monitor the patient's activated partial thromboplastin time or the activated coagulation time at least 5 to 15 minutes after protamine administration to determine its effect. Have equipment readily available to treat shock. Patients with sensitivity to fish and patients who have previously received either protamine or insulins containing protamine are considered at higher risk for hypersensitivity. If protamine is used in these patients, pretreatment with a corticosteroid or antihistamine should be considered. Protamine is contraindicated in patients with a history of allergy to the drug.

Anesthetic considerations

Rapid intravenous injection of protamine is associated with hypotension, bradycardia, and flushing.

PYRIDOSTIGMINE BROMIDE (MESTINON, REGONOL)

Classification

Anticholinesterase agent

Indications

Reversal of nondepolarizing muscle relaxants

Dose

Reversal: intravenous: 10 to 30 mg (0.1 to 0.25 mg/kg), preceded by atropine (0.015 mg/kg) or glycopyrrolate (0.01 mg/kg) intravenously. Myasthenia gravis: oral: 60 to 1500 mg/day; sustained release: 180 to 540 mg daily or twice daily. To supplement oral dosage preoperatively and postoperatively, during labor and post partum, during myasthenic crisis, or when oral therapy is impractical: give $\frac{1}{30}$ the oral dose intramuscularly or very slowly intravenously.

Neonates of myasthenic mothers: 0.05 to 0.15 mg/kg intramuscularly. Differentiate between cholinergic and myasthenic crisis in neonates. Administration 1 hour before completion of the second stage of labor enables patients to have adequate strength during labor and provides protection to infants in the intermediate postnatal stage.

Onset and duration

Onset: reversal: intravenous: 2 to 5 minutes; myasthenia: intramuscular: less than 15 minutes; oral: 20 to 30 minutes. Duration: reversal: intravenous: 90 minutes; myasthenia: oral: 3 to 6 hours; intramuscular: 2 to 4 hours.

Adverse effects

Bradycardia, atrioventricular block, nodal rhythm, hypotension, increased bronchial secretions, bronchospasm, respiratory depression, nausea, vomiting, diarrhea, abdominal cramps, increased peristalsis, increased salivation, muscle cramps, fasciculations, weakness, miosis, diaphoresis

Precautions and contraindications

Use pyridostigmine with caution in patients with bradycardia, bronchial asthma, cardiac arrhythmias, or peptic ulcer and in patients with peritonitis or mechanical obstruction of the intestines or urinary tract.

Anesthetic considerations

Overdosage of pyridostigmine may induce a cholinergic crisis characterized by nausea, vomiting, bradycardia or tachycardia, excessive salivation and sweating, bronchospasm, weakness, and paralysis. Treatment of a cholinergic crisis includes discontinuation of pyridostigmine and administration of atropine (10 mg/kg intravenously every 3 to 10 minutes until muscarinic symptoms subside).

PART III Drugs

RANITIDINE (ZANTAC)

Classification
Histamine (H_2)-receptor antagonist

Indications
Treatment of duodenal or gastric ulcers and gastroesophageal reflux; prophylaxis of aspiration pneumonitis in patients at high risk during surgery

Dose
For patients with normal renal function: 50 mg by intravenous piggyback diluted in at least 25 mL D_5W, normal saline, or suitable diluent, given over 15 to 20 minutes at least 1 hour before induction of anesthesia. The drug may be given with or without a similar dose the preceding evening. For patients with impaired renal function, as evidenced by creatinine clearance less than 50 mL/min: single dose only is needed 1 to 4 hours before induction of anesthesia.

Alternatively, 150 mg ranitidine orally may be substituted for 50 mg by intravenous piggyback. When given orally, however, it is recommended to be given 2 hours preinduction.

Children 2 to 18 years: 0.1 to 0.8 mg/kg/dose by intravenous piggyback at least 1 hour before induction infused over at least 5 minutes. Dilute to concentration of 0.5 to 2.5 mg/mL.

Dosage forms: 150-mg tablets; parenteral injection: 25 mg/mL in 2-mL or 10-mL multidose vials.

Onset and duration
Onset: mean gastric acid concentration significantly decreases 1 hour after intravenous infusion. Duration: gastric acid inhibitory effects persist 8 to 12 hours.

Adverse effects
Most frequent: headache (1.8%), fatigue, dizziness, mild gastrointestinal disturbances; infrequent: reversible hepatitis and potential hepatotoxicity; rarely: reversible leukopenia, thrombocytopenia, granulocytopenia, aplastic anemia

Bradydysrhythmias and hypotension may be associated with rapid intravenous infusion.

Precautions and contraindications
Use ranitidine with caution in patients with hypersensitivity to ranitidine or other H_2-receptor antagonists. Caution is suggested in patients with hepatic insufficiency.

Anesthetic considerations
Ranitidine is useful for gastric preparation in high-risk patients prone to aspiration. Do not use in non–high-risk patients.

REMIFENTANIL (ULTIVA)

Classification
Opiate analgesic

Indications

Perioperative analgesia

Dose

Infusion only: induction: 0.5 to 1 mcg/kg/min; maintenance: 0.05 to 0.8 mcg/kg/min; postoperative pain in postanesthesia care unit: 0.025 to 0.2 mcg/kg/min.

Dosage forms: 1 mg powder in 3-mL vial; 2 mg powder in 5-mL vial; 5 mg powder in 10-mL vial.

Supplemental bolus of 0.05 mcg/kg may be given during induction and maintenance. Supplemental bolus is not recommended postoperatively because of risk of apnea or significant respiratory depression. Changes in infusion rate take 2 to 5 minutes for clinical response to change.

Onset and duration

Onset: 1 to 5 minutes. Duration: continuous infusion effect ceases 5 to 15 minutes after infusion is stopped.

Adverse effects

Similar to those of other opiate agonists and include nausea and vomiting, hypotension, bradycardia, respiratory depression, apnea, muscle rigidity, pruritus

Precautions and contraindications

Oxygen saturation should be continuously monitored throughout remifentanil administration. Resuscitative and airway management equipment must be immediately available. Remifentanil should not be mixed with lactated Ringer's injection or lactated Ringer's/5% dextrose but can be coadministered with these solutions in a freely running intravenous line. Do not run remifentanil in the same line with blood, because this drug is metabolized by esterase enzymes. The intravenous line should be cleared after discontinuation to prevent inadvertent administration. Remifentanil is contraindicated for epidural or intrathecal administration because of glycine in the vehicle formulation.

Anesthetic considerations

The effects of remifentanil rapidly dissipate after discontinuation of the infusion, so preparation for postoperative care may include longer-acting opiates or nonsteroidal antiinflammatory agents. Because remifentanil is metabolized by nonspecific esterases, no change in kinetics has been noted in patients with cholinesterase deficiencies or renal or hepatic disease. Normal kinetics were noted in pediatric, geriatric, and obese patients.

PART III **Drugs**

RITODRINE HCL (YUTOPAR)

Classification

β_2-Adrenergic agonist, tocolytic agent, sympathomimetic

Indications

Management of preterm labor (tocolysis); bronchodilation

Dose

Infusion: prepare in D_5W if clinically appropriate or in sodium chloride 0.9% intravenous solution of 0.3 mg/mL. Start at 0.1 mg/min (20 mL/hour at this concentration) and slowly increase by 0.05 mg/min every 10 to 15 minutes, up to 0.35 mg/min. Continue infusion for at least 12 hours after cessation of uterine contractions at the maximum rate achieved.

Oral: start before discontinuation of the intravenous infusion at 10 mg every 2 hours for 24 hours, then 10 to 20 mg every 4 to 6 hours (maximum dose: 120 mg/day).

Dosage forms: tablet: 10 mg; injection: 10 mg/mL in 5-mL ampules and vials; injection: 15 mg/mL in 10-mL vials and 10-mL prefilled syringe; solution for intravenous infusion: 150 mg in D_5W 500 mL (0.3 mg/mL).

Onset and duration

Onset: intravenous: immediate; oral: 40 to 60 minutes. Duration: intravenous: 3 to 6 hours.

Adverse effects

β_1-Agonist effects (common): tachycardia, arrhythmias, hypertension, hyperventilation, pulmonary edema, tremors, headache, anxiety, nausea, vomiting, diarrhea, hyperglycemia

Reactive hypoglycemia may occur in the postpartum infant.

Precautions and contraindications

Pulmonary edema is common with overhydration, so fluid intake should be closely monitored, especially in patients taking corticosteroids. Monitor glucose and electrolyte levels. Ritodrine is contraindicated before 20 weeks of pregnancy and in preeclampsia, eclampsia, intrauterine fetal death or fetal distress, uncontrolled maternal diabetes, maternal hyperthyroidism and hypertension, and placental detachment. Concern surrounds the clinical benefits related to perinatal morbidity and mortality.

Anesthetic considerations

Patients may experience wide swings in vital signs secondary to β-receptor stimulation. Bradycardia and hypotension may occur after cessation of ritodrine therapy. Glucose, insulin, and potassium levels are commonly altered during therapy and should be evaluated. Mild hypokalemia is usually not treated. Additive hypertension and tachycardia occur when ritodrine is given with other sympathomimetics. Adverse effects may be antagonized by β-blocking agents.

ROCURONIUM (ZEMURON)

Classification

Nondepolarizing neuromuscular blocking agent

Indications

Tracheal intubation and intraoperative skeletal muscle relaxation; in critical care, facilitation of mechanical ventilation

Dose

Adults and children: intubation: 0.6 to 1.0 mg/kg. Maintenance: adults: 0.1 to 0.2 mg/kg; children: 0.08 to 0.12 mg/kg intravenously.

Onset and duration
Onset: 60 to 90 seconds with intubating doses of three to five times the 95% effective dose (0.9 to 1.5 mg/kg; ED_{95} = 0.3 mg/kg). Duration: 30 to 120 minutes, depending on the dose.

Adverse effects
Rare: prolonged effect in patients with hepatic disease

Precautions and contraindications
Rocuronium is contraindicated in patients known to have hypersensitivity to the drug. Proper airway maintenance capabilities must be ensured before administration.

Anesthetic considerations
Use of inhalation agents, antibiotics, and magnesium may prolong the duration of action of rocuronium. Many clinicians consider it the agent of choice for nondepolarizing rapid sequence induction when intubating doses are used. No significant cardiac or histamine-releasing effects occur with clinical doses of rocuronium.

ROPIVACAINE HCL (NAROPIN)

Classification
Amide-type local anesthetic

Indications
Regional anesthesia: epidural, peripheral nerve block; local infiltration

Dose
Epidural: 75 to 250 mg (0.2% to 0.5% solution); obstetric: less than 150 mg (0.5% solution); infiltration: less than 200 mg (0.2% to 0.5% solution); peripheral nerve block: less than 275 mg (0.5% solution). Spinal doses have not been established. Do not exceed 770 mg in 24 hours.

Onset and duration
Onset: epidural: 5 to 13 minutes; obstetrics: 11 to 26 minutes; infiltration: 1 to 5 minutes; peripheral nerve block: 10 to 45 minutes. Duration: epidural: 3 to 5 hours; obstetrics: 1.7 to 3.2 hours; infiltration: 2 to 6 hours; peripheral nerve block: 3.7 to 8.7 hours.

Adverse effects
Hypotension, nausea and vomiting, bradycardia, paresthesia, fetal bradycardia, back pain, chills, fever, headache, pain, dizziness, pruritus, urinary retention, arrhythmias, seizures

Precautions and contraindications
Reduce ropivacaine doses in debilitated, elderly, or acutely ill patients, and in children. Use it with caution in patients with hypotension, hypovolemia, or heart block. It is not for use in paracervical/retrobulbar/intravenous regional/subarachnoid blocks. Ropivacaine is contraindicated in patients with known hypersensitivity to amide-type local anesthetics.

Anesthetic considerations

Considerations with ropivacaine are similar to those with bupivacaine but with less depth and duration of the motor blockade. Its use with epinephrine has only a minor effect on onset and duration. Ropivacaine undergoes liver and renal elimination.

SALMETEROL XINAFOATE (SEREVENT)

Classification

β_2-Adrenergic agonist, antiasthmatic, bronchodilator

Indications

Maintenance treatment of asthma and chronic obstructive pulmonary disease (COPD); prevention of bronchospasm

Dose

Powder: one inhalation (50 mcg) twice daily (morning and evening 12 hours apart); aerosol: two inhalations (42 mcg) twice daily (morning and evening 12 hours apart).

Onset and duration

Asthma maintenance: onset to produce bronchodilation: 10 to 20 minutes. Duration: 12 hours. COPD: onset to bronchodilation: within 30 minutes. Duration: up to 12 hours.

Adverse effects

Sympathomimetic cardiovascular effects, ventricular arrhythmias, electrocardiographic changes (flattening of the T wave, prolonged QT interval, ST-segment depression), laryngospasm, stridor, excitement, aggravation of diabetes mellitus and ketoacidosis

Precautions and contraindications

Use it with caution in patients with hypersensitivity to salmeterol, acute deteriorating asthma, coronary insufficiency, arrhythmias, hypertension, convulsive disorders, or thyrotoxicosis. Safety of salmeterol during pregnancy and in children has not been established. Use it with extreme caution in patients taking monoamine oxidase inhibitors or tricyclic antidepressants—cardiovascular sympathomimetic effects may be potentiated under these circumstances.

Anesthetic considerations

Use of β-antagonists may block the effects of salmeterol and may predispose patients to bronchospasm. Dosing intervals of less than 12 hours may induce bronchospasm.

SCOPOLAMINE (TRANSDERM SCOP)

Classification

Competitive acetylcholine antagonist at muscarinic receptor, antiemetic

Indications

Prevention and treatment of nausea and vomiting induced by motion (motion sickness), premedication, amnesia, sedation, or vagolysis.

It produces greater sedation and amnesia and has greater antisialagogue and ocular effects than does atropine with lesser effects on the heart, bronchial smooth muscle, and gastrointestinal tract.

Dose

Oral: 0.4 to 1.2 mg; usual adult intramuscular, intravenous, or subcutaneous dose: 0.3 to 0.65 mg 30 to 80 minutes before induction; transdermal patch: 1.5 mg/2.5 cm^2; delivers 0.5 mg/72 hours; apply to postauricular skin.

Children: intramuscular or intravenous: 0.006 mg/kg or 0.2 mg/m^2 (maximum dose: 0.3 mg).

Dosage forms: 0.3, 0.4, 0.86, 1 mg/mL parenteral injection; transdermal patch: 1.5 mg/2.5 cm^2.

Onset and duration

Onset: after intravenous administration: 1 to 3 minutes; after oral or intramuscular administration: about 30 minutes. Duration: after intravenous administration: 30 to 60 minutes; after intramuscular administration: 4 to 6 hours. Transdermal systems are designed to provide an antiemetic effect within 4 hours of application with a duration of up to 72 hours.

Adverse effects

Hallucinations, delirium coma in central anticholinergic syndrome (treatment: pyridostigmine, 15 to 60 mg/kg); other effects: paradoxical bradycardia in low doses, mydriasis, blurred vision, tachycardia, drowsiness, restlessness, confusion, anaphylaxis, dry nose and mouth, constipation, urinary hesitancy, retention, increased intraocular pressure, decreased sweating

Children and elderly are more susceptible to adverse effects.

Precautions and contraindications

Use scopolamine with caution when tachycardia would be harmful (i.e., thyrotoxicosis, pheochromocytoma, coronary artery disease). Avoid using scopolamine in patients in hyperpyrexial states because it inhibits sweating. Use it with caution in patients with hepatic or renal disease, congestive heart failure, chronic pulmonary disease (because a reduction in bronchial secretions may lead to formation of bronchial plugs), hiatal hernia, gastroesophageal reflux, gastrointestinal infections, or ulcerative colitis. Scopolamine is contraindicated in patients with acute-angle glaucoma, obstructive disease of the gastrointestinal tract, obstructive uropathy, intestinal atony, or acute hemorrhage when cardiovascular status is unstable.

Anesthetic considerations

Scopolamine potentiates the sedative effects of narcotics, benzodiazepines, anticholinergics, antihistamines, and volatile anesthetics.

SEVOFLURANE (ULTANE)

Classification

Inhalation anesthetic

Indications
General anesthesia

Dose
Titrate to effect for induction or maintenance of anesthesia. Minimum alveolar concentration: 2%.

Dosage forms: volatile liquid.

Onset and duration
Onset: loss of eyelid reflex: 1 to 2 minutes. Duration: emergence time: 8 to 9 minutes.

Adverse effects
Hypotension, arrhythmia, respiratory depression, apnea, dizziness, euphoria, increased cerebral blood flow and intracranial pressure, nausea, vomiting, ileus, malignant hyperthermia.

Precautions and contraindications
Sevoflurane is contraindicated in patients with known or suspected genetic susceptibility to malignant hyperthermia. Causes significant increases in free fluoride ion. Some practitioners avoid in patients with overt renal disease. Reacts with carbon dioxide granulates in the anesthesia machine to produce compound A. A rare fire hazard has been reported when using Sevoflurane under certain anesthesia machine conditions.

Anesthetic considerations
The mostly commonly used inhalation anesthetic in pediatric patients. Safe and effective for inhalation anesthetic induction. May see a short period of restlessness upon emergence.

SODIUM CITRATE (BICITRA)

Classification
Nonparticulate neutralizing buffer

Indications
Prophylaxis of aspiration pneumonitis during anesthesia (metabolizes to sodium bicarbonate and thus acts as systemic alkalinizer)

When given within 60 minutes of surgery, sodium citrate is effective in raising the gastric pH to more than 2.5 in most patients. Theoretically, this decreases the risk of pulmonary damage secondary to aspiration of gastric contents; however, this remains controversial.

Dose
Adults: 15 mL diluted in 15 mL water as a single dose; children: 5 to 15 mL diluted in 5 to 15 mL water as a single dose, or 1 mEq/kg as a single dose.

Dosage forms: sodium citrate dihydrate 500 mg (321.5 mg of citrate)/5 mL and citric acid monohydrate 334 mg/5 mL. Each 1 mL contains 1 mEq sodium and 1 mEq citrate.

Onset and duration
Onset: 2 to 10 minutes. Duration: 60 to 90 minutes. Maximally effective when given less than 60 minutes preoperatively.

Adverse effects

Saline laxative effect (when sodium citrate is given orally); metabolic alkalosis (in large doses in patients with renal dysfunction)

Precautions and contraindications

Sodium citrate is contraindicated in patients with severe renal impairment with oliguria, azotemia, or anuria. It is also contraindicated in patients with Addison's disease, heat cramps, acute dehydration, adynamic episodica hereditaria, or severe myocardial disease.

Anesthetic considerations

Sodium citrate is useful for patients at a high risk of aspiration.

SOMATOSTATIN (ZECNIL)

Classification

Synthetic somatostatin; growth hormone release–inhibiting factor; also inhibitor of glucagon, insulin, secretin, gastrin, and thyroid-stimulating hormone

Indications

Prophylaxis in preoperative management of patients with carcinoid syndrome and treatment of hypotensive episodes associated with surgical manipulation of carcinoid tumor, gastrointestinal bleeding, malignant diarrhea, enterocutaneous and pancreatic fistulas, and short bowel syndrome

Epidural somatostatin is effective in treating postoperative pain; intrathecal and intraventricular somatostatin were employed for the pain of terminal cancer in limited studies.

Dose

Adults: continuous infusion required to sustain therapeutic effects; usual infusion rate: 250 mcg/hour, with or without initial 250-mcg bolus. Dilute 3 mg somatostatin in 50 mL D_5W or normal saline and infuse continuously over 12 hours (250 mcg/hour) on a syringe pump. Octreotide (Sandostatin), a long-acting analogue of somatostatin, may also be used; the initial dose is 50 mcg subcutaneously, but intravenous injection can be used during an emergency.

Dosage forms: somatostatin (Zecnil): 3-mg lyophilized ampules; octreotide (Sandostatin): 0.1, 0.05, 0.5 mg/mL injection.

Somatostatin is currently designated "orphan drug" by the Food and Drug Administration.

Onset and duration

Onset: 5 to 10 minutes after initiation of infusion. Duration: effects decrease rapidly after discontinuance of infusion to baseline in 1 hour; plasma half-life: 1 to 3 minutes. (Half-life of octreotide: after intravenous: 45 minutes; after subcutaneous: 80 minutes).

Adverse effects

Nausea, vomiting, diarrhea, and abdominal cramps during infusion; glucose intolerance in nondiabetic patients and reduced insulin requirements in insulin-dependent diabetic patients; less frequent: arrhythmias, hyponatremia

Precautions and contraindications

Use somatostatin with caution in patients with diabetes. Rebound hypersecretion of growth hormone and other hormones usually occurs after

PART III Drugs

infusion is discontinued. Monitor blood glucose levels during therapy. Rebound fistula output is also noted in patients with enterocutaneous fistulas. Somatostatin is contraindicated in patients with previous hypersensitivity to the drug or with octreotide.

Anesthetic considerations

Sandostatin is indicated for the symptomatic treatment of patients with metastatic carcinoid tumors in which it suppresses or inhibits the severe diarrhea and flushing episodes associated with the disease.

SOTALOL HYDROCHLORIDE (BETAPACE, SOTAGARD)

Classification

Antiarrhythmic, nonselective β-adrenergic blocking agent

Indications

Life-threatening ventricular arrhythmias (i.e., sustained ventricular tachycardia); torsade de pointes or ventricular tachycardia/fibrillation from nonsupraventricular tachycardia or supraventricular tachycardia arrhythmias; atrial fibrillation

Dose

Treatment of sustained ventricular tachycardia: adults: initially, 80 mg orally twice daily (maximum dose: 320 mg/day, given in two divided doses).

Conversion and maintenance of sinus rhythm in patients with atrial fibrillation: adults: 80 to 160 mg orally twice daily; children: safety and efficacy have not been established.

Onset and duration

Onset of action following oral administration: approximately 1 hour. Peak effect: 2.5 to 4 hours. Low lipid solubility; does not cross the blood-brain barrier. Duration: 4 to 6 hours.

Adverse effects

Fatigue, bradycardia, dyspnea, angina, palpitations, dizziness, nausea and vomiting, asthenia, lightheadedness, elevated liver function tests

Overdosage rarely results in death. Treat by hemodialysis due to low protein binding.

Precautions and contraindications

Patients with impaired renal function require dosage reductions. Sotalol is contraindicated in patients with bronchial asthma, bronchitis, sinus bradycardia, second- and third-degree atrioventricular block (may use if patient has functioning pacemaker), uncontrolled congestive heart failure, or cardiogenic shock.

Safety and efficacy have not been established in children. Adequate evaluation for use during pregnancy has not been established.

Anesthetic considerations

Use sotalol with caution when using lidocaine or calcium channel blockers because the additive electrophysiologic effect may cause a pro-arrhythmic event.

SUCCINYLCHOLINE (ANECTINE, QUELICIN, OTHERS)

Classification
Depolarizing skeletal muscle relaxant

Indications
Surgical muscle relaxation for short procedures; facilitation of endotracheal intubation

Dose
Adults: intravenous: 1 to 1.5 mg/kg (maximum: 150 total dose). Children: intravenous: 1 to 2 mg/kg; intramuscular: 2 to 4 mg/kg. Pretreat with atropine because of the incidence of bradycardia.

Dosage form: injection: 20 mg/mL; powder for infusion: 500 mg (mix in 500 mL for 1 mg/mL solution).

Onset and duration
Onset: immediate. Duration: 5 to 10 minutes.

Adverse effects
Effects related to the skeletal muscle depolarizing action of the drug: hyperkalemia, postoperative muscle pain, increased gastric pressure, increased intraocular pressure; cardiac arrhythmias: sudden cardiac arrest and bradycardia with repeat dosing or with any dose in children.

Prolonged paralysis and inadequate recovery may occur with infusion doses. Masseter muscle spasm may be a premonitory sign of malignant hyperthermia along with sudden unexplained tachycardia or an abrupt increase in carbon dioxide elimination.

Precautions and contraindications and anesthetic considerations
Succinylcholine should not be used for routine intubation in children younger than 12 years of age because of reports of sudden cardiac arrest in children with undiagnosed Duchenne muscular dystrophy and with muscle disorders. Succinylcholine is contraindicated in patients with malignant hyperthermia, genetic variants of plasma cholinesterase or cholinesterase deficiencies, myopathies associated with elevated creatine phosphokinase values, muscle disorders or muscular dystrophies, acute narrow-angle glaucoma, severe muscle trauma or muscle wasting, neurologic injury (i.e., paraplegia, quadriplegia, spinal cord injury, or cerebrovascular accident), hyperkalemia, severe sepsis, electrolyte imbalances, or third-degree burns over more than 25% total body surface. Repeated doses at short intervals (less than 5 minutes) are associated with bradycardia.

PART III Drugs

SUFENTANIL CITRATE (SUFENTA)

Classification
Opioid agonist; produces analgesia and anesthesia

Indications
Perioperative analgesia

Dose

Analgesia: intravenous/intramuscular: 0.2 to 0.6 mcg/kg. Induction: intravenous: 2 to 10 mcg/kg; infusion: 0.01 to 0.05 mcg/kg/min. Epidural: bolus: 0.2 to 0.6 mcg/kg; infusion: 5 to 30 mcg/hour (0.2 to 0.6 mcg/kg/hour). Spinal: 0.02 to 0.08 mcg/kg.

Onset and duration

Onset: intravenous: immediate; epidural and spinal: 4 to 10 minutes. Duration: intravenous: 20 to 45 minutes; intramuscular: 2 to 4 hours; epidural and spinal: 4 to 8 hours.

Adverse effects

Hypotension, bradycardia, respiratory depression, apnea, dizziness, sedation, euphoria, dysphoria, anxiety, nausea and vomiting, delayed gastric emptying, biliary tract spasm, muscle rigidity

Precautions and contraindications

Reduce the sufentanil dose in elderly, hypovolemic, or high-risk patients and in patients taking sedatives or other narcotics. Sufentanil crosses the placental barrier; if it is used during labor, depression of respiration in the neonate may result.

Anesthetic considerations

The narcotic effect of sufentanil is reversed with naloxone (intravenously, 0.2 to 0.4 mg). The duration of reversal may be shorter than the duration of the narcotic effect. The circulatory and ventilatory depressant effects of sufentanil are potentiated by other narcotics, sedatives, nitrous oxide, and volatile anesthetics; its ventilatory depressant effects are potentiated by monoamine oxidase inhibitors, phenothiazines, and tricyclic antidepressants. Analgesia is enhanced by α_2-agonists. The skeletal muscle rigidity associated with higher doses of sufentanil is sufficient to interfere with ventilation. Increased incidences of bradycardia occur with the additional use of vecuronium.

TERBUTALINE SULFATE (BRETHINE, BRETHAIRE, BRICANYL)

Classification

β_2-Adrenergic agonist, bronchodilator

Indications

Bronchodilator for treatment of asthma, tocolytic agent

Dose

Bronchodilator: subcutaneous: 0.25 mg (may repeat in 15 to 30 minutes; maximum dose: 0.5 mg in 4 to 6 hours); inhalation: two breaths separated by 60 seconds every 4 to 6 hours; oral: 5 mg three times daily (2.5 to 5 mg, every 6 hours; maximum dose: 15 mg/day).

Children younger than 12 years old: oral: 0.05 mg/kg/dose three times daily (maximum dose: 0.15 mg/kg/dose or 5 mg day); subcutaneous: 5 to 10 mcg/ kg/dose every 20 minutes for three doses.

Dosage forms: injection: 1 mg/mL (1 mL); tablet: 2.5, 5 mg.

Onset and duration
Onset: subcutaneous: 30 to 60 minutes; oral: 2 to 3 hours; inhalation: 1 to 2 hours. Duration: subcutaneous: 1 to 4 hours; oral: 4 to 8 hours; inhalation: 2 to 6 hours.

Adverse effects
Similar to those of other β-agonists: hypertension, tachycardia, arrhythmias, tremors, dizziness, headache, nausea and vomiting, gastrointestinal upset, hypokalemia, hyperglycemia

Precautions and contraindications
Use terbutaline with caution in patients with hypertension, ischemic heart disease, arrhythmias, congestive heart failure, diabetes mellitus, hyperthyroidism, or seizures. The action of terbutaline is antagonized by β-adrenergic blocking agents. Tolerance to terbutaline develops with repeated use.

Anesthetic considerations
Patients may experience wide swings in vital signs secondary to β-receptor stimulation. Bradycardia and hypotension may occur after cessation of therapy. Glucose, insulin, and potassium levels are commonly altered during therapy and should be evaluated. Mild hypokalemia is usually not treated. Additive hypertension and tachycardia occur when terbutaline is given with other sympathomimetics. Adverse effects of terbutaline may be antagonized by β-blocking agents.

TETRACAINE HCL (PONTOCAINE)

Classification
Ester-type local anesthetic

Indications
Local, spinal, and topical anesthesia

Dose
Spinal: 2 to 20 mg adjusted to height (rarely greater than 15 mg). Decrease usual dose in pregnant women. Dilute with equal volume of sterile dextrose 10% (hyperbaric) to control height more easily. Apply topical spray 2% solution in short spurts of less than 2 seconds. Maximum safe dose: 1.5 mg/kg. Inject slowly, not faster than 1 mL/5 second. Pediatric doses have not been established.

Dosage forms: injection: 1% (2 mL) for spinal anesthesia; ointment (ophthalmic): 0.5% (3.5 g); solution (ophthalmic): 0.5% (15 mL); topical: 2% (30 mL, 118 mL).

Onset and duration
Onset: spinal: 5 to 10 minutes; fixing time: 20 to 30 minutes. Duration: 1 to 3 hours, possibly longer if epinephrine is added to spinal bolus.

Adverse effects

Spinal use: hypotension, bradycardia, respiratory depression or apnea, high or total spinal with paralysis, headache

Precautions and contraindications

Avoid the use of tetracaine in patients allergic to ester-type local anesthetics (i.e., procaine, chloroprocaine, and cocaine). Tetracaine contains *para*-aminobenzoic acid, so avoid its use in patients with an allergy to this sunscreen. Tetracaine is reserved for spinal or topical anesthesia only because other local anesthetic drugs are safer for injection or infiltration. Seizures may occur with toxic doses. Monitor vital signs carefully during the initial administration. Tetracaine is not for ocular use.

Anesthetic considerations

Tetracaine is a long-standing agent for spinal anesthesia. Use amide local anesthetics such as lidocaine or bupivacaine if an allergy to tetracaine is suspected. Watch for a high spinal level in patients during use of this drug. Tetracaine produces a stronger motor block and more relaxation than bupivacaine. Adequate hydration during use will minimize hypotension. Reduce the dose in morbidly obese, obstetric, or elderly patients, as well as in patients with increased abdominal pressure.

THIOPENTAL SODIUM (PENTOTHAL)

Classification

Ultrashort-acting barbiturate, anesthesia-inducing agent

Indications

Induction of anesthesia or hypnosis

Dose

Induction: intravenous: 3 to 5 mg/kg. Maintenance: intravenous: 50 to 100 mg whenever the patient moves. Seizures: 75 to 125 mg (3 to 5 mL of 2.5% solution) for seizures from a local anesthetic.

Dosage forms: injection: 250-, 400-, 500-mg syringes; also supplied in vials with diluent, 500 mg, 1 g; also supplied in kits with 1, 2.5, 5 g; rectal suspension: 400 mg/g; mixed as a 2.5% solution or 25 mg/mL.

Onset and duration

Onset: 5 to 20 seconds. Duration: 20 to 30 minutes.

Adverse effects

Inadequate doses: possible increased sensitivity to pain; profound dose-dependent depression of respiration; extravascular injection: possible severe pain, tissue necrosis

Precautions and contraindications

Use it with caution in patients who are lactating, in asthmatic patients, or in patients with hypersensitivity to barbiturates. Thiopental is contraindicated in variegate porphyria and acute intermittent porphyria.

Anesthetic considerations

Thiopental solutions should be freshly prepared; discard them after 24 hours or if a precipitate is present. The effect of thiopental is potentiated by the injection of contrast media. The use of thiopental reduces the minimum alveolar concentration of inhalation anesthetics. Do not mix thiopental with other drugs.

TORSEMIDE (DEMADEX)

Classification
Loop diuretic

Indications
Treatment of edema as a result of cardiac, hepatic, or renal dysfunction; hypertension

Dose
Congestive heart failure: 10 to 20 mg orally or intravenously once daily; may titrate to therapeutic effect. Safety has not been established for doses exceeding 200 mg/day.

Renal dysfunction: 20 mg orally or intravenously once daily; may titrate to effect. Safety has not been established in does exceeding 200 mg/day.

Hypertension: 5 mg once daily; increase to 10 mg as needed, then add another antihypertensive medication if the desired effect has not been achieved.

Onset and duration
Onset: intravenous: 10 minutes. Peak effect: within 1 to 2 hours. Duration: diuresis for all routes lasts 6 to 8 hours.

Adverse effects
Dizziness, headache, nausea and vomiting, hyperglycemia, polyuria; additional effects: hyperuricemia, electrolyte/volume depletions, esophageal bleeding, salicylate toxicity, arrhythmias, dyspepsia

Precautions and contraindications
Contraindicated in patients with hypersensitivity to this drug or sulfonylureas in patients with anuria. Use with caution in hepatic dysfunction. Torsemide can reduce lithium elimination. Safety is not established during pregnancy or in children.

Anesthetic considerations
The patient's electrolyte/volume status should be monitored carefully during torsemide treatment. Electrolyte imbalances may predispose patients taking digitalis to toxicity.

TRIMETHAPHAN (ARFONAD)

Classification
Autonomic ganglion blocking agent; antihypertensive

PART III **Drugs**

Indications

Controlled hypotension during surgery; used during neurologic procedures and abdominal aneurysm repair

Dose

1% solution (500 mg in 500 mL); infuse 0.3 to 2 mg/min and adjust to effect.

Onset and duration

Onset: immediate. Duration: 5 to 30 minutes, depending on the duration of the infusion.

Adverse effects

Hypotension, tachycardia, histamine release, mydriasis, urinary retention, dry mouth

Precautions and contraindications

Avoid using trimethaphan in asthmatic patients because of frequent histamine release. Excessive hypotension and tachycardia may occur, especially in hypovolemic patients. Avoid using trimethaphan in patients with deficiencies of plasma cholinesterase.

Anesthetic considerations

Trimethaphan should be used as a supplement for deliberate hypotensive techniques. Tachyphylaxis develops frequently and is minimized by infusing slowly for brief periods. Nitroprusside and nitroglycerin are more commonly used. Many believe it is the drug of choice for cocaine intoxication–induced hypertensive episodes.

VANCOMYCIN (VANCOCIN)

Classification

Antimicrobial agent

Indications

Treatment of documented or suspected methicillin-resistant *Staphylococcus aureus* or β-lactam–resistant coagulase-negative *Streptococcus;* treatment of documented or suspected staphylococcal or streptococcal infections in penicillin- or cephalosporin-allergic patients; prophylaxis of bacterial endocarditis in high-risk patients (rheumatic heart disease, mitral valve prolapse, valvular heart dysfunction, bioprosthetic and allograft valves) undergoing dental, oral, or upper respiratory procedures and who are penicillin or cephalosporin allergic; prophylaxis in penicillin-allergic patients undergoing gastrointestinal, biliary, or genitourinary tract surgery or instrumentation and who are at risk of developing enterococcal endocarditis; prophylactic therapy for potential infections related to ventricular-peritoneal shunt, vascular graft, or open heart surgery in penicillin-allergic patients

Because vancomycin is not absorbed orally, the only indication for oral vancomycin is pseudomembranous colitis.

Dose

Initial intravenous dosage recommendation: adults: initial intravenous dose 15 mg/kg, followed by 10 mg/kg every 12 hours in patients with normal renal function (maximum dose: 3 g/day). Patients with mild renal failure (creatinine clearance less than or equal to 50 mL/min) should receive vancomycin every 24 to 72 hours; patients with moderate renal failure (creatinine clearance of 10 to 50 mL/min) should receive vancomycin every 72 to 240 hours; patients with severe renal failure (creatinine clearance less than 10 mL/min) should receive vancomycin every 240 hours.

Children: children heavier than 5 kg and older than 7 days postnatal age and younger than 13 years of age: 10 mcg/kg every 6 hours. Children older than 13 years of age: dosed as adults.

Peak and trough serum levels should be monitored if therapy extends beyond 24 hours perioperative prophylaxis. Dosage and dosage interval should be adjusted to produce peak levels of 25 to 40 mcg/mL and trough levels of 5 to 10 mcg/mL.

Dosage forms: Parenteral injection for intravenous use: 500-mg or 1-g vials. Reconstitute sterile powder by adding 10 mL or 20 mL sterile water to 500-mg or 1-g vials, respectively. Reconstituted solution containing 500 mg or 1 g must be further diluted with at least 100 mL or at least 250 mL D_5W or normal saline, respectively. Infuse through an intravenous piggyback over 1 to 1.5 hours.

Onset and duration
Onset: 15 to 30 minutes. Duration: 8 to 12 hours. Half-life varies: 4 to 6 hours reported in patients with normal renal function. Usually given 1 hour before procedure for prophylaxis of endocarditis. Some clinicians suggest the dose should be repeated 8 to 12 hours later in patients with normal renal function; however, the American Heart Association, the American Academy of Pediatrics, and the American Dental Association state that a second dose is unnecessary.

Adverse effects
Rapid infusion: red-man syndrome (erythema, pruritus, and rash involving face, neck, upper trunk, and arms), hypertension, tachycardia; ototoxicity associated with prolonged serum concentrations greater than 40 mcg/mL; other effects: chills, fever, neutropenia, thrombocytopenia, agranulocytosis, phlebitis

Precautions and contraindications
Monitor renal function tests frequently during vancomycin therapy. Use the drug with caution in patients with renal impairment or in patients receiving other nephrotoxic or ototoxic drugs. Vancomycin is contraindicated in patients with hypersensitivity to the drug. Avoid using vancomycin in patients with previous hearing loss.

Anesthetic considerations
Vancomycin potentiation of succinylcholine-induced neuromuscular blockade during has been reported. The drug may increase neuromuscular blockade by nondepolarizing muscle relaxants, whose dose should be titrated. Administer it slowly over a 30-minute period.

VASOPRESSIN (PITRESSIN)

Classification
Antidiuretic hormone

PART III **Drugs**

Indications

Treatment of diabetes insipidus; treatment of bleeding esophageal varices and other types of upper gastrointestinal bleeding; control of refractory operative bleeding in intrauterine procedures

Dose

- Diabetes insipidus or treatment of abdominal distention in postoperative patients: 5 to 10 units three to four times daily as needed.
- Gastrointestinal hemorrhage: 0.2 to 1 unit/min infused intravenously. After 12 hours of hemorrhage control, decrease the dose by half and then stop within the next 12 to 24 hours. Intravenous nitroglycerin should be infused concomitantly to control side effects.
- Locally to operative site: 20 units in 30 mL normal saline as a gauze soak.
- Children: for diabetes insipidus: intramuscular or subcutaneous: 2.5 to 5 units every 6 to 8 hours; titrate based on response.
- Intravenous: infusion pump 0.01 to 0.04 unit/min, or 40 units once for resuscitation in septic shock or cardiac arrest
- Gastrointestinal bleeding: 0.01 unit/kg/min.
- Dosage forms: 20 pressor unit/mL aqueous injection; must be diluted for intravenous infusion in D_5W or normal saline to a concentration of 100 to 1000 units/L.

Onset and duration

Onset: 15 to 30 minutes. Duration: antidiuretic action: intramuscular or subcutaneous: 2 to 8 hours after administration; the pressor effects last 30 to 60 minutes after intravenous injection. Elimination half-life: 10 to 35 minutes.

Adverse effects

Tremor, sweating, vertigo, water intoxication, hyponatremia, metabolic acidosis, abdominal cramps, nausea and vomiting, urticaria, anaphylaxis, angina in patients with preexisting cardiovascular impairment

Precautions and contraindications

Use vasopressin with extreme caution in patients who cannot tolerate rapid retention of extracellular water or who have coronary artery disease. For intravenous infusion use a central vein, preferably, owing to the possibility of tissue necrosis with extravasation. Monitor patients with epilepsy, migraine, asthma, or heart failure closely. Intravenous administration should be used only for emergency treatment of gastrointestinal hemorrhage. Vasopressin is contraindicated in patients with anaphylaxis or hypersensitivity to the drug and in those with chronic nephritis with nitrogen retention, until reasonable nitrogen blood levels are attained.

Anesthetic considerations

Patient should be watched carefully for abrupt cardiac changes following vasopressin injection. Urine monitoring is mandatory.

VECURONIUM (NORCURON)

Classification

Nondepolarizing muscle relaxant

Indications

Intraoperative muscle relaxation; endotracheal intubation; facilitation of mechanical ventilation in critical care

Dose

Intravenous: 0.05 to 0.2 mg/kg for paralysis. Dosage form: powder for injection 10 mg (5, 10 mL).

Onset and duration

Onset: 1 to 3 minutes. Duration: 30 to 60 minutes.

Adverse effects

Prolonged paralysis in patients with hepatic disease; apnea immediately on administration (so appropriate airway management and resuscitative equipment must be immediately available); no significant cardiac effects

Precautions and contraindications

Airway equipment must be on hand for intubation and controlled ventilation in conjunction with the use of vecuronium. The drug's duration of action may be prolonged in patients with liver disease.

Anesthetic considerations

Monitor the patient's response with a nerve stimulator to avoid excessive dosing. Long-term vecuronium infusions in critical care may result in prolonged recovery and an inability to reverse the effects, owing to active metabolites. Corticosteroid therapy in patients with multiorgan failure may exacerbate this effect.

VERAPAMIL (ISOPTIN, CALAN, OTHERS)

Classification

Calcium channel blocker

Indications

Supraventricular arrhythmias; hypertension; angina

Dose

Intravenous: 2.5 to 10 mg slowly; may repeat in 30 to 60 minutes; oral: 120 to 480 mg/day in divided doses.

Dosage forms: injection: 2.5 mg/mL (2 mL); tablet: 40, 80, 120 mg; sustained-release tablet: 120, 180, 240 mg.

Onset and duration

Onset: intravenous: 2 to 5 minutes; oral: 30 to 60 minutes. Duration: intravenous: 30 minutes to 2 hours; oral: 4 to 12 hours.

Adverse effects

Hypotension, heart block, tachycardia, bradycardia; ankle edema and constipation with long-term oral use

Precautions and contraindications

Significant hypotension may occur in patients with poor left ventricular function. Verapamil may exacerbate atrioventricular block or

Wolff-Parkinson-White syndrome. Additive depression occurs with concomitant use of other cardiac depressants.

Anesthetic considerations
Titrate verapamil slowly, owing to significant cardiac depressant effects, which are additive with anesthetics. Diltiazem infusion may be a better option for the treatment of intraoperative atrial arrhythmias. β-Blockers are superior for the treatment of sinus tachycardia.

VITAMIN K, PHYTONADIONE (AQUAMEPHYTON, MEPHYTON)

Classification
Water-soluble vitamin

Indications
Prevention and treatment of hypoprothrombinemia caused by drug- or anticoagulant-induced vitamin K deficiency or hemorrhagic diseases of the newborn

Dose
The intravenous route should be used for emergencies only. Inject slowly intravenously only, not faster than 1 mg/min.

Newborn hemorrhage: intramuscular, subcutaneous prophylaxis: 0.5 to 1 mg within 1 hour of birth. Treat with 1 to 2 mg/day.

Anticoagulant reversal: infants: 1 to 2 mg every 4 to 8 hours; adult: oral, intravenous, intramuscular, subcutaneous: 2.5 to 10 mg, may repeat intravenous, subcutaneous, intramuscular dose every 6 to 8 hours and oral dose in 12 to 48 hours.

Dosage forms: tablet: 5 mg; injection: 2 mg/mL in 0.5-mL ampule and 10 mg/mL in 1-mL ampule and 2.5- and 5-mL vials.

Onset and duration
Onset: intravenous, intramuscular, subcutaneous: 1 to 3 hours; oral: 4 to 12 hours. Duration: 6 to 48 hours, depending on the dose and route of administration.

Adverse effects
Severe anaphylaxis possible with intravenous use; severe hemolytic anemia possible in neonates given large doses (greater than 20 mg)

Precautions and contraindications
Use the intravenous route in emergencies only, owing to possibility of severe anaphylaxis. Vitamin K is ineffective in hereditary hypoprothrombinemia or hypoprothrombinemia secondary to severe liver disease.

Anesthetic considerations
Prothrombin time must be monitored. Transfusion of blood or fresh-frozen plasma may be necessary in severe hemorrhagic states.

WARFARIN (COUMADIN)

Classification
Anticoagulant; depresses formation of vitamin K–dependent clotting factors (II, VII, IX, X) in the liver

Indications
Treatment or prophylaxis of deep vein thrombosis or pulmonary thromboembolism; prophylaxis of thromboembolism in patients with atrial fibrillation who are undergoing cardioversion of atrial fibrillation, those who have prosthetic heart valves, after major surgery requiring prolonged immobilization (total knee or hip replacements), and after myocardial infarction in patients who are at high risk of embolism (those with congestive heart failure, atrial fibrillation, previous myocardial infarction, or history of thromboembolism)

Dose
Warfarin dosing is adjusted according to prothrombin time (PT). Standardization of PT results among laboratories is accomplished with the use of an International Normalized Ratio (INR) equation:

$$INR = (PT_{patient}/PT_{Reference})^{ISI}$$

where ISI is the International Sensitivity Index.

The typical goal INR is 2 to 3, except for patients with prosthetic valves, for whom 2.5 to 3.5 is the desired goal. Commonly, doses of 5 to 10 mg/day are tapered to 2 to 10 mg/day, as indicated by the PT. Consult the pharmacy for institutional guidelines. Multiple drug interactions may increase or decrease the response.

Dosage forms: 2-, 2.5-, 5-, 7.5-, 10-mg tablets; 50 mg for parenteral injection with 2-mL diluent.

Onset and duration
Onset: antithrombogenic effects may not occur for up to 5 to 7 days after initiation of therapy; many clinicians recommend that heparin be administered concurrently for 3 to 7 days until the desired PT is achieved. Duration: single oral dose: 2 to 5 days. Elimination half-life: 0.5 to 3 days.

Adverse effects
Dose-dependent bleeding, ranging from minor local bleeding or ecchymosis (2% to 10%) to major hemorrhagic complications occasionally resulting in death; major hemorrhage usually involving gastrointestinal or genitourinary tract, but possibly involve hepatic, cerebral, or pericardial sites; additional effects: agranulocytosis, leukopenia, thrombocytopenia, necrosis of skin, purple-toe syndrome, neuropathy

Minor bleeding can be treated with vitamin K intramuscularly or intravenously 5 to 10 mg up to 50 mg. Frank bleeding should be treated with administration of fresh whole blood or fresh-frozen plasma (15 mL/kg).

PART III **Drugs**

Precautions and contraindications

Numerous drugs may affect patient response to warfarin, especially hepatic enzyme–inducing or –reducing drugs and highly protein-bound drugs; consultation with a pharmacist or physician regarding all drugs is recommended. Use warfarin with extreme caution in patients with protein C deficiency, congestive heart failure, carcinoma, liver disease, or poor nutritional state. Warfarin is contraindicated in bleeding patients or in patients with hemorrhagic blood dyscrasias, aneurysms, pericarditis or pericardial effusions, uncontrolled hypertension, recent or contemplated surgery of the eye, brain, or spinal cord, or any traumatic surgery resulting in large open surfaces, and in patients with recent cerebrovascular accident. Renal and hepatic function in these patients should be monitored periodically. PT should be monitored daily initially. After PT is stabilized, these patients should be monitored every 4 to 6 weeks. Warfarin is teratogenic and is contraindicated in pregnancy. Risks of hemorrhage may increase with concomitant use of aspirin, nonsteroidal antiinflammatory drugs, cimetidine, amiodarone, steroids, chloral hydrate, metronidazole, streptokinase, urokinase, antibiotics, and heparin. Discontinue warfarin promptly in patients with purple-toe syndrome or skin necrosis. Further use of warfarin is contraindicated in these patients.

Anesthetic considerations

Regional anesthesia is contraindicated. If possible, barbiturates should be avoided because they may decrease warfarin's effect. When emergency surgery is necessary in patients receiving warfarin, fresh-frozen plasma (15 mL/kg) or whole blood can restore coagulation to normal.

Generic Name	Trade Name
adenosine	Adenocard
adrenaline (epinephrine)	
albuterol	Proventil, Ventolin
alfentanil	Alfenta
alprostadil (prostaglandin E_1)	Prostin VR Pediatric
aminocaproic acid	Amicar
aminophylline	Elixophyllin, Theodur, Theolair
amiodarone	Cordarone
amrinone	Inocor
atracurium	Tracrium
atropine	Atropine sulfate, others
bretylium	Bretylol
bumetanide	Bumex
bupivacaine	Marcaine HCl, Sensorcaine
chloroprocaine	Nesacaine
cimetidine	Tagamet
clonidine	Catapres
cocaine	
codeine	
coumarin (warfarin)	Coumadin
cyclosporine	Optimmune, Sandimmune
dantrolene sodium	Dantrium
desflurane	Suprane
desmopressin	DDAVP
dexamethasone	Decadron, Hexadrol
diazepam	Valium
digoxin	Lanoxin
diltiazem	Cardizem
diphenhydramine	Benadryl
dobutamine	Dobutrex
dolasetron	Anzemet
dopamine	Intropin
doxacurium	Nuromax
doxapram	Dopram
edrophonium	Enlon, Tensilon
enalaprilat	Vasotec I.V.
enoxaparin	Lovenox
ephedrine	
epinephrine (adrenaline)	
esmolol	Brevibloc
ethacrynic acid	Edecrin
etidocaine	Duranest
etomidate	Amidate
famotidine	Pepcid
fenoldopam	Corlopam
fentanyl	Duragesic, Oralet, Sublimaze
flumazenil	Romazicon
furosemide	Lasix
glucagon	
glycopyrrolate	Robinul
granisetron	Kytril

Continued

Drugs—cont'd

Generic Name	Trade Name
halothane	Fluothane
heparin	
hetastarch	Hespan
hyaluronidase	Wydase, Vitrase
hydralazine	Apresoline
hydrocortisone	Hydrocort, Solu-Cortef
Ibutilide	Corvert
insulin	Humulin, Novolin
ipratropium	Atrovent
isoflurane	Forane
isoproterenol	Isuprel
ketamine	Ketalar
ketorolac	Toradol
labetalol	Normodyne, Trandate
lansoprazole	Prevacid
levobupivacaine	Chirocaine
lidocaine	Xylocaine
lidocaine/prilocaine	EMLA
lorazepam	Ativan
magnesium sulfate	
mannitol	
meperidine	Demerol
mephentermine	Wyamine Sulfate
mepivacaine	Carbocaine, Polocaine
metaraminol	Aramine
methadone	Dolophine HCl
methohexital	Brevital Sodium
methoxamine	Vasoxyl
methylene blue	Urolene Blue
methylergonovine	Methergine
metoclopramide	Reglan
midazolam	Versed
milrinone	Primacor
mivacurium	Mivacron
morphine	Astramorph PF, Duramorph, Morphine, MS Contin
nalmefene	Revex
naloxone	Narcan
naltrexone	ReVia, Trexan
neostigmine	Prostigmin
nesiritide	Natrecor
nicardipine	Cardene
nifedipine	Adalat, Procardia
nitroglycerin	Nitro-Bid, Nitro-Dur, Nitrogard, Nitrostat, Nitrol, Nitrocine, Nitroglyn, Nitrodisc, Transderm-Nitro, Tridil
nitroprusside	Nipride
nitrous oxide	
nizatidine	Axid
norepinephrine	Levophed
omeprazole	Prilosec, Losic, Omid
ondansetron	Zofran

Drugs—cont'd

Generic Name	Trade Name
oxytocin	Pitocin, Syntocinon
pancuronium	Pavulon
phentolamine	Regitine
phenylephrine	Neo-Synephrine
phenytoin	Dilantin
physostigmine	Antilirium
pipecuronium	Arduan
prilocaine	Citanest
procainamide	Procan SR, Pronestyl
procaine	Novocain
prochlorperazine	Compazine
promethazine	Phenergan
propofol	Diprivan
propranolol	Inderal
prostaglandin E_1 (alprostadil)	Prostin VR Pediatric
protamine	
pyridostigmine	Mestinon, Regonol
ranitidine	Zantac
remifentanil	Ultiva
ritodrine	Yutopar
rocuronium	Zemuron
ropivacaine	Naropin
salmeterol	Serevent
scopolamine	
sevoflurane	Ultane
sodium citrate	Bicitra
somatostatin	
sotalol	Betapace
succinylcholine	Anectine, Quelicin
sufentanil	Sufenta
terbutaline	Brethaire, Bricanyl
tetracaine	Pontocaine
thiopental sodium	Pentothal
torsemide	Demadex
trimethaphan	Arfonad
vancomycin	Vancocin
vasopressin	Pitressin Synthetic
vecuronium	Norcuron
verapamil	Calan, Isoptin
vitamin K (phytonadione)	AquaMEPHYTON, Konakion
warfarin (coumarin)	Coumadin

TABLE 1 Commonly Used Anticholinesterase and Anticholinergic Agents

Dose	Dose Range (mcg/kg)	Onset (min)	Duration	Comment
Neostigmine	25–75	5–15	45–90 min	Most commonly used reversal agent; may increase incidence of postoperative nausea and vomiting
Pyridostigmine	100–300	10–20	60–120 min	Slow onset, long duration of reversal
Edrophonium	500–1000	5–10	30–60 min	Not recommended for deep block; rapid onset, short duration
Atropine	15	1–2	1–2 hr	Should be combined with edrophonium owing to more rapid onset
Glycopyrrolate	10–20	2	2–4 hr	Less initial tachycardia than atropine

TABLE 2 Aminoglycoside Dosages

Aminoglycoside	Usual Loading Doses	Expected Peak Serum Concentrations
Tobramycin	1–2 mg/kg	4–10 mcg/mL
Gentamicin	1–2 mg/kg	4–10 mcg/mL
Amikacin	5–7.5 mg/kg	15–30 mcg/mL
Kanamycin	5–7.5 mg/kg	15–30 mcg/mL

TABLE 3 Macrolide Antibiotic Dosages

Antibiotic	Doses
Erythromycin estolate (Ilosone)	250 mg q6h or 333 mg q8h orally 250 mg q6h orally
Erythromycin ethylsuccinate (E.E.S)	400 mg q6h orally
Erythromycin gluceptate (Ilotycin)	15–20 mg/kg daily in divided doses q6h intravenously
Erythromycin lactobionate (Erythrocin)	15–20 mg/kg daily in divided doses q6h intravenously
Azithromycin (Zithromax)	500 mg single dose on first day followed by 250 mg daily intravenously or orally
Clarithromycin (Biaxin)	250–500 mg q12h orally
Dirithromycin (Dynabac)	500 mg daily orally
Troleandomycin (Tao)	250–500 mg q6h orally

TABLE 4 Proton Pump Inhibitors

Generic Name	Trade Name	Adult Dosage Range	Available Dosage Forms*	Dose Adjustment In Renal Dysfunction	Drug Interactions/Comments
Esomeprazole	Nexium	20 mg daily	Capsule: 20, 40 mg	No	Cefuroxime, cefpodoxime, digoxin, dihydropyridine calcium channel blockers, iron salts, itraconazole, ketoconazole, sucralfate
Lansoprazole	Prevacid	15–30 mg daily or twice daily	Capsule: 15, 30 mg	No	Same as esomeprazole plus theophylline
Omeprazole	Prilosec	20–40 mg daily or twice daily	Capsule: 10, 20, 40 mg	No	Same as esomeprazole plus benzodiazepines, cilostazol, citalopram, clarithromycin, cyclosporine, disulfiram, methotrexate, phenytoin, sulfonylureas, theophylline, warfarin
Pantoprazole	Protonix, Protonix IV	40–80 mg daily	Tablet: 40 mg; Injection: 40 mg/vial	No	Same as esomeprazole
Rabeprazole	Aciphex	20–100 mg daily 60 mg b.i.d.	Tablet: 20 mg	No	Same as esomeprazole plus cyclosporine

*All oral forms are delayed release.
From 2004 Mosby's drug consult, St. Louis, 2004, Mosby.

Appendixes

TABLE 5   Drugs Typically Used during Liver Transplantation

Drug	Induction	Preanhepatic	Anhepatic	Posthepatic
Aprotinin	2 million KI units	150,000 KI units/hr	150,000 KI units/hr	140,000 KI units/hr
Vasopressin	—	0.5 mcg/kg/hr	0	0
Fentanyl	4–6 mcg/kg	4–6 mcg/kg	—	4–6 mcg/kg
Midazolam	10–40 mcg/kg	0–1 mg	0–1 mg	0–1 mg
Pentothal	4–6 mcg/kg	—	—	—
Furosemide	—	10–20 mg	—	—
Mannitol 20%	—	1–1.5 g/kg	—	—
Methylprednisolone	—	—	500 mg	—
Magnesium	—	2–4 g	—	—
Calcium chloride	—	2–4 g	1 g	—
Sodium bicarbonate	—	—	0–100 mEq	—
Protamine	—	—	—	0.50 mg
Phenylephrine boluses	—	—	80 mcg/bolus	80 mcg/bolus
Dopamine (renal)	—	0–2.5 mcg/kg/min	0–2.5 mcg/kg/min	0–2.5 mcg/kg/min
Dopamine (vasopressor)	—	2.5–10 mcg/kg/min	2.5–10 mcg/kg/min	2.5–10 mcg/kg/min

KI, Kallikrein inhibitor.
From Amand MS, and others: Liver transplant. In Sharpe MD, Gelb AW, editors: *Anesthesia and transplantation*, Boston, 1999, Butterworth-Heinemann, p 188.

TABLE 6 Drugs Used in Deep Vein Thrombosis Prophylaxis

Drug	Type	Dose	Comments
Enoxaprin (Lovenox, Clexane)	Low-molecular-weight heparin	30–40 mg subcutaneous twice/day	First dose given immediately after surgery and continued for 7–10 days
Dalteparin (Fragman)	Low-molecular-weight heparin	2500 anti-Xa units subcutaneous/day	First dose 1–2 hr preoperatively and continued for 5 days (5000 anti-Xa units in high-risk patients)
Ardeparin (Normiflo)	Low-molecular-weight heparin	50 anti-Xa units/kg of actual weight subcutaneous twice/day or until ambulatory	First dose in the evening of the day of surgery and continued for 14 days
Heparin	Intravenous anticoagulant	Low dose prophylaxis: 5000 units subcutaneous q8–12h guided by coagulation tests	Pharmacokinetics highly variable; aPTT 1.5–2 times normal is considered adequate; first dose 2hr preoperatively, then q8–12h for 7 days guided by aPPT results; effects may be reversed with protamine
Warfarin (Coumadin)	Oral anticoagulant	2–5 mg/day adjusted to INR	Low-intensity therapy: INR = 2–3; high-intensity therapy: INR = 2.5–3.5; effects may be reversed with vitamin K
Danaparoid (Orgaran)	Subcutaneous anticoagulant	750 anti-Xa units subcutaneous twice/day	First dose given 1–4 hr preoperatively and continued for 7–14 days or until ambulatory in patients undergoing total hip replacement
Desirudin (Iprivask)	Thrombin inhibitor	15 mg q12h; initial dose 5–15 min preoperatively	Caution with neuraxial anesthesia
Anisindione (Miradon)	Prothrombin inhibitor	300 mg day 1, 200 mg day 2, 100 mg day 3, 25–250 mg maintenance	Prothrombin time of 2–2.5 times normal value is therapeutic goal
Tinzaparin (Innohep)	Low-molecular-weight heparin	175 anti-Xa units/kg subcutaneous for 6 days	Caution with neuraxial anesthesia
Fondaparinux (Arixtra)	Factor Xa inhibitor	2.5 mg subcutaneous 6 hr postoperatively	Used following orthopedic surgery

aPTT, Activated partial thromboplastin time; *INR,* international normalized ratio.

Appendixes

TABLE 7 Comparison of Select Corticosteroid Agents

Compound	Equivalent Dose in Milligrams (Oral and Intravenous)	Approximate Relative Potency in Clinical Use		Duration of Action after Oral Dose*	Comments
		Antinflammatory	Sodium-Retaining		
Hydrocortisone† (cortisol)	20	1	1	S	Drug of choice for replacement therapy
Cortisone	25	0.8	0.8	S	Inexpensive; inactive until converted to hydrocortisone; not used as antinflammatory because of mineralocorticoid effects
Prednisolone	5	4	0.8	I	Drug of choice for systemic antinflammatory and immunosuppressive effects
Prednisone	5	4	0.8	I	Inactive until converted to prednisolone
Methylprednisolone	4	5	0.5	I	Antinflammatory and immunosuppressive
Triamcinolone	4	5	0	I	Relatively more toxic than others
Dexamethasone	0.75	25	0	L	Antinflammatory and immunosuppressive, used especially where water retention is undesirable, such as cerebral edema; drug of choice for suppression of corticotropin production
Betamethasone	0.75	30	0	L	Antinflammatory and immunosuppressive, used especially where water retention is undesirable
Fludrocortisone	Not used as glucocorticoid	10	125	I	Drug of choice for mineralocorticoid effects

*Duration of action (hr): S, Short (8–12); I, intermediate (12–36); L, long (36–72).
†Hydrocortisone is the standard for comparison.

Data from Chrousos GP, Margioris AN: Adrenocorticosteroids and adrenocortical antagonists. In Katzung BG, editor: *Basic and clinical pharmacology,* ed 9, New York, 2004, McGraw Hill; and Schimmer BP, Parker KL: Adrenocorticotropic hormone; adrenocortical steroids and their synthetic analogues; inhibitors of the synthesis and actions of adrenocortical hormones. In Hardman JG, and others, editors: *Goodman and Gilman's the pharmacological basis of therapeutics,* ed 10, New York, 2001, McGraw-Hill.

TABLE 8 Monoclonal Antibodies

The monoclonal antibodies (mAbs) are genetically engineered immunoglobulins (IgGs) that react with specific molecular targets. They may be part mouse, part human (termed humanized or chimeric), or fully human. In chimeric mAbs, the antigen-recognizing portion of a mouse antibody is joined to the framework of a human IgG molecule.
- Abciximab: a chimeric mAb against the clotting receptor glycoprotein IIb/IIIa on platelets, used to prevent clotting in patients undergoing coronary angioplasty
- Adalimumab: a humanized mAb against the cytokine tumor necrosis factor-α (TNF-α), used for rheumatoid arthritis
- Alemtuzumab: a humanized mAb against an antigen on T and B lymphocytes, used to treat B-cell leukemia
- Basiliximab: a chimeric mAb against the receptor for the cytokine interleukin-2 on activated T cells, used in acute rejection of kidney transplants
- Daclizumab: a humanized mAb against the receptor for the cytokine interleukin-2 on activated T cells, used in acute rejection of kidney transplants
- Gemtuzumab: a humanized mAb against an antigen on leukemia cells, used to treat relapsed acute myeloid leukemia
- Infliximab: a chimeric mAb against the cytokine TNF-α, used for rheumatoid arthritis and Crohn's disease
- Muromonab (Orthoclone OKT3): a murine mAb to the CD3 antigen of human T cells that functions as an immunosuppressant in heart, kidney, and liver transplants
- Omalizumab: a humanized mAb against the binding of IgE to the high-affinity IgE receptor on the surface of mast cells and basophils for the treatment of asthma
- Palivizumab: a humanized mAb against a protein of respiratory syncytial virus (RSV), used to treat RSV infection in children
- Rituximab: a humanized mAb against the cytokine CD20 receptor on B cells, used in non-Hodgkin's lymphoma
- Satumomab: a conjugate produced from a murine mAb, used for imaging and diagnostics
- Trastuzumab (Herceptin): an mAb against HER2, used for breast cancer treatment

Data from *2004 Mosby's drug consult,* St. Louis, 2004, Mosby; and Rang HP, and others: Pharmacology, ed 5, Edinburgh, 2004, Churchill Livingstone.

Appendixes

TABLE 9 Common Ocular Drugs

Class	Generic Name	Comments
β-Blockers	Timolol Levobunolol Betaxolol Metipranolol Carteolol	First-line therapy; reduce production of aqueous humor; may produce systemic effect. Use with caution in patients with asthma, chronic obstructive pulmonary disease, heart block, heart failure and hypotension.
Carbonic anhydrase inhibitors	Acetazolamide Methazolamide Dorzolamide Brinzolamide	Reduce aqueous production; usually used as second-line therapy for glaucoma
Parasympathomimetic and anticholinesterase miotics	Carbachol Pilocarpine Physostigmine Echothiophate iodide	Promote aqueous outflow; rarely used owing to significant side effects and drug interactions
Prostaglandins	Latanoprost Bimatoprost Travoprost Unoprostone	Promote aqueous outflow; alternative to β-blockers in patients with intolerance to them
Sympathomimetics	Epinephrine Dipivefrin	Contraindicated in patients with narrow-angle glaucoma; reduce aqueous production; contraindicated in patients taking monoamine oxidase inhibitors

α_2-Agonists	Apraclonidine HCI	
	Brimonidine	
Corticosteroids	Dexamethasone	Antiinflammatory; may induce glaucoma with prolonged use.
	Fluorometholone	
	Prednisolone	
	Rimexolone	
Nonsteroidal antiinflammatory agents	Diclofenac	Antiinflammatory; block cyclooxygenase pathway to inhibit prostaglandin-induced inflammation
	Ketorolac	
Mydriatics and cycloplegics	Atropine	Used for eye examination; phenylephrine and tropicamide are mydriatic; the others produce mydriasis and cycloplegia
	Cyclopentolate	
	Homatropine	
	Phenylephrine	
	Tropicamide	

TABLE 10 Topical Anesthetic Drugs

Drug	Concentration	Dose	Notable Features
Cocaine	4%	3 mg/kg	Only local anesthetic with vasoconstrictive ability Blocks reuptake of norepinephrine and epinephrine at adrenergic nerve endings
Lidocaine	2% and 4% solution 2% viscous solution 10% aerosol 2.5% and 5% ointment	4 mg/kg plain 7 mg/kg with epinephrine 250–300 mg	Rapid onset Suitable for all areas of the tracheobronchial tree
Benzocaine	10%, 15%, 20% Cetacaine contains: 14% benzocaine, 2% butamben, and 2% tetracaine		Short duration of action (10 min) Can produce methemoglobinemia
Bupivacaine	0.25%, 0.5%, 0.75%	2.5 mg/kg plain	Slow hepatic clearance Long duration of action
Mepivacaine Dyclonine	1%, 2% 0.5%, 1%	4 mg/kg 300 mg maximum	Intermediate potency with rapid onset Topical spray or gargle Frequent use for laryngoscopy Absorbed through both skin and mucous membranes

TABLE 11 Common Intravenous Agents for Hypotensive Techniques

Drug and Dosage	Advantages	Disadvantages
Sodium nitroprusside Variable age- and anesthetic-dependent effects; 1–5 mcg/kg/min young adults; 6–8 mcg/kg/min children	Potent; reliable; rapid onset and recovery; cardiac output well preserved	Reflex tachycardia; rebound hypertension; pulmonary shunting; cyanide toxicity possible
Adenosine 0.06–0.35 mcg/kg/min	Reliable; rapid onset and recovery; increased coronary blood flow	Reflex tachycardia; possible inadequate cerebral perfusion when combined with hemodilution; greatly reduced urinary output
Esmolol 200 mcg/kg/min to achieve 15% reduction of mean arterial pressure	Particularly useful to control tachycardia	Potential for significant cardiac depression
Nitroglycerin 125–500 mcg/kg/min adults 10 mcg/kg/min children	Preserves myocardial blood flow; reduces preload; preserves tissue oxygenation	Increases intracranial pressure; highly variable dosage requirements
Fenoldopam 0.5–22 mcg/kg/min	Preserves renal blood flow	Reflex tachycardia; rebound hypertension; increased pulmonary shunting
Nicardipine* 5 mcg/kg/min	Calcium channel blocker Preserves cerebral blood flow	
Remifentanil with propofol Remifentanil: 1 mcg/kg intravenously, then continuous infusion 0.25–0.5 mcg/kg/min Propofol: 2.5 mg/kg intravenously, then infusion of 25–100 mcg/kg/min	Remifentanil reduces middle ear blood flow creating a dry surgical field for tympanoplasty Propofol may help reduce postoperative nausea and vomiting	No analgesic effect once remifentanil infusion discontinued

*Tobias JD: Controlled hypotension in children: a critical review of available agents, *Paediatr Drugs* 4:439–453, 2002; and DeGoute CS, and others: Remifentanil and controlled hypotension; comparison with nitroprusside or esmolol during tympanoplasty, *Can J Anaesth* 48:20–27, 2001.
Data from McNulty SE: Induced hypotension during head and neck surgery, *Otolaryngol Head Neck Surg* 11:605, 1993; Kim KH, and others: Nicardipine hydrochloride injectable phase IV open label clinical trial: study on the antihypertensive effects and safety of nicardipine for acute aortic dissection, *J Int Med Res* 30:337–345, 2002.

Appendixes

TABLE 12 Characteristics of Insulin Preparations

Insulin Type	Onset of Action*	Peak Activity	Duration	Route
Short-acting				
Regular	30–60 min	1–2 hr	5–12 hr	IV, SC, IM
Rapid-acting				
Aspart (Novolog)	10–30 min	30–60 min	3–5 hr	SC
Lispro (Humalog)	10–30 min	30–60 min	3–5 hr	SC
Intermediate-acting				
NPH/Lente	1–2 hr	4–8 hr	10–20 hr	SC
Long-acting				
Ultralente	2–4 hr	8–20 hr	16–24 hr	SC
Glargine	1–2 hr	No peak	24 hr	SC

IM, Intramuscular; *IV,* intravenous; *NPH,* neutral protamine Hagedorn; *SC,* subcutaneous.
*Time course is based on subcutaneous administration.
Modified from *Treatment guidelines from the medical letter, vol 1,* 2002.

TABLE 13 Oral Drugs for Type 2 Diabetes

Drug	Usual Daily Dosage
Sulfonylurea: first generation	
Acetohexamide (Dymelor)	500–750 mg once or divided
Chlorpropamide (Diabinese)	250–375 mg once
Tolazamide (Tolinase)	250–500 mg once or divided
Tolbutamide (Orinase)	1000–2000 mg divided
Sulfonylurea: second generation	
Glimepiride (Amaryl)	1–4 mg once
Glipizide	
(Glucotrol)	10–20 mg once or divided
(Glucotrol XL sustained-release tablets)	5–20 mg once
Glyburide	
(DiaBeta, Micronase)	5–20 mg once or divided
(Glynase, micronized tablets)	3–12 mg once or divided
α-Glucosidase inhibitors	
Acarbose (Precose)	50–100 mg tid with meals
Miglitol (Glyset)	50–100 mg tid with meals
Thiazolidinediones	
Rosiglitazone (Avandia)	4–8 mg once or divided
Pioglitazone (Actos)	15–45 mg once
Biguanides	
Metformin	
(Glucophage)	1500–2550 mg divided
(Glucophage XR)	1500–2000 mg once
Metformin/Glyburide (Glucovance)	500 mg/5 mg bid
Nonsulfonylurea secretagogues	
Repaglinide (Prandin)	1–4 mg tid before meals
Nateglinide (Starlix)	60–120 mg tid before meals

bid, Twice daily; *tid,* three times daily.
Modified from *Treatment guidelines from the medical letter, vol 1,* 2002.

TABLE 14 Cephalosporins, Parenteral

Generic Name (Generation)	Usual Adult Dose (g)	Adjust Dose for Renal Insufficiency	Comment
Cefazolin (1)	0.25–2 q6–12h	Yes	Commonly used for surgical prophylaxis
Cephapirin (1)	0.5–2 q4–6hr	Yes	
Cefamandole (2)	0.5–2 q4–8h	Yes	
Cefmetazole (2)	2 q6–12h	Yes	Intraabdominal infections
Cefonicid (2)	0.5–2 q24h	Yes	May be useful in outpatient therapy of endocarditis
Cefotetan (2)	1–2 q12–24h	Yes	Covers gastrointestinal anaerobes
Cefoxitin (2)	1–2 q4–8h	Yes	Covers gastrointestinal anaerobes
Cefuroxime (2)	0.75–1.5 q8h	Yes	Crosses blood-brain barrier
Cefepime (3)	0.5–2 q8–12h	No	
Cefoperazone (3)	1–2 q8–12h	Yes	
Cefotaxime (3)	1–2 q4–12h	Yes	Crosses blood-brain barrier
Ceftazidime (3)	0.5–2 q8–12h	Yes	
Ceftizoxime (3)	1–12 g/day divided q4–8h	Yes	Crosses blood-brain barrier
Ceftriaxone (3)	1–2 q12–24	No	May be useful in outpatient therapy of endocarditis; single-dose (250 mg intramuscularly) therapy for gonococcal genital and pharyngeal infections; crosses blood-brain barrier

From 2004 Mosby's drug consult, St. Louis, 2004, Mosby.

Appendixes

TABLE 15 Penicillins, Parenteral

Generic Name	Brand Name	Usual IV Adult Dose	Available Dosage Forms	Comments
Natural penicillins				
Penicillin G benzathine	Bicillin L-A	Given IM never IV; 1.2–2.4 million units as a single dose	300,000 units/mL	Provides low, long-lasting blood levels of penicillin G
Penicillin G benzathine and procaine combined	Bicillin C-R	Given IM never IV; 2.4 million units as a single dose	300,00 units/mL (150,000 units each of penicillin G benzathine and penicillin G procaine)	Provides low, long-lasting blood levels of penicillin G
Penicillin G procaine	Wycillin	Given IM never IV; 300,000-1,000,000 units/day as 1–2 doses/day	600,000 units/mL in 1, 2 mL syringes	Indicated for infections that respond to low, long-lasting penicillin G blood levels
Penicillin G potassium	Pfizerpen	1–24 million units/day in divided doses q4h, depending on severity of infection and microbial sensitivity	Injection: 5 million units; frozen premixed bag: 1, 2, 3 million units; powder for injection, 1, 5, 10, 20 million units	Infuse over 1–2 hr; Note: 250 mg = 400,000 units; sodium content of 1 million unit = 2 mEq; potassium content of 1 million unit = 1.7 mEq; often called "aqueous" penicillin
Broad-spectrum penicillins				
Ampicillin	Omnipen	1–12 g/day divided q4–6h	Powder for injection: 250, 500 mg, 1, 2, 10 g*	Infuse over at least 10–15 min
Ampicillin/Sulbactam	Unasyn	1.5–3 g q6–8h (equivalent to 1–2 g of ampicillin)	Powder for injection: 1.5 g (ampicillin 1 g + sulbactam 0.5 g), 3 g (ampicillin 2 g + sulbactam 1 g): 10 g*	Infuse over 15–30 min

Ticarcillin	Ticar	4–24 g/day in divided doses q4–6h	Powder or injection: 1, 3, 5, 20, 30 g*	Infuse over at least 30 min; sodium content of 1 g = 5.2–6.5 mEq;
Ticarcillin/Clavulanate	Timentin	12–24 g/day in divided doses q4–6h	Powder for injection and frozen premixed bags; ticarcillin disodium 3 g + clavulanate potassium 0.1 g	Infuse over 30 min; sodium content of 1 g = 4.75 mEq; potassium content of 1 g = 0.15 mEq
Mezlocillin	Mezlin	6–24 g/day in divided dose q4–6h	Powder for injection: 1, 2, 3, 4, 20 g*	Infuse over 30 min; sodium content = 1.85 mEq/g
Piperacillin	Pipracil	18–24 g/day divided q4–6h, depending on severity	Powder for injection: 2, 3, 4, 40 g*	Infuse over at least 20 min; sodium content = 1.85 mEq/g
Piperacillin/Tazobactam	Zosyn	3.375 g q6h or 4.5 g q8h	Powder for injection (piperacillin/tazobactam): 2/0.25, 3/0.375, 4 g/0.5 g, 36 g/4.5 g*	Infuse over 30 min
Penicillinase-resistant penicillins				
Nafcillin	Unipen	500 mg: 2 g q4–6h	Powder for injection: 500 mg, 1, 2, 4, 10 g*	Infuse over 30–60 min
Oxacillin	Bactocill, Prostaphlin	250 mg: 2 g q4–6h	Powder for injection: 250, 500 mg, 1, 2, 4, 10 g*	By direct IV injection over 10 min

IM, Intramuscularly; *IV*, intravenously.
From 2004 Mosby's drug consult, St. Louis, 2004, Mosby.
*Bulk package intended for pharmacy use only.

Appendixes

TABLE 16 Fluoroquinolones, Parenteral

Generic Name	Brand Name	Usual Intravenous Adult Dose	Available Dosage Forms	Comments
Ciprofloxacin	Cipro	200–400 mg q12h	Injection: 200, 400 mg, in glass vials and premixed bags	Infuse over 60 min
Gatifloxacin	Tequin	200–400 mg q24h	Injection: 200, 400 mg; premixed bags; 400 mg/250 mL	Infuse over 60 min
Levofloxacin	Levaquin	500 mg q24h (for urinary tract infection, 250 mg q24h)	Injection: (24 mg/mL) 500, 750 mg; premixed bags; (5 mg/mL) 250, 500, 750 mg	L-Isomer of the racemate ofloxacin (another commercially available fluoroquinolone antibiotic); infuse over 60 min
Moxifloxacin	Avelox IV	400 mg q24 h	Premixed bags; 400 mg/250 mL	Infuse over 60 min
Ofloxacin	Floxin	200–400 mg q12h	Injection: 200, 400 mg	Not effective for syphilis; infuse over 60 min
Trovafloxacin	Trovan	200–300 mg/day	Injection (as alatrofloxacin mesylate): (5 mg/mL) 250, 300 mg	Intravenous formulation contains alatrofloxacin, a trovafloxacin prodrug; infuse over 60 min; case reports of fatal hepatic reactions; use only in cases of life- or limb-threatening infections, and begin therapy in inpatient setting

TABLE 17 Sulfonamides, Parenteral

Generic Name	Brand Name	Usual Adult Dose	Available Dosage Forms	Comments
Sulfamethoxazole/trimethoprim (SMZ/TMP), Co-trimoxazole	Bactrim IV; Septra IV	8–20 mg of TMP/kg/day, in divided doses q6h, depending on type and severity of infection	Injection: 80 mg SMZ and 16 mg TMP per mL	Infuse over 60-90 min; first-line therapy for *Pneumocystis carinii* pneumonia; pay special attention to complaints of skin/mucosal rash; could signify early Stevens-Johnson syndrome

From *2004 Mosby's drug consult*, St. Louis, 2004, Mosby.

Appendixes

TABLE 18 Pediatric Drug Doses

Drug	Route	Dose
Emergency (resuscitation) drugs		
Atropine	IV	0.02 mg/kg/dose (minimum 0.1 mg/dose; maximum 1 mg)
Calcium chloride	IV	10–20 mg/kg
Calcium gluconate	IV	50–100 mg/kg
Epinephrine	IV	0.01 mg/kg (0.1 mg/kg via endotracheal tube)
Lidocaine	IV	1 mg/kg
Sodium bicarbonate	IV	1 mEq/kg/dose 0.3/kg/base deficit
Opiates		
Codeine	IM/PO	0.5–1 mg/kg
Meperidine	IV	0.2–1 mg/kg
	IM	1–2 mg/kg
Midazolam	IV	0.05–0.1 mg/kg
	IM	0.2–0.3 mg/kg
	PO	0.5–0.75 mg/kg
Morphine	IV	0.05–0.2 mg/kg
	IM/subcutaneous	0.1–0.2 mg/kg
Remifentanil	Infusion	0.5–1 mcg/kg/min (induction) 0.05–0.08 mcg/kg/min (maintenance)
Sufentanil	IV	0.1–0.5 mcg/kg with nitrous oxide; 5–10 mcg/kg alone
Fentanyl	IV	1–5 mcg/kg
Induction agents		
Propofol	IV	2–3 mg/kg
Ketamine	IV	1–2 mg/kg
	IM	5–10 mg/kg
Methohexital	IV	1–2 mg/kg
Thiopental	IV	3–6 mg/kg
Muscle relaxants		
Atracurium	IV	0.2–0.5 mg/kg
Cisatracurium	IV	0.1 mg/kg
Mivacurium	IV	0.1–0.2 mg/kg
Pancuronium	IV	0.04–0.15 mg/kg
Succinylcholine	IV	1–2 mg/kg
	IM	2.5–4 mg/kg
Rocuronium	IV	0.6–1 mg/kg (intubation) 0.08–0.12 mg/kg (maintenance)
Vecuronium	IV	0.04–0.2 mg/kg
Reversal agents		
Edrophonium	IV	0.5–1 mg/kg
Neostigmine	IV	0.05–0.07 mg/kg
Pyridostigmine	IV	0.2 mg/kg
Naloxone	IV/IM/subcutaneous	5–10 mcg/kg
Nalmefene	IV	0.25 mcg/kg

IM, Intramuscularly; *IV,* intravenously; *PO,* orally.

TABLE 19   Potential Drug Interactions Affecting Perianesthesia Care

Drug Category	Perianesthesia Concern
Drugs affecting the cardiovascular system	
Angiotensin-converting enzyme inhibitors	*Intraoperative concerns:* hypotension with or without bradycardia; intolerance to hypovolemia *Management:* maintenance of hydration; moderate doses of vasopressor *Discontinuation issues:* (1) brief interruption well tolerated; (2) continuation possibly improving regional blood flow and oxygen delivery and preserving renal function; (3) consideration of withholding in patients taking amiodarone, taking multiple antihypertensives, or in whom even a brief period of hypotension is unacceptable
Diuretics	*Intraoperative concerns:* hypokalemia; hypovolemia *Management:* monitoring of potassium levels preoperatively; maintain hydration *Discontinuation issues:* (1) patients rarely symptomatic if morning dose withheld; (2) patients appreciate lack of urinary urgency while awaiting surgery; (3) may be desirable to continue in patients receiving diuretics for chronic renal failure
Antiarrhythmics	*Intraoperative concerns:* cardiac depression; prolonged neuromuscular blockade; amiodarone: hypotension and atropine-resistant bradycardia requiring ventricular pacing *Management:* monitoring of serum drug levels as needed; amiodarone: large doses of vasopressors or inotropes and pacemaker capability *Discontinuation issues:* discontinuation rarely recommended because usually not prescribed for benign arrhythmias; amiodarone: impractical to discontinue because half-life is weeks to months; withhold concurrent medications (e.g., angiotensin-converting enzyme inhibitors)
Drugs affecting hemostasis	
Nonsteroidal antiinflammatory drugs	*Perioperative concerns:* impaired platelet function, altered renal function, gastrointestinal bleeding *Discontinuation issues:* unless surgery puts patient at particular risk for increased or catastrophic bleeding or impaired renal function, reasonable to continue up to morning of surgery
Anticoagulants (heparin, warfarin [Coumadin])	*Intraoperative concern:* increased hemorrhage *Management:* possible to reverse heparin with intravenous protamine; possible to reverse warfarin with vitamin K or fresh-frozen plasma *Discontinuation issues:* heparin: discontinue intravenously 4–5 hr and check partial thromboplastin time; warfarin: discontinue 3–5 days and check prothrombin time

Continued

TABLE 19 Potential Drug Interactions Affecting Perianesthesia Care—cont'd

Drug Category	Perianesthesia Concern
Drugs affecting hemostasis—cont'd	
Fibrinolytic drugs (streptokinase, urokinase, tissue plasminogen activator)	*Intraoperative concern:* hemorrhage *Management:* antifibrinolytic agent (aprotinin) possibly indicated *Discontinuation issues:* discontinuation usually not an option when administered for life-threatening conditions (e.g., acute myocardial infarction, massive pulmonary embolus)
Hypoglycemic agents	
Insulin	*Intraoperative concerns:* hyperglycemia, hypoglycemia *Management:* monitoring of serum glucose; insulin supplementation protocol *Discontinuation issues:* morning dose either withheld or reduced and adjustments in therapy based on periodic serum glucose determinations
Oral hypoglycemic agents	*Intraoperative concerns:* hyperglycemia, hypoglycemia *Management:* monitoring of serum glucose; avoidance of dehydration *Discontinuation issues:* withholding of oral hypoglycemic agents beginning on the day of surgery.
Drugs affecting the central nervous system	
Monoamine oxidase inhibitors	*Intraoperative concerns:* hypertension secondary to indirect-acting sympathomimetic drugs causing release of norepinephrine; excitatory state (from meperidine) or depressive phenomenon secondary to opioid administration *Management:* avoidance of known triggering agents such as meperidine and indirect-acting sympathomimetic agents (e.g., ephedrine) *Discontinuation issues:* (1) older, nonselective, irreversible monoamine oxidase inhibitors: discontinue for 2–3 wk with risk of serious psychiatric consequences; (2) newer, reversible inhibitors of monoamine oxidase A have short half-life, thus stop drug on morning of surgery

Modified from Marley RA: Preoperative preparation. In Zaglaniczny K, Aker J, editors: *Clinical guide to pediatric anesthesia,* Philadelphia, 1999, WB Saunders.

TABLE 20	Commonly Used Neuromuscular Terminology

- Onset time: time from drug administration to maximum effect
- Clinical duration: time from drug administration to 25% recovery of the twitch response
- Total duration of action: time from drug administration to 90% recovery of twitch response
- Recovery index: time from 25% to 75% recovery of the twitch response
- Train-of-four (TOF) ratio: compares the fourth twitch of a TOF with the first twitch; when the fourth twitch is 90% of the first, recovery indicated

TABLE 21	General Guidelines for Successful Neuromuscular Monitoring

- During onset, paralysis begins with the eye muscles followed by the extremities, trunk (from the neck muscles downward through the intercostals), abdominal muscles, and, finally, the diaphragm. Recovery returns in the opposite manner. Protective reflex muscles of the pharynx and upper esophagus recover later than the diaphragm, larynx, hand, or face.
- Monitoring the facial nerve for determination of onset/intubation may be preferable than monitoring the ulnar nerve.
- Monitoring the offset/recovery from neuromuscular blockade is probably better at the ulnar nerve.
- Tactile evaluation of double-burst stimulation may be better to differentiate "fade" than is train-of-four.
- When there is only one response to train-of-four stimulation, successful reversal may take as long as 30 minutes.
- At a train-of-four count of two to three responses, recovery may take up to 10 to 12 minutes following administration of long-acting relaxants and 4 to 5 minutes after intermediate-acting drugs.
- When the fourth response to train-of-four stimulation appears, adequate recovery can be achieved within 5 minutes of reversal with neostigmine or 2 to 3 minutes after use of edrophonium.

TABLE 22 Neuromuscular Blockers: Dose, Onset, and Duration*

Intubating Agent	ED$_{95}$ (mg/kg)	Intubating Dose (mg/kg)	Time to Onset (min)	Duration of Action (min)
Succinylcholine	1	1–1.5	30–60 sec	Ultrashort, 5–15
Mivacurium	0.25	0.75	2–4	Short, 20–30
Atracurium	0.15	0.5	2–4	Intermediate, 30–60
Cis-Atracurium	0.05	0.1	2–4	Intermediate, 30–60
Rocuronium	0.3	0.6–1	1–1.5	Intermediate, 30–60
Vecuronium	0.05	0.1	2–4	Intermediate, 30–60
Pancuronium	0.05	0.08–1.8	2–4	Long, 60–90
Pipecuronium	0.05	0.08–1	2–4	Long, 60–90
Doxacurium	0.025	0.075	2–4	Long, 60–90

ED_{95}, Effective dose for 95% paralysis.
*All data are for adult patients without significant disease.

TABLE 23 Neuromuscular Blockers: Elimination Mechanism

Agent	Elimination Mechanism	Comments
Mivacurium	Plasma cholinesterase	Prolonged in patients with cholinesterase deficiency
Atracurium	Hofmann elimination, plasma cholinesterase	Non–organ-dependent elimination produces consistent duration in patients with significant hepatic and renal disease, as well as the elderly
Cis-Atracurium	Hofmann elimination	Similar to atracurium but without the histamine release
Rocuronium	Renal	May be prolonged with hepatic and renal disease
Vecuronium	Renal (20%–30%); hepatic (40%–80%)	May be prolonged with hepatic disease
Pancuronium	Renal	May be prolonged with renal disease
Pipecuronium	Renal	May be prolonged with renal disease
Doxacurium	Renal; possibly hepatic	May be prolonged with renal disease
Succinylcholine	Plasma cholinesterase	Prolonged in patients with cholinesterase deficiency

TABLE 24 Response of Neuromuscular Blocking Agents in Select Muscle Disorders

Neuromuscular Disorder	Succinylcholine	Nondepolarizing Neuromuscular Blocking Agents
Multiple sclerosis	Contraindicated	Increased sensitivity; anesthesia stress may increase the rate of relapse
Motor neuron disease (amyotrophic lateral sclerosis [ALS; Lou Gehrig's disease])	Contraindicated	Increased sensitivity
Guillain-Barré syndrome	Contraindicated	Increased sensitivity; avoid agents with cardiac side effects
Charcot-Marie-Tooth disease	Contraindicated	Response to atracurium and mivacurium normal; all others, increased sensitivity
Muscular dystrophies	Contraindicated	Increased sensitivity
Myotonias	Contraindicated	Increased sensitivity; anticholinesterase agents may precipitate myotonia
Myasthenic syndromes	Resistant; prolonged duration of action may be present with plasmapheresis or anticholinesterase therapy	Extreme sensitivity
Mitochondrial myopathies	Contraindicated	Increased sensitivity
Hyperkalemic periodic paralysis	Contraindicated	Normal response
Hypokalemic periodic paralysis	Contraindicated	Normal response
Malignant hyperthermia	Contraindicated	Normal response
Myasthenia gravis	Resistant	Increased sensitivity
Huntington's chorea	Increased sensitivity	Increased sensitivity
Up-regulation of acetylcholine receptors from spinal cord trauma, stroke, or prolonged immobility	Contraindicated	Usually resistance, but depends on time since injury

TABLE 25 Factors That May Prolong Paralysis

Pathophysiologic Causes	Pharmacologic Causes
Acid maltase deficiency	Aminoglycoside toxicity
Adrenocortical dysfunction	Penicillin toxicity
Acute intermittent porphyria	Steroid myopathy
Amyotrophic lateral sclerosis	
Anoxia/ischemia	**Antihypertensives**
Carcinomatous polyneuropathy	Ganglionic blockers
Cholinesterase deficiency or genetic variance	Calcium channel blockers
Compressive neuropathy	β-blockers
Critical illness polyneuropathy	Furosemide
Diphtheria	
Eaton-Lambert syndrome	**Antidysrhythmics**
Guillain-Barré syndrome	Quinidine
Hypokalemia and hypocalcemia	Bretylium
Hypomagnesemia	Procainamide
Hypophosphatemia	Local anesthetics in large doses
Hypothermia	
Motor neuron disease	**Antibiotics**
Multiple sclerosis	Aminoglycoside antibiotics
Muscular dystrophy	Polymyxin B
Myasthenia gravis	Clindamycin
Myotonic syndromes	Tetracycline
Neurofibromatosis	
Nonspecific nutritional deficiency	**Miscellaneous drugs**
Poliomyelitis	Cyclosporine
Porphyria	Steroids
Pyridoxine abuse	Volatile anesthetics
Polymyositis	Dantrolene
Renal failure (variable prolongation)	Magnesium
Respiratory acidosis	Lithium
Sepsis	Azathioprine
Thiamine deficiency	Organophosphate poisoning
Tick bite paralysis	
Trauma	
Vitamin E deficiency	
Wound botulism	

TABLE 26 Drugs Affecting Blood Coagulation

Clinical uses of anticoagulants
- Heparin or the low-molecular-weight heparins are used acutely for short-term action.
- Warfarin is used for long-term therapy.
- Anticoagulants are given to prevent: perioperative deep vein thrombosis, extension of deep vein thrombosis or recurrence of a pulmonary embolism, thrombosis, and embolization in patients with atrial fibrillation, thrombosis on prosthetic heart valves, clotting during extracorporeal circulation such as dialysis or cardiopulmonary bypass, or unstable angina.

Procoagulant drugs (e.g., vitamin K)
- The reduced form of vitamin K is a cofactor in the posttranslational γ-carboxylation of a cluster of glutamic acid residues in each of factors II, VII, IX, and X; vitamin K is oxidized during the reaction. The γ-carboxylated glutamic acid residues are essential for the interaction of these factors with calcium and negatively charged phospholipid.

Injectable anticoagulants (e.g., heparin, low-molecular-weight heparins)
- These increase the rate of action of antithrombin III, a natural inhibitor that inactivates Xa and thrombin.
- They act both in vivo and in vitro.
- Anticoagulant activity results from a unique pentasaccharide sequence with high affinity for antithrombin III.
- The effect of heparin is monitored by the activated partial thromboplastin time, and the dose is individualized.
- Low-molecular-weight heparins have the same effect on factor X as heparin but less effect on thrombin; however, their anticoagulant effects are similar to those of heparin.
- Low-molecular-weight heparins are given subcutaneously or intravenously, and the onset of action is rapid. A standard dose (on a body weight basis) is given without the need for monitoring or individual dose adjustment. Patients can administer these agents at home.

Oral anticoagulants (e.g., warfarin [Coumadin])
- These inhibit the reduction of vitamin K, thus inhibiting the γ-carboxylation of glutamic acid in factors II, VII, IX, and X.
- They act only in vivo, and the effect is delayed.
- Many factors modify their action; drug interactions are especially important.
- There is wide variation in response; their effect is monitored by measuring the prothrombin time and international normalized ratio, and the dose is individualized accordingly.

Antiplatelet drugs (e.g., aspirin)
- Aspirin, dipyridamole, and clopidogrel have different actions, but their effects are additive.
- Their uses mainly relate to arterial thrombosis and include the following: acute myocardial infarction; prevention of morbidity after myocardial infarction, angina, transient ischemic attacks, intermittent claudication, coronary bypass, angioplasty with stenting; transient cerebral ischemic attack; and atrial fibrillation.
- Their effects are monitored by measuring bleeding time.

Appendixes

TABLE 27 Common Pediatric Premedications and Dosages

Medication	Dose	Route	Onset	Duration
Benzodiazepines				
Midazolam	0.1–0.15 mg/kg up to 10 mg	IM	5–10 min	0.5–2 hr
	0.2 mg/kg	IN	10 min	0.5–2 hr
	0.025–1 mg/kg	IV	1–3 min	0.5–2 hr
	0.25–1 mg/kg up to 20 mg	PO	15–30 min	0.5–2 hr
	0.3–1 mg/kg	PR	10–20 min	0.5–2 hr
Diazepam	0.1–0.5 mg/kg	IM, PO, PR	60 min	>24 hr
Narcotics				
Fentanyl	1–3 mcg/kg	IM	5–15 min	30–60 min
	0.5–1 mcg/kg	IV	1–3 min	30–60 min
	5 mcg/kg	OT	5–30 min	30–60 min
Sufentanil	1.5–4.5 mcg/kg	IN	7–10 min	30–60 min
Morphine sulfate	0.1–0.2 mg/kg	IM	30–45 min	4–5 hr
	0.05–0.1 mg/kg	IV	3–10 min	3–6 hr

Dissociative anesthetics

	Dose	Route	Administration time	Notes
Ketamine	1–2 mg/kg	IM	30 sec–2 min	12–25 min
	3 mg/kg	IN	20 min	???
	0.2–1 mg/kg	IV	30 sec–1 min	
	6–10 mg/kg	PO	10–20 min	
	10 mg/kg	PR	10 min	

Reversal agents

	Dose	Route	Administration time	Notes
Flumazenil	Adult: 0.2 mg	IV	Over 15 sec	Wait 45 sec; if necessary give 0.2 mg; repeat at 60-sec intervals; maximum dose: 3 mg/kg
Naloxone	Child: 10 mcg	IV		Up to 1 mg cumulative dose
	Adult: 0.4–2 mg	IV, subcutaneous, IM	Over 60 sec	Repeat q2–3min if needed
	Child: 0.5–2 mcg/kg	IV, subcutaneous, IM		Repeat q1min if needed

IM, Intramuscular; *IN*, intranasal; *IV*, intravenous; *OT*, oral transmucosal; *PO*, by mouth; *PR*, per rectum.

Appendixes

Standards for Nurse Anesthesia Practice

INTRODUCTION

These standards are intended to:

1. Assist the profession in evaluating the quality of care provided by its practitioners.
2. Provide a common base for practitioners to use in their development of a quality practice.
3. Assist the public in understanding what to expect from the practitioner.
4. Support and preserve the basic rights of the patient.

These standards apply to all anesthetizing locations. Although the standards are intended to encourage high-quality patient care, they cannot ensure specific outcomes.

STANDARD I

Perform a thorough and complete preanesthesia assessment.

Interpretation

The responsibility for the care of the patient begins with the preanesthetic assessment. Except in emergency situations, the certified registered nurse anesthetist (CRNA) has an obligation to complete a thorough evaluation and to determine that relevant tests have been obtained and reviewed.

STANDARD II

Obtain informed consent for the planned anesthetic intervention from the patient or legal guardian.

Interpretation

The CRNA shall obtain or verify that informed consent has been obtained by a qualified provider. Discuss anesthetic options and risks with the patient and/or legal guardian in language the patient and/or legal guardian can understand. Document in the patient's medical record that informed consent was obtained.

STANDARD III

Formulate a patient-specific plan for anesthesia care.

Interpretation

The plan of care developed by the CRNA is based on comprehensive patient assessment, problem analysis, anticipated surgical or therapeutic procedure, patient and surgeon preferences, and current anesthesia principles.

STANDARD IV

Implement and adjust the anesthesia care plan based on the patient's physiologic response.

Interpretation

The CRNA shall induce and maintain anesthesia at required levels. The CRNA shall continuously assess the patient's response to the anesthetic and/or surgical intervention and intervene as required to maintain the patient in a satisfactory physiologic condition.

STANDARD V

Monitor the patient's physiologic condition as appropriate for the type of anesthesia and specific patient needs.

A. *Monitor ventilation continuously.* Verify intubation of the trachea by auscultation, chest excursion, and confirmation of carbon dioxide in the expired gas. Continuously monitor end-tidal carbon dioxide during controlled or assisted ventilation. Use spirometry and ventilatory pressure monitors as indicated.

B. *Monitor oxygenation continuously* by clinical observation, pulse oximetry, and, if indicated, arterial blood gas analysis.

C. *Monitor cardiovascular status continuously* via electrocardiogram and heart sounds. Record blood pressure and heart rate at least every 5 minutes.

D. *Monitor body temperature continuously* in all pediatric patients receiving general anesthesia and, when indicated, in all other patients.

E. *Monitor neuromuscular function and status* when neuromuscular blocking agents are administered.

F. *Monitor and assess the patient positioning* and protective measures.

Interpretation

Continuous clinical observation and vigilance are the basis of safe anesthesia care. The standard applies to all patients receiving anesthesia care and may be exceeded at any time at the discretion of the CRNA. Unless otherwise stipulated in the standards, a means to monitor and evaluate the patient's status shall be immediately available for all patients. As new patient safety technologies evolve, integration into the current anesthesia practice shall be considered. The omission of any monitoring standards shall be documented and the reason stated on the patient's anesthesia record. The CRNA shall be in constant attendance of the patient until the responsibility for care has been accepted by another qualified health care provider.

STANDARD VI

There shall be complete, accurate, and timely documentation of pertinent information on the patient's medical record.

Interpretation

Document all anesthetic interventions and patient responses. Accurate documentation facilitates comprehensive patient care, provides information for retrospective review and research data, and establishes a medical-legal record.

STANDARD VII

Transfer the responsibility for care of the patient to other qualified providers in a manner that ensures continuity of care and patient safety.

Interpretation

The CRNA shall assess the patient's status and determine when it is safe to transfer the responsibility of care to other qualified providers. The CRNA shall accurately report the patient's condition and all essential information to the provider assuming responsibility for the patient.

STANDARD VIII

Adhere to appropriate safety precautions, as established within the institution, to minimize the risks of fire, explosion, electrical shock, and equipment malfunction. Document on the patient's medical record that the anesthesia machine and equipment were checked.

Interpretation

Before use, the CRNA shall inspect the anesthesia machine and monitors according to established guidelines. The CRNA shall check the readiness, availability, cleanliness, and working condition of all equipment to be utilized in the administration of the anesthesia. When the patient is ventilated by an automatic mechanical ventilator, monitor the integrity of the breathing system with a device capable of detecting a disconnection by emitting an audible alarm. Monitor oxygen concentration continuously with an oxygen supply failure alarm system.

Appendixes

STANDARD IX

Precautions shall be taken to minimize the risk of infection to the patient, the CRNA, and other health care providers.

Interpretation

Written policies and procedures in infection control shall be developed for personnel and equipment.

STANDARD X

Anesthesia care shall be assessed to ensure its quality and contribution to positive patient outcomes.

Interpretation

The CRNA shall participate in the ongoing review and evaluation of the quality and appropriateness of anesthesia care. Evaluation shall be performed based on appropriate outcome criteria and reviewed on an ongoing basis. The CRNA shall participate in a continual process of self-evaluation and shall strive to incorporate new techniques and knowledge into practice.

STANDARD XI

The CRNA shall respect and maintain the basic rights of patients.

Interpretation

The CRNA shall support and preserve the rights of patients to personal dignity and ethical norms of practice.

June 2002

This *Scope of Practice* statement, slightly modified for style, was previously published in the 1980, 1983, 1989, and 1992 predecessors of this document, which were respectively titled: *The American Association of Nurse Anesthetists Guidelines for the Practice of the Certified Registered Nurse Anesthetist* (1980, 1983), *Guidelines for Nurse Anesthesia Practice* (1989), and *Guidelines and Standards for Nurse Anesthesia Practice* (1992).

LATEX AVOIDANCE PRECAUTIONS

By touching any latex object, the health care worker can transmit the allergen by hand to the patient. Caution should be taken to keep the powder from the gloves away from the patient, because the powder will act as a carrier for the latex protein. Therefore, to reduce the possibility of the latex protein's becoming airborne, care must be taken not to snap gloves on and off.

Patients should be identified as being *latex sensitive*. The room should be labeled *latex free* to avoid personnel from bringing rubber products (e.g., wrist bands, chart labels, bed, room signs) into the room. A master list of latex-free devices and products is readily available from several Internet Web sites including:

Kendall's health care products: Search their latex-free database: http://www. kendallhq.com/catalogs. asp

Hudson RCI: Latex-free respiratory care and anesthesia products: http://www.hudsonrci. com/

Establish a latex consultant in your institution; an allergist is recommended. Develop programs to educate health care workers in the care of *latex-sensitive* patients. Develop educational programs for patients and their families in the care and precautions that should be taken to prevent latex exposure. This should encompass a first aid protocol in the event a severe reaction should arise. Encourage latex-sensitive patients to obtain and carry with them, at all times, some type of identification such as a medical alert bracelet and to have an epinephrine autoinjection kit if warranted.

Resource articles on latex allergy and a sample letter to manufacturers requesting latex information and resource articles are available in a *Latex Packet* from the Practice Department, American Association of Nurse Anesthetists, 222 South Prospect Avenue, Park Ridge, IL 60068-4001. Telephone: 847-692-7050, ext. 3016.

RECOMMENDATIONS FOR PATIENT CARE

Patients with Latex Allergy or Latex Risk

Schedule *latex-allergy* and/or *latex-risk* patients as the first cases in the morning. This approach will allow later dust (from the previous day) to be removed overnight.

The operating room

- Remove all latex products from the operating room.
- Bring a *latex-free* cart (if available) into the room.
- Use *latex-free* reservoir bag, airways, and endoctracheal tubes and laryngeal mask airways.
- Use *nonlatex* breathing circuit with plastic mask and bag.
- The ventilator must have *nonlatex* bellows.
- Place all monitoring devices, cords/tubes (oximeter, blood pressure, electrocardio-graph wires) in a stockinet and secure with tape to prevent direct skin contact. Items sterilized in ethylene oxide must be rinsed before use. Residual ethylene oxide reacts and can cause an allergic response in a latex-allergic patient.

Intravenous line preparation

- Use intravenous tubing without latex ports; utilize stopcocks if available.
- If you are unable to obtain intravenous tubing without latex ports, cover the latex ports with tape.
- Cover all rubber injection ports on intravenous bags with tape and label in the following way: *Do not inject* or *withdraw fluid through the latex port.* Note: Pulmonary artery catheters (especially the balloon), central venous catheters, and arterial lines may all contain latex components.

Appendixes

Operating room patient care

- Use nonlatex gloves. (Use caution when selecting nonlatex gloves. Not all substitutes are equally impermeable to blood-borne pathogens; care and investigation should be taken in the selection of substitute gloves.)
- Use *nonlatex* tourniquets or use *nonlatex* examination gloves or polyvinyl chloride tubing.
- Draw medication directly from opened multidose vials (remove stoppers) if medications are not available in ampules.
- Draw up medications immediately before the beginning of the case or their administration. The rubber allergen could leach out of the plunger of the syringe and cause a reaction. The intensity of this reaction appears to increase over time.
- Utilize *latex-free* or glass syringes.
- Use stopcocks to inject drugs rather than latex ports.
- Minimize mixing/agitating lyophilized drugs in multidose vials with rubber stoppers.
- Notify pharmacy and central supply that the patient you are caring for is latex sensitive so these departments can use appropriate procedures when preparing preparations and instruments for the patient. Also notify radiology, respiratory therapy, housekeeping, food service and postoperative care units so the appropriate precautions can be made to protect the patient.
- Place clear and readily visible signs on the doors of the operating room to inform all who enter that the patient has a latex allergy.

SIGNS AND SYMPTOMS OF ALLERGIC REACTIONS TO LATEX

Symptoms usually occur within 30 minutes following anesthesia induction; however, the actual onset can range from 10 to 290 minutes.

Awake Patient

- Itchy eyes
- Generalized pruritus
- Shortness of breath
- Feeling of faintness
- Feeling of impending doom
- Nausea
- Vomiting
- Abdominal cramping
- Diarrhea
- Wheezing

Anesthetized Patient

- Tachycardia
- Hypotension
- Bronchospasm
- Cardiorespiratory arrest
- Flushing
- Facial edema
- Laryngeal edema
- Urticaria

EMERGENCY RESPONSE AND MANAGEMENT

- Remove all latex-containing products and agents, if possible. Do not delay immediate emergency therapy.
- Inform the surgical team to stop treatment or abort the procedure.
- Assess and sustain ABCs of resuscitation.
- Maintain the airway and administer 100% oxygen.
- Discontinue inhalational halogenated agents (they are cardiovascular depressants that sensitize the myocardium to catecholamines, which may be required for therapy).
- Start intravascular volume expansion with Ringer's lactate or normal saline (10 to 50 mL/kg if hypotension is present and the patient has no history of congestive heart failure or any volume-related contraindication).
- Treat pharmacologically as indicated by presentation and clinical course. Administer epinephrine; start with a 0.5 to 1 mcg/kg bolus (10 mcg/mL dilution). Escalate to higher doses depending on the patient's response. If an intravenous line has not been established, epinephrine can be given subcutaneously in doses larger than would be administered intravenously (10 mcg/kg dose). Endotracheal administration may be necessary if intravenous access has not been established.

SECONDARY PHARMACOLOGIC TREATMENT

- Hydrocortisone, 0.25 to 1 g, or methylprednisolone, 1 mg/kg intravenously
- Diphenhydramine, 0.5 to 1 mg/kg (maximum dose, 50 mg)
- Epinephrine infusion, 2 to 4 mcg/min or more, titrate to effect
- Aminophylline, 5 to 6 mg/kg over 20 minutes for persistent bronchospasm
- Ranitidine 0.5 to 2 mg/kg intravenously (maximum dose, 150 mg)
- Sodium bicarbonate, 0.5 to 1 mEq/kg for persistent hypotension with acidosis diagnosed with laboratory confirmation

NONPHARMACOLOGIC CONSIDERATIONS

- Obtain allergy, pulmonary, pediatric consultations as indicated.
- Draw and send a blood sample for immunoglobulin E radioallergosorbent testing and tryptase level (1 hour after the reaction).
- Report the incident to the appropriate institutional entities (e.g., pharmacy, therapeutics, UR (utilization review) quality control.
- Document events thoroughly and succinctly to examine at a morbidity and mortality review at a later date.

Postreaction stabilization should include appropriate monitoring by dedicated providers well versed in managing postanaphylaxis patients. The pediatric, intensive, or special care area should be used when appropriate.

PRETREATMENT

Debate regarding the efficacy of premedication agents to treat patients with confirmed latex allergy remains somewhat controversial. Individual consideration for each patient undergoing elective operation or diagnostic and therapeutic procedures who has a known latex allergy should be initiated with the involvement of his or her primary care provider or allergy specialist. Premedication with steroids and antihistamines, including H_2 blockers, before general anesthesia or deep sedation may be preferred for children with a known and documented latex allergy. Although these agents will not *prevent* an allergic reaction, they may attenuate such a response by lessening the severity of a reaction. The patient's regular provider or specialist managing the allergy should be consulted to recommend appropriate pretreatment when warranted.

LATEX AVOIDANCE AND ALTERNATIVE MANAGEMENT OPTIONS

Common latex medical devices used in perioperative areas include the following:

- Mattresses on stretchers
- Rubber gloves
- Adhesive tape (porous)
- Urinary catheters and drainage systems
- Electrode pads
- Wound drains
- Eye shields
- Stomach and intestinal tubes
- Chest tubes and drainage systems
- Condom urinary collection devices
- Protective sheets
- Enema tubing kits
- Instrument pads
- Intravenous solutions and tubing systems
- Fluid-circulating thermal blankets
- Hemodialysis equipment
- Ambu (bag-valve) masks
- Medication syringes
- Bulb syringes

Appendixes

- Elastic bandages, wraps
- Medication vial stoppers (multidose)
- Stethoscope tubing
- Band-Aids and other similar bandage products
- Gloves: examination and sterile
- Dental dams
- Surgical drapes
- Patient-controlled analgesia syringes
- Tourniquets

ANESTHESIA EQUIPMENT AND PRODUCTS CONTAINING LATEX

- Stethoscope tubing
- Rubber masks
- Electrode pads (e.g., electrocardiogram, peripheral nerve stimulator, contact pads)
- Head straps
- Rubber tourniquets, esmarch bandages
- Rubber oral, nasal, and pharyngeal airways
- Teeth guards, eye shields, and bite blocks
- Blood pressure cuffs (inner bladder and tubing)
- Breathing circuits containing rubber
- Reservoir breathing bags, disposable oxygen masks, and nasal cannulas
- Rubber ventilator hoses and bellows
- Rubber endotracheal tubes
- Latex cuffs on plastic endotracheal tubes
- Latex injection ports on intravenous tubing and stopcocks
- Certain epidural catheter injection adapters
- Multidose-vial stoppers
- Patient-controlled analgesia syringes
- Rubber suction catheters and specimen traps
- Intravenous solutions and tubing systems (injection ports)

Developed in 1993 by the Infection and Environmental Control Task Force. Revised by the Occupational Safety and Hazard Committee and approved by the American Association of Nurse Anesthetists Board of Directors on July 31, 1998; slightly modified for style.

DIAGNOSIS

- The most sensitive indicator of potential malignant hyperthermia (MH) in the operating room is an unanticipated increase (e.g., doubling or tripling) of end-tidal carbon dioxide (CO_2) when minute ventilation is kept constant. The increase in CO_2 may occur over a brief period or may develop over longer periods (minutes to hours). If upward adjustments of minute ventilation (tidal volume and frequency) are required to maintain normal end-tidal CO_2, the possibility of MH should be considered and promptly evaluated.
- If sudden, unexpected cardiac arrest occurs, especially in a young male patient, hyperkalemia should be considered immediately and therapy started with calcium, hyperventilation, and glucose and insulin. Plasma potassium concentration should be measured immediately or as soon as possible.
- Unexpected tachycardia, tachypnea, and jaw muscle rigidity (masseter spasm) are often common signs of MH that follow the CO_2 increase.
- Respiratory and metabolic acidosis usually occurs in fulminant MH.
- A specific sign of MH is body rigidity (i.e., limbs, abdomen, and chest). When there is a suspicion of MH, attempts should be made to determine whether peripheral muscle rigidity is present.
- Temperature elevation is often a late sign of MH. Temperature change during MH is best detected by core temperature measurement (tympanic, nasopharyngeal or oropharyngeal, esophageal, rectal, or pulmonary artery). Forehead skin temperature is acceptable, but it is slower in reflecting changes in core temperature. *We recommend that core temperature be measured whenever general anesthesia is administered for procedures lasting more than 30 minutes.*
- Postoperative rhabdomyolysis without intraoperative signs of MH should be treated with hydration, mannitol, and bicarbonate. Plasma potassium concentration should be measured immediately or as soon as possible. The patient should be referred to an MH testing center to determine the need for evaluation of MH susceptibility.
- In the event of an acute MH episode, coagulation profile should be obtained in addition to electrolytes, arterial blood gas, and creatine kinase determinations.
- MH may occur at any time during anesthesia, including emergence and in the immediate postoperative period.

TREATMENT OF ACUTE MALIGNANT HYPERTHERMIA

- Call for additional experienced help.
- Do not administer volatile anesthetics or succinylcholine once MH has been diagnosed or considered.
- Hyperventilate at two to three times predicted minute ventilation with 100% oxygen.
- Give 2.5 mg/kg of dantrolene sodium for injection. Repeat as often as necessary titrated to control clinical signs of MH. Sometimes more than 10 mg/kg (up to 30 mg/kg) is necessary. Continue intravenous dantrolene for at least 24 hours after control of the episode (approximately 1 mg/kg every 6 hours).
- Dantrolene sodium does not produce significant cardiac or pulmonary complications when administered acutely. Therefore, there is little harm in administering dantrolene where MH is suspected, but not yet proved.
- Treat acidosis with bicarbonate if the acidosis is not promptly reversed by dantrolene.
- *Avoid calcium channel blockers.* Persistent arrhythmias may be treated with any other standard antiarrhythmics. Most arrhythmias respond to correction of hyperkalemia and acidosis by hyperventilation, dantrolene, and bicarbonate.
- Monitor core temperature.

Appendixes

- Treat hyperkalemia with glucose, insulin, and calcium.
- If the patient is hyperthermic or the core temperature rises rapidly, cool the patient; when possible, use nasogastric lavage, rectal lavage, and/or surface cooling, but avoid overcooling.
- Continue intravenous dantrolene for at least 24 hours after control of the episode (approximately 1 mg/kg every 6 hours). Continue dantrolene administration for at least 36 hours after an event.
- Watch for recrudescence by monitoring the patient in an intensive care unit for at least 24 hours. Recrudescence occurs in about 25% of MH cases. Core temperature should be monitored throughout.
- Avoid parenteral potassium, if possible, during ongoing rhabdomyolysis. Following control of the acute episode, persistent hypokalemia may be treated with careful monitoring of the serum potassium level.
- Ensure adequate urine output by hydration and diuretics because myoglobinuria is common.
- Follow the patient's coagulation profile; dissemination intravascular coagulation may occur.
- Measure creatine kinase levels every 6 hours until decreased. Creatine kinase may remain elevated for 2 weeks if event was severe. After the patient has improved and stabilized, creatine kinase should be measured on a declining time basis until it is normal (e.g., every 4 hours during the acute episode to every week during convalescence). This is important because it is elevated normally in some myopathies, and this should be recognized as a part of overall evaluation and treatment.
- For consultation to help with patient management, call the MH Hotline: 1-800-MH-HYPER (1-800-644-9737) or 1-315-464-7079 if outside the United States.
- Report patients who have had acute MH episodes to the North American MH Registry of the MH Association of the United States (MHAUS): 1-412-692-5464.
- Refer patients and families to MHAUS for information.

DRUGS AND MALIGNANT HYPERTHERMIA

- All volatile inhalation anesthetics (halothane, enflurane, isoflurane, desflurane, sevoflurane, ether, methoxyflurane and cyclopropane) and succinylcholine are MH triggers. Nitrous oxide is not a trigger.
- Calcium channel blockers should not be administered when dantrolene has been given.
- All other currently used anesthetics and life-support drugs are considered safe.

SUCCINYLCHOLINE IN CHILDREN

- Routine use of succinylcholine for elective surgery is best avoided in children.
- The pharmaceutical companies that manufacture succinylcholine have changed the package insert to indicate that the drug should not be used routinely in children. Some indications for succinylcholine are airway emergencies, risk of aspiration, and procedures in which it is advisable that paralysis be induced within 60 seconds of induction of anesthesia. The reason for the change relates to the complications such as masseter muscle rigidity (MMR), rhabdomyolysis, and sudden hyperkalemic cardiac arrest in patients with undiagnosed myopathies (i.e., may be in the preclinical stage). Rhabdomyolysis may occur in as many as 40% of children given intravenous succinylcholine, whether clinical or "subclinical."

MANAGEMENT AND PRETREATMENT OF PATIENTS SUSCEPTIBLE TO MALIGNANT HYPERTHERMIA

- A treatment plan for MH should be available in every anesthetizing location.
- All facilities, including ambulatory surgery centers and offices, where MH-triggering anesthetics (halothane, enflurane, isoflurane, desflurane, sevoflurane, ether, methoxyflurane, cyclopropane and succinylcholine) are administered, should stock a minimum of 36 vials of dantrolene sodium for injection. If potent volatile agents are not used, and succinylcholine is available for an emergency situation such as to facilitate obtaining an airway that is lost or difficult, a minimum of 36 vials of dantrolene sodium

for injection should be available. If none of the triggering agents are used or available, then dantrolene sodium for injection need not be present.

- Do not use MH-triggering agents in patients susceptible to MH or in their undiagnosed relatives.
- Dantrolene prophylaxis is not recommended for most MH-susceptible patients. Dantrolene can worsen muscle weakness in patients with muscle disease and should be used with caution. For most procedures, even those requiring general anesthesia, dantrolene prophylaxis may be omitted.
- The anesthesia machine to be used for a patient susceptible to MH should be prepared in the following way: Ensure that anesthetic vaporizers are disabled by removing, draining, or taping in the "OFF" position. Some consultants recommend changing CO_2 absorbent (soda lime or baralyme). Flow 10 L/min O_2 through the circuit via the ventilator for at least 20 minutes. If a fresh gas hose is replaced, 10 minutes is adequate. During this time, a disposable, unused breathing bag should be attached to the Y-piece of the circle system, and the ventilator should be set to inflate the bag periodically. Use a new or disposable breathing circuit.
- The patient susceptible to MH who is undergoing outpatient surgery may be discharged on the day of surgery if the anesthetic has been uneventful. A minimum of 4 hours observation is suggested.

TESTING FOR SUSCEPTIBILITY

- There are a few testing centers in North America. A complete list is available from MHAUS *(www.mhaus.org)*.
- Muscle specimens for MH testing must be harvested at the biopsy center.
- Muscle biopsy centers in the United States, Canada, and Europe have standardized the contracture test and determined its sensitivity and specificity. The muscle biopsy is highly sensitive for the detection of MH and currently is the only valid definitive test for MH.
- Molecular genetic testing for MH susceptibility is progressing slowly. To date, there are about 30 mutations identified as being causal for MH, but specific genotypes have been identified for fewer than 50% of MH-susceptible persons. In some families in which a specific gene is associated with MH susceptibility in several family members, DNA testing may be used for determining susceptibility in other family members. Such testing is gradually becoming available in the United States on a research basis. In vitro muscle biopsy contracture testing is still the gold standard for MH diagnosis.

MUSCLE DISEASE ISSUES

- Several muscle diseases may predispose to MH or to hyperkalemic reactions to MH-triggering agents. MH susceptibility is definitely associated with central core disease. Patients with central core disease should not be given MH-triggering anesthetics.
- Patients with Duchenne or Becker muscular dystrophy are at risk for developing life-threatening hyperkalemia when they are administered succinylcholine or potent volatile agents. Subtypes of myotonia, specifically sodium channel forms of myotonia and cold-induced myotonia, may predispose to MH. Hyperkalemic and hypokalemic paralyses have also been associated with MH susceptibility. Mitochondrial myopathies do not appear to predispose to MH.

MASSETER MUSCLE RIGIDITY

- MMR is a sustained contracture of the jaw muscles following the administration of succinylcholine and, if considered abnormally long in duration, may be a forewarning of MH. A mild increase in masseter muscle tone with limb flaccidity following succinylcholine may be a normal response. It is not possible to determine, clinically, whether that increase in tone represents an MH reaction or some other myopathic response.

Appendixes

However, if generalized rigidity also occurs, then MH is highly likely. Immediately check the patient's potassium and blood gas values.

- MMR occurs more frequently in children, with or without inhalation agents.
- Clinical signs of MH occur in about 20% of patients with MMR. These signs may follow immediately or be delayed. Temperature monitoring should be employed, if not yet done so.
- Experts are divided on how to proceed after MMR: either continue with anesthetic agents that will not trigger MH or discontinue the anesthetic regimen and postpone elective surgery.
- Unless clinical signs of MH appear, dantrolene is not recommended following the occurrence of MMR only.
- Because of the likelihood of rhabdomyolysis and the possibility of an undiagnosed myopathy, creatine kinase and urine color should be checked every 6 hours until they return to normal. Also test electrolytes; rapidly developing rhabdomyolysis causes rapid increases in potassium, and slowly developing rhabdomyolysis is less dangerous, because potassium is redistributed more quickly than blood levels can increase.
- Hyperkalemic cardiac arrhythmias may follow MMR and presage severe rhabdomyolysis. Myoglobinuria may occur within a few hours after MMR and should be sought and treated to prevent acute tubular necrosis and obstructive nephropathy.
- Patients experiencing MMR with associated clinical signs or symptoms of MH should be observed closely (temperature monitoring) for at least 24 hours.
- Discuss muscle biopsy with an MH expert.

SUDDEN, UNEXPECTED CARDIAC ARREST: MALIGNANT HYPERTHERMIA OR AN OCCULT MYOPATHY

- Sudden cardiac arrest, especially soon after the use of succinylcholine in young or adolescent male patients, is likely caused by hyperkalemia in a patient with an undiagnosed myopathy. Many such cases have been described since 1990, most with the use of intravenous or intramuscular succinylcholine. Initial reports indicated a high mortality. Muscle rigidity and/or hyperthermia may also be present.
- Therapy should be directed at treatment of hyperkalemia: calcium chloride, bicarbonate, insulin, glucose, and hyperventilation. Dialysis and cardiopulmonary bypass may be required.
- If hyperkalemia is successfully treated, a good outcome may be attained even after prolonged resuscitation.
- Even though hyperkalemic cardiac arrest is uncommon, because of the extremely high mortality in such cases, the inability to predict which child may be at risk, and the availability of alternative neuromuscular blocking agents, anesthesia providers have been warned against elective use of succinylcholine in children.

INFORMATION RESOURCES

MHAUS provides educational and technical information to patients and health care providers. Contact MHAUS at 607-674-7901 or e-mail to *info@mhaus.org*. Information is available on the Internet at *http://www.mhaus.org*.

NORTH AMERICAN MALIGNANT HYPERTHERMIA REGISTRY OF MHAUS

The North American MH Registry, an operating unit of MHAUS, registers information about specific patients and their families. The Registry is now located at Children's Hospital of Pittsburgh at the University of Pittsburgh, and Dr. Barbara Brandom is the director. Health care providers are encouraged to report MH and MH-like episodes to the Registry. Contact the Registry office at 1-888-274-7899 for forms or information.

Reprinted, with slight modifications for style, with permission from the Malignant Hyperthermia Association of the United States, P.O. Box 1069, 11 East State Street, Sherburne, NY 13460.

APPENDIX 5 **Difficult Airway Algorithm**

1. Assess the likelihood and clinical impact of basic management problems.
   A. Difficult ventilation
   B. Difficult intubation
   C. Difficulty with patient cooperation or consent
   D. Difficult tracheostomy

2. Actively pursue opportunities to deliver supplemental oxygen throughout the process of difficult airway management.

3. Consider the relative merits and feasibility of basic management choices.

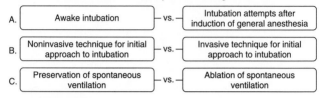

A. Awake intubation — vs. — Intubation attempts after induction of general anesthesia

B. Noninvasive technique for initial approach to intubation — vs. — Invasive technique for initial approach to intubation

C. Preservation of spontaneous ventilation — vs. — Ablation of spontaneous ventilation

4. Develop primary and alternative strategies.

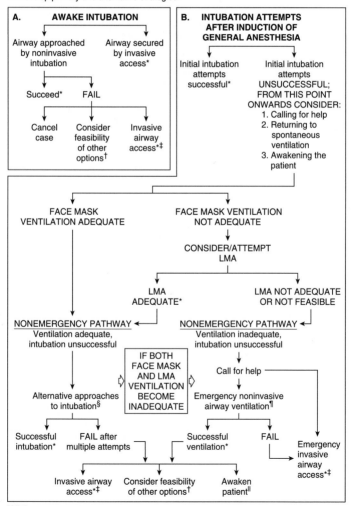

From American Society of Anesthesiologists, Park Ridge, IL.

LMA, Laryngeal mask airway.

* Confirm tracheal intubation or LMA placement with exhaled CO_2.

† Other options include (but are not limited to) surgery utilizing face mask or LMA local anesthesia infiltration, or regional nerve block. Pursuit of these options usually implies that mask ventilation will not be problematic. Therefore, these options may be of limited value if this step in the algorithm has been reached via the Emergency Pathway.

‡ Invasive airway access includes surgical or percutaneous tracheostomy or cricothyrotomy.

§ Alternative noninvasive approaches to difficult intubation include (but are not limited to) use of different laryngoscope blades, LMA as an intubation conduit (with or without fiberoptic guidance), fiberoptic intubation, intubating stylet or tube changer, light wand, retrograde intubation, and blind oral or nasal intubation.

‖ Consider repreparation of the patient for awake intubation or canceling surgery.

¶ Options for emergency noninvasive airway ventilation include (but are not limited to) rigid bronchoscope, esophageal-tracheal combitube ventilation, or transtracheal jet ventilation.

Appendixes

Hemodynamic Formulas

Parameter	Formula	Normal Range
CO	HR × SV	4–8 L/min
CI	CO ÷ BSA	2.5–4 L/min/m^2
CVP	cm H$_2$O = mm Hg × 1.34	2–6 mm Hg
PCWP	—	8–12 mm Hg
MAP	[(DBP × 2) + SBP] ÷ 3	70–105 mm Hg
SVR	[(MAP − CVP) ÷ CO] × 80	700–1400 dynes/cm/sec^{-5}
PVR	[(PAM − PCWP) ÷ CO] × 80	50–350 dynes/cm/sec^{-5}
SV	(CO × 1000) ÷ HR	60–100 mL/beat
SVI	SV ÷ BSA	33–47 mL/beat per m^2
LVSWI	[SVI × (MAP − PCWP)] × 0.0136	40–60 g × m/beat/m^2
RVSWI	[SVI × (PAM − PAD)] × 0.0136	7–12 g × m/beat/m^2
RVEDV	SV ÷ EF	100–160 mL
RVESV	EDV − SV	50–100 mL
RVSV	(CO × 1000) ÷ HR	60–100 mL
EF	(EDV − ESV) ÷ EDV or SV ÷ EDV	55%–70%
CPP	MAP − CVP or MAP − ICP	70–80 mm Hg

CI, Cardiac index; *CO,* cardiac output; *CPP,* cerebral perfusion pressure; *CVP,* central venous pressure; *EF,* ejection fraction; *LVSWI,* left ventricular stroke work index; *MAP,* mean arterial pressure; *PAD,* pulmonary artery diastolic; *PAM,* pulmonary artery mean; *PCWP,* pulmonary capillary wedge pressure; *PVR,* pulmonary vascular resistance; *RVEDV,* right ventricular end-diastolic volume; *RVESV,* right ventricular end-systolic volume; *RVSV,* right ventricular stroke volume; *RVSWI,* right ventricular stroke work index; *SV,* stroke volume; *SVI,* stroke volume index; *SVR,* systemic vascular resistance.

APPENDIX 7 | Pulmonary Function Test Values

Test	Normal Values
Vital capacity (VC)	60–70 mL/kg
Tidal volume (VT) (spontaneous ventilation)	6–8 mL/kg
Minute ventilation (VE)	80 mL/kg
Functional residual capacity (FRC)	28–32 mL/kg
Forced expiratory volume in 1 second (FEV_1)	>75%
Forced vital capacity (FVC)	60–70 mL/kg
Dead space (VDS)	2 mL/kg
VDS/VT	33%
FEV_1/FVC	>75%

Age	Weight (kg) 50th Percentile	Respiratory Rate (breaths/min)	Heart Rate (beats/min)	Systolic Blood Pressure (mm Hg)
Premature	<3	50–60	120–180	40–60
Newborn	3–4	35–40	100–180	50–70
1 mo	4	35–40	100–180	50–70
3 mo	5	24–30	100–180	60–110
6 mo	7	25–30	100–180	60–110
12 mo	10	20–25	90–150	65–115
2 yr	12	16–22	90–150	75–125
3 yr	15	16–22	90–150	75–125
5 yr	20	14–20	60–140	80–120
7 yr	30	14–20	60–140	90–120
10 yr	40	12–20	60–100	90–120

Estimating weight in kilograms
<1 yr: (age [mo]) $\times$ 0.5 + 3.5
>1 yr: (age [yr]) $\times$ 2 + 1

Estimating endotracheal tube (ETT) size*

Age	ETT Size	Laryngoscope Blade	Distance (cm)
Premature	2.5	0 Miller	According to weight: 500 g @ 6 cm 1000 g @ 7 cm 2000 g @ 8 cm 3000 g @ 9 cm
Newborn	3–3.5	0 Miller	10
6 mo	3.5–4	1 Miller	10–11
1 yr	4	1 to Miller/Mac	11
2 yr	4.5–5	1 or 2 Miller/Mac	12.5

>20 mo: 4 + age (yr) $\div$ 4
Length of insertion (>1 yr: 12 + age $\div$ 2)

*This is only a guide; prepare an ETT one size larger and one size smaller than the ETT size selected.

Estimated blood volume (EBV)

Age	Volume (mL/kg)
Premature	90
Full-term	90
0–2 yr	80
2 + yr	70

Maximum allowable blood loss (MABL)

$$MABL = \frac{EBV \times (\text{Initial hematocrit} - \text{Target hematocrit})}{\text{Initial hematocrit}}$$

Nothing by mouth (NPO) time

Age (mo)	Clear liquids (hr)	Milk/Solids (hr)
0–6	2	4
6–36	2–4	4–6
>36	2–4	6–8

Calculation of maintenance fluid requirements

Weight (kg)	Requirement
0–10	4 mL/kg/hr
10–20	40 mL + 2 mL/kg >10
>20	60 mL + 1 mL/kg >20

NPO deficit

NPO hours × Maintenance: Replace 50% the first hour, 25% the second hour, and 25% the third hour.

Appendixes

APPENDIX 9 · Preoperative Laboratory Tests

Test	Normal Serum Values
Activated coagulation time	80–120 sec
Alanine aminotransferase, female	9–24 units/L
male	10–32 units/L
Albumin, total	6.6–7.9 g/dL
fractional	4.4–4.5 g/dL
Alkaline phosphatase	45–125 units/L
Ammonia	80–110 mcg/dL
Amylase	20–110 units/L
Anion gap	8–14 mEq/L
Arterial blood gases: pH	7.35–7.45
Carbon dioxide pressure	35–45 mm Hg
Oxygen pressure	80–100 mm Hg
Bicarbonate	22–26 mEq/L
Aspartate aminotransferase	8–20 units/L
Bilirubin, direct	0–0.4 mg/dL
indirect	0.1–1.2 mg/dL
Blood urea nitrogen	8–20 mg/dL
Calcium	4.5–5.5 mEq/L
Chloride	100–108 mEq/L
Creatine kinase, total	
female	15–57 units/L
male	24–100 units/L
MB	0–7 units/L
MM	6–70 units/L
Creatinine	0.2–1.5 mg/dL
Fibrin split product/fibrin degradation product	<3 mcg/mL
Fibrinogen	195–365 mg/dL
Glucose, fasting	70–100 mg/dL
Hematocrit, female	37%–47%
male	42%–52%
Hemoglobin, female	15–16 g/dL
male	14–18 g/dL
glycosylated	5.5%–9%
International Normalized Ratio	1
Lactate dehydrogenase (LDH), total	48–115 international units/L
LDH_1	17.5%–28.3% of total LDH
LDH_2	30.4%–36.4% of total LDH
	($LDH_1 < LDH_2$)
Magnesium	1.5–2.5 mEq/L
Phosphorus	1.8–2.6 mEq/L
Platelets	130,000–370,000/mm^3
Potassium	3.8–5.5 mEq/L
Pseudocholinesterase	8–80 units/mL
Prothrombin time	11–13.2 sec
Partial thromboplastin time	22.5–32.2 sec
Red blood cell count, female	4.2–5.4 million/dL
male	4.7–6.2 million/dL

Sodium	134–145 mEq/L
Triiodothyronine	90–230 ng/dL
Thyroxine	5–13 mcg/dL
Thyroid-stimulating hormone	0.406 microunits/mL
White blood cell count	4100–10,900/microliter

Therapeutic drug level

Amitriptyline	160–240 ng/mL
Digoxin	0.8–2 ng/mL
Lidocaine	1–5 mcg/dL
Lithium	0.7–1.5 mEq/L
Phenobarbital	10–30 mcg/mL
Phenytoin	10–20 mcg/mL
Theophylline	5–20 mcg/mL

Anesthetic Considerations for Herbal Medicines

Clinical Effect	Herbal Drugs
Anticoagulant (discontinue 2 wk before elective surgery)	Alfalfa, chamomile, dong quai root, echinacea, feverfew, garlic, ginger, ginkgo, ginseng, goldenseal, guarana, horse chestnut, willow bark
Serum glucose alteration (monitor preoperative serum glucose level)	*Decrease:* akee fruit, alfalfa, aloe, argimony, artichokes, barley, bitter melon, burdock root, carrot oil, chromium, coriander, dandelion root, devil's club, eucalyptus, fenugreek seeds, fo-ti, garlic, ginseng, grape seed, guayusa, gymnena, juniper, neem seed oil, onions, periwinkle, yellow root *Increase:* ephedra
Central nervous system stimulation (consider potential vasoactive agent interactions)	Feverfew, goldenseal, gotu kola, guarana, ma huang, milk thistle, Saint John's wort, yohimbine
Central nervous system depressant (may potentiate the central nervous system depressant effects of barbiturates, benzodiazepines, and opioids)	Hawthorn, kava, lavender, lemon balm, lemon verbena, mugwort, passion flower, rauwolfia, valerian
Antidepressant (caution when coadministered with tricylic antidepressants, selective serotonin reuptake inhibitors, and monoamine oxidase inhibitors)	Ginseng, lemon balm, ma huang, mugwort, passion flower, Saint John's wort, yohimbine

Modified from Zaglaniczny K: An introduction to herbal medicine and anesthetic considerations, *Nurs Anesth Forum* 2:11, 1999.

Preoperative Examination	Acceptable End Points	Significance of End Points
Length of upper incisors	Qualitative; short incisors	Long incisors; blade enters mouth in cephalad direction
Involuntary: maxillary teeth anterior to mandibular teeth	No overriding of maxillary teeth anterior to the mandibular teeth	Overriding maxillary teeth; blade enters mouth in a more cephalad direction
Voluntary: protrusion of mandibular teeth anterior to the maxillary teeth	Anterior protrusion of the mandibular teeth relative to the maxillary teeth	Test of temporomandibular joint function; indicates good mouth opening and jaw will move anteriorly with laryngoscopy
Interincisor distance	>3 cm	2-cm flange on blade can be easily inserted between teeth
Oropharyngeal class	Class II	Tongue small in relation to size of oropharyngeal cavity
Narrowness of palate	Should not appear very narrow or highly arched	Narrow palate decreases the oropharyngeal volume and room for both blade and endotracheal tube
Mandibular space length (thyromental distance)	5 cm or three ordinary-size fingerbreadths	Larynx relatively posterior to other upper airway structures
Mandibular space compliance	Qualitative; palpation of normal resilience/softness	Laryngoscopy retracts tongue into the mandibular space; compliance of the mandibular space determines if tongue fits into mandibular space
Length of neck	Qualitative; quantitative index not yet available	Short neck decreases the ability to align the upper airway axes
Thickness of neck	Qualitative; quantitative index not yet available	Thick neck decreases the ability to align the upper airway axes
Range of motion of head and neck	Neck flexed on chest 35 degrees plus head extended on neck 80 degrees is sniff position	Sniff position aligns oral, pharyngeal, and laryngeal axes to create favorable line of sight

Modified from Benumof JL: The ASA difficult airway algorithm: new thoughts and considerations, *Curr Rev Nurs Anesth* 22:103, 1999.

Appendixes

APPENDIX 12 Fasting Guidelines for Healthy Patients (All Ages) Undergoing Elective Surgery

No chewing gum or candy after midnight (foreign body aspiration concern)

    Clear liquids up to 2 hours before surgery*

    Breast milk allowed until 4 hours before surgery

    No infant formula, nonhuman milk,[†] or light meal[‡] for at least 6 hours before surgery

    Prescribed medications (e.g., premedication) administered with a sip of water or prescribed liquid mixture (up to 150 mL for adult; up to 75 mL for children) up to 1 hour before anesthesia

---

*Consider the possibility of the case proceeding earlier than scheduled.

[†]Because nonhuman milk is similar to solids in gastric emptying time, the amount ingested must be considered when determining an appropriate fasting period.

[‡]A light meal typically consists of toast and clear liquids. Meals that include fried or fatty foods or meat may prolong gastric emptying time. Both the amount and the type of foods ingested must be considered when determining an appropriate fasting period.

Consensus Formula for Fluid Resuscitation and Urine Output in Burn Patients (American Burn Association)

Adults: Ringer's lactate 2–4 mL × kg body weight x percent body surface area (BSA) burned*

Children: Ringer's lactate 3–4 mL × kg body weight x percent BSA burned*†

*One half of the estimated volume of fluid should be administered in the first 8 hours after burn injury. The remaining half should be administered over the subsequent 16 hours of the first postburn day.

†Infants and young children should receive fluid with 5% dextrose at a maintenance rate in addition to the resuscitation fluid noted previously.

MINIMUM URINARY OUTPUT IN BURN PATIENTS

Adults: 0.5 mL/kg/hour

Children weighing less than 30 kg: 1 mL/kg/hour

Patients with high-voltage electrical injuries: 1–1.5 mL/kg/hour

From American Burn Association: *Advanced burn life support course provider's manual,* Chicago, 2001, American Burn Association.

APPENDIX 14 — Prevention of Human Immunodeficiency Virus Infection after Occupational Exposure*

Setting	Eligible Patients	Recommended Regimen	Alternative Regimens
Percutaneous exposure to blood	Persons with highest and increased-risk exposure	Zidovudine 300 mg PO bid or 200 mg PO tid plus lamivudine 150 mg PO bid plus either indinavir 800 mg PO bid ii. I. D. or nelfinavir 750 mg PO tid for 4 wk	
	Persons with exposure of no increased risk	Not recommended	Offer zidovudine 300 mg PO bid or 200 mg PO tid plus lamivudine 150 mg PO bid
Other percutaneous exposure	Persons exposed to fluid containing blood, other fluid, or tissue	Not recommended	Offer zidovudine 300 mg PO bid or 200 mg PO tid plus lamivudine 150 mg PO bid; addition of indinavir or nelfinavir is optional
	Persons exposed to other fluid (e.g., urine)	Not recommended	
Exposure of mucous membrane or skin	Persons exposed to blood	Not recommended	Offer zidovudine 300 mg PO bid or 200 mg PO tid plus lamivudine 150 mg PO bid
	Persons exposed to fluid containing blood, other fluid, or tissue	Not recommended	Do not offer
	Persons exposed to other fluid (e.g., urine)	Not recommended	

bid, Twice daily; *PO*, orally; *tid*, three times daily.

*Highest- and increased-risk exposures involve a larger volume of blood (e.g., deep injury with large-diameter hollow needle previously in source patient's vein or artery, especially involving an injection of source patient's blood) or blood containing a high titer of human immunodeficiency virus (HIV). A high titer of HIV is defined as blood from a person with acute retroviral illness or end-stage acquired immunodeficiency syndrome (AIDS): viral load measurement may be considered, but its use in relation to prophylaxis has not be evaluated.

Alternative regimens with other nucleoside reverse transcriptase inhibitors, protease inhibitors, or nonnucleoside reverse transcriptase inhibitors may be required. Alternative regimens may be required in certain situations (e.g., resistance of source's virus to standard regimen). Other regimens have not been approved by the CDC.

There is no increased risk if exposure was to neither a large volume of blood nor blood with a high titer of HIV (e.g., solid suture-needle injury from source patient with asymptomatic HIV infection. Other fluids include semen, vaginal secretions, and cerebrospinal, synovial, pleural, peritoneal, pericardial, and amniotic fluids.

For skin exposures, the risk is increased if the fluid contains a high titer of HIV, there is prolonged contact, the exposed area is large, or the integrity of the exposed skin is visibly compromised. For skin exposures without increased risk, the risk of drug toxicity outweighs the benefit of postexposure prophylaxis.

Modified from recommendations of the United States Centers for Disease Control and Prevention (CDC). American Society of Health-System Pharmacists. ASHP therapeutic guidelines for nonsurgical antimicrobial prophylaxis. *Am. J. Health-Sys Pharm.* 56: 1201–50. 1999.

TABLE 1 Postanesthesia Discharge Scoring System for Determining Home Readiness

Criterion	Score*
Vital signs	
Vital signs must be stable and consistent with age and preoperative baseline	
Blood pressure and pulse within 20% of preoperative baseline	2
Blood pressure and pulse 20%–40% of preoperative baseline	1
Blood pressure and pulse >40% of preoperative baseline	0
Activity level	
Patient must be able to ambulate at preoperative level	
Steady gait, no dizziness, or meets preoperative level	2
Requires assistance	1
Unable to ambulate	0
Nausea and vomiting	
The patient should have minimal nausea and vomiting before discharge	
Minimal: successfully treated with oral medication	2
Moderate: successfully treated with intramuscular medication	1
Severe: continues after repeated treatment	0
Pain	
The patient should have minimal or no pain before discharge	
The level of pain should be acceptable to the patient	
Pain should be controllable by oral analgesics	
The location, type, and intensity of pain should be consistent with anticipated postoperative discomfort	
Acceptability:	
Yes	2
No	1
Surgical bleeding	
Postoperative bleeding should be consistent with expected blood loss for the procedure	
Minimal: does not require dressing change	2
Moderate: up to two dressing changes required	1
Severe: more than three dressing changes required	0

*Total possible score is 10. Patients who score 9 or 10 are considered fit for discharge.

TABLE 2 Aldrete's Phase II Postanesthetic Recovery Score

Patient Sign	Criterion	Score*
Activity	Able to move four extremities (voluntarily or on command)	2
	Able to move two extremities (voluntarily or on command)	1
	Able to move no extremities (voluntarily or on command)	0
Respiration	Able to breathe deeply and cough	2
	Dyspnea, limited breathing, or tachypnea	1
	Apneic or on mechanical ventilator	0
Circulation	Blood pressure ±20% of preanesthesia level	2
	Blood pressure ±20%–49% of preanesthesia level	1
	Blood pressure ±50% of preanesthesia level	0
Consciousness	Fully awake	2
	Arousable on calling	1
	Not responding	0
Oxygen saturation	SpO_2 >92% on room air	2
	Requires supplemental oxygen to maintain SpO_2 >90%	1
	SpO_2 <90% even with oxygen supplement	0
Dressing	Dry and clean	2
	Wet but stationary or marked	1
	Growing area of wetness	0
Pain	Pain free	2
	Mild pain handled by oral medications	1
	Severe pain requiring intravenous or intramuscular medications	0
Ambulation	Can stand up and walk straight[†]	2
	Vertigo when erect	1
	Dizziness when supine	0
Fasting-feeding	Able to drink fluids	2
	Nauseated	1
	Nauseated and vomiting	0
Urine output	Has voided	2
	Unable to void but comfortable	1
	Unable to void and uncomfortable	0

*Total possible score is 20. A score of 18 or greater is required before patient discharge.
[†]May be replaced by Romberg's test, or picking up 12 clips in one hand.

TABLE 1 Neuromuscular Monitoring Modalities

Monitoring Test	Definition	Comments
Single twitch	A single supramaximal electrical stimulus ranging from 0.1–1 Hz	Requires baseline before drug administration; generally used as qualitative rather than quantitative assessment
Train-of-four	A series of four twitches at 2 Hz every half-second for 2 sec	Reflects blockade from 70%–100%; useful during onset, maintenance, and emergence
Tetanus	Generally consists of rapid delivery of a 30-, 50-, or 100-Hz stimulus for 5 sec	Should be used sparingly for deep block assessment; painful
Posttetanic count	50-Hz tetanus for 5 burst sec, a 3-sec pause, followed by single twitches of 1 Hz	Used only when train-of-four or double-stimulation response is absent; count less than eight indicates a deep block, and prolonged recovery is likely
Double-burst stimulation	Two short bursts of 50 Hz tetanus separated by 0.75 sec	Similar to train-of-four; useful during onset, maintenance, and emergence; may be easier to detect fade than with train-of-four; tactile evaluation

Modified from Savarese JJ and others: Pharmacology of muscle relaxants and their antagonists. In Miller RD, editor: *Anesthesia*, ed 5, Churchill Livingstone, 2000, Philadelphia.

TABLE 2 Key Points Related to Tests of Neuromuscular Transmission and Reversal

Test	Acceptable Clinical Result to Suggest Normal Function	Approximate Percentage of Receptors Occupied When Response Returns to Normal Value (%)	Comments/Advantages/Disadvantages
Tidal volume	At least 5 mL/kg	80	Necessary but insensitive as an indicator of neuromuscular function
Single twitch strength	Qualitatively as strong as baseline	75–80	Uncomfortable; need to know twitch strength before relaxant administration; insensitive as an indicator of recovery, but useful as a gauge of deep neuromuscular blockade
Train-of-four (TOF)	No palpable fade	70–75	Uncomfortable, but more sensitive as indicator of recovery than is single twitch; useful as a gauge of depth of block by counting the number of responses perceptible
Sustained tetanus at 50 Hz for 5 sec	No palpable fade	70	Very uncomfortable, but a reliable indictor of adequate recovery
Vital capacity	At least 20 mL/kg	70	Requires patient cooperation, but is the goal for achievement of full clinical recovery
Double-burst stimulation	No palpable fade	60–70	Uncomfortable, but more sensitive than TOF as an indicator of peripheral function; no perceptible fade indicates TOF of at least recovery of 60%
Inspiratory force	At least −40 cm H$_2$O	50	Difficult to perform with endotracheal intubation, but a reliable gauge of normal diaphragmatic function
Head lift	Must be performed unaided with patient supine and sustained for 5 sec	50	Requires patient cooperation but remains the standard test of normal clinical function
Hand grip	Sustained at a level qualitatively similar to preinduction	50	Sustained strong grip, although requires patient cooperation, another good gauge of normal function
Sustained bite	Sustained jaw clench on tongue blade	50	Very reliable with patient cooperation. Corresponds with TOF of 85%

Modified from Savarese JJ and others: Pharmacology of muscle relaxants and their antagonists. In Miller RD, editor: *Anesthesia*, ed 5, Churchill Livingstone, 2000, Philadelphia.

Thoracic Surgery Considerations

TABLE 1 **Initial Preanesthetic Assessment for Thoracic Surgery**

Patient Type	Assessments
All patients	Assess exercise tolerance, estimate ppoFEV₁%*, discuss postoperative analgesia, discontinue smoking
Patients with ppoFEV₁ <40%	DLCO, V/Q scan, Vo₂ max
Patients with cancer	Consider the "4 Ms": mass effects, metabolic effects, metastases, medications
Patients with COPD	Arterial blood gas, physiotherapy, bronchodilators
Increased renal risk	Measure creatinine and blood urea nitrogen

COPD, Chronic obstructive pulmonary disease; *DLCO,* diffusing capacity for carbon monoxide; *Vo₂ max,* maximum oxygen consumption; *V/Q,* ventilation-perfusion ratio.

*ppoFEV₁%, Preoperative percentage of forced expiratory volume in 1 sec (FEV₁ %) × (1–% functioning lung tissue removed/100). Values >40% indicate that postoperative complications are rare; values between 30% and 40% indicate that postoperative problems are possible; values <30% indicate that postoperative ventilation will likely be required.

TABLE 2 Summary of Lung Separation Devices and Recommendations for Placement

Device	Indication	Tube Size	Placement and Confirmation
Left-sided double-lumen tube	Majority of elective left or right thoracic surgical procedures	Determined by measurements of the tracheal width from chest radiograph	Fiberoptic bronchoscopy
Right-sided double-lumen endotracheal tube	Left bronchus–distorted anatomy Left pneumonectomy		Fiberoptic bronchoscopy with guided technique
Fogarty occlusion catheter	Critically ill patient Small bronchus Difficult airway Nasotracheal intubation	Standard endotracheal tube at least 6-mm inner diameter	Fiberoptic bronchoscopy
Univent blockers	Selective lobar blockade bronchoscopy Difficult airway requiring lung separation		Fiberoptic
Wire-guided endobronchial blockers	Critically ill patient Selective lobar blockade Difficult airway Nasotracheal intubation requiring lung separation	Standard endotracheal tube at least 8-mm inner diameter	Fiberoptic bronchoscopy with guided technique

TABLE 3 Evaluation of Candidates for Thoracotomy

FACTORS THAT IDENTIFY "LOW-RISK" PATIENTS

- FEV_1 >2 L
- Maximal ventilatory volume >50% predicted
- Predicted postoperative FEV_1 >0.8 L and 40% predicted
- Absence of cardiac disease

PROPOSED FACTORS THAT IDENTIFY "HIGH-RISK" PATIENTS

- Partial carbon dioxide pressure >45
- Partial oxygen pressure <50
- Predicted postoperative FEV_1 <0.7 L and/or 40% predicted
- Age <70 yr
- Poor exercise performance

FEV_1, Forced expiratory volume in 1 second.

TABLE 4 Evidence-Based Preoperative Evaluation of Candidates for Thoracotomy

- All patients considered for thoracotomy should have preoperative spirometry.
- Patients meeting the following criteria should also have quantitative radionuclide perfusion scanning: significant obstructive lung disease (FEV_1 <60% predicted), known or suspected endobronchial obstruction, significant hilar disease (mass or adenopathy), significant pleural disease, or selected patients who have had prior resections
- Patients believed to be at high risk on the basis of predicted postoperative FEV_1 should be considered for exercise assessment.
- If exercise assessment is performed, an MVO_2 of <10–15 mL/kg/min or a predicted postoperative MVO_2 <10 mL/kg/min identifies a patient at very high risk for complications and mortality.
- Limited available data support the use of preoperative risk indices to identify patients at high risk
- Lung volume–reduction surgery may provide new approaches in selected patients with significant obstructive lung disease and concomitant lung cancer.

FEV_1, Forced expiratory volume in 1 second; MVO_2, maximal oxygen uptake.

TABLE 5 Indications for One-Lung Ventilation

SURGICAL PROCEDURES

- Lung resection: lobectomy, segmental resection, pneumonectomy
- Drainage of lung abscess or cyst
- Video-assisted thoracoscopic surgery using general anesthesia
- Bronchopleural fistula
- Bronchial tumors
- Lung transplant
- Esophageal surgery
- Anterior approach to the thoracic spine
- Bronchopulmonary lavage (unilateral)
- Pericardial procedures
- Select open heart procedures
- Repair of thoracic aortic aneurysm
- Pulmonary artery rupture or embolism
- Pleural procedures: pleurectomy, decortication

IMPROVED PATIENT OUTCOME

- Restriction of infection or bleeding to one lung
- Desire to ventilate each lung differentially such as with bronchopleural fistula, tracheobronchial mass, trauma, or postoperatively

TABLE 1 Blood Coagulation Factors

Factor*	Synonym	Biologic Half-life (hr)	Blood Product Source
I	Fibrinogen	100–150	Cryoprecipitate (200–300 mg/bag)
II	Prothrombin	50–80	FFP, PCC
V	Proaccelerin	24	FFP
VII	Proconvertin	6	Recombinant VIIa, FFP, PCC
VIII	Antihemophilic factor	12	FFP, PCC, factor concentrates, cryoprecipitate
IX	Christmas factor	24	FFP, PCC, factor concentrates
X	Stuart-Prower factor	25–60	FFP, PCC
XI	Plasma thromboplastin antecedent	40–80	FFP
XII	Hageman factor	50–70	
XIII	Fibrin-stabilizing factor	150	FFP, cryoprecipitate

FFP, Fresh-frozen plasma; *PCC*, prothrombin-complex concentrate.

*Coagulation factors are numbered with Roman numerals in order of their discovery. Factor III (tissue factor) and factor IV (calcium ions) have been omitted. There is no factor VI.

Modified from Bickert B, Kwiatkowsky JL: Coagulation disorders. In Dipiro JT and others, editors: *Pharmacotherapy: a physiological approach,* ed 5, New York, 2002, McGraw-Hill.

Appendixes

TABLE 2   Hematology Laboratory Procedures

Procedure	Identifies	Causes of Prolonged Value	Clinical Manifestations
Bleeding time	Platelet function: adhesion, aggregation, and release	Thrombocytopenia Inherited qualitative platelet defects, von Willebrand's disease Uremia Collagen defects Antiplatelet drugs (i.e., aspirin) Factor V deficiency Afibrinogenemia	Bleeding from the gums Easy bruising Bleeding following surgery or tooth extraction Nosebleeds
Prothrombin time (PT)	Factors of common pathway: I, II, V, X Factor of extrinsic pathway: VII	Newborn status Vitamin K deficiency Inherited factor deficiencies Warfarin therapy Liver disease Lupus anticoagulant Afibrinogenemia	Bleeding, uterine surgery, childbirth, trauma Bleeding in newborn: umbilical cord, intracranial, gastrointestinal
Activated partial thromboplastin time (aPTT)	Factors of contact phase: HMWK, XII, prekallikrein Factors of intrinsic pathway: VIII, IX, XI Factors of common pathway: I, II, V, X	Inherited factor deficiencies Lupus anticoagulant Heparin therapy Liver disease Afibrinogenemia von Willebrand's disease	Increased incidence of thrombotic disease with lupus anticoagulant Joint and muscle bleeding with factor deficiencies Mucosal bleeding with von Willebrand's disease
Thrombin time (TT)	Fibrinogen Inhibitors of fibrin aggregation	Afibrinogenemia Heparin therapy	Life-long hemorrhagic disease

HMWK, High-molecular-weight kininogen.
Modified from Bickert B, Kwiatkowsy JL. Coagulation disorders. In Dipiro JT, Talbert RL, Yee GC et al, editors: *Pharmacotherapy: a physiological approach,* ed. 5, McGraw Hil, 2002, New York.

List of Available Equipment and Supplies Compatible with Magnetic Resonance Imaging

Anesthesia machine compatible with magnetic resonance imaging
Pulse oximeter
Intravenous bag pole
Liquid crystal temperature monitoring strip
Respiratory rate monitor
Noninvasive blood pressure monitor
Pulse oximeter
Electrocardiogram
Electrocardiogram patches
Electrocardiogram cable
Capnograph
Laryngoscope with lithium batteries and aluminum spacers
Laryngoscope blades
Nerve stimulator
Intravenous infusion pump
Oxygen tanks
Precordial stethoscope
Esophogeal stethoscope
Patient carts
Tables and trays

Checklist of Requisites for Performance of Anesthesia in Remote Locations

UTILITIES

Adequate work space
Adequate overhead lighting
Adequate numbers and current-carrying capacity of electrical outlets
Two-way communication devices: telephone, intercom
Back-up power
(All building and safety codes and facility standards must be met)

EQUIPMENT
Local Infiltration, Intravenous Sedation, Regional and General Anesthesia

Patient monitors to include: pulse oximeter, electrocardiogram, blood pressure monitor with a selection of adequate-sized cuffs, capnography, and body temperature
Oxygen supplies: a minimum of two oxygen sources available, with regulators attached (compressed oxygen should be the equivalent of an E cylinder)
Positive-pressure ventilation sources including an Ambu bag and a mouth-to-mask unit
Defibrillator (charged)
Suction source or suction machine, tubing, suction catheters, and Yankauer suction devices
Anesthesia cart to provide for organization of supplies including endotracheal equipment, laryngeal mask airways, Combitubes, face masks, nasal cannulas, Connell airways, disposable face masks with oxygen tubing, oral and nasal airways, syringes (3, 5, 10, 20, 60 mL), needles, intravenous catheters, tourniquet, intravenous fluids and tubing, alcohol pads, adhesive tape, disposable gloves, face mask, stethoscopes, and appropriate anesthetic medications
Battery-powered flashlight
Syringe pump
Warm blankets or forced-air warming devices and the appropriate blanket
Emergency medications to include, at a minimum, atropine, epinephrine, ephedrine, lidocaine, diphenhydramine, cortisone, and a bronchial dilator inhaler such as albuterol
Preoperative anesthesia evaluation forms
Anesthesia charts/black ink pens, indelible ink pens

Additionally for General Anesthesia

Oxygen fail-safe system
Oxygen analyzer
Waste gas exhaust scavenging system
End-tidal carbon dioxide analyzer
Vaporizers: calibration and exclusion system
Alarm system

Anesthetic medications

In addition to the emergency medications listed above, consider:
Induction drugs: propofol, etomidate, methohexital, thiopental
Maintenance drugs: bottles of sevoflurane, isoflurane, desflurane, propofol
Narcotics: midazolam, diazepam, fentanyl, alfentanil, sufentanil, remifentanil
Muscle relaxants: succinylcholine, mivacurium, rocuronium, cisatracurium, vecuronium
Muscle relaxant reversal agents: edrophonium, neostigmine, atropine, glycopyrrolate
Cardiovascular drugs: labetalol, esmolol, verapamil, hydralazine

Narcotic reversal drugs: naloxone, flumazenil
Antiemetic drugs: ondansetron, dolasetron, granisetron, droperidol

Emergencies
Emergency cart and equipment

Basic airway equipment (adult and pediatric)
Nasal and oral airways
Face mask (appropriate for patient)
Laryngoscopes, assortment of laryngoscope blades, endotracheal tubes (adult and
    pediatric), laryngeal mask airways, Combitube
Ambu bag
Difficult Airway Equipment (laryngeal mask airway, light wand, cricothyrotomy kit)
Defibrillator
Supplemental oxygen and nitrous oxide tanks
Emergency medications
Succinylcholine
Compression board
Suction equipment (suction catheter, Yankauer type)
Malignant hyperthermia drugs, equipment, and the telephone number of the Malignant
    Hyperthermia Association of the United States

A policy must be developed that outlines the organization of emergency services for
either in-hospital or office-based facilities. Office-based facilities should have a plan for
emergency transportation to the nearest hospital emergency department.

Note: An anesthesia machine and portable anesthesia cart with the previously listed
equipment, supplies, and medications should be dedicated strictly for use in remote
locations. This can save preparation time whenever a procedure is required in a remote
location. It will also decrease the risk of a mishap's resulting from lack of necessary
equipment and materials.

Appendixes